Cases in Field Epidemiology
A Global Perspective

Edited by

Mark S. Dworkin, MD, MPH&TM, FACP
Associate Professor
Division of Epidemiology and Biostatistics
University of Illinois at Chicago School of Public Health
Chicago, Illinois

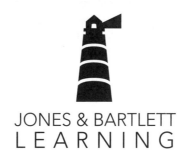

World Headquarters
Jones & Bartlett Learning
5 Wall Street
Burlington, MA 01803
978-443-5000
info@jblearning.com
www.jblearning.com

Jones & Bartlett Learning books and products are available through most bookstores and online booksellers. To contact Jones & Bartlett Learning directly, call 800-832-0034, fax 978-443-8000, or visit our website, www.jblearning.com.

> Substantial discounts on bulk quantities of Jones & Bartlett Learning publications are available to corporations, professional associations, and other qualified organizations. For details and specific discount information, contact the special sales department at Jones & Bartlett Learning via the above contact information or send an email to specialsales@jblearning.com.

Copyright © 2011 by Jones & Bartlett Learning, LLC, an Ascend Learning Company

All rights reserved. No part of the material protected by this copyright may be reproduced or utilized in any form, electronic or mechanical, including photocopying, recording, or by any information storage and retrieval system, without written permission from the copyright owner.

This publication is designed to provide accurate and authoritative information in regard to the Subject Matter covered. It is sold with the understanding that the publisher is not engaged in rendering legal, accounting, or other professional service. If legal advice or other expert assistance is required, the service of a competent professional person should be sought.

Some images in this book feature models. These models do not necessarily endorse, represent, or participate in the activities represented in the images.

Production Credits
Publisher: Michael Brown
Associate Editor: Catie Heverling
Editorial Assistant: Teresa Reilly
Production Manager: Tracey Chapman
Production Assistant: Rebekah Linga
Senior Marketing Manager: Sophie Fleck
Manufacturing and Inventory Control Supervisor: Amy Bacus
Composition: Publishers' Design and Production Services, Inc.
Cover Design: Kristin E. Parker
Photo Research and Permissions Manager: Kimberly Potvin
Associate Photo Researcher: Jessica Elias
Cover Image: © Image Team/ShutterStock, Inc.
Printing and Binding: Edwards Brothers Malloy
Cover Printing: Edwards Brothers Malloy

Library of Congress Cataloging-in-Publication Data
Cases in field epidemiology : a global perspective / [edited by] Mark S. Dworkin.
   p. ; cm.
Rev. ed. of: Outbreak investigations around the world. c2010.
Includes bibliographical references and index.
ISBN-13: 978-0-7637-7891-0 (pbk.)
ISBN-10: 0-7637-7891-5 (pbk.)
1. Epidemiology—Case studies. I. Dworkin, Mark S. II. Outbreak investigations around the world.
   [DNLM: 1. Disease Outbreaks—Personal Narratives. 2. Epidemiologic Methods—Personal Narratives. WA 105]
RA652.4.O98 2011
614.4—dc22

2010030009

6048

Printed in the United States of America
17 16 14 14 13   10 9 8 7 6 5 4 3 2

DEDICATION

To my wife, Renee, and daughters, Josie and Julie.
And to my mother, Una, and to Henry and Frieda,
for having made me feel like each good work I try to do
has made them proud.

Acknowledgments

I wish to recognize the chapter authors who graciously donated their time to contribute to this book because of their strong commitment to public health education. I know that they are all very busy; thus, taking on writing a chapter of an investigation that, in some cases, occurred decades ago was a true labor of love. They are really special people who have spent most or all of their careers in public health and I feel honored that they accepted my request for their contributions. I also appreciate the review of the Preface and Chapter 1 by Frank Sorvillo and Bill Keane, respectively. Additionally, many persons have directly and indirectly helped me to develop an understanding of field epidemiology, including teachers, supervisors, coworkers, colleagues, public health personnel, infection control practitioners, microbiologists, and the many others I interacted with during and after these events. I am especially grateful to the Centers for Disease Control and Prevention's Epidemic Intelligence Service program for providing me with training that opened my eyes to the exciting career that is public health. Finally, I acknowledge the students, fellows, and EIS officers I have had the privilege to instruct and the many students and public health workers for whom I hope this book will become a useful complement to the study and practice of epidemiology.

Table of Contents

Preface   xi

About the Editor   xv

Contributors   xvii

PART I   Outbreak Investigations   1

CHAPTER 1
An Overview of Outbreak Investigation   3
Mark S. Dworkin, MD, MPH&TM, FACP

CHAPTER 2
How an Outbreak is Investigated   7
Mark S. Dworkin, MD, MPH&TM, FACP

PART II   Outbreak Investigations of Infectious Diseases   17

CHAPTER 3
Leptospirosis at the Bubbles   19
Kenrad E. Nelson, MD, PhD

CHAPTER 4
Cholera for a Dime   29
Paul A. Blake, MD, MPH

CHAPTER 5
Legionnaire's Disease: Investigation of an Outbreak of a New Disease   43
Steven B. Thacker, MD, MSc

CHAPTER 6
The Investigation of Toxic Shock Syndrome in Wisconsin, 1979–1980 and Beyond
Jeffrey P. Davis, MD

CHAPTER 7
The Early Days of AIDS in the United States: A Personal Perspective   65
Harold W. Jaffe, MD, MA, FFPH

CHAPTER 8
Verify the Diagnosis: A Pseudo-Outbreak of Amebiasis in Los Angeles County   73

Frank Sorvillo, PhD

CHAPTER 9
Measles Among Religiously Exempt Persons   83

Charles E. Jennings

CHAPTER 10
An Outbreak of Fulminant Hepatitis B in a Medical Ward in Israel   91

Ronald C. Hershow, MD, MPH

CHAPTER 11
What Went Wrong? An Ancient Recipe Associated with Botulism in Modern Egypt   101

J. Todd Weber, MD

CHAPTER 12
Controlling an Outbreak of Shigellosis with a Community-Wide Intervention in Lexington County, Kentucky   109

Janet Mohle-Boetani, MD, MPH

CHAPTER 13
Pork Tapeworm in an Orthodox Jewish Community: Arriving at a Biologically Plausible Hypothesis   115

Peter M. Schantz, VMD, PhD and Mary E. Bartlett, BA

CHAPTER 14
The Massive Waterborne Outbreak of *Cryptosporidium* Infections, Milwaukee, Wisconsin, 1993   121

Jeffrey P. Davis, MD

CHAPTER 15
A Community Outbreak of Hepatitis A Involving Cooperation Between Public Health, the Media, and Law Enforcement, Iowa, 1997   145

Patricia Quinlisk, MD, MPH; Yvan J.F. Hutin, MD; Ken W. Carter; Thomas M. Carney; and Kevin Teale, MA

CHAPTER 16
Tracking a Syphilis Outbreak Through Cyberspace   163

Jeffrey D. Klausner, MD, MPH

CHAPTER 17
Eschar: The Story of the New York City Department of Health 2001 Anthrax Investigation   173

Don Weiss MD, MPH and Marci Layton, MD

CHAPTER 18
Ebola Hemorrhagic Fever in Gabon: Chaos to Control   191

Daniel G. Bausch, MD, MPH&TM

CHAPTER 19
Whipping Whooping Cough in Rock Island County, Illinois   203

Mark S. Dworkin, MD, MPH&TM, FACP

CHAPTER 20
Emergency Yellow Fever Mass Vaccination in Post–Civil War Liberia   217

Gregory Huhn, MD, MPH&TM

CHAPTER 21
A Mumps Epidemic, Iowa, 2006   245

Patricia Quinlisk, MD, MPH

PART III   Outbreak Investigations of Intoxications and Other Noninfectious Causes   259

CHAPTER 22
Something Borrowed, Something Blue: A Wedding to Remember   261

Cortland Lohff, MD, MPH; Tom Boo, MD; and Patricia Quinlisk, MD, MPH

CHAPTER 23
Toxic School Lunch: Chemical Poisoning of Elementary School Children in Joliet, Illinois   273

Alpesh Patel, MBBS, MPH, CERC, CPHA and Mark S. Dworkin, MD, MPH&TM, FACP

CHAPTER 24
When Your Food Glows Blue   287

Eduardo Azziz-Baumgartner, MD, MPH

CHAPTER 25
What Do People Eat When They Have No Food? A Tragic Story of Poverty, Monsoon Floods, and Weeds 301

Emily S. Gurley, MPH

CHAPTER 26
Toxic Tryptophan? Investigating the Eosinophilia Myalgia Syndrome in Minnesota 313

Edward A. Belongia, MD

CHAPTER 27
A Mystery Illness in Panama 337

Lauren S. Lewis, MD, MPH

CHAPTER 28
"We're Prepared to Believe You"—Investigating Cancer Cluster Reports 349

Tim E. Aldrich, PhD, MPH

PART IV Cases in Environmental and Occupational Health 371

CHAPTER 29
Fine Wines and Cohorts Take Time: The History of a Cohort Study of Workers Exposed to Ethylene Oxide 373

Leslie Stayner, PhD and Kyle Steenland, PhD

CHAPTER 30
Why Have the Children of Chernivtsi Lost All of Their Hair? 389

Daniel Hryhorczuk, MD, MPH

CHAPTER 31
Not in My Backyard: An Investigation of the Health of a Community Living Near a Landfill 401

Preethi Pratap, PhD

PART V Investigating Hard-to-Reach and Special Populations 413

CHAPTER 32
Back to School: Using Basic Epidemiologic Data on Asthma in Urban School Children to Improve Respiratory Health 415

Victoria Persky, MD

CHAPTER 33
Sex, Drugs, and Community-Based Ethnography: Field Investigations Involving Difficult-to-Reach Populations Around the World 421

W. Wayne Wiebel, PhD

CHAPTER 34
Investigation of Attitudes Toward Immunization in an Old-Order Amish Community 439

Jonathan S. Yoder, MSW, MPH

CHAPTER 35
Performing a Seroprevalence and Ocular Study in Rural Guatemala—Toxoplasmosis, a Chronic Infectious Disease 449

Jeffrey L. Jones, MD, MPH and Beatriz López, QB

Index 461

Preface

Field epidemiology is the most exciting epidemiological work. That may be a bold statement, but I can't think of any other public health activity that gets more people excited while they are doing their work and talking about it long after they have returned from the field. Reading field investigations in scientific publications is often very interesting. Personal stories and media coverage of field epidemiology are sometimes responsible for students deciding on public health as a career, even changing from one long-planned career to this useful and rewarding type of work. At public health conferences, it is not unusual for presentations of field investigations to attract large and enthusiastic audiences. However, what is not usually conveyed in these presentations or their subsequent scientific publications are the many challenges and unique circumstances that the investigators had to deal with along the way. There is much to be learned from what lies between the lines of the introduction, methods, results, and conclusions.

The term "epidemiology" is defined as the distribution and determinants of disease. The term "field" is used to reflect that an epidemiological investigation involved some degree of getting out of the office and into the environment where the disease distributed or gaining a firsthand account or understanding of the factors that may have been responsible for or associated with the disease. As a result, investigations of disease that involve field epidemiology have taken their investigators to all parts of the world—from urban homeless shelters to refugee camps and distant tropical islands where there may be no electricity. I think that this is one of the great benefits of a career practicing field epidemiology. It is a ticket to places that you would never otherwise have gone. In my own public health career, for one reason or another, I have gotten to work and learn inside a ham processing plant, numerous restaurants, many hospitals, many schools, a county jail, a facility for the developmentally disabled, a hotel, a recreational water park, sports competition and work out areas, sunny docks on the northern Washington state coastline, rural snow-blanketed cabins, a Catholic shrine, a village in India, abandoned houses, and the homes of the Amish. I could go on, but it is not necessary. Equally remarkable is that the list of another epidemiologist is likely to be different, but not less diverse. What makes it possible to work in so many completely different environments is a good grounding in basic epidemiological principles, including the steps of outbreak investigation and other epidemiological methods, as well as healthy doses of common sense, perseverance, and humility.

Outbreak investigations are a type of field epidemiology. However, an epidemiologist working in the field need not be involved in an outbreak. If the epidemiologist is involved in an outbreak, it does not have to be caused by an infectious disease. This book provides a spectrum of investigations from many countries that illustrate the unique and genuinely interesting world of field epidemiology, while teaching and reviewing scientific and epidemiological methods and facts that derive from a broad spectrum of investigations and careers investigating public health problems in the field. Compared to many other countries, field epidemiology is highly developed within the United States. As a result, this book includes more examples from the United States than elsewhere. However, excellent work is performed throughout the world and training programs are emerging that are helping to bridge the gap.

This book is not intended to replace an epidemiology textbook, but rather to complement it. Given its unique style, it does not and cannot realistically review all epidemiological methods. The methods that are reviewed are those that happen to be relevant to the investigations included. In fact, some methods are mentioned but not explained because to do so would interrupt the flow of the case study too much and the methods are better addressed in authoritative epidemiology or biostatistics textbooks. This book is intended to illustrate the application of epidemiologic methods and to demonstrate to its readers how interesting epidemiology can be. It also provides readers who have not yet selected their career path with an idea of what this work can be like. As I have read and reread each of these chapters in the preparation of this book, I found myself drawn to the story and excited by each example of a real-world application of information that may have been taught during the acquisition of a public health degree or would need to be learned afterwards in the work world. It was common for authors to tell me how much they enjoyed writing the chapter. The enjoyment of experiencing these investigations comes through in their writing and illustrates how special this kind of work can be.

It is my intention to reach out to both the experienced and less experienced investigator, students interested in any of the applications of field epidemiology, as well as anyone interested in the study of epidemics by presenting extraordinary and illustrative investigations. It is my hope that these outbreak descriptions will clarify what was involved in the investigation beyond what is found in a published scientific article. The first-person style is intended to create a reader friendly format that is more like a story that can entertain while instructing. They also provide a context for the investigations by introducing the reader to where the authors were in their careers at the time, with whom they were working, and the real-world conditions they had to face while practicing field epidemiology. In an article titled "In Philadelphia 30 Years Ago, an Eruption of Illness and Fear" written for *The New York Times* by Lawrence K. Altman recalling the Legionnaires' disease outbreak of 1976, he described an interview with a patient that left the epidemiologic team unable to explain why that patient developed the disease, but four other Legionnaires, with whom he spent a great deal of time, did not develop the disease. He goes on to recognize that dead ends like these in epidemiologic investigations are not what scientific journals publish. The concise and focused scientific article that becomes what most persons know of the outbreak investigation (along with other factors) "creates a false impression that investigations and discoveries are simpler than they really are." (*The New York Times*, August 1, 2006). These investigations are typically very complex and bring together many challenges, including recalling and applying epidemiologic knowledge; making numerous decisions, often quickly and under stressful conditions; working as a team that includes team members one has never worked with before; working in an environment away from the office where most of one's resources are located; and many more.

These examples of applied field epidemiology are appropriate for students interested in infectious disease outbreaks and students interested in noninfectious disease topics such as environmental health, cancer, substance abuse, and other chronic diseases. In fact, it is healthy for an education in infectious disease epidemiology to include exposure to the approach and tools used by persons who investigate chronic disease and environmental health problems and vice versa. A broader understanding of investigation can lead to creative and useful ideas during future investigations. Within these chapters, one finds the intersection of behavioral, environmental, and political factors that influence real public health decisions.

It is a privilege to be able to access this information because some issues that are relevant to epidemiologic investigation do not arise during epidemiology training through traditional textbooks. Yet the speed of an investigation and even its success could be influenced by the level of the investigators' familiarity with these issues. Many field epidemiologists gain such exposure only through practice, including trial and error, or through exposure to great mentors. This book intends to bridge the gap between the inexperienced and the experienced by offering more complete information about what happened, why decisions were made in a certain way, and even the working conditions and little pains or pleasures of the investigator. Candid accounts should not be taken for granted, because sometimes not everyone involved feels comfortable revealing how things unfolded. In fact, in the preparation of this book, one investigation was completely written in an entertaining and educational fashion, but was not cleared by the agency with the authority to do so. There were many valuable lessons from that investigation, but it is uncertain if and when those lessons will ever be shared. Because clearance was not given, it was not published in this book.

Some of these chapters deal with events that unfolded quickly (like poisonings and most infectious disease outbreaks), while other chapters review a career with selected experiences presented and lessons learned along the way or an investigation that took many months or years to complete. Not every investigation results in a slam-dunk definitive answer or involves cooperation from those who have a stake in the results. That's the real world, as opposed to a television episode. This book desires to present the real world. Therefore, such investigations are included despite their possible limitations or loose ends. And finally, some chapters simply reveal how certain kinds of applications of epidemiology were carried out, whether it involved recruiting children to be bled as part of a seroepidemiologic study, creating a survey intended for a difficult to access population, or experiencing work within a unique setting like a school system.

Readers will likely recognize that a few chapters are much longer than others. This was not an accident of editing, but a conscious decision to have certain topics expanded to allow a fuller discussion of the investigation or the circumstances in which it took place. Therefore, instructors might choose to teach or assign reading from the longer chapters into two parts.

At the end of the chapters are learning questions. The authors or I have written these questions to stimulate review of important material presented in the chapter and class discussion. They are not intended to be a complete review of all the material presented. Therefore, students or instructors will find it beneficial to identify other epidemiologic issues or methods, judgment calls, and lessons learned in the chapters as both a teaching tool and possibly a way of testing from the book.

How do you enter a career that includes field epidemiology? Many of the authors share a glimpse into their entry into this work. Often, it includes training or working for local, state, or federal government. The most famous training program in the United States is the Centers for Disease Control and Prevention's two-year Epidemic Intelligence Service (EIS) program (http://www.cdc.gov/eis/index.html). This program is mentioned in many of the chapters because it is an excellent program for learning surveillance and field epidemiology methods while applying them to current important public health problems. Typically, persons accepted into the EIS have a professional degree, such as a PhD, MD, VMD, or equivalent. The Council of State and Territorial Epidemiologists, in partnership with other organizations including the CDC, also has a program known as the CDC/CSTE Applied Epidemiology Fellowship (http://www.cste.org). Persons who are recent masters- or doctoral-level graduates in epidemiology or a related field are placed with mentors (much like the EIS program) in state or federal programs. Some programs are offered elsewhere in the world. For example, the European Centre for Disease Prevention and Control has the European Programme for Intervention Epidemiology Training program and many countries around the world now offer epidemiology training similar to the EIS program through collaboration with the CDC's Field Epidemiology Training Program (FETP http://www.cdc.gov/globalhealth/FETP/). There are other opportunities to get experience and readers are encouraged to speak to their local and state health departments to explore possible training, employment, and volunteer opportunities. Enjoy reading this book. I hope that it will stimulate many students to pursue the exciting and challenging work of field epidemiology and that it will be helpful to the many public health professionals who work in the field.

Mark S. Dworkin, MD, MPH&TM, FACP

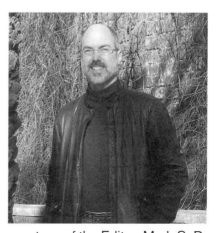

Photo courtesy of the Editor, Mark S. Dworkin

About the Editor

Mark S. Dworkin, MD, MPH&TM, FACP, is a medical epidemiologist and is board certified in internal medicine and infectious diseases. After receiving his medical degree from Rush Medical College (Chicago), he trained in Internal Medicine at Rush Presbyterian St. Luke's Medical Center and in Infectious Diseases at Tulane University Medical Center, he also obtained a Master's Degree in Public Health and Tropical Medicine from the Tulane University School of Tropical Medicine and Public Health in New Orleans. He then served for two years in the Centers for Disease Control and Prevention's (CDC) Epidemic Intelligence Service stationed at the Washington State Department of Health where he investigated many outbreaks including those due to pertussis, *Salmonella, Cryptosporidium, Trichinella,* and measles. Dr. Dworkin worked at the CDC in Atlanta for four years in the Division of HIV/AIDS Prevention and performed many epidemiologic analyses related to opportunistic infections. During 2000 to 2006, he was the Illinois Department of Public Health State Epidemiologist in the Division of Infectious Diseases and team leader for the rapid response team (an outbreak investigation team). He is now an associate professor in the Division of Epidemiology and Biostatistics at the University of Illinois at Chicago School of Public Health and an attending physician at the HIV outpatient Core Center of the John H. Stroger, Jr. Hospital of Cook County (formerly Cook County Hospital) and provides on-call coverage to a private practice infectious disease group in the Chicago area. Dr. Dworkin lectures at Northwestern University and the University of Chicago. He has authored or co-authored many scientific publications on various topics including outbreak investigations, surveillance, HIV/AIDS opportunistic infections, salmonellosis, tick-borne illnesses, and vaccine-preventable infections. Current research interests include food safety education of restaurant food handlers, persons with AIDS, and a variety of consumer populations. Additional information may be viewed at this web page: http://tigger.uic.edu/~mdworkin/Dworkinweb.htm. Dr. Dworkin has been awarded both the Commendation Medal and the Achievement Medal by the United States Public Health Service.

Contributors

Tim E. Aldrich, PhD, MPH
East Tennessee State University College of Public Health
Johnson City, Tennessee

Eduardo Azziz-Baumgartner, MD, MPH
Centers for Disease Control and Prevention
Atlanta, Georgia

Mary E. Bartlett, BA
Division of Parasitic Diseases
National Center For Zoonotic,
Vectorborne and Enteric Diseases
Centers for Disease Control and Prevention
Atlanta, Georgia

Daniel G. Bausch, MD, MPH&TM
Associate Professor
Tulane School of Public Health and Tropical Medicine
New Orleans, Louisiana

Edward A. Belongia, MD
Director
Epidemiology Research Center
Marshfield Clinic Research Foundation
Marshfield, Wisconsin

Paul A. Blake, MD, MPH
Salem, Oregon

Tom Boo, MD
Family Practice Northern Inyo Hospital
Bishop, CA

Thomas M. Carney
President
Carney Consulting, LLC
Johnston, Iowa

Ken W. Carter
Adjunct Instructor
Des Moines Area Community College
Des Moines, Iowa

Jeffrey P. Davis, MD
Chief Medical Officer and State
Epidemiologist for Communicable Diseases
Wisconsin Division of PublicHealth
Madison, Wisconsin

Emily S. Gurley, MPH
International Centre for Diarrhoeal Disease Research
Programme on Infectious Diseases and Vaccine
  Sciences
Dhaka, Bagladesh

Ronald C. Hershow, MD, MPH
Associate Professor of Epidemiology
Clinical Associate Professor of Medicine
University of Illinois at Chicago School of Public Health
Chicago, Illinois

Daniel Hryhorczuk, MD, MPH
Professor, Division of Environmental and Occupational Health Sciences
University of Illinois at Chicago School of Public Health
Chicago, Illinois

Gregory Huhn, MD, MPH&TM
Assistant Professor
Section of Infectious Diseases
John H. Stroger, Jr. Hospital of Cook County
Rush University Medical Center
Chicago, Illinois

Yvan J.F. Hutin, MD
Medical Field Officer
Field Epidemiology Training Programme
WHO India country office
New Delhi, India

Harold W. Jaffe, MD, MA, FFPH
Department of Public Health
University of Oxford
Oxford, England

Charles E. Jennings
CEO
Inject-Safe Bandages, LLC
Jacksonville, Illinois

Jeffrey L. Jones, MD, MPH
Division of Parasitic Diseases and Malaria Center for Global Health
Centers for Disease Control and Prevention
Atlanta, Georgia

Jeffrey D. Klausner, MD, MPH
Associate Clinical Professor of Medicine
Division of AIDS and Infectious Diseases
Department of Medicine
University of California, San Francisco

Marci Layton, MD
Assistant Commissioner
Bureau of Communicable Disease
The City of New York
Department of Health and Mental Hygiene
New York, New York

Lauren S. Lewis, MD, MPH
Chief, Health Studies Branch
National Center for Environmental Health, Centers for Disease Control
Chamblee, Georgia

Cortland Lohff, MD, MPH
Medical Director, Environmental Health
Chicago Department of Public Health
Chicago, Illinois

Beatriz López, QB
Universidad del Valle de Guatemala
Guatemala, Guatemala

Janet Mohle-Boetani, MD, MPH
Chief Medical Officer
Public Health Unit
California Prison Health Care Services
Sacramento, California

Kenrad E. Nelson, MD, PhD
Department of Epidemiology
Bloomsburg School of Hygiene and Public Health
Johns Hopkins University
Baltimore, Maryland

Alpesh R. Patel, MBBS, MPH, CERC, CPHA
Coordinator for Epidemiology & Communicable Disease Program
Will County Health Department
Joliet, Illinois

Victoria Persky, MD
Professor
Division of Epidemiology and Biostatistics
University of Illinois at Chicago School of Public Health
Chicago, Illinois

Preethi Pratap, PhD
Research Assistant Professor
Division of Environmental and Occupational Health Sciences
University of Illinois at Chicago School of Public Health
Chicago, Illinois

Patricia Quinlisk, MD, MPH
Medical Director and the State Epidemiologist
Iowa Department of Public Health
Adjunct Professor
College of Public Health
The University of Iowa
Iowa City, Iowa

Peter M. Schantz, VMD, PhD
Department of Global Health
Rollins School of Public Health
Emory University
Atlanta, Georgia

Frank Sorvillo, PhD
Associate Professor in Residence
University of California Los Angeles
School of Public Health
Los Angeles, California

Leslie T. Stayner, PhD
Division of Epidemiology & Biostatistics
University of Illinois at Chicago School of Public Health
Chicago, Illinois

Kyle Steenland, PhD
Professor
Environmental Health
Rollins School of Public Health
Emory University
Atlanta, Georgia

Kevin Teale, MA
Senior Communications Consultant
Media Relations
Wellmark Blue Cross and Blue Shield
Des Moines, Iowa

Stephen B. Thacker, MD, MSc
RADM (Ret.), USPHS Director
Office of Workforce and Career Development
Centers for Disease Control and Prevention
Atlanta, Georgia

J. Todd Weber, MD
CDC Liaison
European Centre for Disease Prevention and Control
Stockholm, Sweden
U.S. Department of Health and Human Services
Centers for Disease Control and Prevention
Atlanta, Georgia

Don Weiss, MD, MPH
Director of Surveillance
Bureau of Communicable Disease
New York City Department of Health and Mental Hygiene
New York, New York

W. Wayne Wiebel, PhD
Division of Epidemiology & Biostatistics
University of Illinois at Chicago School of Public Health
Chicago, Illinois

Jonathon S. Yoder, MSW, MPH
Centers for Disease Control
Atlanta, Georgia

PART I

Outbreak Investigations

CHAPTER 1

An Overview of Outbreak Investigation

Mark S. Dworkin, MD, MPH&TM, FACP

An outbreak (or epidemic) is a unique public health event and poses many challenges and opportunities to those tasked with the response. It occurs when more cases of a disease are recognized than would normally be expected at a given time among a specific group of people, whether it is a dozen persons with gastroenteritis that attended a church supper or the occurrence of a marked rise in cases of a disease among the population of an entire country. Unlike a research experiment where you try to control many things, such as precisely how the study subjects are exposed to some health-related variable, the responder to an outbreak has had no control over the exposure and may not even know what the exposure was. Rather, the focus is on investigating and describing this natural experiment that nature or man (intentionally or unintentionally) has caused with the hope of mitigating its consequences. The investigator might only be confronted with a syndrome (such as an outbreak of diarrheal illness) without knowing which agent has specifically caused this outbreak. They may even be challenged with the cause of the outbreak being a novel organism that has not previously been described. In the case of the many thousands of public health employees working in health departments in units or sections that are responsible for more than one disease (such as those dealing with communicable or immunization preventable diseases), they never know what will be the next outbreak, and are challenged to master the information about each of what can be 40, 60, or more reportable conditions. And regardless of whether the disease is named on the list of reportable conditions, usually if it causes an outbreak it is automatically reportable.

In an outbreak, there is typically an urgent need to control the public health outcome and minimize its impact, especially through prevention of further cases. One of the first things that is needed by the public health responder is some familiarity with what is already known about how to deal with the problem. For example, when one is confronted with a Salmonella outbreak, it is useful to have had experience investigating previous outbreaks of salmonellosis and to have read the literature of Salmonella outbreaks to gain familiarity with methods of investigation and issues that can arise. The scientific literature has many publications of outbreak investigations. Some of these are descriptive and others focus on one or more aspects of the outbreak, such as laboratory issues or infection control. These publications are wonderful resources, but may be less accessible to those not trained in epidemiology, the laboratory science, or biostatistics. Such reports are also limited by journal word count and scientific writing requirements that may make them less accessible to some public health employees and students.

Outbreaks are fascinating stories. They are real-life events that sometimes weave together all the drama any Hollywood producer could wish for in a blockbuster: the baker vomiting in the kitchen sink and then resuming his work duties; a casual or even celebratory meal out at a restaurant followed days later by hospitalization and death, only because the deceased decided that he would have the Caesar salad with the entrée for a small additional price; or perhaps a family reunion at a hotel followed by a family cluster of illnesses with fever because the whirlpool they enjoyed may have been aerosolizing *Legionella* species. Some outbreaks, including several in this book, are even more dramatic, making national headlines, as when previously unrecognized organisms hospitalize and kill, or when massively large numbers of persons are sickened, or when a relatively small number of persons is sickened or killed but an entire nation is fearful for their own safety. Some outbreaks are fascinating puzzles for the epidemiologist to solve. How do Orthodox Jews who never eat pork become sick from the pork tapeworm? Why do children in a Ukrainian town go bald?

A pessimist that studies outbreaks finds reason not to drink, swim, relax in, or even shower in water, and not to eat shellfish, meat, chicken, pork, fried rice, home canned vegetables, fresh spinach, tomatoes, alfalfa sprouts, peanut butter, apple cider, and even pasteurized milk! Beware hotels, any banquet (especially at a wedding), any catered meal, and flying on an airplane or taking a cruise. Heaven forbid your child goes to a daycare, plays on an athletic team, visits a petting zoo, or just plain goes to school at all. Just when you thought it might be good to get away, you had better avoid beaver dams and rivers, caves, well water, and rustic cabins where ticks are hiding to bite you and your friends or family painlessly in the night. Don't get sick with anything so you won't need any medicine or sleeping aids and so you can avoid the hospitals and surgicenters. And don't even think of having sex!

But the optimist recognizes the incredible potential to learn and apply public health skills while performing useful and rewarding work. It is no coincidence that some of the most important outbreak investigations have had lead investigators who lacked subspecialty knowledge of the disease that they were investigating (before they began the investigation). However, the reason that they were so suitable for the investigation was due in large part to their epidemiologic skill set. They brought their "epidemiologic tool kit" with them to the outbreak and, in the midst of investigating, attempted to master relevant knowledge of the disease and, whenever possible, to partner with others who had disease-specific knowledge. I have seen many successful epidemiologists move their careers from one area of study to a seemingly unrelated area of study. How can someone who worked on AIDS for 8 years transfer to work on cancer or air pollution or smoking cessation, and then some years later transfer to work on influenza? Why do such programs hire that person? The answer is that these individuals have a highly valuable "epidemiologic tool kit," and those that hire them understand the value of this. A well-rounded epidemiologist has been involved in a diversity of epidemiologic analyses; a great way to develop and polish these epidemiologic skills is through outbreak investigation.

An outbreak is both a negative public health event and an opportunity. Although people are ill, there are many benefits to outbreak investigation. Outbreak investigations identify populations at risk for a disease, allow for modes of disease transmission to be characterized, and provide information that can be used to control the outbreak (thus preventing further disease transmission) as well as to prevent similar occurrences in the future. Outbreak investigations also provide the opportunity to evaluate public health programs or policies (such as a requirement for universal immunization against a particular disease) and whether they have been effective. In the course of an outbreak investigation, laboratory methods might reveal if there is something new about the causative organism (such as a strain that is novel and not well covered by the current vaccine), or if the strain is usual and therefore immunity from the vaccine may be less long lasting than hoped or believed. These investigations allow for the evaluation of new control measures that might be introduced in the course of the outbreak and are derived from the data analysis. They also allow for an improved understanding of the disease, especially when the disease is relatively uncommon. Whereas a disease might occur only sporadically throughout the country and get reported occasionally as a case report, the outbreak creates a series of cases under the thoughtful observation of an investigator or team of investigators who may recognize epidemiological, clinical, or laboratory features not previously observed. The outbreak also generates what can be relatively large numbers of samples (such as stool or blood) or isolates of an organism that can allow for advancement of the scientific knowledge related to that disease or organism.

Outbreak investigations are also an opportunity for public health staff training. It is common for outbreaks to occur where staff have little to no experience dealing with them (such as outside of a city or county with a very large population). As a result, the administrative staff may wisely request assistance from the state or federal health department. The arrival of experienced staff under real-world conditions can lead to training that advances the skills of the staff in the jurisdiction requesting the help and the individual(s) who provide assistance to them. The Centers for Disease Control and Prevention's Epidemic Intelligence Service (EIS) is a wonderful example of this benefit. There have been numerous deployments of the EIS officers into outbreaks of all kinds throughout the United States, its territories, and to other countries. Many of the chapters in this book derive from EIS officer experiences. I have heard numerous former EIS officers describe their time in the EIS as the best 2 years of their career.

Outbreak investigations also allow for the fulfillment of legal obligations and duty of care for the public. State legislatures have passed rules and regulations establishing what should happen under certain circumstances, such as the reporting of a disease or outbreak. Outbreaks allow for the fulfillment of these legally mandated control measures, such as removing a food handler from food preparation activities while they have diarrheal illness or are shedding *Salmonella* species in their stool despite recovery from diarrhea. Other legislative mandates, such as the authority to close down a business (such as a restaurant) or to isolate or quarantine a patient may be fulfilled as the public health authority responding to the outbreak carries out its control efforts.

An outbreak investigation offers a unique opportunity to educate the public about disease prevention. Although the media is sometimes an investigative watchdog and can be overzealous or less than scientific in its approach to a public health problem, it can also be a terrific partner of the health department with the mutual goal of informing the public with what they need to know. As a result, while information about hand washing, covering your cough, receiving immunizations, or cooking meat or chicken to a certain temperature might not be news on any given day, during an outbreak it might be a critical control measure and can even become front page news. Contact with the media can also be very useful to calming fears, combating rumors, directing the public to where they can access special assistance (such as antibiotics, immunizations, or information) and promoting the single overriding communication objective (SOCO). The SOCO is very important, because while a thoughtful investigator can talk about many features of the outbreak that may be of interest, the journalist is limited by the space and focus of their article. Therefore, it is helpful to be concise and focused with what is being shared with the journalist, even to the point of being redundant, such as saying "We really want to emphasize that thorough hand washing after using the bathroom is an essential way to prevent the spread of this disease", "Parents need to help their children wash their hands thoroughly to minimize risk of spread of this disease", and "The public does not need to be afraid of this disease. Something as simple as hand washing can protect themselves and others from getting it".

Public health departments often go unnoticed by many in the community. The public might be aware of influenza or other immunization services offered by them, but a lot of the very important functions of the local public health department are performed quietly and without fanfare. As a result, when there is an outbreak investigation, it is an opportunity for the public health department to improve and promote its credibility in dealing with a health emergency. As mentioned previously, while not every health department can take an active lead in such an investigation due to the heterogeneous distribution of epidemiologic skills from health department to health department, even inexperienced staff can provide vital support roles to those invited in to take the lead. A public health department can be praised for calling in needed assistance, just as it can be condemned for not realizing when it has delayed getting help, to the detriment of the community. It is a difficult balance that should be kept in mind, as it impacts the credibility of the health department to its stakeholders, including the community it serves.

An outbreak also provides an opportunity to intelligently direct laboratory resources. I have heard laboratory workers on more than one occasion in my career recoil or ridicule the outbreak investigator who, when asked "What do you want us to test for?" about food or environmental samples, replies "Test for everything". While testing for everything might eventually find the pathogen, it is an unrealistic use of laboratory personnel and financial resources, and can create a great deal of unfocused busy work for the laboratory. Laboratory testing should

Laboratory testing should ideally follow epidemiologic information and test a hypothesis.

ideally follow epidemiologic information and test a hypothesis. However, there are circumstances where less targeted testing is reasonable, such as when mortality is high, time is of the essence, and the laboratory results might inform hypothesis generation.

Finally, an outbreak is an opportunity for sharing information with other health professionals, scientists, the public, and many others (such as our elected leaders). In addition to a written report that might sit for years in a file drawer, some outbreaks are published. These published outbreaks may be disseminated worldwide as their journals circulate to subscribers, including libraries where many persons gain access to them. With the Internet, some of these outbreak investigations are available for study without any subscription through free access or access granted through academic institutions. There is great value in many of these publications, as they can provide useful background information about the disease, summaries of methods used to perform part or all of the investigation, ways to display and interpret the results, and references to other publications that might be useful to future outbreak investigators.

Outbreak investigation would be considered beneficial even if only one or two of the above mentioned reasons applied. However, the benefits of outbreak investigation are many and substantial. Outbreak investigation is a vital public health duty and, as this book demonstrates, can also be a fascinating and instructive drama.

LEARNING QUESTIONS

1. Make a list of the benefits of outbreak investigation and consider who is the beneficiary with each one.
2. Define the acronym "SOCO" and explain its purpose.

CHAPTER 2

How an Outbreak is Investigated

Mark S. Dworkin, MD, MPH&TM, FACP

INTRODUCTION

It is worth summarizing and elaborating briefly on the steps (or activities) of outbreak investigation (Exhibit 1-1). Although the steps may not always occur in exactly this order, this is the general pattern of events. It is not unusual for more than one step to be occurring at the same time. Not all lists of outbreak investigation steps are identical, as some steps may be combined into one overarching step or may not be listed as a step but included in a discussion of outbreak methods. It is important to recognize that a list of outbreak investigation steps is less of a recipe to be followed precisely than it is guidance. Also, as the investigation progresses, knowing where one is at within the outbreak investigation steps can make it easier to stay organized and plan ahead for what may need to occur next. (The reader is also encouraged to examine other good reviews of outbreak investigation referenced at the end of this chapter.)[1–3]

> *It is important to recognize that a list of outbreak investigation steps is less of a recipe to be followed precisely than it is guidance.*

VERIFY THAT AN OUTBREAK IS OCCURRING

Often a telephone call reports the suspicion of an outbreak. Someone has noticed something out of the ordinary, such as an unexpectedly high number of cases of a disease or syndrome. The call might come from someone who attended a group function, like a wedding, and now they and others they know are ill. It might come from a hospital infection-control nurse or hospital microbiologist who notices that they have more than typical numbers of a particular bacterial isolate in the laboratory or infectious disease among the patients. It could arise, however, from a thoughtful review of surveillance data (perhaps from a public health laboratory) demonstrating an unexpected rise. Whether the recognition arises from a community member, a health professional, or an astute public health employee, the first step of an outbreak investigation is to verify that there is indeed an outbreak occurring. This is the first, but not the only, time during an outbreak investigation that one must be careful not to assume anything and to have a healthy skepticism about the information that one is receiving.

> **EXHIBIT 1-1 The Steps of an Outbreak Investigation**
>
> 1. Verify that an outbreak is occurring.
> 2. Confirm the diagnosis.
> 3. Assemble an investigation team.
> 4. Create a tentative case definition.
> 5. Count cases.
> 6. Perform epidemiologic analysis.
> 7. Perform supplemental laboratory or environmental investigation (if indicated).
> 8. Develop hypotheses.
> 9. Introduce preliminary control measures.
> 10. Decide whether observation or additional studies are indicated.
> 11. Perform additional analyses or plan and perform additional study.
> 12. Perform new (investigation-derived) control measures, and/or ensure the compliance of existing control measures.
> 13. Communicate prevention information and findings.
> 14. Monitor surveillance data.

A common method of verifying that an outbreak exists is to examine surveillance data (if the condition is a reportable disease). One of the important uses of surveillance data is outbreak detection. It can quickly be determined whether the suspicion of a high number of case reports of salmonellosis, shigellosis, or pertussis bears out as accurate by comparing the report to a median number of reported cases during a similar time period historically. In some cases, the disease is not known but the outbreak is initially recognized as a sudden rise in the onset of a sign or symptom, such as rash or diarrhea. A report might be that someone attended a group event where food was served and that many persons are ill; however, until it has been confirmed that more than one person is truly ill with a similar illness, and that they consumed food in common, it is premature to declare that a foodborne outbreak has occurred.

CONFIRM THE DIAGNOSIS

Another early step of the investigation is to confirm the diagnosis. A classic example of this would be when a hospital laboratory reports that they have several isolates of an uncommon bacteria or virus. Because the isolate is unusual, the laboratory might not have substantial expertise in identifying it; therefore, it is necessary to confirm the diagnosis by forwarding the isolates to a reference laboratory, such as at the state health department or Centers for Disease Control and Prevention (CDC). In such reference laboratories, it can be determined, for example, whether the *Salmonella* outbreak is really five isolates of *Salmonella* (and which serotype is involved), or actually one or even no *Salmonella* at all.

ASSEMBLE AN INVESTIGATION TEAM

Depending on the outbreak and the public health jurisdiction(s) involved, an investigation team may need to be assembled. This is especially likely if it is an outbreak of such a remarkable size or complexity that it needs a more formal group to work on it. Sometimes the investigation is conducted by an individual for whom this is an occasional duty and there is not a team per se, but individuals who react to the reports coming in and deal with them as needed. In other words, not every outbreak receives a full formal investigation. In some settings, a team is already assembled and on call for the next outbreak, whenever it may occur. In that case, this step would actually be the first step, as the public health jurisdiction recognizes that outbreaks occur with a great enough frequency to have planned ahead; however, more commonly, outbreak teams are assembled based on the unique issues surrounding the outbreak.

Considerations in assembling the team include determining a team leader. This determination is based on experience and expertise of the team leader; therefore, it might be a communicable disease section chief if there is an outbreak of salmonellosis, whereas it might be an immunization section chief for an outbreak of measles. Alternatively, there could be a program staff level individual (ideally with epidemiologic training) who is well suited to this task, or an epidemiologist might be invited in from a higher level jurisdiction (such as state or federal government) when necessary skills are lacking locally or when an investigation was attempted but was unsuccessful and still needs resolution. A higher profile investigation or one involving multiple jurisdictions might be led by a state epidemiologist or other senior epidemiology personnel. The team leader may not always be an epidemiologist but may be a skilled administrator or environmental health worker. The most important thing is that it should make sense that someone in the lead belongs there, as there is much to be gained with a well run outbreak investigation and much to be lost when it is poorly run.

Team members should be considered based on their experience, abilities, and availability. A team is best comprised of one or more members with experience, as the activities are likely to proceed much more smoothly with fewer misunderstandings or errors along the way; however, some team members may be inexperienced but need on-the-job training, or they may be needed to ensure that certain activities (such as interviewing) are adequately staffed to gather quickly the data needed for analysis. If they have the needed abilities (such as interviewing, data entry, or analysis skills), they can become useful contributing members once provided with the appropriate guidance or training. However, providing guidance or training in the setting of an urgent outbreak investigation can pose quite a challenge with many priorities competing for one's time.

If medical record abstraction or other clinical-related work is needed as part of an investigation, a healthcare provider, such as someone with nursing or medical training, may be essential.

Given that outbreaks do not schedule themselves when it is convenient to staff them, an additional consideration is who can be available for the duration needed. Personnel are typically diverted off their routine duties (which may also be essential and can only be delayed briefly). They may need to travel, including staying overnight for several days or longer. It is best to staff an outbreak with personnel who can remain with their outbreak duties without interruption, although this just may not be possible at times.

CREATE A TENTATIVE CASE DEFINITION

Once convinced that an outbreak is really occurring and having confirmed the diagnosis (or syndrome) that is involved, a tentative case definition is needed to begin to determine the extent of the outbreak in a systematic way. Essentially, this is a surveillance system that one is creating within the outbreak investigation. If a reportable disease is responsible for the outbreak, much of the outbreak definition may already be available. The case definition should involve elements of person, place, and time. Routine reporting of a reportable disease would not include the wedding, church supper, or other cohort information, nor would it necessarily include any geographic boundaries that might be needed to define the outbreak; therefore, a reportable disease case definition is often adapted, but it is not just used without any modification at all in an outbreak setting.

The case definition is tentative because, as additional information is learned, there may be a need to modify it so that it is most accurate and useful for analysis. It is important when communicating with the media and others, such as administrators who may not have epidemiologic training, that the preliminary information is just that—preliminary. An outbreak investigation needs to remain flexible, including the possibility of revising the case definition to achieve its goals of disease control and prevention.

The creation of a case definition may involve a thoughtful discussion of sensitivity and specificity. In an attempt to identify every case of a disease that might lead to death or severe morbidity, a highly sensitive case definition might be needed; however, when performing data analysis of reported cases, a more specific case definition is desired to limit the influence that inclusion of those without the disease of interest that happen to meet the case definition may have on the analysis results. As an illustrative but extreme example, if an investigation wanted to identify nearly every case of influenza, the case definition might include anyone with fever; however, such a definition also captures cases of numerous other illnesses and thus lacks the specificity needed to trust any data analysis intended to be specific to the control of influenza. Alternatively, if the case definition required the isolation of the influenza virus, there would be a high degree of certainty about the cases reported, but because most persons with influenza do not have laboratory procedures performed that lead to isolation of the virus, relatively few cases would be reported. A case definition should avoid including any potential risk factors within it, as that would prevent the analysis of whether those risk factors are statistically associated with the exposure.

> *The creation of a case definition may involve a thoughtful discussion of sensitivity and specificity.*

> *A case definition should avoid including any potential risk factors within it, as that would prevent the analysis of whether those risk factors are statistically associated with the exposure.*

A case definition often has more than one category within it, such as confirmed versus probable or primary versus secondary. Confirmed cases typically represent cases that have been laboratory confirmed. It is important to make this distinction of "laboratory confirmed" versus just saying "confirmed" because some surveillance systems, such as the one used for pertussis in the

United States, include cases without laboratory confirmation as confirmed cases if they are epidemiologically linked to a laboratory confirmed case. Probable cases usually refer to cases that have not met the relatively specific criteria of laboratory diagnostic testing but have other information that makes their likelihood of being true cases high.

The case definition is for the investigator's benefit. It is intended to assist the investigator with counting the cases and best determining the associated factors and source. This can madden the media, who are following some of these investigations, and even public health officials, who do not understand why the case count is changing, but keep in mind that its usefulness is in helping the investigator to provide a sound explanation for what has happened and why. The case definition in this setting is not designed to count exactly how many people got that disease. That number is likely to get underestimated in the race to solve and control the outbreak.

Primary cases are the cases that were exposed to the implicated source, whereas secondary cases usually arise from their contact with an infectious primary case. For example, a restaurant may be implicated in an outbreak. The cases that ate a *Salmonella*-contaminated food develop gastroenteritis and are called primary cases. They will shed the organism in their stool, and if they do not practice good hand hygiene after using the bathroom, they may transfer the organism to a family member or friend (such as if they prepared sandwiches for them). These new cases of salmonellosis may never have been to the implicated restaurant and are secondary cases. Unfortunately, sometimes you can have cases in the same household where the second case could have been exposed to the implicated source but had a long enough delay after the first case to have been caused by secondary transmission as well. This needs to be kept in mind when designing the case definition.

When later performing analysis of the cases ascertained through outbreak investigation, it is important to exclude the secondary cases from the analysis of risk factors, especially when the goal is to identify the primary source of the outbreak. In addition, if there are sufficient numbers of laboratory-confirmed cases, probable cases may be excluded to increase the likelihood that an association is real and to avoid the possibility of bias against a true association if probable cases include some persons who met the case definition but do not (unknown to the investigation staff) have the outbreak disease. Thus, while chasing down laboratory specimens (sputum, vomit, feces, blood, or others) from many of the cases can involve a lot of work, it can pay off if it yields a big enough number of cases that you are confident really are cases.

COUNT CASES

After a case definition has been created, the work of identifying as many cases as is feasible follows. In some situations, like a commercial product outbreak or one that has substantial morbidity or mortality and is not readily being solved, that means trying to get all of the exposed ill persons reported, often by announcing the outbreak through a variety of means, including electronic, fax, and press release, although there may be situations where the outbreak is so massive that efforts are eventually best directed toward prevention and control. In the uncommon situation where an outbreak is massive, an estimate of the case burden may be performed. It is a judgment call whether resources are to be expended on reporting tens of thousands of cases versus allowing passive reporting to decline naturally without active and persistent efforts. Broadcasting the existence of an outbreak may be indicated when there is a good prevention intervention (like an effective vaccine or immunoglobulin), and thus, raising awareness could help exposed persons prevent the onset of illness (such as in the case of hepatitis A exposure).

PERFORM EPIDEMIOLOGIC ANALYSIS

After there are data from cases to analyze and those data are entered into a computer database, it is time to perform descriptive epidemiology. This allows for many basic questions to be answered, especially when the number of cases on the initial "line list" (where the first reports were summarized on paper or in spreadsheets) has become numerous. The initial analysis might include frequencies of all the variables, thus demonstrating basic patterns of the outbreak, such as age, gender, racial, occupational, clinical manifestations, and exposure information. Cases may be examined for their geographical distribution, and the results may lead to a hypothesis regarding a suspected exposure site. If an onset of illness date and an exposure date are known, a mean or median incubation period might be calculated that can be compared with what is already known for suspected pathogens (most useful when the pathogen is unknown). Depending on the type of outbreak (such as respiratory or foodborne) and whether the number of persons who have been exposed is known, preliminary overall or food-specific attack rates can be determined. Several computer statistical software packages are available for analyzing outbreak data, but one of the more commonly used and freely accessible epidemiological software packages is Epi Info (available for free download from the CDC at http://www.cdc.gov/epiinfo/). Epi Info is particularly convenient for investigators with limited epidemiologic and analysis skills because it has many functions that do not involve writing any programming code.

PERFORM SUPPLEMENTAL LABORATORY OR ENVIRONMENTAL INVESTIGATION

Environmental or laboratory studies may be recognized as potentially useful early in some outbreak investigations. For example, in foodborne outbreak investigations where a food establishment, such as a restaurant, is implicated by several of the cases, a restaurant inspection by the local health authority is a routine response. This would typically occur even if that food establishment had received a routine inspection some time in the recent past. The inspection could reveal useful clues that may help with use or interpretation of the epidemiologic data (such as learning of ill food handlers or discovery that there was a recent plumbing problem). It may simply reveal sooner (rather than after data are entered and analyzed) that there are violations of required food sanitation practices that must be remedied for that restaurant to stay in business. In other words, a control measure such as closing down a restaurant should not have to wait until epidemiologic analysis if an onsite inspection of an implicated site reveals the need for such actions. Alternatively, an implicated site may not be recognized as being in need of inspection until epidemiologic analysis provides the hypothesis of such a site. This might be the case for an outbreak of sporadic cases of a disease (such as travel-associated Legionnaire's disease) where cases are not becoming recognized all at one time and the outbreak is picked up by a central repository of cases, such as a national or international surveillance system.[4] Alternatively, sporadic cases may become linked by a laboratory surveillance system that identifies identical bacterial strains referred from cases in disparate locations reported to different health jurisdictions.[5]

DEVELOP HYPOTHESES

The development of a hypothesis is usually a very early step in outbreak investigation. The first hypothesis may even come from a case, and it's possible that it could be correct ("My husband, daughter, and I are all sick and so is my sister's family. We both attended my cousin's wedding and I'm sure it was the chicken because it wasn't fully cooked.") Alternatively, a hypothesis may be difficult to develop, as the information may not be revealing enough. This might occur when the questions that need to be asked simply have not been asked yet; however, enough is known of many diseases that cause outbreaks to lead experienced investigators to at least some hypothesis to explore with the descriptive data. For example, there have been many outbreaks of diarrheal disease attributed to *E. coli* O157:H7, and among the potential sources, undercooked ground meat is a well recognized source; therefore, it is common for cases of this disease to be asked whether ground meat was consumed. An examination of the frequency of having eaten ground meat among the cases is helpful because when many of the cases have this exposure it leads to a biologically plausible hypothesis that ground meat was the source of the outbreak. Although it is reasonable to consider ground meat in every *E. coli* O157:H7 outbreak (and therefore to inquire about it), the absence of a majority of the cases with such an exposure should raise the issue of alternative hypotheses; however, recall of an exposure can be poor, whether early or late in an investigation, leading those questioned about the true exposure that caused the outbreak to respond at a rate not reaching 50% with a yes answer (William Keene, PhD, personal communication). Efficiency in solving outbreaks comes with increased familiarity with the most common pathogens that cause them and emerging information about these pathogens.

INTRODUCE PRELIMINARY CONTROL MEASURES

As early as possible, preliminary control measures should be introduced. Some of these control measures may already be established and incorporated into legislated rules and regulations for a reportable disease. In the case of botulism, removing any suspected product (such as a batch of a suspected home canned vegetable) might be performed immediately on the recognition of this source before any data analysis has occurred, and possibly before any data have even been entered into a database. Similarly, there need not be an outbreak of meningococcal meningitis for the control measure of providing prophylactic antibiotics to close contacts of a case to occur. When more than one person with gastroenteritis implicates having eaten at the same restaurant and becoming ill within a biologically plausible time period, an inspection of that restaurant by the local health department is reasonable, although it is uncertain whether that restaurant is the source at this early time; therefore, a restaurant inspection is a reasonable preliminary control measure, but closing the restaurant might be premature.

This brings up the important issue of when to pursue an extreme control measure, such as closure of a business, where the economic implications could be substantial for the business and are being weighed against the public health implications of delaying such an action. Each decision should be made on a case-by-case basis. If the decision is made to take extreme action and it is wrong, there is risk for litigation and loss of credibility. If the decision is made not to take extreme action and it is wrong, again there is risk for litigation and loss of credibility. Thus, with such a dilemma, what is one to do? Essentially, the basis for this decision should be made by weighing factors such as the severity of the illness, the vulnerability of the population exposed, and whether the suspected exposure is ongoing. An illness that is killing its victims is certainly worthy of a heavier hand than one that causes an inconvenient gastroenteritis with very rare mortality. If the exposure is threatening persons at higher risk for clinically severe manifestations, such as infants, older individuals, or immunocompromised persons, it increases the weight of considering a more extreme measure (at least temporarily, until more evidence comes in). If the exposure is a food, and the product has been discarded or its preparation has been discontinued, then closure of a restaurant with the aim of controlling the outbreak would be of little benefit after this activity has already occurred. In the case of a business, it may be possible to reason with the owner or manager, leading to his or her enacting the control measure of closure on a voluntary basis. It may be decided that they have less to lose by closing voluntarily and appearing cooperative than by being closed involuntarily or announced in a press release from the health department.

Other preliminary control measures might involve public education about the mode of transmission and prevention methods that are recognized about the outbreak disease from previous experience. Alternatively, a more expensive or difficult outbreak control measure, such as mass vaccination, may need to wait for clear evidence from additional studies or supplemental laboratory testing that demonstrates whether the vaccination is appropriate. For example, in an outbreak of invasive meningococcal disease, the vaccine covers four of the five most common serotypes of the organism (types A, C, Y, and W135 of *Neisseria meningitidis*); therefore, if the laboratory investigation determines that the outbreak is due to serotype B, mass vaccination with the quadrivalent vaccine would not be expected to impact on the outbreak.

Finally, political considerations can trump everything as a decision may be made by a high-level administrator who has determined that there is a right side and a wrong side of this issue to be on and they have decided to get on what they consider to be the right side. At a minimum, the investigators can offer wise counsel to the administrator based on the evidence and any other information, but sometimes these decisions are out of the investigators' hands.

DECIDE WHETHER OBSERVATION OR ADDITIONAL STUDIES ARE INDICATED

Before launching into additional studies, such as case control or cohort studies to test hypotheses, a decision should be made whether further studies are warranted. Sometimes these additional studies may be done with the existing data depending on the question. In some situations, an outbreak has "burnt out." No further cases are being reported and it seems that whatever the exposure was, it may have all been consumed. The pursuit of additional study at this time may be of little public health use compared with the resources needed to carry it out. Sometimes a case control study may be possible as with an *E. coli* O157:H7 outbreak where one or two dozen cases have been reported over a few months in a geographic area where that is unexpected. Preexisting outbreak investigation questionnaires are available from the Internet (an example can be found at http://www.oregon.gov/DHS/ph/acd/keene.shtml). It may be tempting to pursue a case control study because there are well-recognized risk factors and asking these questions of controls is feasible; however, in the absence of a sound hypothesis, there is little chance for success with such an approach compared with the likelihood of wasting personnel resources.

One of the authors of a chapter in this book, Dr. Paul Blake, was formerly the head of the Foodborne and Diarrheal Diseases Branch at the CDC in Atlanta. Back in 1984, he authored a memorandum that provided guidance at the CDC on this issue. He emphasized the importance of interviewing the initial cases and that if such interviews did not lead to a hypothesis about the exposure that it would be best to have a more experienced interviewer reinterview them. If that still did not lead to a hypothesis, rather than pursue a study not based on a sound hypothesis, one could try to bring the cases together (with their consent, either in person or perhaps by conference call) to discuss possible exposures that could weave a common thread among them. Their interaction with each other could lead to information that an interviewer might not have thought to ask.

The in-depth and open-ended hypothesis-generating interview can be very useful to lead to the discovery of unexpected vehicles for disease. A single investigator would be best to perform each of these hypothesis-generating interviews. The interviews should be performed as soon as possible after the report of the case because recall may diminish with time. Recalling one Louisiana outbreak of cholera that Dr. Blake investigated, he said this:

> It was not until I interviewed the fourth case and he mentioned eating cooked crabs which the first three had also mentioned, that a chill went up my spine and I thought, "Cooked crabs could be the cause of this outbreak." We would never have otherwise included cooked crabs on a case control questionnaire because we did not consider cooked crabs to be a possible vehicle for cholera because they were cooked.[6]

PERFORM ADDITIONAL ANALYSES OR PLAN AND PERFORM ADDITIONAL STUDY

If a sound hypothesis exists, additional analysis may be performed, such as a cohort or case control study. Entire books can be written on these study methods. The cohort study gets its name from the convenience of having the entire population exposed clearly defined, as with a church supper, catered banquet, or persons who share the same well for their drinking water. In the latter example, it can be difficult to demonstrate an association because everyone may have had the exposure, and thus, you do not know whether the well water drinkers are ill because they drank the well water or because they have some other common exposure. In this type of situation, it can be helpful if a dose-response relationship can be demonstrated. The more well water those exposed drank, the more likely they became ill. In the case of a heavily contaminated vehicle, this may be more difficult to show.[7]

Multiple studies may be needed to derive final conclusions. In the case of an Illinois outbreak caused by the parasite Cryptosporidium, the first study performed was a community case control study to determine whether a popular water park was the exposure site. Other possibilities considered included other recreational water exposure such as a lake, contact with animals, and drinking a possibly contaminated beverage. After exposure to the water park was strongly associated with having cryptosporidiosis, a cohort study was performed among water park attendees to determine the exposure within the water park. This study demonstrated the importance of ingesting the pool water. Finally, supplemental laboratory investigation involving testing of the water filter system for the presence of the parasite was also performed.[8] These studies taken together made a strong case for the source being the water at the water park.

Selecting controls for a case control study can be a challenge. Controls should not have had

> *Selecting controls for a case control study can be a challenge.*

the outbreak disease but should have had a similar likelihood of having been exposed as the cases (as best one can establish this). This may be handled by picking controls that live in the same neighborhood as the cases or are referred by controls (friends and family). They may be matched to cases by age group or gender to control for behavioral differences that are influenced by these factors, some of which may be unknown to the investigator. After a control is identified and the interviewing has begun, it should be established right away whether the control could meet the case definition completely or even partially (perhaps qualifying as a probable or suspect case). Exclusion criteria should be established to ensure that any controls could not actually be cases. Although this might ideally be done with laboratory testing, this is often not realistic, and thus, screening them with questions that determine whether they satisfy the case definition is more feasible. Controls that may meet the case definition should be investigated further and reclassified as cases as needed.

A variety of biases could be introduced when selecting cases and controls for further study.[7] These include sampling bias if there is a need to select among the cases, as when there are a very large number but a large number of interviews are not feasible or statistically necessary to evaluate a hypotheses (an uncommonly fortuitous situation to be in). Diagnostic suspicion bias may occur if the cases are well aware of the suspected vehicle, perhaps from widespread media attention. Diagnostic access bias may interfere with selection of controls because cases may have (by definition) had access to diagnostic tests and thus been recognized as cases while controls may include persons who, for reasons that could be relevant to the analysis, were less likely to access such diagnostic testing. Misclassification bias can be dealt with by the screening of controls for any similar illness to cases as stated previously here. Other biases such as recall bias or interviewer bias must also be considered. A good outbreak investigation will consider these biases and interpret the results with them in mind.

Several factors may support a decision to perform additional analytic studies even when the outbreak appears to be over when it is first recognized. These include a high morbidity or mortality of the disease, high visibility of the outbreak with substantial media attention, enthusiasm by those affected by the outbreak (where their cooperation and/or their desire for an answer to what happened is high), and the novelty of the pathogen, its mode of transmission, or its clinical manifestations such that it provides an opportunity to learn something new about the organism or disease. Another important factor is the availability of personnel and financial resources to continue with the investigation.

Sometimes outbreak investigation studies are referred to as "quick and dirty" because biases are not substantially dealt with in the study design and the number of cases and controls is not derived from any power calculations based on the hypothesis and assumptions. This is a reality of outbreak investigation because, as they are essentially experiments of nature, there is no control over how many cases will have occurred. The best one can do is pursue case ascertainment aggressively to attempt to populate the database with as many cases as may be needed to lead to statistically significant findings. It should also be recognized that even statistically significant findings are not the same thing as cause and effect. Simply stated, if it is 95% likely that an association did not occur by chance, it is still 5% likely that it could have; therefore, for any results from these studies, there should be biologic plausibility. Also, the finding (or association) should account for most of the cases if the source of the outbreak will be attributed to that finding and be of a sufficiently high magnitude to be relevant.

Outbreak investigators should also be familiar with the binomial probability method. When enough information is available, this method can allow for estimation of the probability that a particular exposure was present among cases by chance alone. Without performing a case control study, the results of such a study can be estimated. For example, in an outbreak caused by *Salmonella enterica* serotype enteritidis, routine food exposure interviews had not indicated a common exposure. A much expanded questionnaire was then used, and it led to a hypothesis concerning consumption of raw almonds. Using the binomial probability method, the rate of consumption of almonds (and other foods) was compared with the background rates of consumption of these foods based on available Oregon survey results. It was helpful that background information on the expected rate of consumption of almonds was available for the Oregon population. In that survey, 9% of 921 Oregon residents had consumed raw almonds in the preceding week; however, all five of the sporadic cases had consumed raw almonds in the week before illness. These and other data from this investigation contributed to a recall of 13 million pounds of almonds![9] Additional information on this method can be found on the Internet (http://www.oregon.gov/DHS/ph/acd/outbreak/binomial.xls and http://faculty.vassar.edu/lowry/binomialX.html), and "A Population Survey Atlas of Exposures" that is available from the CDC (http://www.cdc.gov/foodnet/reports.htm).

PERFORM NEW CONTROL MEASURES AND/OR ENSURE THE COMPLIANCE OF EXISTING CONTROL MEASURES

Depending on the outbreak, new control measures may derive from the investigation results. If identification of an exposure such as a food item or activity like swimming is revealed as the source of the outbreak only after additional studies were performed, a food may need to be recalled and product embargoed, or perhaps a swimming pool or lake may need to be closed to the public. New environmental and laboratory investigations may follow as an attempt is made to explain more fully the origin of the outbreak. In the case of a foodborne outbreak, a trace back might help to explain where an imported product became contaminated. Alternatively, when monkeypox was imported to the United States, a trace back determined that the outbreak likely began from giant Gambian rats imported from Ghana that later mixed with highly susceptible United States prairie dogs sold (unknowingly infected) to lovers of "pocket pets."[10]

It is an important practical matter to ensure that control measures put into place are being carried out. This is usually not an issue unless the persons who are directly responsible for carrying out the control measure (such as closing a restaurant or catering business) fail to accept that the control measure is sound or perhaps if they do not trust the source of the prevention information. If a publicly accessible area is restricted, such as when a beach is closed because it is a risk, it should be a routine matter that someone is assessing that there are no swimmers and that the sign(s) posted is readily visible and posted in the appropriate languages to make sure that the message is readily understood.

COMMUNICATE PREVENTION INFORMATION AND FINDINGS

Communication is a key issue from the beginning to the end of the outbreak. Within the outbreak investigation team, information such as telephone and fax numbers and e-mail addresses are all basic information to be exchanged. Regularly, the team should be meeting either in person or by conference call to update each other, and it is beneficial to summarize the update in a written format such as an e-mail circulated internally among those with direct or indirect responsibility for the investigation, such as high-level administrators. It is especially important for no assumptions to be made related to communication. In other words, it can be an unwise gamble to assume that someone else is sharing important information with the team leader or an administrative person in a central office if that is not known with certainty. Redundancy of communication may be inefficient, but it is a far lesser sin than lack of communication.

The public and other stakeholders of the outbreak are important communication targets as well. These may include hospital staff such as emergency room physicians or infection control workers, day care workers, school principals or teachers, parents, and the media. Depending on what information is being released, those responsible at the site of the outbreak (such as a restaurant or hotel manager or hospital administrator) should be made aware of basic developments, as their level of anxiety can be very high and their cooperation may be linked to the trust that can come from good communication. Partnering organizations, such as the U.S. Department of Agriculture or the Food and Drug Administration as well as state or local equivalents, should also be updated. Those who need to be informed and what they need to be told may vary based on the specifics of the outbreak investigation.

What is said in oral versus written communication is also worth considering because written word typically becomes part of a permanent record. It may be read or reread, sometimes with unintended negative intonation. E-mails may be sent to one party and forwarded to another. Written communication may be released to attorneys if legal action follows. It is a practical matter for any investigator to be open and honest in all of their communication, but to be concise and clear without unneeded unbalanced accusation or risk of breeching confidentiality by recording names unnecessarily. An example of this could be when the investigation staff might name a person or restaurant they are investigating in an e-mail that is forwarded to someone outside of the investigation team who then reveals this name prematurely to the media. The person to whom this e-mail was forwarded may have had too little information about the details of the outbreak or too little experience with these situations. The use of terms "Hotel X," "Product A," "Nurse B," or "Restaurant Y" arose to help protect the unnecessary release of identities where that information could be damaging and would not benefit public health. Alternatively, if protection of public health warrants it, communication broadly of the name of a person, institution, or other exposure source may be needed. Investigators should be aware of legal requirements in their jurisdictions concerning matters that involve confidentiality.

Communicating the prevention message of the outbreak and the findings through internal report or scientific publication is also important. In the case of the latter, agreement early on concerning who will be assigned the lead authorship is very important to avoid conflict or resentment later on. This is especially important when more than one person on the team might be qualified to lead the investigation or to undertake the writing of a scientific article describing it. It is also especially important when multiple public health jurisdictions are involved, including when federal assistance is performed at the state or local level.

> *Communicating the prevention message of the outbreak and the findings through internal report or scientific publication is also important.*

MONITOR SURVEILLANCE DATA

Finally, it is important to continue to monitor surveillance data as the outbreak ends. This may reveal that the control measures were inadequate and that new hypotheses and new investigation may be needed. Also, secondary outbreaks may arise. For example, after the massive cryptosporidiosis outbreak in Wisconsin (described in this book), additional smaller outbreaks were recognized as the parasite was shed by persons with cryptosporidiosis in a variety of settings such as a swimming pool.[11]

CONCLUSION

The steps of outbreak investigation are extremely useful to keep in mind during an outbreak to help provide some order to what can be a stressful, fast moving, and complicated process. Outbreak work is reactive. Although some outbreaks are actually over when they are recognized, many are in progress and have an urgency to them. The hours can be long but some of an epidemiologist's best work actually is performed in this intense setting. The examples in this book will hopefully provide the reader with an illustration of how some of these steps have played out in real outbreaks of infectious diseases. Keep in mind, however, that sometimes not all of the steps need to get done before a press release comes out to announce the concern. There is an art to making the decision of how far to go with an investigation, and that comes with much experience. Nonetheless, it is a gamble every time.

REFERENCES

1. Reingold AL. Outbreak investigations: a perspective. *Emerg Infect Dis* 1998;4:21–27.
2. Gregg MB. Conducting a field investigation. In Gregg MB, ed. *Field Epidemiology*, 2nd ed. New York: Oxford University Press, 2002:62–77.
3. Magnus M. Outbreak investigations. In *Essentials of Infectious Disease Epidemiology*. Sudbury: Jones and Bartlett, 2008:43–61.
4. Ricketts KD, Yadav R, Joseph CA. European Working Group for Legionella Infections. Travel-associated Legionnaires disease in Europe: 2006. *Euro Surveill* 2008;13:18930.
5. Jones TF, Scallan E, Angulo FJ. FoodNet: overview of a decade of achievement. *Foodborne Pathog Dis* 2007;4:60–66.
6. Yoder J, Ritger K, Dworkin MS. Foodborne outbreak investigation: how do I find the implicated food when I have few cases and no good hypothesis? *Illinois Infectious Disease Report* (Volume 3, Spring 2006). Retrieved June 25, 2008, from www.idph.state.il.us/health/infect/ID_Report_Spring06.pdf.
7. Palmer SR. Epidemiology in search of infectious diseases: methods in outbreak investigation. *J Epidemiol Com Health* 1989;43:311–314.
8. Causer LM, Handzel T, Welch P, et al. An outbreak of Cryptosporidium hominis infection at an Illinois recreational waterpark. *Epidemiol Infect* 2006;134:147–156.
9. Keady S, Briggs G, Farrar J, et al. Outbreak of *Salmonella* serotype enteritidis infections associated with raw almonds: United States and Canada, 2003–2004. *MMWR* 2004;53: 484–487.
10. Reed KD, Melski JW, Graham MB, et al. The detection of monkeypox in humans in the Western Hemisphere. *N Engl J Med* 2004;350:342–350.
11. Mac Kenzie WR, Kazmierczak JJ, Davis JP. An outbreak of cryptosporidiosis associated with a resort swimming pool. *Epidemiol Infect* 1995;115:545–553.

LEARNING QUESTIONS

1. How do public health investigators verify if a suspected outbreak is a true outbreak?
2. After obtaining descriptive data in an outbreak investigation, what are the considerations when deciding whether to perform additional analyses or studies such as a case-control study?

PART II

Outbreak Investigations of Infectious Diseases

CHAPTER 3

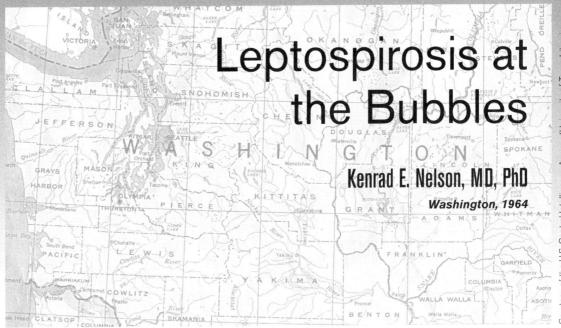

Leptospirosis at the Bubbles

Kenrad E. Nelson, MD, PhD

Washington, 1964

INTRODUCTION

After completing a rotating internship and Internal Medicine residency at Cook County Hospital in Chicago, I joined the Epidemic Intelligence Service (EIS) at the Centers for Disease Control (CDC) in Atlanta in 1963. The EIS provides a 2-year experience in applied public health and field epidemiology for health professionals who have recently completed their training. Most EIS officers were physicians, who like me had just completed residency training, but the EIS program also included other health professionals, such as veterinarians, nurses, dentists, biostatisticians, and public health specialists.

I became interested in the EIS program during my year as chief resident in Internal Medicine at Cook County Hospital. When I was on the pulmonary rotation, I cared for many patients with tuberculosis (TB), a very common disease in the 1960s in Cook County. Although some patients with TB responded well to therapy, it was very frustrating that many did not. It was common in those days for TB patients to leave the hospital against medical advice after having received a week or two of anti-TB drugs, especially if they were asked to undergo bronchoscopy, which was done then using a rigid bronchoscope. Unfortunately, the director of the chest surgery service in the hospital viewed training surgery residents to do bronchoscopy on TB patients as his most important teaching responsibility. Patients who left the hospital were often readmitted several months later with more advanced, active TB after having stopped their treatment as soon as they became afebrile or felt better.

When I did a follow-up study of the outcome of TB treatment of about 120 patients with positive cultures 2 years earlier, the results were very discouraging. Only about a third of these patients were cured of their TB and still alive. About a third had died, often with active TB because they had discontinued their therapy and resumed drinking alcohol or injecting drugs or were just lost to follow-up by the Chicago TB clinics. This was long before directly observed treatment became the standard of care in Chicago.

The results of this study peaked my interest in public health and epidemiology. When I visited the CDC before joining the EIS I became interested in public health and epidemiology because of its more comprehensive and inclusive analysis of the sociocultural and environmental determinants, as well as the biological factors, related to disease and health problems. Also, the investigation of outbreaks of disease was a fascinating and important responsibility of an epidemiologist in the EIS program, and this interested me as well.

When I joined EIS in 1963, I was assigned to the Washington State Health Department. The position included reviewing and analyzing the reports of diseases submitted by the county health departments, communicating with the public and health professionals about public health issues and prevention programs, and performing field epidemiology whenever an outbreak or cluster of illness was reported. There were many opportunities for evaluating possible outbreaks because the state epidemiologist was very competent and had established a good working relationship with most of the local health officers and practicing physicians in the state. Consequently, I investigated outbreaks of foodborne illnesses (i.e., salmonellosis, *Clostridium perfringens*, and botulism), measles, vaccine-associated polio, influenza, diphtheria, and other diseases. One of the more memorable and interesting outbreak investigations is described here.

THE BUBBLES OUTBREAK

In August 1964, I received a call from the director of the Benton-Franklin County Health Department in southeastern Washington asking for assistance in investigating a cluster of cases of a febrile illness in adolescents. Several local physicians had cared for teenaged children who had become ill with a fever, headache, and muscle aches that seemed to be clinically similar. Several of these patients had been hospitalized. Some patients had a stiff neck, but respiratory or gastrointestinal symptoms or a skin rash was uncommon.

I agreed to come and help with the investigation. I was aware that several arboviruses that cause encephalitis and meningitis, including Western equine and St. Louis Encephalitis viruses, had been frequently isolated from patients with central nervous system infections living in central and eastern Washington in the past. No horse deaths had been reported, however. All of the ill persons seemed to have recovered, and these patients seemed to be somewhat older than most reported arbovirus encephalitis cases in the past. Another possible consideration could have been a systemic fungal infection; however, central Washington was north of the area of endemicity of coccidioidomycosis (Valley Fever). Another consideration was an enterovirus infection, as these viruses are common in the summer and may cause aseptic meningitis, sometimes as outbreaks. Another, less likely possibility was amebic encephalitis. Thus, I packed my copy of Benenson's *Infectious Diseases of Man* (a public health book that has been essential to communicable disease investigators in health departments for decades, although its editor has changed over the years) and flew to eastern Washington.

When I arrived, I met with the director of the health department, and together we outlined a plan to investigate the outbreak. By that time, about 35 to 40 cases had been reported. Although we did not know which diagnosis we were dealing with, we believed an outbreak was occurring because this was a much higher number of similar illnesses in the adolescent population than any of the local practitioners or the health department routinely recognized. An initial look at the descriptive epidemiology of the cases revealed that the dates of illness onset extended back a couple of months to the middle of June. Since then, several cases had been reported each week, without obvious temporal clustering; therefore, it did not appear to be a single exposure, common source outbreak, but perhaps an ongoing epidemic of an arbovirus or enterovirus infection should be considered. Another curious feature was that most of the cases (about 80%) were in boys. This appeared to be evidence against the outbreak being an arbovirus or an enterovirus because we were unaware of any gender predilection for illnesses caused by those viruses.

My first step after reviewing the data available at the health department was to go to the local hospital and review the charts of several typical cases who had been hospitalized. This was long before the HIPPA legislation had been enacted, which might have complicated this approach. I took the list of names of the reported cases to the hospital and asked the record librarian to pull the charts for me. I discovered that a typical illness characteristically included fever, myalgia, headache, and shaking chills with a stiff neck reported in about half the cases (Tables 3-1 and 3-2). The illness lasted about 5 to 7 days, and respiratory symptoms, diarrhea, and rash were uncommon. Some patients had a recurrence of their symptoms a few days after they had recovered. Lumbar punctures had been done in four cases; three were normal, but one had 798 white blood cells/mm^3, of which 53% were polymorphonuclear cells and 47% were mononuclear cells. In this patient, the protein was elevated at 130 per 100 ml, and the sugar was normal (50 mg/100 ml). The normal glucose was evidence against TB or fungal meningitis. All cultures of blood, urine, and cerebrospinal fluid were sterile. There was a modest

TABLE 3-1 Symptoms of 61 Children with Leptospirosis

Symptom	No.	Percentage
Fever	61	100.0
Myalgia	60	98.4
Headache	58	95.1
Shaking Chills	56	91.8
Nausea	55	90.2
Vomiting	33	54.1
Arthralgia	19	31.1
Diarrhea	7	11.5

Reprinted with permission from Nelson KE, et al. *Am J Epidemiol* 1973;98:336–347.

increase in the peripheral white blood cell count. Urinalysis performed on 26 patients revealed that 22 had more than five white blood cells per high-power field with a slight proteinuria (1 to 2+) in 10 cases. These clinical data were peculiar and unexpected for any common seasonal infection in a presumably healthy adolescent population.

I decided that the next step should be to interview a few typical cases as a way toward generating a hypothesis of what was going on. My colleagues at the health department said this could be arranged. Thus, I met with several recently reported cases and a couple of those who had become ill in June. These cases did not report any common meals, gatherings, or special associations or common exposures with other children who had been ill; however, they usually knew several other children who had experienced similar illnesses. Finally, one of them said, "Doc, you should check out 'the Bubbles,'" after which I asked what and where were the Bubbles? He offered to take me there.

> *Finally, one of them said, "Doc, you should check out 'the Bubbles,'" after which I asked what and where were the Bubbles? He offered to take me there.*

The next day we went to the Bubbles. It was a concrete block structure a few miles out in the country in the field between the three surrounding towns of Kennewick, Pasco, and Richland (Figure 3-1). Connected to the small concrete structure at the Bubbles were two concrete walls about 5 feet high. These walls extended out about 7 feet. The Bubbles was a part of the irrigation system that divided the stream of irrigation water into two directions with a pump, which created bubbles when the water was pumped forcefully from below the surface. The structure was known by irrigation specialists as a "bifurcator." It was used to distribute the water in two directions and keep it flowing downstream. We were told that about 800 gallons of water passed through the bifurcator every 1 to 2 seconds. This caused the water to bubble and churn forcefully when the bifurcator was operating at full speed.

To the junior and senior high school students, however, the Bubbles was a great place to go swimming

TABLE 3-2 Abnormal Physical Findings in 46 Leptospirosis Patients Seen by a Physician

Finding	Number Affected	Percentage
Fever	46	100.0
Stiff neck	23	50.0
Throat injection	14	30.4
Biphasic course	10	21.7
Adenopathy	8	17.4
Flank tenderness	5	10.9
Conjunctivitis	5	10.9
Splenomegaly	1	2.2

Reprinted with permission from Nelson KE, et al. *Am J Epidemiol* 1973;98:336–347.

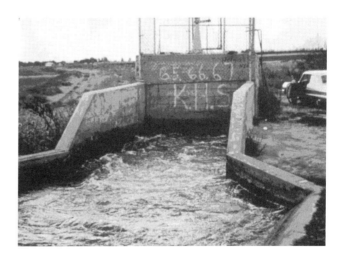

FIGURE 3-1 "The Bubbles." The depth of the water at this point was 2.1 meters, the walls rose 1.1 meter above the water and were 3 meters apart. The churning of the water was caused by subsurface feeding. Reprinted with permission from: Nelson KE, et al. *Am J Epidemiol* 1973;98:336–347.

during the summer. During that summer, as was not uncommon in southeastern Washington, the temperature often exceeded 95°F to 100°F. The local swimming pool was often closed and very crowded when it was open. Thus, the Bubbles was a great and special place to swim for teenagers. Students could stand on the concrete wall and jump into the bubbling water to be swirled around and often careen into the walls of the structure. Swimming at the Bubbles combined the joy of a swimming pool with the thrill of a ride at an amusement park. Swimming at the Bubbles often caused small skin abrasions, but it was described as "fun" and "exciting."

After learning about the Bubbles, I contacted several adolescents that I had decided were typical "cases" of the mysterious illness based on their reported symptoms of fever, headaches, muscle aches, and stiff neck. Interestingly, all of the typical cases reported swimming at the Bubbles before they became ill. It then became clear to me that swimming at the Bubbles was a very important exposure that occurred before the onset of this febrile illness. The water at the Bubbles appeared clean, although it was not potable but used only for irrigation. The ultimate source was the Columbia River, which was very nearby. We found later that the water at the Bubbles had a very high coliform count (>240,000 colonies per ml) and was alkaline (pH, 8.3).

We then decided to explore the irrigation canal upstream from the Bubbles for potential sources of contamination. The most effective way to do this was to hire a small plane that was used for crop dusting and fly over the irrigation canal, as there were no roads running parallel to the canal. This was an exciting trip, which resembled a roller coaster ride, as the plane was flying quite low and at slow speeds so that we could observe the canal and take pictures. This trip was quite revealing in that about 300 yards upstream from the Bubbles we noticed a herd of cattle, some of whom were also using the irrigation ditch as a watering hole to cool off (Figure 3-2). These were the only animals that we found to have direct access to the irrigation canal between the Bubbles and the origin of the canal a couple of miles upstream at the Yakima River. Thus, after the plane landed we decided to investigate the herd further. By then, we had decided that it was likely that the outbreak was due to leptospirosis. The exposure of cases to water that may have been contaminated by cattle and the clinical epidemiology made this diagnosis biologically plausible. This was confirmed when we obtained blood specimens from several of the typical cases and sent them to the CDC laboratory in Atlanta for testing.

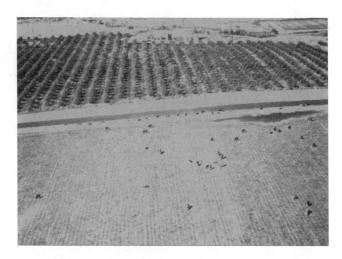

FIGURE 3-2 Aerial view of site of epidemic of leptospirosis among swimmers in irrigation canal. Note numerous cattle upstream from irrigation canal site used for swimming. Reprinted with permission from: Nelson KE, et al. *Am J Epidemiol* 1973;98:336–347.

There are very few laboratories in the United States or worldwide that test for leptospirosis. The assays are not commercially available, nor are they included in the standard screening panel for meningoencephalitis screening. (Because of the limited availability of laboratory confirmation of suspect cases and the protean clinical manifestations, the disease was removed from the list of officially reportable diseases by the Council of State and Territorial Epidemiologists in 1995.) The definitive serological assay is the Microscopic Agglutination Test (MAT). In this assay, various serogroups of pathogenic leptospiral organisms are incubated with dilutions of sera from persons or animals with suspected infection, and the maximal dilution of sera that will cause 50% of the organisms to agglutinate when viewed under the microscope is reported to be the MAT titer. The MAT titers are read using serial dilutions of sera and live or formalinized organisms from several different leptospiral organisms, that is, serovars, to make the diagnosis and to estimate which organism might have caused the infection. The need for live or formalin treated antigens from several leptospiral organisms explains why so few laboratories test for infection. There is a significant risk of infection among laboratory workers when the organisms are subcultured. Nevertheless, the definitive serological assay for leptospirosis and the specific organism

> *There are very few laboratories in the United States or worldwide that test for leptospirosis.*

responsible for the infection are reported as the MAT titer.

In our study, MAT antibodies against leptospires from 18 serovars were evaluated, and the titers against *Leptospira pomona* were generally highest. This was consistent with the literature, as *L. pomona* and *L. hardjo* serovars from the *L. pomona* serogroup have been reported to be the predominant organisms infecting cattle and among persons who had acquired their infection from cattle worldwide. Since we now had evidence that the leptospirosis infections were acquired by swimming at the Bubbles, we needed to take action to prevent further infections; therefore, we posted warnings and publicly advised persons against swimming in the water at the Bubbles or other areas of the irrigation canal, especially downstream from the cattle herd. Also, the cattle were screened off to prevent them having direct access to the irrigation canal.

We also wanted to evaluate the cattle and the environment further; therefore, we collected water samples for culture from the irrigation canal and from water standing in the field where the cattle were herded. We cultured the blood samples from the children who had been ill, although all of the children had recovered from their illness before we obtained a blood specimen. *L. pomona* was recovered by guinea pig inoculation from water standing in the cattle pasture at three sites; however, cultures of water from the irrigation canal and sera from the students who had been ill were all negative (Figure 3-3).

Culturing blood and urine from the cattle was also a priority. We clearly needed assistance from a veterinarian to obtain these cultures. Fortunately, my colleague Dr. Everett (Ted) Baker, DVM, also an EIS officer, was available to help obtain these specimens for culture. I was not experienced with the methods for getting a urine specimen from a cow! I knew I could not be successful if I just asked the animal to provide it, which is how I usually got a urine sample from my patients. I was told that often urine appeared after you massaged the cow's under belly. If this failed, you could poke or push the area firmly, but I do not know how Ted eventually managed to obtain the samples from the cattle.

Eventually, we found that 9 of 43 cattle (21%) were shedding *L. pomona* in their urine in September, about a month after the last human case, and 21 of 25 sera (84%) from the cattle herd were seropositive in the MAT test with the highest titers to *L. pomona*. The herd of 300 cattle had been purchased locally in the spring before the outbreak. There had been no reports of illness or

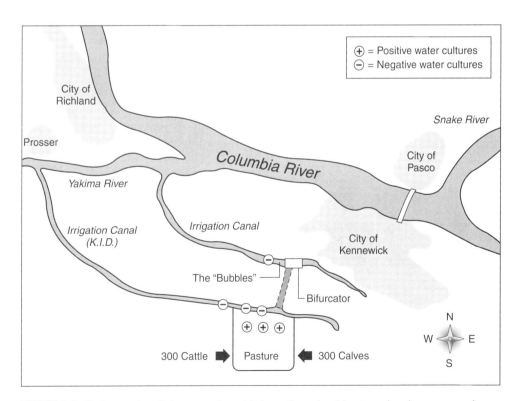

FIGURE 3-3 Schematic of the area in which outbreak of leptospirosis occurred during the summer of 1964. Reprinted with permission from: Nelson KE, et al. *Am J Epidemiol* 1973;98:336–347.

unexpected deaths in the cattle and no abortions, which have commonly been reported as a consequence of animal leptospirosis. The animals had not been vaccinated for leptospirosis. We obtained blood specimens from 305 additional cattle entering two local sales yards between August 31 and October 31; 26 of these sera (8.5%) were positive for leptospiral antibodies.

In addition to warning the students and the public about the dangers of swimming or other exposures to the irrigation canal, we recognized the need for other public health measures to prevent additional cases. These included restricting the cattle from direct access to the canal and stopping the process of rill (flooding) irrigation of the pasture where the cattle were located. This could lead to contamination of the standing water with cattle urine, which could then be washed back into the irrigation canal when it rained. Leptospires can survive for considerable periods, especially in an alkaline environment. As mentioned previously, we had isolated *L. pomona* from the standing alkaline water in the pasture by guinea pig inoculation.

We made an effort to locate all of the cases in order to further define the risk exposures. Although this swimming hole was quite small, it clearly was a major site of exposure. There was also a possibility of infections occurring from exposures to the irrigation water at other areas, as the canal was several miles long winding between the fields. In order to detect additional (unreported) cases, we asked all of the known cases the names of everyone they knew who visited the Bubbles or who had swum elsewhere in the irrigation canal that summer. Another source of possible exposed persons was the signatures on the concrete wall of the Bubbles. We made certain that we interviewed each of the persons who had left their name on the wall of the Bubbles (i.e., had "signed in" at the site).

We decided to do a larger survey after the schools reopened in September. We designed a questionnaire that included questions about having had a compatible illness during the summer, swimming anywhere in the irrigation canal during the summer, and swimming at the Bubbles during the summer. This questionnaire was distributed to the 6,062 students attending the three high schools and two junior high schools in the three neighboring towns of Kennewick, Pasco, and Richland. We found that 594 of the students (9.8%) in these five schools reported swimming at the Bubbles, and 60 had an illness confirmed serologically to be leptospirosis, for an attack rate of 10.1% among Bubbles swimmers (Table 3-3). We used a clinical definition of "suspected cases" (compatible illness), which included the reported symptoms of fever, myalgia, and headache, that were reported by over 95% of the serologically confirmed cases for our epidemiological survey. We also put notices in the local newspaper, and our interest in locating additional cases was mentioned by the local news media. We supplemented the request for reporting illnesses by reviewing local hospital and clinic records of febrile illnesses. When our case-finding efforts had been completed, we had identified 61 serologically confirmed cases (Table 3-4). All were between the ages of 12 and 19 years; 53 were male (86.9%) and 8 were female (13.1%). The numbers of cases increased with increasing age between 12 and 17 years (Table 3-4). In our school surveys, we found that 594 students (10.3%) reported swimming at the Bubbles during the summer; 16.0% of boys and 4.3% of girls reported swimming at the Bubbles. The proportion who reported swimming at the Bubbles also

TABLE 3-3 Number of Students Who Swam at the Bubbles During the Summer of 1964 and Leptospirosis Attack Rates by School

	Enrollment	Swam at "Bubbles" Number (1%)	Leptospirosis Cases	Swimmers' Attack Rate (%)
Kennewick High School	1,420	184 (13.0)	31	16.8
Park Jr. High School	994	54 (5.4)	6	11.1
Highland Jr. High School	746	58 (7.8)	6	10.3
Pasco High School	1,284	100 (7.8)	7	7.0
Columbia High School	1,618	198 (12.2)	10	5.1
Total	6,062	594 (9.8)	60*	10.1

* One of the 61 cases occurred in a nonstudent.
Reprinted with permission from Nelson KE, et al. *Am J Epidemiol* 1973;98:336–34

TABLE 3-4 Distribution of 61 Patients with Leptospirosis by Age and Gender

Age (Years)	Male	Female	Total
12	2	0	2
13	2	1	3
14	6	0	6
15	8	1	9
16	14	3	17
17	18	2	20
18	3	0	3
19	0	1	1
Total	53	8	61

Reprinted with permission from Nelson KE, et al. *Am J Epidemiol* 1973;98:336–347.

increased with age between 12 and 18 years; the distribution of those who reported swimming was similar to the age and gender distribution of the cases (Table 3-5).

The highest attack rate of leptospirosis (16.8%) was experienced by the students attending Kennewick High School. Students at Kennewick High School and Columbia High School in Richland had the highest rates of exposure to the Bubbles, 13.0% and 12.2%, respectively (Table 3-3); however, because the Bubbles was located closer to Kennewick, we believe that exposures were more frequent among students living in Kennewick than those from Richland or Pasco, but we did not collect data on the frequency or specific dates that students swam at the Bubbles.

We did not detect any laboratory-confirmed cases of leptospirosis in those who had not swum at the Bubbles; however, a few children with leptospirosis reported swimming elsewhere in the irrigation canal in addition to the Bubbles. Nevertheless, several features of exposure to water when swimming at the Bubbles may have been important in increasing the risk of leptospirosis among these swimmers. First the churning, swirling water at the Bubbles often resulted in abrasions when the swimmers were thrown against the concrete walls of the structure, providing a source of entry for *L. pomona* organisms. Second, diving into the water usually resulted in immersion of the swimmers head, exposing the conjunctiva as a site of entry of the organisms. Cases often reported recurring exposure; only three of the confirmed cases reported swimming at the Bubbles only

TABLE 3-5 Students' History of Swimming at the Bubbles by Age and Gender, Summer 1964*

Age (Years)	Male			Female			Both Genders		
	Total	Swam	% Swam	Total	Swam	% Swam	Total	Swam	% Swam
<11	1	0		0	0		1	0	
11	21	2	9.5	20	1	5.0	41	3	7.3
12	224	14	6.3	278	3	1.1	502	17	3.4
13	278	24	8.6	265	15	5.7	543	39	7.2
14	320	36	11.3	302	4	1.3	622	40	6.4
15	646	84	13.0	637	22	3.5	1,283	106	8.3
16	716	122	17.0	646	38	5.9	1,362	160	11.7
17	650	161	24.8	598	33	5.5	1,248	194	15.5
18	101	30	29.7	36	4	11.1	137	34	24.8
>18	8	0		6	0		14	0	
Unknown	3	1	33.3	2	0		5	1	20.0
Total	2,968	474	16.0	2,790	120	4.3	5,758	594	10.3

* Based on questionnaires answered by 5,758 students.
Reprinted with permission from Nelson KE, et al. *Am J Epidemiol* 1973;98:336–347.

once during the summer. Their illnesses had onset 7 to 10 days after their exposure. In addition, the number of cases increased about 10 days after the warmest day in June, when the ambient temperature reached 97°F and a similar period after the temperatures exceeded 100°F between July 10 and July 14 (Figure 3-4). We also learned that the water flow was slowed on July 13 and July 14 to facilitate repairs to the Bubbles. We suspect that the number of students exposed to the Bubbles was high during these very warm days and that the risk of infection among swimmers may have increased when the rate of water flow decreased, but we could not confirm this level of detail in our interviews.

LABORATORY STUDIES OF THE OUTBREAK

We were very fortunate to have access to the excellent Leptospirosis Reference Laboratory at the CDC in the investigation of this outbreak. Many suspected outbreaks of leptospirosis have not had laboratory confirmation of the cases or the animal reservoir as detection of the organisms or the serological response to leptospiral infection is highly specialized and available in only a few reference laboratories.

Recovery of leptospiral organisms in culture requires special media and often very long incubation times. Primary cultures are retained for up to 13 weeks before being discarded, if there is no growth. When there is growth, it usually occurs within 10 to 14 days in liquid media.[1] Growth of contaminants is inhibited by adding 5-fluorouracil to the media.

Serologic investigation of cases also requires specialized laboratories. The traditional gold-standard method of detecting a specific antibody response is the MAT, which has been described previously here. Several other genus-specific serological diagnostic assays have been described, but they are not well standardized or widely available.

In this outbreak the Leptospirosis Reference Laboratory at the CDC performed the MAT test on all suspect cases that resulted in the 61 laboratory-confirmed cases mentioned previously here. The CDC laboratory also tested the sera with a microscopic slide test, which is a less sensitive test than the MAT but is easier to perform in the laboratory and sometimes used as a screening assay. Among the 61 students that were positive on the MAT, only 48 were positive on the microscopic slide test. The highest titers and most frequent reactions were to *L. pomona* antigens. We did follow-up testing of 45 ill students 200 to 264 days after the outbreak. At this time,

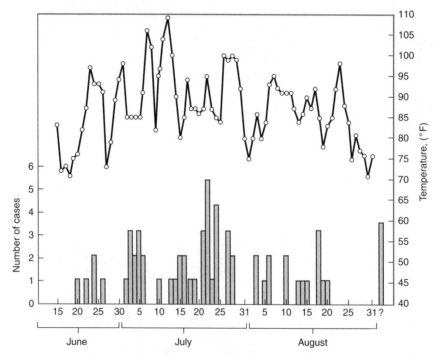

FIGURE 3-4 Cases of leptospirosis by date of onset of symptoms and daily maximum temperature, June 15–August 31, 1964. Reprinted with permission from: Nelson KE, et al. *Am J Epidemiol* 1973;98:336–347.

only 10 sera were MAT positive for antibodies to *L. pomona*. This decline of reactivity in the MAT test was evidence against chronic infection or re-exposure.

LEPTOSPIROSIS HISTORY, EPIDEMIOLOGY, AND CAUSATIVE ORGANISMS

The clinical features of leptospirosis in humans have been known since 1886 when Adolph Weil reported cases of febrile jaundice among sewer workers in Heidelberg, Germany.[2] Although there were other earlier reports of this syndrome,[3] the clinical disease became known as "Weil's Disease." A spirochetal organism, identified in the kidney tubules of a patient with the disease by silver staining, was reported by Stimson in 1909.[4] The spirochetes had hooked ends and Stimson called them Spirochete interrogans because of their resemblance to a question mark. The importance of rats as a carrier of the organism, which was excreted chronically in their urine, was recognized and reported by Japanese investigators in 1917.[5] After these seminal discoveries, Weil's disease came to be known as an occupational disease of sewer workers throughout the world, especially in Europe. The disease also occurred frequently among persons harvesting rice in China and other countries in Asia. The Japanese called the disease "Akiyami," or Autumnal fever. Spirochetes were detected by injecting guinea pigs with blood from infected patients by German investigators.[6] Leptospirosis in livestock was recognized several decades later.[7]

> *In the last couple of decades, it has been recognized that leptospirosis is a very common disease globally.*

In the last couple of decades, it has been recognized that leptospirosis is a very common disease globally. The clinical picture and epidemiology of leptospirosis in humans is quite variable. The disease is quite common in the tropics and has been estimated to be one of the most common zoonotic infectious diseases of humans globally.[8] Leptospirosis has been reported not only as an occupational disease but among other populations as well. Human infections have been acquired by occupational or recreational exposures to a wide range of infected animals or their urine. A wide range of exposures have been reported to transmit the organisms. High-risk groups include miners, veterinarians, farmers, abattoir workers, sugar cane cutters, fish workers, soldiers, and other occupations having direct or indirect exposures to animals. During World War II, an outbreak of a febrile illness with a pretibial rash and splenomegaly occurred among troops at Fort Bragg, North Carolina, which became known as "Fort Bragg fever" or pretibial fever. This illness was later found to be leptospirosis caused by the *L. autumnalis* infection.[9]

In addition, several outbreaks of leptospirosis among swimmers after exposure to contaminated water have been reported. A recent comprehensive review found 26 reported water-borne outbreaks among swimmers or rafters that have occurred between 1931 and 1998.[10] Most of these outbreaks were small; however five, including this one, involved more than 60 cases. In over half of the outbreaks, the source of infection was unknown, and the serogroup of the infecting organism was estimated based on serologic evidence. The water had been contaminated by urine from cattle, pigs, dogs, or rodents in most of these outbreaks.

Human leptospirosis is acquired by direct contact with infectious material, generally water contaminated with urine from an infected animal; however, subculturing the organism in the laboratory can cause infection among laboratory personnel by direct contact or possibly by aerosol. The organism is thought to enter the body through abrasions in the skin or through the conjunctiva; however, drinking of contaminated water also has been reported to transmit infection.[10]

The protean clinical features of leptospirosis in humans include clinical Weil's disease manifested by jaundice, sepsis, and renal failure, but also aseptic meningitis, as in this outbreak, pulmonary disease, cardiac involvement, and ocular disease. In addition, animals and also humans may have abortions if the infections occur during pregnancy. Cattle can develop mastitis, and ocular disease has been seen in animals.[10]

Recently, international interest in leptospirosis has been generated by several large clusters of cases that have occurred in South and Central America after flooding from storms.[11,12] It has been recognized in the past decade that human exposures to animals have caused the emergence and re-emergence of many infectious diseases, including SARS (severe acute respiratory syndrome), hantavirus, monkeypox, HIV/AIDS, avian influenza, and many others. In fact, cross-species transmission of infectious agents may be the most significant of the many factors leading to the emergence of important infections in humans in recent times. In reality, our experience in investigating the Bubble's outbreak of leptospirosis could have been viewed as a "seminal" experience of newly emerging infections on the horizon.

LESSONS FROM THIS OUTBREAK

1. Although the most commonly reported infectious etiology of aseptic meningitis cases and outbreaks in the summer time are enteroviruses and arboviruses, other organisms contribute, such as leptospires, whose importance may be underappreciated because of the hurdles of laboratory diagnosis.
2. Zoonotic infections appear to have become increasingly important in the emergence of new infectious diseases in humans.
3. It is often an excellent idea to determine which exposures the infected patients believe might have caused their illness and then follow-up on their suggestion(s). Epidemiologists should "listen to their patients."
4. Recreational activities, such as swimming, hiking, and rafting, may expose persons to a wide variety of infectious risks.
5. Outbreak investigation is interesting and challenging but often requires support from several disciplines, including laboratory scientists, veterinarians, and other professionals with special skills, such as irrigation experts as in the case of this outbreak.

REFERENCES

1. Nelson KE, Ager EA, Galton MM, Gillespie RW, Sulzer CR. An outbreak of leptospirosis in Washington State. *Am J Epidemiol* 1973;98:336–347.
2. Weil A. Ueber eine eigentümliche, mit Milztumor, Icterus und Nephritis einhergehende akute Infektionskrankheit. *Dtsche Arch Klin Med* 1886;39:209–232.
3. Landouzy LT. Typhus hépatique. *Gaz Hospital* 1883;56:913.
4. Stimson AM. Note on an organism found in yellow-fever tissue. *Public Health Rep* 1907;22:541.
5. Ido Y, Hoki R, Ito H, Wani H. The rat as a carrier of *Spirochaeta icterohaemorrhagiae*, the causative agent of Weil's disease (spirochetosis icterohaemorrhagiae). *J Exp Med* 1917;26:341–353.
6. Huebner EA, Reiter K. *Dtsche Med Wochenschr* 1915;41:1275–277.
7. Alston JM, Broom JC. *Leptospirosis*. Edinburgh, UK: Livingston Ltd., 1958.
8. Bhort AR, Nally JE, Ricaki JN, et al. Leptospirosis: a zoonotic disease of global importance. *Lancet Infect Dis* 2003;3:757–771.
9. Gochenour WS, Smadel JE, Jackson EB, Evans LB, Yager RH. Leptospiral etiology of Fort Bragg fever. *Public Health Rep* 1952;67:811–812.
10. Levett PN. Leptospirosis. *Clin Micro Rev* 2001;34:296–326.
11. Epstein PR, Pena OC, Racedo JB. Climate and disease in Colombia. *Lancet* 1995;346:1243–1244.
12. Ko AI, Galvao Reis M, Ribeiro Dourado CM, Johnson WD, Riley LW, the Salvador Leptospirosis Study Group. Urban epidemic of severe leptospirosis in Brazil. *Lancet* 1999;354:820–825.

LEARNING QUESTIONS

1. The author concludes that this was an outbreak of leptospirosis. List all the pieces of information that the author presents that support that conclusion.
2. Case ascertainment is an important part of outbreak investigation. What were the ways in which the author attempted to find as many cases as he could?

NOTE

We learned several months after this outbreak had been investigated and controlled that a spill of radioactive waste into the Columbia River from the Hanford Nuclear Energy facility had occurred just before this outbreak. There was some concern among officials at the facility and the Department of Energy that the epidemic might have been related to the spill.

CHAPTER 4

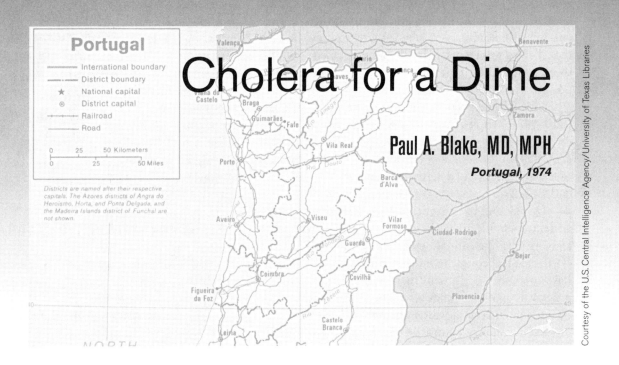

Cholera for a Dime

Paul A. Blake, MD, MPH

Portugal, 1974

INTRODUCTION

Listening to the radio late one night in Boston in May, 1974 while taking a break from studying for my master's degree in public health finals from the Harvard School of Public Health, I was riveted by the news that cholera had broken out in Portugal. Might I be sent to Portugal? I would soon be an epidemiologist in the enteric diseases branch of the Centers for Disease Control (CDC) and would be an obvious candidate for an investigation in Portugal because I could speak Portuguese, having lived as a child in a Portuguese colony, Angola. On the other hand, my epidemiologic skills were weak. I had joined the Epidemic Intelligence Service (EIS) at the CDC because of my international public health interests and to avoid military service in Vietnam* and had been sent to Puerto Rico. My 2 years there had been rich in public health experience but devoid of on-the-job supervision in traditional CDC "shoe-leather epi-

demiology." In those days, communication with my supervisors at the CDC in Atlanta required hours, even days, of struggles with the much-loathed Federal Telecommunications System. I was buffing up my fledgling epidemiologic expertise with a master's in public health, but I still felt inadequate. Within days, however, the CDC called to ask whether I was interested in going to Portugal, and I was indeed. My wife, who would be left with two small boys in a new neighborhood in Atlanta, was less enthused.

Cholera is a diarrheal disease caused by toxigenic *Vibrio cholerae* O-group 1 or O-group 139. The infection is often

> *Cholera is a diarrheal disease caused by toxigenic* Vibrio cholerae *O-group 1 or O-group 139.*

mild or subclinical, but in the worst cases, severe diarrhea and vomiting can cause death within 24 hours. The incubation period ranges from a few hours to 5 days. In the Northern Hemisphere, cholera usually peaks in August to September. The main source of infection is human feces. The infectious dose is very high, requiring about 1 million organisms in food and even more in water. The organisms are very sensitive to acid, and

---

* We occasionally referred to ourselves as the "Yellow Berets" (in contrast to the Green Berets, elite troops who fought in Vietnam), although in truth our work could be dangerous, and one of my classmates died in the line of duty when his plane crashed in Africa.

persons with low gastric acid are at greater risk for cholera. Back in 1974, few analytic studies of cholera transmission had been performed. The disease was thought to be caused largely by polluted drinking water, with food playing a minor role. Fish and shellfish had been reported to cause cholera, but the evidence was circumstantial until 1973, when studies in Italy showed that cholera was associated with eating mussels thought to be contaminated after harvest by "freshening" with polluted harbor water.[1]

Portugal had been free of cholera for many decades until 1971, when it reported 89 cases caused by *V. cholerae* O-group 1 serotype Ogawa, mostly in the Lisbon area. Neither the source of introduction nor the vehicles of transmission were determined; however, the outbreak ended, and no cases were detected in 1972 and 1973.

Throughout the summer of 1974 I was kept on alert, and the epidemic grew while the CDC worked with officials in Washington, DC to secure an invitation from Portugal. Most countries understandably are reluctant to have foreigners document their public health failures, and few invitations materialize. The situation was complicated by uncertainty after Portugal's virtually bloodless leftist military coup (the "Carnation Revolution") in April 1974 against the right-wing dictatorship of President Américo Thomaz and Prime Minister Marcelo Caetano, successor to António Salazar. There was ongoing infighting in the government and military. Remarkably, an invitation arrived on Friday, September 6, perhaps prompted by the escalating epidemic, which peaked in late August. My departure was delayed until Monday so that I could fly to Washington to be briefed on Portuguese politics at the State Department's "Portugal Desk"; however, the briefer was taking a 3-hour lunch break, and I proceeded unbriefed.

My CDC supervisors had instructed me thoroughly on cholera, and I was crammed with advice and laden with reference material. Most useful was Bill Baine's CDC report on his investigation of cholera in Italy the year before,[1] when his matched-pair case control studies incriminated ingestion of raw shellfish. The matched-pair case control technique had been used in chronic disease investigations, but to our knowledge, Bill was the first to use it in an infectious disease investigation outside of a hospital. It was particularly useful in investigating scattered, apparently unrelated cases because each case was matched to an age- and gender-matched neighborhood control subject (rather than a hospital control—Bill's innovation), and the matching was maintained in the analysis; thus, the results would not be distorted by age, gender, or socioeconomic (as reflected by neighborhood) status. My supervisors expected me to have a study of new Lisbon cases using Bill's technique underway by the end of the week. My objectives were to learn how cholera transmission was occurring to guide prevention and control measures in Portugal and to gain a better understanding of cholera transmission that would help cholera control worldwide.

> *My objectives were to learn how cholera transmission was occurring to guide prevention and control measures in Portugal and to gain a better understanding of cholera transmission that would help cholera control worldwide.*

FIRST INVESTIGATION–LISBON

I arrived in Lisbon at dawn on Tuesday, September 10, with little sleep, a headache, and no luggage (it arrived 36 hours later), but fearing the worst, I had my papers in a carry-on bag. Black and green taxis drumming along cobblestone streets, streetcars, double-decker buses, red tile roofs, colorfully tiled facades, palm trees, cascading bougainvilleas, Portuguese voices, and the smell of grilling sardines and diesel exhaust in the air—despite my fatigue, it was exhilarating to be in Lisbon! I checked into my hotel and hurried to the U.S. Embassy; immediately, however, I faced the first of many delays as I discovered that not everyone shared my sense of urgency. I had to wait all day to see the deputy ambassador and used the time to work with consular officials to get statistics for Portugal, newspaper clippings on the cholera epidemic, a desk, and access to a mimeograph machine and a massive mechanical calculator that used metal parts rather than electronics to add and subtract (these were the olden days). For division and multiplication, I had a slide rule.

The embassy arranged for me to meet with three national Portuguese officials, including Portugal's director general of health and the national epidemiologist, on Wednesday afternoon. They had only descriptive information. The first known cholera case had onset of illness on April 24 in Tavira on Portugal's southern coast. The 33-year-old man had diarrhea and dehydration so severe that he suffered a cardiac arrest, and the national laboratory isolated *V. cholerae* O-group 1 biotype El Tor serotype Inaba from his stool. The disease spread 300 km to Lisbon within 16 days and 600 km to Porto in the far north within 20 days and eventually was reported

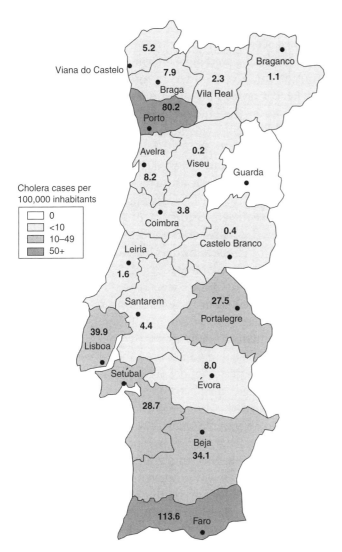

FIGURE 4-1 Hospitalized cholera patients in Portugal, by district of residence, April–October, 1974. Reprinted with permission from Blake P, et al. Cholera in Portugal 1974. II Transmission by bottled mineral water. *Am J Epidemiol* 1977;105:344–348.

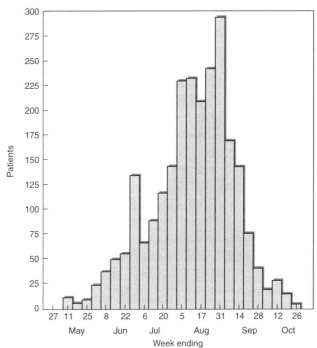

FIGURE 4-2 Patients with cholera, by date of hospitalization, Portugal, 1974. Reprinted with permission from Blake P, et al. Cholera in Portugal 1974. II Transmission by bottled mineral water. *Am J Epidemiol* 1977;105:344–348.

from 17 of 18 districts (Figure 4-1). When I arrived in Portugal in early September, approximately 2,000 laboratory-confirmed cases and several dozen deaths had been reported. The epidemic had peaked the last week in August and was now declining rapidly (Figure 4-2), but a few new widely scattered cases were still occurring in Lisbon. I began to worry that while an investigation of cases that were part of the peak of the epidemic might incriminate one or more important vehicles that caused the bulk of the cases, the last few scattered cases at the tail end of the epidemic might be caused by many different exposures (e.g., food contaminated by an infected household member), making successful incrimination of any one vehicle unlikely; however, I had arrived primed to concentrate on new cases and did not yet have the self-confidence or experience to deviate from the plan.

From anecdotes, cultures of food and the environment, and educated guesses, the Portuguese officials suspected several vehicles—cooked snails collected from sewage-contaminated gullies, lettuce irrigated with human sewage during the dry summer, watercress, Lupini beans sold by street vendors, raw shellfish, and well water. Later I learned that spring water and commercially bottled mineral water were also suspected, but were not mentioned initially because they involved an important company and thus were politically sensitive.

The national officials made it clear that they were too understaffed and overburdened to find staff to work with me, but they referred me to the Lisbon District Health Department. I went there Thursday morning; the Director was on vacation until Friday, but I met with an elderly physician who specialized in waterborne disease.* While waiting to meet the Director, I worked

---

* Dr. Leopoldo de Figueiredo gave me his publications on water and sewer systems in Portugal. My mother later told me (and he confirmed) that he was our family doctor in 1947 when I was 4 and my parents were in Lisbon learning Portuguese—a small world!

on a draft questionnaire and included the suspect foods, other plausible foods, and various sources of water, as well as possible risk factors such as gastric surgery and the use of antacids. I planned to ask the cases about exposures during the 5 days before onset and to ask age- and gender-matched neighbor controls about the 5 days before interview. The Portuguese had been doing a good job of culturing suspect cases, and in this and all subsequent investigations, we were able to define cases as persons with *V. cholerae* O1 isolated from their stools. In this investigation, we defined our cases as any culture-confirmed case from Lisbon or the adjacent city of Oeiras diagnosed on or after September 13.

Writing the questionnaires was doubly difficult because although I could speak Portuguese, I had never learned to read or write the language; I had to write the questions phonetically and get help from Portuguese staff in the embassy. I then struggled until nearly midnight to type stencils and mimeograph questionnaires. I returned to my hotel with inky hands and clothes but enough questionnaires to get started.

The next morning the director told me about the Lisbon District cholera activities. Eight nurses in four teams worked on cholera. One team interviewed new cases in hospitals, whereas the other three visited recent cases and their families. World Health Organization (WHO) epidemiologists had visited Portugal several months earlier. At their recommendation, the Lisbon District had begun to complete a new cholera case-investigation form for all cholera patients in July. It included questions about exposures, including recent travel and sources of drinking water. The questionnaires lay unanalyzed in stacks destined, as is so often the case, for the archives rather than for analysis and use in disease control. They were to prove useful, however, in the weeks ahead.

I went out with a team the same day and completed questionnaires on three cases and two controls. On Saturday, the work went more smoothly as the nurses (and I) gained experience and our team interviewed three case control pairs in 6 hours. Being naturally diffident, it was stressful for me to knock on the doors of complete strangers, try to explain why I was there, and ask them personal questions in a language that I had hardly used in 17 years. Each interview was easier than the last, however, and the experience of going into private homes all over Lisbon was vastly more interesting than being a tourist. The case and control subjects were cooperative, and I enjoyed talking with them. One woman control looked at me quizzically as I stumbled through questions in my rusty Portuguese and finally said, "Ah! You are from Mozambique!" She recognized the African colonial accent but had the wrong colony.

Despite the seemingly interminable delays, the case control study was underway on schedule. Over the weekend I revised the questionnaires to fix problems turned up by the interviews and retyped and mimeographed them. I decided that the same person should interview both subjects in each case control pair so that the questions would be asked similarly. I worried that we needed more rigorous methods to select neighbor controls because investigators might unknowingly introduce bias if left to their own devices. Thus, I improved on the Italian studies, which selected neighbor controls from passers-by or other conveniently accessible neighbors, by adapting methods learned in a chronic disease course to create a scheme that I used in all subsequent investigations. The investigators would start at the case's house and go door to door following a printed schematic map (go right until the corner, then return to the case's house and go left until the corner, etc.) until they located a person of the same gender and within the same age range. After I amended the schematic map to include apartments, it failed only once, when the patient was a railroad crossing operator who lived in a hut by the rails—his residence was not part of a block.

I intended to train and enlist all three field teams, but although most of the nurses quickly learned proper techniques, one was overenthusiastic; she pressed patients to admit that they had eaten suspect foods and suggested to controls that they had *not* eaten those foods. Also, her suicidal driving caused a minor crash, and thus, we dropped her team from the investigation.

These were politically turbulent times in Portugal. Early one Sunday morning as I was walking up an empty cobblestone street, President (and General) António Spínola swept past in a small white car surrounded by National Republican Guards—impressive, solidly built, middle-aged men on eerily quiet motorcycles. Shortly afterward, there were mass demonstrations in Lisbon and an attempted coup, and President Spínola was forced to resign on September 30. Despite the unrest, I never felt threatened, even though an American consular official chilled me by saying that as a Portuguese-speaking American I would be suspected of being a Central Intelligence Agency operative.

Each week brought fewer new cases in Lisbon; they were widely scattered and difficult to locate in the labyrinthine streets. We visited the addresses of many subjects repeatedly and at odd hours before we caught them at home. Over 3 weeks our strenuous efforts interviewed just 34 case control pairs, 59% of the 58 reported new cases. On analysis of the data, I had my worst fears realized. My effort for almost 4 weeks had failed to associate cholera with any exposure. My CDC supervisors were dissatisfied. Portuguese officials were losing interest, and some nurses returned to their precholera duties. I was dejected and wanted to go home; however, I was learning how to operate in Portugal. My Portuguese was improving daily, and I was learning the limitations of case control studies. I wanted to try again with cases that had occurred earlier in the epidemic when single vehicles might have been important.

On September 20, in the midst of the Lisbon investigation, I was joined by Mark Rosenberg, an Afrocoifed, Earth Shoe-shod, first-year EIS officer from my branch (this was the 1970s, after all—I sported a bushy C. Everett Koop beard) (Figure 4-3). We quickly adapted to each other's work styles, and although he did not know Portuguese, he could communicate with many Portuguese professionals in French. He plunged into the work but helped the most by being an epidemiologist with whom I could discuss the details of our investigations face to face; he was the quintessential devil's advocate, sometimes to a fault.

As the Lisbon case control study of current cases limped to a close, Mark and I explored possibilities for other studies. The Lisbon cholera nurses told us in late September that back in August they began to see cases in the upper and upper-middle classes for the first time. Many of these patients reported recent travel to Vimeiro Thermal Springs, a spa in Lisbon District but 50 km north of Lisbon in Torres Vedras County, and others had drunk Agua do Vimeiro, commercially bottled water from the same springs. At about the same time, prompted by two cholera cases in a nearby village, a sanitarian cultured water from the springs as part of a sanitation inspection of the area. On August 22, *V. cholerae* was isolated from the spring water samples. On the 23rd, the springs and the bottling plant were closed, and the bottled water was recalled. A press release was issued on August 24.

We painstakingly reviewed the Lisbon government cholera questionnaires for August; there was no bottled water question, but the nurses asked about it on their own initiative (smart nurses!) after they learned of the potential problem. Torres Vedras County had 16 cases in persons who worked at (4), visited (1), or lived near (11) the springs within 5 days before onset. In Lisbon District, excluding Torres Vedras County, 29 of 418 cases reported visiting the springs, and at least 81 reported drinking Vimeiro bottled water within 5 days before onset. The peak number of cases appeared in all three groups (Torres Vedras county residents, spa visitors, and Vimeiro water drinkers) at about the same time—the last 2 weeks of August.

Our interest was piqued. We asked the Lisbon Health Director for a car and a sanitarian to visit the Vimeiro springs and bottling plant. He agreed, but for several days, there was one delay after another—car trouble, illness, and so forth. Finally, the light dawned—because a large business was involved, the situation was politically sensitive, and they did not want us to visit the springs but did not want to tell us that directly. We had been careful not to rock the political boat, but we decided it was time to take risks. Accordingly, I told the authorities that we understood how difficult it was to free up a car and a sanitarian for a day and that Mark and I would just hire a taxi and visit the plant without a health department escort. I feared that they might forbid it, but suddenly they found a car and a sanitarian to take us. Sr. João Florencia, the wiry, chain-smoking, espresso-fueled sanitarian who had collected the Vimeiro water samples, drove us sedately to the springs, giving us no hint of the driving style that he would exhibit on the ride back to Lisbon; in retrospect, he was still sizing us up.

The spa's owner gave us some statistics. In 1973, the previous year, about 20,000 people visited the spa during August, and about 70% of these were from Lisbon District. Approximately half of the bottled water was carbonated, and half was untreated. Usually about 10.5 million liters of water were bottled annually, but in 1974, production increased about 50%, apparently because people turned to bottled water for fear of cholera. The uncarbonated water was distributed in 5-gallon jugs and in smaller capped bottles (Figure 4-4) that sold for 3 escudos (10 cents). In August, the month of greatest

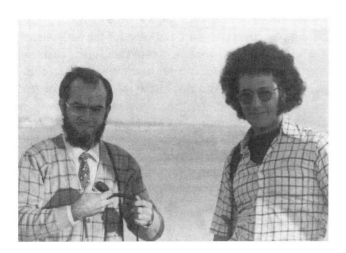

FIGURE 4-3 Paul Blake and Mark Rosenberg in the Algarve, October 1974.

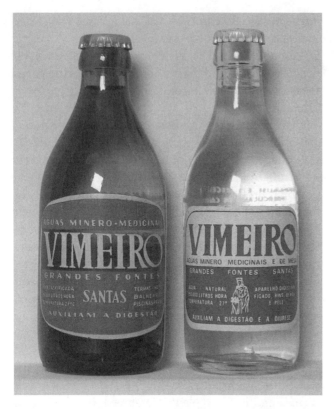

FIGURE 4-4 Carbonated and noncarbonated Agua do Vimeiro.

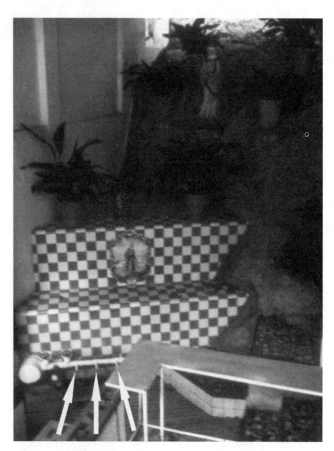

FIGURE 4-5 Termos do Vimeiro grotto with drinking water outlets (bottom).

demand, bottles could be on Lisbon store shelves within 4 hours after production. Approximately 42% of the bottled water was distributed outside of Lisbon District.

We visited the two springs, the spa, and the bottling plant. Most interesting was the Fonte Santa Isabel (Santa Isabel Spring), the source of most of the water. The Fonte lay less than 50 feet from a small river, the Ribeira de Alcabrichel, which carried sewage from upstream towns; cultures of river water samples collected on August 13 and August 26 yielded *V. cholerae* O1. The Fonte originally welled up spontaneously from the underlying limestone rocks, but subsequently, a large chamber was dug into the limestone and covered with concrete, creating an underground reservoir. Untreated water was pumped from this reservoir to the baths, drinking water spigots (Figure 4-5), a swimming pool, and the bottling plant. Limestone aquifers are infamous for having underground fissures and channels through which water can flow rapidly. Five of six water samples collected from the Fonte on August 13, 22, 26, and 28 yielded *V. cholerae*. The springs were closed to the public on August 23 and were still closed when we were there.

In the midst of our tour, we had soft drinks, but the spa's bartender said he had been ordered not to charge us. We insisted that we could not appear to be "bought," but he looked shaken and resisted. Finally we just left money on the bar.

We finished late and had a wild ride back to Lisbon through the gathering night. João careened the VW beetle at up to 90 km/h through town and country on the narrow winding roads, flashing the high beams and passing on curves. He compensated for the car's anemic acceleration by not slowing for anything other than certain catastrophe. He said he had been a paratrooper until recently and did not know the meaning of fear, but we certainly did. Fortunately, I was in the back seat (my invariable choice), but Mark sat in the front passenger seat which, João told him with relish, the Portuguese refer to as "o lugar do morto" (the place of the dead). João stopped half a block short of our hotel—to let us out, or so we thought. Instead, we were out of gas. We pushed the car to a gas station.

We planned a case control study in Lisbon to find out whether Agua do Vimeiro was associated with cholera, but our CDC supervisors vetoed it, pointing out that bottled water was a highly unlikely vehicle because it had never been shown to cause cholera or any other disease. They directed us toward Faro District (the Algarve), Portugal's southern coast where the epidemic had begun and the incidence was highest to see whether we could implicate shellfish. Mark left for Faro on October 8 to see whether studies there were feasible, and I followed 2 days later after tying up loose ends.

My calls to Atlanta to brief and consult with my supervisors were always challenges. Public telephones were invariably in noisy public places where I found it difficult to hear and to think, and I had to watch what I said in public. At the CDC end, a crowd would gather on a bad speaker phone, making the acoustics even worse, and interruptions were frequent, breaking trains of thought. Our study's progress was slow, and I was asked by someone at the CDC, "Are you working nights and weekends?" This implied that I was loafing—I could barely contain my rage. I could not explain all of the details and subtleties by telephone, and I was plied with advice that I thought was misguided; however, I could not say that to my new bosses. I felt at a great disadvantage because I was new to the branch and had no significant publications from my EIS experience, although the branch was one of the most "academic," prestigious, and publication-oriented units at the CDC. I was afraid that I would return to the CDC a failure and would have no future in the branch. Thus, I was noncommittal on the phone and once off did what I thought was best. I wrote this to my wife: "I'm going to avoid calling Atlanta—they are trying to solve the problems without understanding the situation, and I can't explain it all to them at $2 a minute ($8 in today's dollars) standing in the embassy lobby surrounded by a dozen noisy people, shouting into the telephone, and barely able to hear. It takes me a couple of hours to calm down after every call. When Bill Baine investigated cholera in Italy he called them once in 2 months, and that sounds about right to me!" Nevertheless, I kept on calling as instructed.

SECOND INVESTIGATION— TAVIRA, FARO DISTRICT

We had a warm welcome in Faro, the capital of Faro District, although we had to "waste" a lot of time building relationships by enduring well-meant distractions—for example, a 7-hour tour of the district's many hotels and seemingly endless irrelevant (although entertaining) stories. The district health director gave us a key to the health department for after-hours access and found nurses to help us.

We discussed the cholera epidemic with local health officials and pored over their lists of cases to chart the course of the epidemic in the various municipalities. The first case had been detected in Tavira, a coastal town in Faro District near the Spanish border. Founded by the Phoenicians over 2,700 years ago, Tavira is known for its "Roman" bridge (actually Moorish from the 12th century) over the Gilão River. The river flows through the town into the Ria de Faro, a coastal strip of mud flats and islands 50 km long and up to 5 km wide that separates Tavira and Faro from the open sea and supplied most shellfish consumed in Portugal. Raw sewage from coastal towns emptied into the Ria, where water and shellfish had been known to have high coliform bacteria counts for at least a decade. After anecdotal reports of shellfish causing cholera, the Maritime Biology Institute in Faro isolated *V. cholerae* from 24% of seawater and 42% of shellfish samples from the Ria between May and August 1974.

We went to Tavira to try to find out how the epidemic began. Local health officials pointed out elements that might have contributed to the outbreak—raw sewage flowing into the tidal river, people gathering shellfish near the sewage outlets ("where the cockles are fattest"), sewage and water lines under repair, and two closed springs. Although chlorinated, Tavira's municipal water supply was suspect because the water lines were old, ruptured frequently, and ran beside leaking sewage lines. Water and sewer system renovation began in 1973, and we found excavated streets and wooden plugs in exposed pipes. We were told that when cholera first occurred heavy rain filled the excavations with sewage-contaminated water, enhancing the potential for sewage to contaminate potable water. Two suspect springs within the town were closed on May 10 and May 11.

The first detected case in Tavira (this was also the first case detected in Portugal, as described previously) had onset of illness on April 24. No other cases were identified for 13 days, but then a cluster of 14 cases in Tavira had onset between May 6 and May 15, followed by other clusters within the town over the succeeding months. Review of Tavira hospitalization records revealed an increase in diarrheal illnesses the second half of April; thus, there may have been some undetected cholera in April, and there may have been cases before the first detected case. We decided to focus on the first 15 culture-proven cases in Tavira, hoping that our findings would help us to understand how the Portuguese epidemic began.

In planning an investigation, we worried that recall of specific exposures 6 months before would be difficult for cases and worse for control subjects who had no illness as a reference point; however, we guessed (correctly, as we found out) that subjects would be able to recall their usual practices and unusual experiences like travel. Our questionnaire asked about demographic data; travel; frequency of eating raw vegetables, fruits, and seven varieties of shellfish; shellfish cooking methods; and drinking water sources. We asked all subjects about exposures during April and May and also asked the cholera patients about exposures during the 5 days before the onset.

Working with two nurses, we located and interviewed 14 of the 15 initial cases and matched controls in 2 days (October 14 and 15). The work went quickly because of short distances and relative ease in locating the patients. Our excitement mounted as case after case said that they liked the flavor of the water from one of the two local springs, the Fonte do Bispo, so much that they regularly walked across town to fill their jugs. Furthermore, they were angry that it was closed because decades of drinking that water had never made them sick. Eleven of 14 cases and none of 14 control subjects recalled drinking water from the Fonte do Bispo. We constructed a table that shows how matched-pair case control data are analyzed (Table 4-1). It maintains the matching, and the numbers refer to case control pairs of individuals rather than just to individuals. The probability that the result of our interviews occurred by chance is calculated using just two cells: pairs in which the case drank but the control did not (11) and pairs in which the control drank but the case did not (0). The two-tailed exact test for matched pairs testing our hypothesis that having cholera was associated with drinking water from the Fonte do Bispo yielded a P value of 0.001, and the relative risk (11/0) was infinite. More than a month after arriving in Portugal, we had a significant P value!

Our epidemiologic analysis failed to explain the index case in which the person did not drink water from the Fonte do Bispo or travel outside Portugal in 1974. Although our analysis had not demonstrated that having cholera was statistically associated with eating raw or partially cooked shellfish, the story from the index case suggested that they played a role. Three days before onset of illness, he gathered cockles from the Ria near the mouth of the Gilão and heated them only until they opened, and then he and two others ate them. Only the patient, who took antacids, developed diarrhea. There was no suggestion that any cases were related to drinking municipal water, and thus, the broken pipes appeared to be a red herring.

> *There was no suggestion that any cases were related to drinking municipal water, and thus, the broken pipes appeared to be a red herring.*

How might *V. cholerae* O1 El Tor serotype Inaba, the epidemic strain, have been introduced into Portugal? Soldiers traveled back and forth from a military training base 120 meters uphill from the Fonte do Bispo to the wars in Portugal's three African colonies—Angola, Mozambique, and Portuguese Guinea—where El Tor Inaba cholera was endemic. Sewage from the base emptied into the Gilão and flowed to the Ria. Thus, vibrios from an infected soldier could be taken up by filter-feeding shellfish in the Gilão and the Ria. Then people infected by eating contaminated shellfish would discharge more vibrios down the river, and the epidemic would be underway. Even though they were thousands of miles away, the African colonies were a much more likely source than nearby North Africa, where only El Tor Ogawa cholera was being reported. Subsequently, phage typing, a more sensitive method than serotyping to detect differences between cholera strains, showed that the 1974 Portuguese Inaba strains were indistinguishable from Angolan Inaba strains. Angola is a south-

TABLE 4-1 Distribution of 14 Case Control Pairs by History of Drinking Fonte do Bispo Water During April and May, 1974, Tavira, Portugal

	Control		
Case	Drank	Did Not Drink	Total Pairs
Drank	0	11	11
Did not drink	0	3	3
Total pairs	0	14	14

The other local spring was not implicated.

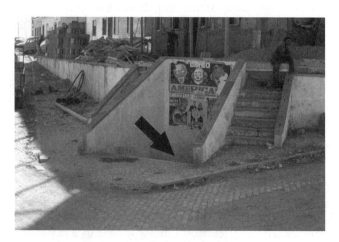

FIGURE 4-6 Fonte do Bispo, Tavira, Portugal, October 1974.

central African country that was a Portuguese colony until 1975.

Health officials had suspected that the Fonte do Bispo (a pipe emerging from the side of a hill through a concrete wall on a street corner) (Figure 4-6) caused a typhoid outbreak long before the advent of cholera; however, the public would not let them close it because they did not believe that it had caused the outbreak and they liked the flavor of the water. The officials said the spring produced clear water until September 1973, when, after construction blasting of the rock behind the spring followed by a heavy rain, the emerging water was muddy for a few days. A sewer line running down the hill beside the spring could have been damaged during the blasting. The sewer line was renovated in 1973, but it was unclear whether that occurred before or after the blasting. Perhaps damage from the blasting allowed sewage from persons infected by shellfish or from troops up the hill to pollute the spring. Unfortunately, dye testing was not politically feasible.

THIRD INVESTIGATION—FARO

There is nothing like a significant P value to raise epidemiologists' spirits. Now that we knew how the epidemic began, we wanted to examine the vehicles of transmission during the rest of the epidemic. We decided to try to continue our investigations in Faro District because we had good working relationships there and it had the highest incidence of cholera in Portugal. We immersed ourselves in analyses of Faro District data to pick our next target. We chose as our subjects the 59 cases identified in the city of Faro during the 5 months of May through September. Only eight cases occurred during May through July, but there were 51 cases during August through September. Compelling anecdotes pointing to shellfish abounded. In one instance, four small boys found a pile of cockles by the shore, heated them on a flattened tin can over a small fire until they opened, and ate them. All four developed diarrhea, and stool from one was cultured and yielded *V. cholerae*. Our questionnaire asked cases and individually matched controls about exposures during a 2-month period—the month of onset of illness and the nearest adjacent month. On October 18, as the study began, Mark was recalled to the CDC because the branch was so shorthanded that our supervisors feared (horrors!) that they would have to investigate the next outbreak themselves. Two nurses and I interviewed and matched 53 cases over the next several days and showed that eating raw or semi-

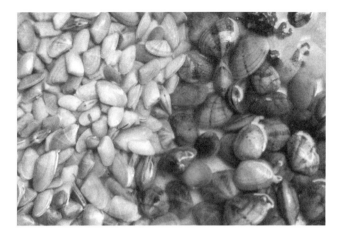

FIGURE 4-7 Live cockles (above) and clams in a Lisbon bar.

cooked cockles was significantly associated with cholera. I was ecstatic. These findings added credence to the theory that distribution of contaminated live shellfish from the Ria throughout Portugal could explain the rapid spread of cholera nationwide (Figure 4-7).

Now I had been in Portugal for over 6 weeks, and I ached to go home; however, on my next call to Atlanta (the worst yet, from a bar packed with rowdy tourists), my supervisors changed their minds about the plausibility of bottled water as a vehicle for cholera. Now, after Mark briefed them in person, they wanted me to conduct a case control study of Agua do Vimeiro in Lisbon. I finished up in Faro, flew back to Lisbon on October 26, and plunged into planning the investigation.

FOURTH INVESTIGATION— BOTTLED WATER

I was able to use the available data from the Lisbon Health Department's cholera case investigation forms in a retrospective cohort approach to show that visiting the springs was associated with cholera. During August, 36 (2.57/1,000) of the estimated 14,000 visitors to the springs from Lisbon District, excluding Torres Vedras County, had cholera, but only 382 (0.25/1,000) of 1,530,831 who did not visit the springs had cholera. The cholera risk was 10.3 times greater for visitors than for nonvisitors. The big question, however, was whether bottled Agua do Vimeiro had caused cholera.

I decided to study Lisbon District cases with onset during the week ending August 24 for several reasons: The government's cholera questionnaires showed the number of new cases in persons who recalled drinking

Agua do Vimeiro in the 5 days before onset peaked during that week; it was the last week when bottled Agua do Vimeiro was available in stores (it was recalled on August 23). A news release on August 24 said that the bottled water was suspect, and thus, after that date, the public would be less likely to drink bottled water they bought before the recall. Also, water collected from the Fonte Santa Isabel on August 22 was positive for *V. cholerae* O1. When I reviewed the government's cholera case investigation forms more carefully to identify the cases for study, I found that some cases had date of positive culture but not date of onset. Allowing for delay between onset and positive culture, I included cases with no recorded onset date if the patient's positive culture was between August 22 and 28. That gave me 47 symptomatic cases. I then excluded six who visited the springs (they might have been infected by drinking the water directly from the springs), three less than 10 years of age (their recall might be inaccurate), one who was not the first case of cholera in the family (cholera can spread through multiple vehicles within households), and two nonresidents who were ill before arriving in Lisbon (they were not infected in Lisbon District), leaving 35 for the investigation. Planning the study was the easy part, however; now I had to get help.

When I approached the Lisbon District Health Director, it was clear that I had worn out my welcome. Lisbon had been cholera-free for 8 days, and cholera was old news. Even though 4 days earlier he had told me by telephone that he would provide nurses to investigate Agua do Vimeiro, he now said rather brusquely that he could not. I did not know if he really could not, if he just wanted to get rid of me, or if cholera from bottled water was so politically sensitive that he had been told to not let me touch it. I suspected the last. One official told me confidentially that under the dictatorship, before the Carnation Revolution, the public would never have known about the contamination at Termos do Vimeiro because it was a big business—it would have been hushed up. Although the revolutionary government had recalled the water and issued a press release in late August, now more than 2 months had passed, and there was reluctance to bring fresh attention to the problem through an epidemiologic investigation by a foreigner.

I visited the national epidemiologist with all of the results to date and made the case for the investigation. I told him that all I needed was a car and driver—no nurses—so that I could track down cases nights and weekends when they were most likely to be home and that when it was done I would stop bothering him and go back to Atlanta. Somehow he was able to get me the best help possible—the sanitarian João Florencia and a car. We began the study the next day.

Investigating cases with João was a revelation. With no previous experience in epidemiology, he quickly grasped the investigation's logic and techniques and worked enthusiastically far into the night, over the weekend, and on All Saints Day even though he was not paid for overtime. Finding cases in Lisbon was often exceedingly difficult. Addresses were incomplete. There were multiple streets with the same name, and some streets were only a few houses long; however, with the aid of a detailed street guide in tiny print and his experience as a sanitarian, João found almost all of them. He also proved to be an excellent interviewer, maintaining rapport and eliciting information without "leading" the interviewees. Throughout my career, I was to find that one of the pleasures of working in the field with local coworkers was serendipitous encounters with extraordinary people.

> *Throughout my career, I was to find that one of the pleasures of working in the field with local coworkers was serendipitous encounters with extraordinary people*

Interviewing cases at night led to awkward situations. At 10:30 one night we sat in our VW on a dark street waiting for a 17-year-old schoolgirl to return home. A person with high thick-heeled shoes, long hair, and bell-bottoms came clopping down the street and approached the door with a young man, so I got out to interview her. At the door I asked, "Are you Constância Engrácia?" Unfortunately, the person was a young man, and I asked the question while looking him full in the face. His friend exploded with laughter while I tried to blame the darkness.

Another night we traced an older woman with cholera to a palatial mansion and were interrogated on the marble steps politely but suspiciously by the patient's son, an admiral. Apparently he checked us out with the authorities because the next day the national epidemiologist said with a knowing smile, "So you have been visiting admirals late at night?"

We tracked down 32 of the 35 patients (91%) and found neighborhood control subjects matched by age (within 5 years), gender, ethnic group, and approximate socioeconomic status. The cases and controls were asked whether, during August, they drank carbonated or uncarbonated bottled Agua do Vimeiro or visited the springs. As the investigation progressed, it became increasingly obvious that bottled water would be associated with cholera, and I worked in an advanced state of euphoria.

My fear of failure was gone. I knew that I would be going home soon, and I reveled in the opportunity to immerse myself in Lisbon and all things Portuguese. It was a privilege to talk with people at every social level in their homes and in their language. I found places that I dimly remembered from having lived in Lisbon for 8 months in 1947–1948 when I was 4 years old—our basement apartment at 22 Abaracamento de Peniche, a small park with a spreading tree under which I had played, and the botanical garden. I savored Portuguese food and music; I had café com leite and superbly crusty and chewy pães pequenos for breakfast, bife a Portuguesa for lunch, and concoctions of potato, onion, tomato, and fish with olive oil for dinner. I drank one brand of orange soft drink almost exclusively and then learned at the end from João that it had the worst coliform counts among the soft drinks. I continued, however, to add iodine to my drinking water, did not have a salad in 9 weeks, and stayed well.

The results were clear-cut: 13 cholera patients, but only two control subjects had consumed bottled non-carbonated Agua do Vimeiro ($P = 0.003$) (relative risk = 12). Interestingly, cholera was not associated with drinking carbonated Agua do Vimeiro, which made sense because carbonated water is acidic and *V. cholerae* cannot tolerate a low pH. The bottled water had infected all levels of society from an admiral's mother living in a mansion to someone living under metal roofing leaning against a wall. As I pored over the national data, I began to suspect that Agua do Vimeiro caused many cases all over Portugal because the epidemic peaked in the north (Porto), middle (Lisbon), and south (Faro) and in some other districts during the last 2 weeks of August, coinciding with contamination of the bottled water. Although 42% of the bottled water was distributed outside of Lisbon District, I wondered if vibrios could survive being trucked long distances at ambient temperature. It was too late to do more investigations, but I returned to our incompletely analyzed Faro case control data and discovered that we had implicated Agua do Vimeiro in Faro without realizing it! In Faro, nine cases and two control subjects reported having drunk Agua do Vimeiro ($P = 0.046$), and the association remained significant ($P = 0.031$) when controlling for eating cockles. Because the spa and the bottled water plant were closed on August 23 but the spring remained culture positive until at least August 28, stopping access to the spring water clearly prevented many cases of cholera. The Portuguese government did not allow the bottled water plant to reopen until the water source was changed to a deep well drilled in the same area as the Fonte Santa Isabel; however, at a higher altitude, the well water was shown to contain no pathogenic bacteria, and the plant began to treat the water with ultraviolet light before bottling.

WRAP-UP

I prepared a report for my exit interviews with Portuguese officials, and after 9 weeks, my work in Portugal was finally done. I felt, however, that I had barely scratched the surface of the possibilities that the cholera epidemic in Portugal presented for understanding cholera transmission. Once *V. cholerae* O1 is widely distributed by a vehicle of transmission (in Portugal raw shellfish), each infected person excretes enormous numbers of vibrios that can then contaminate foods (where they can multiply) and water and cause other outbreaks. Thus, the epidemic curve describing the course of an epidemic may represent the combined effects of many outbreaks, large and small, caused by a variety of vehicles, with only the largest outbreaks (such as the bottled water outbreak) having enough cases to cause marked distortion of the overall epidemic curve. Bits and pieces of information from across Portugal suggested that further investigations could have been fruitful. I mourned the lost opportunities—among others, a large inland outbreak attributed to a contaminated well in Portalegre, a sharp and massive outbreak in Porto affecting all age groups equally that may have been caused by public water, and a daycare center outbreak in Portimão that may have been caused by the diaper washer reconstituting powdered milk.

> *Bits and pieces of information from across Portugal suggested that further investigations could have been fruitful.*

I returned to Atlanta through Geneva at the request of the WHO. Epidemiologists often feel that the value of outbreak investigations is self-evident; however, that is not true, and it was certainly not the case at the WHO in the early 1970s. Our data, however, impressed the WHO officials, and they asked me to write a simple description of how to perform matched-pair case control studies to determine vehicles of transmission for use and publication by the WHO. Subsequently I complied, thinking it would help the WHO provide critical assistance to countries with epidemics, but in fact, it was buried in an appendix of a WHO monograph on shellfish hygiene.[2]

Sic transit gloria mundi (thus passes the glory of the world). Nevertheless, at the WHO, the successful cholera investigations in Portugal and Italy lent credibility to CDC investigations and may have helped ease the way for future requests from the WHO for CDC epidemiologists to investigate outbreaks worldwide.

On November 29, 1974, Portugal was declared free of cholera. In all, 2,467 culture-confirmed cases and 48 deaths were reported to the WHO. The case-fatality ratio was 1.9%, remarkably low considering that only the more severe cases were likely to be culture confirmed. Cholera did not reappear the following year. In 1974, five European countries reported 10 cases of cholera imported from Portugal. By writing to a case's physician in England, I learned that the patient visited Vimeiro Thermal Springs in mid August and drank spring water there.

Back in Atlanta, I struggled to find time to complete the analyses and write up the results, and I quickly discovered that my work had just begun and that the "fun" part was over. Over the years, I have seen many exquisite investigations (some of them, sadly, my own) that failed to achieve their potential public health impact and faded from memory because the investigators lacked the self-discipline to publish them. I had little experience in scientific writing, and organizing the results from our multiple studies in Portugal was particularly difficult. Now any resentment I harbored against my supervisors from our difficult communications in Portugal faded as they provided superb mentoring one on one. With help from my supervisors and coworkers, I eventually produced two papers (with five Portuguese coauthors) that we thought were ready for publication, and in September 1975, I sent them to the Portuguese director general of health for approval.

Two months dragged by with no response from Portugal, and thus, I sent the papers again stating that we planned to submit them to a journal on December 15 but could not include the Portuguese coauthors without written permission. That provoked a reply. On December 11, the director general wrote that he would not agree to publication of the papers in their present form because they could harm tourism. I was crushed. With my supervisors' coaching, however, I painfully made many small changes in the papers that I should have made in the first place, trimming some place and brand names and stressing (accurately) the Portuguese government's vigorous and appropriate response to the epidemic: case investigations; tetracycline treatment of contacts; no mass vaccinations; public health education; chlorinating water; closing the Fonte do Bispo and the Vimeiro springs, spa, and bottled water plant; recalling the bottled water; monitoring bottled water quality; and accepting CDC collaboration. I sent the director general the revised papers, a detailed list of the changes, and a properly humble letter, and by May 1976, he approved publication. The papers were finally published in 1977.[3,4]

Our investigations' impact on Portugal is difficult to judge. The 1974 cholera epidemic was ending as we arrived, and thus, we could not take any credit for controlling that epidemic; however, we showed how epidemiologic investigations could systematize and quantitate the things that health officials had suspected, proving some and disproving others. Unlike 1971, when the cause of the cholera outbreak in Lisbon remained a mystery, our investigations in 1974 showed that cholera may have been imported from Angola by the military, that contamination of the Fonte do Bispo infected many people and helped amplify the number of organisms in the environment, that contaminated shellfish caused many cases in southern Portugal and could have disseminated cholera throughout Portugal, and that pollution of two springs north of Lisbon caused many cases in visitors to the springs and in people in Lisbon, Faro, and possibly throughout Portugal who drank bottled uncarbonated spring water. We hope that statistical incrimination of these vehicles helped stiffen prevention measures and thus helped prevent future epidemics.

Our investigations contributed to scientific knowledge about transmission of cholera, including the most conclusive evidence ever presented that cholera could be transmitted by shellfish contaminated before harvest, the first reports that spring water contaminated before it emerges from the ground can transmit cholera, and the first report that bottled uncarbonated mineral water can transmit cholera. Because investigators sometimes focus on known vehicles and disregard possible vehicles that have not been implicated previously, publishing this information may have saved lives by alerting health authorities to these potential vehicles in prevention and control of cholera worldwide. It also had one tangible impact: The CDC changed its recommendation for international travelers to areas where chlorinated

> *I have seen many exquisite investigations (some of them, sadly, my own) that failed to achieve their potential public health impact and faded from memory because the investigators lacked the self-discipline to publish them.*

> *Carbonated mineral water is still on the list of recommended beverages for travelers.*

tap water is not available or where hygiene and sanitation are poor. Until 1974, the CDC recommended that one option for such travelers was to drink bottled water. After 1974, the recommendation was changed to bottled carbonated water. Carbonated mineral water is still on the list of recommended beverages for travelers.[5] Dramatic advances—many from the CDC's Enteric Diseases Branch—in understanding vehicles for cholera transmission have occurred since our investigations.[6] Foods have proven to be more important vehicles than was thought previously and include raw and cooked seafood, cooked grains and legumes, and frozen coconut milk.

This 9-week investigation shaped the rest of my career in epidemiology. It improved my epidemiologic skills and self-confidence and gave me a record of accomplishment that helped secure my career in the CDC's Enteric Diseases Branch, where I worked for the next 20 years, eventually as branch chief. Cholera and other vibrio-related diseases became my special interest. The investigation made me acutely aware of the limitations of supervision by telephone and pushed me toward letting field epidemiologists use their own judgment. It enhanced my Portuguese*, leading to subsequent work in Angola, Mozambique, Brazil, and Portugal. Most important, it taught me valuable lessons—and gave me a rich source of anecdotes—that I used in mentoring EIS officers, preventive medicine residents, and other epidemiologists:

1. Matched-pair case control studies with neighborhood controls can be a powerful tool, and people with the right temperament can be trained quickly to interview subjects and select matched controls; however, supervise them carefully, and do not send them out alone until they have demonstrated competence.
2. Take pains to develop good hypotheses before plunging into an investigation.
3. Keep an open mind about possible vehicles of transmission—the fact that a vehicle seems to be unlikely (e.g., spring water) or has not been implicated before (e.g., bottled water) does not rule it out, and experts, scientific articles, and textbooks can be wrong.
4. Without conclusive evidence, do not assume that any potential source of infection, no matter how logical and likely (e.g., decrepit water pipes and sewers in Tavira), is actually a source.
5. Scattered cases at the end of an epidemic may not provide useful information; focus on the heart of the epidemic curve, any unusual peaks, and the beginning.
6. Although it is best to investigate soon after illnesses occur, you can get a history of exposures even months later if you ask about usual practices like customary sources of water or memorable one-time exposures like travel.
7. Local investigators will tire before you do—they have different motivations and their usual work is backing up. Thus, work as quickly and efficiently as possible, and treat local investigators as colleagues and coworkers rather than as errand runners.
8. Try to understand the local officials' point of view, and adapt to it as much as possible without distorting the science—they will be dealing with the consequences of the investigation (and any publications) long after you are gone.
9. Resisting the urge to cut corners and go home can really pay off; it is better to stay in the field until you have completed the studies and preliminary analyses and identified and filled gaps in knowledge such as the distribution of incriminated products.
10. Do not pack an unused jar of thiosulfate citrate bile salts sucrose agar powder, a culture medium for *V. cholerae*, with your precious papers on your trip home; when it breaks, your papers will have a sticky green crust forever.

My experience in Portugal hooked me on epidemiologic investigations for life, and even now in retirement, I get a rush when I can contribute to an investigation. To me, the greatest joy of epidemiologic investigation is trying to solve the mystery. Initially, the situation often appears chaotic, with people becoming ill for no apparent reason; however, there is always order beneath the chaos, with everything happening for a reason. It is our fascinating job as epidemiologists to investigate, tease out the truth, and describe what happened and why it happened so that it can be stopped now and prevented in the future. The satisfaction that comes with finding out why things happen is immense.

---

* I wrote to my wife: "For two months I thought people were telling me that they were constipated, and I tried not to listen, but now I learn that 'constipado' means 'congested,' as in stuffy nose."

REFERENCES

1. Baine WB, Mazotti M, Greco D, et al. Epidemiology of cholera in Italy in 1973. *Lancet* 1974;2:1370–1381.
2. Blake PA, Martin SM, Gangarosa EJ. Simple case-control studies for determining the mode of transmission of cholera. In Wood PC, ed. *Guide to Shellfish Hygiene*. Geneva, World Health Organization Offset Publication No. 31, 1976:73–77.
3. Blake PA, Rosenberg ML, Costa JB, Ferreira PS, Guimaraes CL, Gangarosa EJ. Cholera in Portugal, 1974. I. Modes of transmission. *Am J Epidemiol* 1977;105:337–343.
4. Blake PA, Rosenberg ML, Florencia J, Costa JB, Quintino LDP, Gangarosa EJ. Cholera in Portugal, 1974. II. Transmission by bottled mineral water. *Am J Epidemiol* 1977;105:344–348.
5. Centers for Disease Control and Prevention. *Health Information for International Travel 2008*. Atlanta: U.S. Department of Health and Human Services, Public Health Service, 2007.
6. Mintz ED, Popovic T, Blake PA. Transmission of *Vibrio cholerae* O1. In Wachsmuth IK, Blake PA, Olsvik O, eds. *Vibrio cholerae and Cholera: Molecular to Global Perspectives*. Washington, DC: American Society for Microbiology, 1994:345–356.

LEARNING QUESTIONS

1. When the author and his colleague were planning to investigate shellfish consumption as a risk factor in Tavira (a coastal town in the Faro District), they worried that there would be poor recall of specific exposures by cases (and worse recall by controls) that had occurred six months before the case-control study was launched. How did they deal with this problem of anticipated poor recall?
2. The author excluded several cases from his case-control study of bottled water. These included six cases that visited the springs (Fonte Santa Isabel or Santa Isabel Springs), three younger than 10 years of age, one who was not the first case of cholera in his family, and two nonresidents of Lisbon who were ill before arriving in Lisbon. What was the rationale for excluding each of these groups?
3. What is a matched pair case control study?

CHAPTER 5

Legionnaires' Disease: Investigation of an Outbreak of a New Disease

Stephen B. Thacker, MD, MSc

Pennsylvania, 1976

INTRODUCTION

Late on a Monday afternoon in 1976, my first day at the Washington, DC health department, I received a telephone call from my supervisor at the Centers for Disease Control (CDC) in Atlanta, Georgia. The Friday before, I had completed 3 weeks in Atlanta in an intensive training course for the Epidemic Intelligence Service (EIS) as a field epidemiologist, whose responsibility is to detect and control epidemic disease. An epidemic of what appeared to be pneumonia was occurring in Pennsylvania, and I was to be in Harrisburg early the next morning to join the team that had assembled on Monday. Although a number of cases had been reported and deaths had occurred, all I knew was that the cause of the problem was unknown and that cases were being reported from across the state.

Already, epidemiologists, laboratory scientists, and statisticians were on the team, and they were ultimately joined by specialists in toxicology, pathology, environmental health, and environmental engineering. The major concern initially was the possibility of swine influenza ("swine flu"), as the initial call from a nurse at the Veterans Administration Hospital in Philadelphia was to the influenza program, which had been established in response to the threat of a new pandemic strain of the virus. Also, because of the concern about biologic terrorism—the nation was celebrating its bicentennial and Pope Paul VI was scheduled to visit the city in August—the state and local police were involved, and investigators from the Federal Bureau of Investigation and the military had been called in to assist.

The major concern initially was the possibility of swine influenza

During the training course, I learned the basic steps of an epidemic investigation.[1] I was to spend the next 3 weeks in Harrisburg and Philadelphia learning on the job how to investigate an epidemic.

THE INVESTIGATION

By the time I arrived in Harrisburg, the number of cases was already in the dozens. The majority of illnesses were among men who had attended a statewide convention of the American Legion in Philadelphia in late July that had been headquartered at the Bellevue-Stratford Hotel, an elegant old building on Broad Street. To determine a baseline and gather evidence about the epidemic, the investigation team had already begun to review death certificate data, hospital data, and visits to emergency rooms for a pneumonia-like illness (Figures 5-1, 5-2, and 5-3).

On that first day, we developed a case definition of the unknown disease, trying to balance concerns about sensitivity and specificity. A case was defined as having onset during July 1 to August 18, 1976, of fever and having chest radiograph evidence of pneumonia or temperature of ≥102°F and cough *and* attendance at the American Legion convention on July 21–24, 1976, or entry into the Bellevue-Stratford Hotel since July 1, 1976.

> *On that first day, we developed a case definition of the unknown disease, trying to balance concerns about sensitivity and specificity.*

On day 2, I was assigned to interview men and women with the disease, as well as their families, friends, and physicians. I also reviewed clinical and laboratory records, as well as pathology and autopsy reports. All of the information was collected on forms developed and copied the night before. EIS officers were sent throughout the state that day to gather information on what was then approximately 50 reports of the disease, and the information was being analyzed by other team members as it came in.

That same day I was introduced to another role of an EIS officer (and anyone else in public health practice)—meeting the press. I had been assigned to room with David Fraser, MD, an EIS alumnus and chief of the CDC's Special Pathogens Branch, who I had met for the first time that day and who was leading the investigation. In the late morning, I received a message to call Dr. Fraser, and between visits to hospitals, we were able to connect. He indicated that he was under pressure to have an EIS officer meet with the media. I was relatively close by, and thus, he asked if I would be willing to meet with a half-dozen members of the media at the community hospital in Chambersburg, about an hour away from Harrisburg. Arriving at Chambersburg about 30 minutes early, I proceeded to the pathology department to review the files on a deceased patient, when I was soon approached by Lawrence Altman, MD, who identified himself as a medical reporter from the *New York Times* and an EIS alumnus. Although not an official member of the press team, he proceeded to ask questions while I spoke with the pathologist and reviewed the records.

When I arrived at the hospital director's conference room, I quickly realized that Dr. Altman's unofficial presence was not well received by the other members of the press and television media. As I reviewed what I was doing, I learned two things: The media really wanted to understand what was going on, and I already knew a substantial amount that would be of help to them without speculating. Afterward, wearing a mask, I proceeded to examine and interview a patient who had been critically ill but was recovering despite the distraction of the media cameras. Mr. Thomas Payne was resting comfortably on his back in a typical hospital bed when I walked in, his left hand behind his head. He was alert and comfortable and seemed less nervous than his physician and the hospital nurse. As with each visit that day, patients, their families, as well as the physicians and hospital staff were friendly and eager to be helpful, clearly looking to me as a representative of the CDC

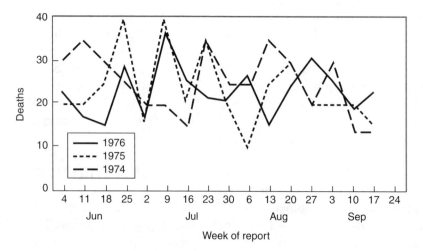

FIGURE 5-1 Pneumonia and influenza deaths, by week of report, Philadelphia, 1974–1976.

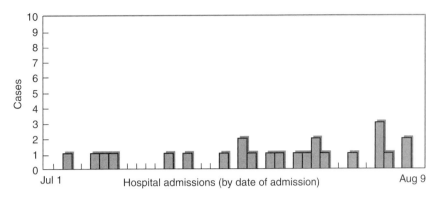

FIGURE 5-2 Number of cases of illness resembling Legionnaires' disease seen in three center city Philadelphia hospitals July 1–Aug. 9, 1976.

and the state health department for help with a perplexing and frightening epidemic. The patient answered the long list of questions that we had developed the night before. Through this visit, I also learned how fearful people were about the disease; the media's reluctance to enter patient rooms exacerbated this fear. After the patient interview, I traveled to the university hospital in Hershey where I visited a patient in intensive care and was met by EIS alumnus Dr. Robert Aber who had recently joined the faculty in infectious disease. Then I returned to Harrisburg to debrief the team.

Beginning the following day, I was asked to maintain the line listing of all confirmed cases on a large wall chart that included epidemiologic, clinical, and laboratory information. At this time, before computers were routinely used in public health investigations, large pieces of poster board and pencil, ink, or a marker worked just as well for this purpose. Each time the team met in the morning and evening the line listing was used to summarize the information gathered to date and to provide a visual backdrop for the investigators as we planned the next investigative steps. Different hypotheses were rapidly generated and tested by the team with the data laid out in this way. Hypotheses ranged from psittacosis (parrot fever) to intentional poisoning.

The descriptive data gathered to determine the existence of the epidemic helped establish the time frame of the outbreak, which is best depicted by an epidemic curve in which all cases are entered by the date of symptom onset (Figure 5-4).[2] Because this was a state con-

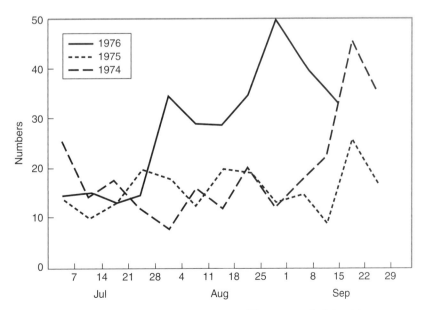

FIGURE 5-3 Emergency room visits for "Pneumonia" in 11 Philadelphia hospitals.

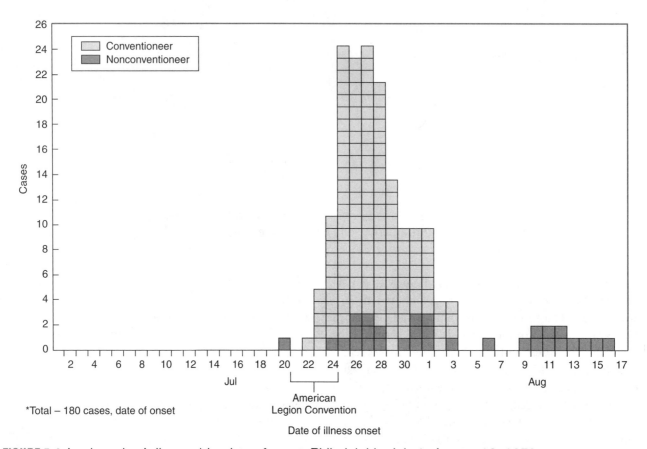

FIGURE 5-4 Legionnaires' disease,* by date of onset, Philadelphia, July 1–August 18, 1976.
From Fraser DW, Tsai TR, Orenstein W, Parkin WE, Beecham HS, Sharrer RG, et al. Legionnaires' disease: description of an epidemic of pneumonia. *N Engl J Med* 1977;297:1189–97. Copyright ©1977 Massachusetts Medical Society. All rights reserved.

vention, cases were displayed on a map divided into American Legion districts, which depicted the geographic scope of the epidemic (Figure 5-5). The epidemic was linked to all four hotels that had housed conventioneers; however, all convention functions had occurred at the Bellevue-Stratford Hotel, and the investigation therefore led to the primary role of that hotel where delegates had spent on average more time (56.5 vs. 51.6 hours). The common site of exposure was the hotel, but no one location within the hotel or any event at the convention was recognized as a unique common exposure.

Analysis of the data collected demonstrated that delegates had higher attack rates than family members and other nondelegates who attended the convention. Men had higher attack rates than women (5.4% vs. 1.9%), and attack rates increased with patient age. It was especially

> *We were dealing with a pneumonia that killed approximately one of seven patients, despite the use of powerful antibiotics and supportive care.*

concerning that this was not a mild illness. We were dealing with a pneumonia that killed approximately one of seven patients, despite the use of powerful antibiotics and supportive care. In addition, even persons who had not attended the convention were among the cases. There was a pilot who came in about noon one day, slept a few hours, and then left. There was even an older woman (at least 80 years old) who came in to use the toilet (for about 20 minutes at most) and died a couple of weeks later.

Meanwhile, this outbreak had become national news, hitting television news broadcasts, as well as the front pages of newspapers and the covers of *Time* and *Newsweek* magazines. Dr. Altman, who had interviewed me on day 2, published a daily *New York Times* column about the investigation. The CDC was already in the limelight because of the threat of a global influenza pandemic, and this attention only intensified when this mysterious outbreak became a political concern during this, a presidential election year. Headlines like the *New York Times*' "20 flu-like deaths in Pennsylvania. 115 ill. A mystery" captured the public's attention.

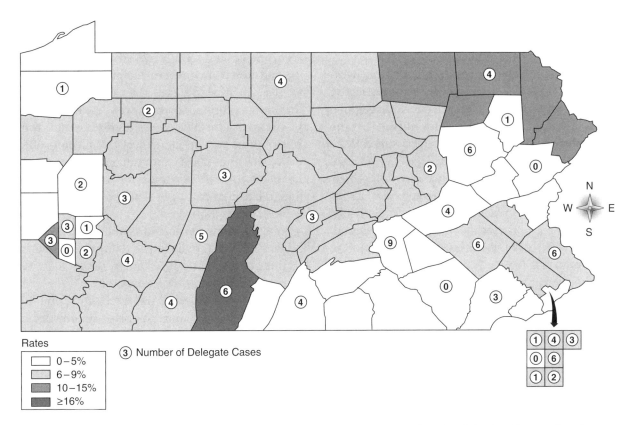

FIGURE 5-5 Legionnaires' disease cases and attack rates, by American Legion District, Pennsylvania, 1976.

As previously noted, clearly, delegates to the convention and their families were at risk, but other cases were emerging. One at-risk population included those who had nothing to do with the convention but who had stayed at the hotel at the same time. Eventually, 20 such persons received diagnoses of the disease. Only one case in a hotel employee fit the case definition, although later serologic tests identified a limited number of others with antibodies. Possibly, this younger, healthier employee population was not at high risk. Most interesting were persons with signs and symptoms of the disease who had passed by the hotel but never even entered the facility. Our investigation team nicknamed the illness in these persons as "Broad Street pneumonia," after the street on which the hotel was located, and their data were maintained on a separate line listing. Eventually, data regarding 37 persons were placed on this list, and their illnesses were confirmed. The investigators also looked at conventions that had previously been at the hotel, seeking possible missed cases.

As we intently studied the data brought back by the EIS officers on the second and third days of the investigation, as well as data telephoned in from throughout the state by veterans, clinicians, local health departments, and the general public, the team generated hypotheses about the nature of the illness, risk factors for illness and death, sources of the exposure, modes of transmission, and potential causes. Clinical specimens were already being tested at the state and CDC laboratories for infectious agents and known chemical causes of respiratory disease. During the next weeks, specialists in infectious disease and in natural and manmade biologic and chemical toxins were brought in to consult, as were specialists in pathology, environmental engineering, and even biologic and chemical weapons. A CDC engineer collected specimens from all parts of the hotel, including sleeping quarters, convention rooms, offices, the lobby air conditioner, the elevators, and the cooling tower on top of the hotel. Not all locations for sampling were based on epidemiologic data.

The immediate challenge was to design and conduct a case control study to test the multiple hypotheses that were being generated. In addition to the hotel registration records and the relevant hotel floor plans, we obtained the calendar of events for the 3-day convention. We designed a questionnaire that included basic demographic information; such behaviors as smoking, drinking, medication, and drug use; eating practices both in and outside the hotel, including local restaurants and street vendors; water drinking, including sources and amounts; time spent in different parts of the hotel, including the lobby and the elevators; and such potential exposures as pigeons.

After approximately 10 days, the focus of the investigation moved to Philadelphia. The team in Harrisburg was reduced, and some of us traveled to Philadelphia, where we stayed at the Bellevue-Stratford Hotel. As the case control study was being implemented, surveillance continued. More cases were identified. New hypotheses were proposed, and the investigation adapted to the new information. For example, to test the hypothesis that this might be a psittacosis epidemic, a woman regularly observed feeding pigeons near the hotel was interviewed. Because nickel carbonyl was a suspected cause and the metal alloys in use for scalpels and forceps contained nickel, autopsy teams were provided plastic tools.

At the end of 3 weeks, we had described an epidemic that involved more than 220 persons, including 34 deaths. Every known infectious pathogen had been sought, but none was identified. Different toxins and environmental agents had been considered, but none was identified as the causal agent. Hypotheses had been proffered, tested, and rejected. No new cases were being identified, despite active surveillance for disease. We knew a substantial amount about the epidemic, but we had not uncovered what had caused it, why it had happened when it did, why it had happened where it did, and why the Legionnaires and others exposed at the hotel were victims. In summary, the epidemic had ended without our intervention, and we had nothing to recommend specifically to prevent another occurrence. The team returned to their regular jobs but still remained actively engaged in the work both in Pennsylvania and Atlanta.

In summary, the epidemic had ended without our intervention, and we had nothing to recommend specifically to prevent another occurrence.

After any field investigation requested by a state, EIS officers are required to submit a written summary of their work to the state and to the CDC director. During that fall, a detailed report of the investigation was developed, eventually totaling 71 pages; however, a discovery late in the calendar year delayed publication of the report and marked a turning point in the investigation.

The causal agent was discovered during the Christmas holidays of 1976 when Joseph McDade, PhD, who worked in the CDC's Rickettsial Disease Laboratory, was motivated to reexamine cultures after hearing criticism of the CDC's efforts in the investigation voiced at a party he attended. Hen's eggs are used to culture *Rickettsia*, and as Dr. McDade looked one more time at the egg cultures from the Philadelphia investigation, he noted a consistent contamination among the specimens. The contamination, however, was located only among the specimens from persons with disease, not from the control subjects. This Gram-negative pleomorphic rod turned out not to be a contaminant, but instead, it was the bacterium that caused the epidemic, the first human bacterial pathogen that had been discovered in decades.[3] The pathogen was confirmed as the etiologic agent of the epidemic, including the Broad Street pneumonias.[2,4] It was rapidly linked to unsolved CDC investigations in 1965[5] and 1968[6] and was later identified as the cause of other unsolved epidemics.[7,8]

Isolation of the agent led to a series of groundbreaking publications and, more importantly, provided investigators with clues to sources in the environment and airborne transmission, and ultimately uncovered the means to detect, control, and treat the disease. In fact, I was asked to review a large cardboard box full of files from 1965 and to write up the unsolved investigation of an epidemic of pneumonia at a chronic disease hospital in Washington, DC, where I was assigned as the EIS officer. It turned out this 1965 epidemic was an unsolved Legionnaires' outbreak. Legionnaires' disease has now been recognized as a much more common cause of illness, resulting in an estimated 20,000 cases of pneumonia each year. It is spread through the air and has been identified in such places as cooling towers, fresh water, and shower heads. It is also treatable with antibiotics that were available at the time of the investigation.

The approach to this groundbreaking epidemic differs little from the standard approach to any epidemic. The size and scope of the investigation, as well as the publicity surrounding it, serve to dramatize the challenging and important work undertaken every day by the practicing epidemiologist in the field. It also underscores the reality of the critical roles that members of the public health team play at every step of the investigation—from recognition of the problem to control of the epidemic and publication of the results.

The size and scope of the investigation, as well as the publicity surrounding it, serve to dramatize the challenging and important work undertaken every day by the practicing epidemiologist in the field.

PERSONAL REFLECTIONS

This investigation introduced me to the application of epidemiology to real problems in public health. My experience as an EIS officer led to a career in epidemiology and public health at the CDC (now the Centers for Disease Control and Prevention). At the CDC, I have had the opportunity to apply the tools of epidemiology to a range of public health problems, including not only infectious diseases (e.g., the initial studies of AIDS), but also toxic chemicals in the environment (e.g., dioxin exposures of soldiers and childhood lead poisoning), environmental disasters, violence and unintentional injuries, as well as chronic conditions (e.g., breast cancer and heart disease).

As the director of the CDC's epidemiology program since 1989, I have been involved in critical public health problems, including the discovery of hantavirus pulmonary syndrome in the southwestern United States, introduction of West Nile virus to the United States and its spread across the country, the emergence of the *Escherichia coli* O157:H7 bacterium as the cause of local and national epidemics, the response to the threat of Ebola virus in Central Africa, and the impending crisis of antibiotic resistance. Recently, the epidemics of severe acute respiratory syndrome (SARS), monkeypox, and avian influenza have engaged CDC epidemiologists throughout the world. The health effects of disasters, most dramatically the 2004 tsunami in Asia and Hurricanes Katrina and Rita in the United States in 2005, but also earthquakes in Central America, drought and starvation in Africa, and refugee crises related to other natural disasters and war, have involved CDC epidemiologists. Any of the leading causes of morbidity, mortality, and disability have been subject to the analytic insights of epidemiologists for both understanding the processes leading to disease and injury and for implementing effective prevention programs.

On the afternoon of September 11, 2001, a CDC team was flown from Atlanta to assist the New York City Department of Health and Mental Hygiene in responding to the tragedy of the World Trade Center terrorist attack. Included on that team were two EIS officers who were assigned to establish that night a surveillance system at ground zero to document as rapidly as possible the health consequences for both victims and workers; their immediate actions helped target New York City's emergency response. By Friday of that week, an additional team of EIS officers were flown to the city to establish a surveillance system in 17 city hospitals to monitor the effects of the attack and to look for disease related to chemical or biologic terrorism.

On October 4, 2001, the EIS officer assigned to the Florida Department of Health was joined by the CDC staff to assist the state in investigating a case of anthrax in a 63-year-old man in Boca Raton, the first known victim of anthrax transmitted through the U.S. mail. Epidemiologists became involved in surveillance and investigation activities throughout the United States and countries around the world. All 140 EIS officers became involved, with 133 being deployed away from their assignment for weeks during the response.

Epidemiology has been called the basic science of public health. The tools of the epidemiologist help investigators extract useful information from complex data that leads to effective public health action. The work is challenging and can sometimes be risky. The rewards, however, are sizable, as one uses the best available science to work with others in addressing the major health problems that face the world's population. Although not all of my work has been as dramatic as my first investigation in Philadelphia, the gratification of seeing improvements in health stemming from the efforts of epidemiologists at the CDC and elsewhere around the world is enormous.

> *Epidemiology has been called the basic science of public health.*

REFERENCES

1. Gregg MB. Conducting a field investigation. In Gregg MB, ed. *Field Epidemiology*, 2nd ed. New York, NY: Oxford University Press, 2002:62–67.
2. Fraser DWD, Tsai TR, Orenstein W, et al. Legionnaires' disease: description of an epidemic of pneumonia. *N Engl J Med* 1977;297:1189–1197.
3. McDade JE, Shepard CC, Fraser DW, et al. Legionnaires' disease: isolation of a bacterium and demonstration of its role in other respiratory disease. *N Engl J Med* 1977;297:1197–1203.
4. Chandler FW, Hicklin MD, Blackmon JA. Demonstration of the agent of Legionnaires' disease in tissue. *N Engl J Med* 1977;297:1218–1220.
5. Thacker SB, Bennett JV, Tsai TF, et al. An outbreak in 1965 of severe respiratory illness caused by the Legionnaires' disease bacterium. *J Infect Dis* 1978;138:512–519.
6. Glick TH, Gregg MB, Berman B, et al. Pontiac fever: an epidemic of unknown etiology in a health department. I. Clinical and epidemiological aspects. *Am J Epidemiol* 1978;107:149–160.

7. Terranova W, Cohen ML, Fraser DW. 1974 outbreak of Legionnaires' disease diagnosed in 1977: clinical and epidemiologic features. *Lancet* 1978;2:122–124.
8. Osterholm MT, Chin TDY, Osborne DO, et al. A 1957 outbreak of Legionnaires' disease associated with a meat packing plant. *Am J Epidemiol* 1983;117:60–67.

LEARNING QUESTIONS

1. The CDC invested substantial personnel resources into providing assistance with this outbreak investigation. Considering the time period and circumstances, why did such a prioritization of this particular outbreak investigation make sense?
2. What was "Broad Street pneumonia" and why were those cases maintained on a separate line list?
3. The case-control study had several hypotheses including a possible role for smoking, alcohol consumption, medication use, drug abuse, time spent in different areas of the hotel, and exposure to pigeons. What is the biological plausibility of each of these possible factors being associated with becoming a case of the (at that time) unknown etiology of Legionnaires' disease?

CHAPTER 6

The Investigation of Toxic Shock Syndrome in Wisconsin, 1979–1980 and Beyond

Jeffrey P. Davis, MD

Wisconsin, 1979–1980

INTRODUCTION

In early December 1979, I had just completed my first 13 months of employment after joining the (later renamed) Wisconsin Division of Health (DOH) as the State Epidemiologist and Chief of the Section of Acute and Communicable Disease Epidemiology (ACDE). During the 5 years before beginning my tenure in the DOH, I served as an Epidemic Intelligence Service (EIS) officer assigned as a field services officer to the South Carolina Department of Health and Environmental Control and then completed the third year of my pediatrics residency and a pediatric infectious diseases fellowship at Duke University. All were formative experiences that resulted in the shaping of my career as an infectious diseases physician focused on infectious diseases epidemiology using applied methods.

In addition to wonderful staff in categorically funded programs (immunization, sexually transmitted diseases, and tuberculosis), the ACDE section included three general epidemiologists, all of whom were newly hired: Martin LaVenture, Wendy Schell, and me. Although few in number, my epi team colleagues were young, bright, and eager. I actually interviewed Marty during my first visit to the DOH during the recruitment process for my position. Although this would be considered unusual procedure, I remember thinking that they better take my advice and hire this guy. Wendy was already in the state system as an employee at the State Laboratory of Hygiene.

The probationary period for a new employee with supervisory responsibilities was 12 months, but those 12 months flew by rapidly. Our epi team revised reporting procedures, developed a new reporting form in triplicate (copies for the local health department, DOH, and the patient's medical record), began publication of the *Wisconsin Epidemiology Bulletin*, and planned and conducted training activities. The media became interested in our investigations and recommendations as a result of the *Wisconsin Epidemiology Bulletin* distribution to 7,000 physicians, public health professionals, and media representatives.

During July and August 1979, I was directing our epi team's first large-scale investigation, which involved an outbreak of 13 cases of Legionnaires' disease in Eau Claire. After an intensive several days of initial and hypothesis-generating investigation by our team that focused us on a likely source of a cooling tower on the roof of a hotel, I invited a team from the Centers for Disease Control (CDC) to join us in an epidemic aid (Epi-Aid) investigation to help determine the extent of the outbreak and the precise mechanism of transmission of *Legionella* from the associated cooling tower. The outbreak occurrence and investigation was very visible, particularly after the CDC team arrived, and our interactions with the media were daily and generally at the same time each day, which was a valuable process. The investigation involved my first experiences with using credit card receipts as a case finding tool, isolating *Legionella pneumophila* from an environmental source (cooling tower water), and watching the application of air tracer studies to provide information regarding where the cooling tower aerosols went. In this case, it was used to demonstrate the inadvertent intake of the cooling tower exhaust down a chimney with an open damper and into a meeting room via the fireplace.[1] It was quite exciting to be involved with the successful application of these neat techniques. Our investigation team was thrilled that their epidemiologic data were supported by the laboratory findings.

In 1979, the report of a cluster of three cases of Lyme disease occurring in 1978 in individuals who cleared brush at a site in Washburn County in northwestern Wisconsin represented the first known cluster of Lyme disease to occur west of the Eastern seaboard.[2] Dick Kaslow, who at the time was working at the National Institute of Allergy and Infectious Diseases, and I initiated surveys of the distribution of *Ixodes dammini* (at that time considered to be the vector of the agent that caused Lyme disease) and another established prevalent tick (used as a control) on white tailed deer. The survey involved our epi team and additional National Institute of Allergy and Infectious Diseases, Wisconsin Department of Natural Resources, and Rocky Mountain Laboratory colleagues and numerous volunteers willing to pick ticks off of freshly killed deer at the beginning of the deer hunting season. This represented a different type of challenge: a collaborative, multiagency investigation involving detailed prospective planning. We completed the field work of our first of four surveys (1979–1982) in 1979[3] shortly after Thanksgiving and were working on shipping live ticks to Willy Burgdorfer at the Rocky Mountain Laboratory for speciation and with the intent to establish tick colonies to look for the causative agent of Lyme disease.

In the midst of this phase of our Lyme disease work, I was called by a resident in the Department of Pediatrics, University of Wisconsin Medical School, on behalf of Joan Chesney who was a colleague of mine, regarding two currently hospitalized young women from Madison with rapid onset of fever, rash, and hypotension among other findings, including acute renal failure. Joan was an infectious diseases specialist, and her husband, Russ Chesney, was a nephrologist. Both were faculty in the University of Wisconsin Department of Pediatrics and consulted on these cases from their different clinical perspectives. In essence, Joan had seen a patient with high fever, hypotension, and a rash who had acute renal failure, and Russ had seen a patient with acute renal failure who had high fever, hypotension, and a rash. While serendipitously discussing details of their cases during a dinner at home, they concluded these patients may have toxic shock syndrome (TSS), although neither had previously seen a case. After speaking with the resident, I called Joan, and she provided me with more clinical details of these two cases and told me about a third case, also in a currently hospitalized individual.

Although first reported in the 1920s, TSS is a condition initially described and named by Jim Todd of the University of Colorado and his colleagues in an article published in the *Lancet* in 1978.[4] They described a severe acute disease associated with strains of *Staphylococcus aureus* of phage group I that produced a unique epidermal toxin. His series involved seven children, 8 to 17 years old who presented between June 1975 and November 1977 with sudden onset of high fever, headache, sore throat, diarrhea, and erythroderma (a diffuse sunburn-like rash) with associated findings of acute renal failure, hepatic abnormalities, and confusion. All had refractory hypotension. One patient died, and each survivor had desquamation (peeling of the skin) of the hands and feet during convalescence.

> They described a severe acute disease associated with strains of **Staphylococcus aureus** of phage group I that produced a unique epidermal toxin.

THE OUTBREAK

Fortunately, I was familiar with TSS before publication of the article by Todd and his colleagues. I had participated in the care of an extremely ill adolescent female with TSS while I was a pediatric ID fellow in the Department of Pediatrics at Duke University. I told Joan that I felt the current three patients' clinical and laboratory findings were highly consistent with TSS. I recalled that

Jim Todd's series involved sporadic cases accumulated over a prolonged period, at least 2 years. In the absence of any existing surveillance for TSS to use to estimate the expected number of cases, the Todd article was used to judge whether this was an outbreak (even if it involved only two cases at the time). I concluded that this was likely a departure from an expected number of cases because of the rarity of this condition and apparent clustering of cases in time and space. An immediate field investigation began. The next day Bill Taylor, an EIS field officer assigned to the Wisconsin DOH, and I interviewed the three patients and reviewed their medical records in an effort to begin the process of understanding host and risk factors and generating a hypothesis. We asked about a variety of work, exercise, and social activities, social venues, restaurants visited, where their groceries were purchased, whether they had traveled, and many other things. Apart from Madison-area residence, the only readily apparent common factor among these patients was being a young woman. I was struck by this. I wondered whether any of these three patients had onset of illness during menstruation. I recalled that at multiple junctures during my training I was taught of the importance of the often overlooked menstrual history, which could provide important clues regarding a variety of disease processes. Naturally, the medical records of the three patients did not contain this information, but additional interviews of the patients revealed all three had their illness onsets during a menstrual period. I immediately thought this was more than a coincidence. An aggressive case finding surveillance was established and began expeditiously.

Local surveillance was facilitated in part by Joan Chesney's contacts with hospital colleagues and a grand rounds presentation made by Joan and I. Surveillance in four Madison hospitals generated four more cases by early January 1980. All seven cases occurred since July 1979 in women. Six were menstruating at illness onset, and one premenarchal adolescent had infected figure skating-induced blisters. Of note, two had similar but milder illnesses during prior menstrual periods, suggesting that the syndrome could recur. I generated a case report form that included data on demographic features, clinical findings, clinical management and course of illness, presence and course of recurrences, and laboratory data. The form was also used to collect data on potential risk factors that included presence of skin lesions and detailed information on menstruation (onset, duration, intensity) and factors related to menstruation (catamenial and oral contraceptive product use).

Because of the striking severity and novelty of this syndrome, I prepared a mailing sent on January 31, 1980, to 3,500 internists, pediatricians, and family practice physicians licensed in Wisconsin to inform them of TSS and the currently reported case illnesses, provide management recommendations based on what we knew about these first seven case patients, establish statewide TSS surveillance with expeditious reporting to DOH, and generate appropriate specimens for culture and serologic testing to be sent to the Wisconsin State Laboratory of Hygiene (WSLH) for processing (Exhibit 6-1).[5]

Concurrently, I called Merlin Bergdoll at the University of Wisconsin Food Research Institute to discuss whether TSS could be caused by a staphylococcal enterotoxin. Merlin was the foremost authority on staphylococcal enterotoxins, and his lab was just a few miles away from our offices. At that time, there were five known staphylococcal enterotoxins (A-E), which were heat stable and primarily known for their ability to cause foodborne illnesses. Merlin thought a staphylococcal enterotoxin would be a good candidate and was most willing to collaborate and test specimens from case patients.

While expanding TSS surveillance in Wisconsin, I received a call one Sunday in January 1980 from Andy Dean, the State Epidemiologist in Minnesota. Andy learned of five cases, two cases initially and a subsequent three cases, in women hospitalized with an unusual acute illness. I said, "Let me describe it to you," which I did. The illness I described was identical to those occurring in Minnesota. Andy asked what the illness was. I said that it was TSS and further described our cases, the association with menstruation, and the potential for recurrence. By the next day, these 12 cases from the two states were reported to the CDC by Andy and I.

In February 1980, while planning an initial case control study, I called Jim Todd, the chief of pediatric infectious diseases at the University of Colorado Medical School, to discuss our findings. My call to him must have seemed as though it came out of left field. By then Jim knew of 35 cases from multiple states that occurred since 1975. These included 25 females with a mean age of 20 years of whom 20 had vaginitis and 10 males with a mean age of 11 years of whom 7 had focal bacterial infections. All had toxigenic strains of *S. aureus* isolated; however, one third were not associated with the unique epidermal toxin noted in his initial report and one third involved nonphage group I *S. aureus*. Jim had not studied risk factors. He could recall only one potential recurrence, and he

EXHIBIT 6-1 The Initial Memorandum on TSS Mailed to Physicians in Wisconsin on January 31, 1980

State of Wisconsin/Department of Health and Social Services
January 31, 1980

TO: Physician in the State of Wisconsin
FROM: Jeffrey P. Davis, MD
State Epidemiologist and Chief
Section of Epidemiologic Surveillance and Assessment
SUBJECT: Toxic Shock Syndrome

The detailed information which is to follow is intended to describe a clinical entity which has recently been seen in patients in Wisconsin. The information is detailed as certain physicians in the state may not be familiar with this entity. Most physicians that will take care of such cases will manage them in a tertiary care setting. I feel that a broad description of the illness might stimulate a higher index of suspicion, facilitate any needed referrals, and enhance reporting of these cases and the communication involved with management of these patients.

Between July, 1979 and January 6, 1980 seven patients with a syndrome of toxic shock have been directly hospitalized in or transferred to Madison area hospitals. All seven patients have been women between the ages of 14 and 44, and all but one have been between the ages of 14 and 28. Each of these patients had a strong similarity in clinical onset and in clinical course, a composite clinical description follows:

Onset:	high fever (39–41 degrees C)
	vomiting (profound)
	watery diarrhea (profuse)
	headache
	myalgias that may include abdominal guarding
	sore throat
	confusion
	the onset seems to be associated with an ongoing menstrual period
Admission findings:	shock that is seemingly refractory requiring dopamine or other agents and massive fluid therapy
	acute renal failure (oliguria and azotemia with elevated creatinine)
	proteinuria
	elevated serum glutamic-oxaloacetic transaminase, serum glutamic-pyruvic transaminase, LDH, bilirubin
	prolonged protime
	hypoalbuminemia
	rhabdomyolysis (extreme elevations of serum CPK)
	leukocytosis with predominance of bands and juvenile forms (extreme shift to the left)
	thrombocytopenia
	anemia–at first seemingly hemolytic
	blood cultures are sterile
Additional manifestations:	diffuse erythematous, nonpruritic scarlatiniform rash (erythroderma) prominent on the trunk and extremities
	early fine desquamation and late peripheral desquamation
	nonpitting, subcutaneous edema
	vaginitis
	conjunctivitis, several with hemorrhages
	stomatitis, several with vesicles
	mild jaundice
	evidence if DIC in several patients
Further supportive measures:	one patient required dialysis
	three patients had evidence of the adult respiratory distress syndrome, and one required ventilatory assistance
	one patient required a D and C to control vaginal bleeding
Outcome:	All seven patients have recovered

The five patients with onsets since late November 1979 have all had staphylococci recovered from either a mucosal site (throat, NP, or vagina) or a sequestered site; further studies of toxigenicity are pending. Two of these five patients have had herpes simplex virus type I isolated from throat or oral lesion cultures; the others have had multiple site viral cultures during the acute phase of the illness which were negative. Studies of paired sera completed in two patients have been negative for antibodies to a broad series of respiratory viruses and coxsackie B viruses are pending.

EXHIBIT 6-1 (Continued)

A clinical entity that is identical to that just described has been reported by Todd et al in 1978 (*Lancet*; 1116–1118, November 25, 1978). Todd reported seven cases ranging from 8 to 17 years of age, all of whom had isolates of staphylococci from mucosal or sequestered sites that were noted to produce an exfoliative exotoxin (a unique epidermal toxin detected by a positive Nikolsky sign in neonatal mice). Viral cultures completed on five of these patients were negative, but the sites cultured were not stated. Each of the toxigenic strains of staphylococci were phage group I organisms. The entity was called a toxic shock syndrome-associated phage group I staphylococci. In Todd's series, five patients recovered, one patient had gangrene of the toes, and one patient died.

All seven of the patients in Wisconsin have recovered. Each of the five most recent patients has received specific antistaphylococcal antibiotic therapy as part of broad spectrum antibiotic coverage. It appears that clinical improvement has been noted after the initiation of specific antistaphylococcal therapy. This is not to say that these Wisconsin patients had toxic shock syndrome-associated with staphylococci: the diagnosis is suspected but has not been proven. Other etiologies must still be considered as potentially associated with this syndrome.

Among other diseases to consider in the differential diagnosis as bacterial sepsis; severe systemic viral infections associated with adenovirus, coxsackie B virus, herpes virus, or other viruses; Kawasaki disease (mucocutaneous lymph node syndrome); hemolytic uremic syndrome; ingestion of preformed staphylococcal enterotoxin or other exogenous toxin; and other staphylococcal syndromes. This does not represent a comprehensive list.

While the current series of Wisconsin patients are all women, the entity may not be limited to women. Males have been reported to experience this syndrome and they tend to be in the pediatric age range with evidence of focal staphylococcal disease prior to the onset of these symptoms.

Recommendations:

A. Laboratory

We strongly suggest the following laboratory studies to further investigate the possibility of toxic shock syndrome and its association with staphylococci or with other etiologic agent.

1. Bacterial cultures:

    Nasopharynx and anterior nares, trachea, vagina, stool, urine, blood, and focal lesions. Blood cultures have been uniformly negative in TSS, but are needed to rule out bacterial sepsis.

    Please have your laboratory save each separate colony type of any coagulase positive or coagulase negative staphylococcus isolated from any cultured site from any patient in whom toxic shock is considered. Please call Dr. Jeffrey Davis or Dr. William Taylor at the Bureau of Prevention, 608/266-1251 to inform us of such isolates. Further arrangements will then be made with the State Laboratory of Hygiene to facilitate further studies.

2. Viral Cultures:

    These are needed to rule out the possibility of a wide range of systemic viral etiologic agents disease. Suggested sites include respiratory (throat or nasopharynx), stool, lesion cultures (most likely to be oral or genital), vagina, and urine. Please forward all material for viral isolation to the Viral Laboratory, State Laboratory of Hygiene.

3. Serum:

    Acute and convalescent phase sera are needed to diagnose viral disease and potentially screen for the presence of staphylococcal exotoxin and any potential antibody to such a toxin. Please obtain the following specimens:

    1. acute phase—as soon as possible after admission;
    2. 14 days after onset;
    3. one month after onset.

    Please obtain at least 5 cc of serum per specimen. Forward all serum specimens to the Viral Laboratory, State Laboratory of Hygiene.

Please indicate on any specimens that are sent to the State Laboratory of Hygiene that you are interested in ruling out toxic shock syndrome. Please provide the requested clinical information.

B. Management

Because the syndrome has been associated with staphylococci, institution of empiric antistaphylococcal therapy with a penicillinase-resistant penicillin or another appropriate antistaphylococcal antibiotic as part of broad spectrum coverage seems warranted as part of the patients' management. Patients in our series placed on specific antistaphylococcal regimens have demonstrated clinical improvement, but it is not clear how significant antistaphylococcal therapy is relative to other components of supportive therapy. Full attention to ruling out all clinical possibilities and maintaining full supportive management is stressed.

C. Reporting

Please call Dr. Jeffrey Davis (Wisconsin Division of Health, Bureau of Prevention) 608/266-1251 or Dr. William Taylor 608/266-1251 or 608/266-9783 as soon as you become clinically aware of any potential case of toxic shock syndrome. If you recall seeing a similar case at any point in time in the past we would greatly appreciate learning of such cases. Please feel free to call if you have any questions pertaining to any facet of this syndrome.

Further information as it becomes available will appear in the *Wisconsin Epidemiology Bulletin*.

agreed that a case control study to examine risk factors was needed.

In February 1980, Kathy Shands, an EIS officer in the Special Pathogens Branch, began the CDC's work on TSS by collaborating to generate a clinical case definition with Jim Todd and Neil Halsey of the University of Colorado, Mike Osterholm of the Minnesota DOH, and me.[6] At that time, Mike was an assistant state epidemiologist who had been investigating the Minnesota TSS cases. By April, we concurred on the case definition criteria, which became very durable in its application over time (Table 6-1).[7]

Fortunately, the response to our January 30 mailing was rapid and dramatic, particularly by physicians. After subsequent publication of my office phone number in a newspaper article about TSS by Neil Rosenberg of the *Milwaukee Journal*, a widely circulated newspaper, a large number of cases were self-reported (parenthetically, Neil developed a keen interest in TSS and Lyme disease). We received numerous physician generated and self-reports of potential cases and laboratory specimens. Clinical and laboratory data were systematically collected using a case report form that I had generated. Line lists were created and maintained using long-hand entry—no computers yet. Phil Wand, a bacteriologist at the WSLH, received all submitted subcultures of *S. aureus* isolates from mucous membranes of case patients to characterize, split for Dr. Bergdoll's laboratory and also stored at the WSLH. In addition, he stored paired samples of sera from case patients for future testing. It is always critical to anticipate future testing, and storing isolates and paired sera is most valuable. A very large bank of specimens evolved.

> *It is always critical to anticipate future testing, and storing isolates and paired sera is most valuable.*

TABLE 6-1 TSS Case Definition

Clinical Case Definition
An illness with the following clinical manifestations:
Fever: temperature greater than or equal to 38.9°C (102.0°F)
Rash: diffuse macular erythroderma
Desquamation: 1 to 2 weeks after onset of illness, particularly on the palms and soles
Hypotension: systolic blood pressure less than or equal to 90 mm Hg for adults or less than fifth percentile by age for children aged less than 16 years; orthostatic drop in diastolic blood pressure greater than or equal to 15 mm Hg from lying to sitting, orthostatic syncope, or orthostatic dizziness
Multisystem involvement (three or more of the following):
Gastrointestinal: vomiting or diarrhea at onset of illness
Muscular: severe myalgia or creatine phosphokinase level at least twice the upper limit of normal
Mucous membrane: vaginal, oropharyngeal, or conjunctival hyperemia
Renal: blood urea nitrogen or creatinine at least twice the upper limit of normal for laboratory or urinary sediment with pyuria (greater than or equal to 5 leukocytes per high-power field) in the absence of urinary tract infection
Hepatic: total bilirubin, serum glutamic-oxaloacetic transaminase, or serum glutamic-pyruvic transaminase at least twice the upper limit of normal for laboratory
Hematologic: platelets less than 100,000/mm^3
Central nervous system: disorientation or alterations in consciousness without focal neurologic signs when fever and hypotension are absent
Negative results on the following tests, if obtained:
Blood, throat, or cerebrospinal fluid cultures (blood culture may be positive for *S. aureus*)
Rise in titer to Rocky Mountain spotted fever, leptospirosis, or measles
Case classification
Probable: a case with five of the six clinical findings described previously here
Confirmed: a case with all six of the clinical findings described above, including desquamation, unless the patient dies before desquamation could occur

From Wharton M, Chorba TL, Vogt RL, et al. Case definitions for public health surveillance. *MMWR* 1990;39(RR-13):1–43.

I also received numerous calls from physicians in other states who had read or heard of our mailing and wanted to discuss suspect cases and send clinical specimens to the WSLH for processing. I reported confirmed cases of TSS to Kathy at the CDC, as did other state epidemiologists. National surveillance was initially established after a description of TSS and its recent occurrence in an *MMWR* article published on May 23, 1980.[8] Fifty-five cases had been reported to the CDC, including 31 cases from Wisconsin; 95% of cases occurred in women, and 95% of 40 women with known histories had onsets during menses. The case fatality rate was 13% among all cases, but it was 3.2% among the 31 cases in Wisconsin where surveillance had been heightened for more than 4 months and 25% among 24 cases occurring in other states. This difference can be explained in part by rapid dissemination of extensive clinical and epidemiologic information to a broad group of stakeholders who included physicians, infection control practitioners, public health partners, and the media. The letter to physicians was particularly important because it had detailed description of the illnesses and known risk factors, which facilitated rapid disease recognition, including recognition of milder cases. These materials also included detailed recommendations for patient management, which facilitated rapid and appropriate clinical management that in turn enhanced outcomes and reduced mortality.

After publication of this *MMWR* article, reporting of TSS continued to be voluntary and passive, and it was further heightened by media coverage, enthusiasm regarding a newly described condition, and concern regarding its severity. Indeed, the national media response to this *MMWR* article was intense. Shortly thereafter, a group of CDC-based EIS officers, including Kathy Shands, George Schmid, Bruce Dan, and Debbie Blum supervised by Dave Fraser (who previously directed the CDC's initial investigation of Legionnaires' disease) and John Bennett, officially became the CDC TSS Task Force. During ensuing months, they would be joined by many others.

THE INITIAL WISCONSIN CASE CONTROL STUDY AND CLINICAL AND LABORATORY FINDINGS

Facilitated by the strong response to our mailing and the reporting of cases that met criteria in our case definition, I planned and we (our epi team) conducted a case control study in Wisconsin during winter and early spring 1980. Each case patient was matched to three gynecology clinic patients as controls. These controls had to be not more than 2 years of age younger or older than their respective case patients and had to be nonpregnant at the time of survey administration. All participants were Wisconsin residents. Based on information from case reports and my phone conversations with case patients, their physicians, and Joan, I created a survey instrument. This survey was used to examine potential risk factors and host factors and hypotheses, including demographic features (marital status, other), characteristics of menstruation (flow duration and intensity), catamenial products (tampons, napkins, pads) used during menstruation (including type and brand, deodorant containing or not), exertion and its extent, birth control and contraceptive methods used, and presence of herpes infection. Because all patients, except for two, had TSS associated with menstruation, the survey was focused on menstrual TSS. In late spring, we balanced the concern about the need for a sufficiently large population to assess adequately differences in the use of commonly used products with the need for important information on risk factors of a serious widespread illness. I conducted a preliminary analysis of case control data to help inform discussions of menstrual TSS occurrence. At that time, nearly all women (30 of 31 [97%]) with confirmed menstrual TSS used tampons during every menstrual period compared with a significantly smaller proportion of controls (71 of 93 [76%], $P < 0.01$). This significant difference demonstrated the initial association of tampon use with menstrual TSS occurrence.

Our study inclusive of cases with onsets through June 30, 1980, was published in the *New England Journal of Medicine*.[5] Among 38 cases meeting our case definition, 37 occurred after January 1, 1979. Thirty seven occurred in women, and 35 case illnesses had onsets during menses. We found the median time from the onset of menses to the onset of illness was 3 days (mode, 2 days; range, 0 to 9 days). Among the women with nonmenstrual TSS, one was the premenarchal girl with *S. aureus* skin lesions on her heels, and the other was a patient who had undergone menopause 5 years earlier, was bleeding from a dilation and curettage procedure performed 10 days prior to onset, and was using tampons at the onset. One patient (2.6%) died. All case patients were white. Although the minority population proportion in Wisconsin was relatively small at the time, this complete absence of minorities among the case patients was a striking finding.[5]

We found that 34 of 35 case patients (97.1%) versus 80 of 105 controls (76.2%) used tampons during every menstrual period ($P < 0.01$) (Table 6-2), findings

TABLE 6-2 Results of a Case Control Study to Evaluate Potential Risk Factors for TSS Associated with Menses

Characteristic	Cases	Controls	Chi-Square*	P Value†
Number	35	105	—	—
Mean age (yr.)	24.1 ± 8.6	24.8 ± 8.0	—	NS‡
Married (no.)	12	51	3.06	NS
Menses				
Flow duration (days)	5.38 ± 1.3	5.18 ± 1.4	—	NS‡
Flow intensity (no. moderate)	22	74	0.65	NS
Birth control				
Using any method	9	64	11.70	< 0.001
Using oral contraceptives	6	38	3.58	0.05 < P < 0.10
Married only: use of any method	5/12	38/51	—	0.028§
Physical exertion pattern, moderate to active**	22	66	0.00	NS
Tampon or napkin use				
Case episode period vs control pattern††	34	80	7.56	< 0.01
Deodorant tampon use	7	32	1.53	NS
Napkin usage (case episodes vs. control pattern)	6	17	0.02	NS

* The Mantel-Haenszel method for multiple controls was used unless otherwise specified.
† NS, not significant.
‡ Statistical inference for two means, unpaired core.
§ Fisher's exact test.
** "Moderate to active" denotes that a person participates in at least two vigorous exercise activities per week.
†† Number of cases using tampons during the menstrual period associated with an episode of TSS versus number of controls who always use tampons during menstrual periods.
From Davis JP, Chesney PJ, Wand PJ, LaVenture M, Investigation and Laboratory Team. Toxic-shock syndrome: epidemiologic features, recurrence, risk factors and prevention. *N Engl J Med* 1980;303:1429–1435, Copyright ©1980 Massachusetts Medical Society. All rights reserved.

virtually identical to those noted in the preliminary analysis. Our analysis of tampon brand data did not implicate a specific brand. We also found the practice of contraception (any method) was protective (9 of 35 cases vs. 64 of 105 controls, $P < 0.001$), and this difference remained significant when the rates were adjusted for marital status. Additionally, fewer case patients used oral contraceptives (6 of 35 vs. 38 of 105 controls, $P < 0.10$), but no single method accounted for the difference. We waxed eloquently on the meaning of this finding in our discussion that included the difference in marital status (34% of case patients were married vs. 49% of controls). We also discussed the physiology of oral contraceptives but did not understand its role.[5]

Another important finding arose when I analyzed (the old-fashioned way, with calculator and pencil and paper) the clinical and laboratory data. Only 1 of 19 women who received beta-lactamase–resistant antibiotics (principally antistaphylococcal penicillins such as oxacillin, methicillin, and cloxacillin) during management of their first episode had recurrences of TSS within the ensuing 2 months compared with more than half (9 of 13) the women not receiving such antibiotics ($P = 0.0002$).[5] Similar findings were noted when the analysis involved treatment during any episode of TSS. Besides a means to prevent recurrences by encouraging the treatment of this condition with these beta-lactamase resistant antibiotics, this provided indirect evidence that staphylococci were involved in the etiology of TSS. More directly, however, 74% of 23 women tested before antibiotic treatment had *S. aureus* isolated from vaginal or cervical sites, far greater than rates of 0% to 17% cited in previously published colonization studies of healthy women.[5]

In addition to recommending treatment with beta-lactamase resistant antibiotics during the initial and recurrent episodes of TSS, we recommended that until the association of TSS was further clarified, the avoidance of tampon use for at least several menstrual cycles by women who had TSS was warranted. We recognized the need for a broader recommendation as well and advised that women who have not had TSS might reduce their probability of having an episode of TSS even further by minimizing their use of tampons.[5]

We also reported results of state and university laboratory testing of isolates of *S. aureus* from 15 patients with TSS (11 with cervical or vaginal isolates) that demonstrated 11 to be resistant to penicillin or ampicillin but sensitive to other antibiotics. Eleven were lysed by group I bacteriophages, including 10 lysed by phage 29, and 7 of 13 produced enterotoxins A or C, whereas 6 produced none of the known enterotoxins A–E.[5] These data indicated a unifying causative toxin had not yet been detected; however, more than half of these bacterial isolates produced enterotoxins that were already known to enhance susceptibility to lethal shock. I felt confident that Merlin and his laboratory team would soon isolate the causative toxin of TSS.

Parallel to our epidemiologic and laboratory investigations was a comprehensive examination of the clinical manifestations of TSS. Joan was the lead of this clinical investigation that involved a series of 22 cases of TSS among 22 women hospitalized in Madison during August 1977 through September 1980. This study provided an extraordinary compendium of the presence, emergence, and course of the many specific clinical features and laboratory alterations of TSS and an assessment of its clinical management.[9] During our TSS investigations, I was communicating almost daily with Joan regarding our findings, and virtually every conversation was marked with the observation of a new, previously unknown clinical or epidemiologic feature. Although we were working extraordinary hours for such a lengthy time and would expect to generate new information, we were amazed at the rapidity of the emergence of so much new information.

For example, before this outbreak, it had not been recognized that patients with TSS typically develop hypocalcemia (a low calcium level in their blood). Some of the other previously undescribed features of TSS noted in this study included hypophosphatemia, hyponatremia, hypocholesterolemia, lymphocytopenia, hypoferrinemia, vulvar cellulitis, and a disorder called telogen effluvium that is hair- and nail-loss occurring when the patient is convalescing.[9] These findings and associated data in the study were important to the development of the criteria in the TSS case definition. Members of our team and academic colleagues at the University of Wisconsin were also involved with a variety of associated specific studies focused on many of the clinical criteria noted in the TSS case definition.[10–12] All of the significant findings in our early studies, whether positive or negative, were valuable and lead to additional focused collaborative studies involving our epi team to understand further risk and host factors associated with TSS occurrence.

THE CDC CASE CONTROL STUDIES

In June 1980, the use of tampons as a risk factor for TSS was corroborated in a case control study (CDC-1) involving 52 cases and 52 age- and gender-matched acquaintance controls conducted by the CDC TSS Task Force and colleagues. This study did not include cases occurring in Wisconsin, Minnesota, or Utah, and it included only one case among those reported in the May *MMWR* article. All 50 case patients with onsets during menstruation used tampons compared to 86% of 50 controls.[13] Among other findings, the CDC study also showed no significant differences in tampon brand use, and 94% of 17 women with pretreatment specimens had vaginal cultures positive for *S. aureus*.

In a separate, smaller case control study conducted in Utah by Bob Latham, Mark Kehrberg, and colleagues, all 12 cases and 80% of 40 neighborhood-matched controls used tampons. A trend was demonstrated, but it was not statistically significant.[14]

Because of the common use of tampons among young women and the association of tampon use with TSS, the number of persons possibly at risk for TSS was huge. Thus, this was an extremely important public health issue. In late June, officials from each tampon manufacturer in the United States traveled to Atlanta to be advised of all case control study findings by CDC staff and me. An article presenting updated TSS surveillance data and findings of the CDC, Wisconsin, and Utah case control studies was published in the June 27, 1980, *MMWR*.[14] The article included recommendations that women who had menstrual TSS avoid tampon use for at least several menstrual cycles afterward, that beta-lactamase resistant antibiotics be administered during acute TSS episodes after appropriate specimens for culture were obtained, and that supportive therapy was important. Virtually immediately after this *MMWR* article was published, tampons became a household word, and menstruation became the topic of dinnertime conversation.

Intense investigation continued to reveal further the risk factors associated with TSS occurrence. In September 1980, Wally Schlech and many CDC colleagues conducted the second CDC case control study (CDC-2) that addressed concerns regarding study size, recall accuracy, friend controls, and dynamic changes in tampon products. CDC-2 corroborated earlier findings regarding tampon use as a menstrual TSS risk factor.[15] Cases occurred in association with multiple brands of tampons; however, among women who were exclusive users of a single tampon brand, significantly more case patients compared with age-matched acquaintance controls reported using Rely brand tampons. Rely tampons were a recently introduced and rather unconventional product that had rapidly been gaining market share. Of note, the early-phase rollout of this product in 1979 included Wisconsin. I recalled receiving free samples of Rely in the mail at my home on two occasions, which was unusual because I was single at the time.

The preliminary results of the CDC-2 were reported in the September 19 *MMWR*.[16] On September 22, Proctor and Gamble, the manufacturer of Rely, voluntarily withdrew the product from the market.

THE TRI-STATE CASE CONTROL STUDY

More pieces were soon fit into the puzzle. In August, Mike Osterholm in Minnesota, Vern Wintermeyer, the state epidemiologist in Iowa, and I, along with university and health department colleagues in each of our states, initiated a three-state collaborative comprehensive case control study of menses-associated and other potential TSS risk factors (the Tri-State TSS Study). Mike coordinated and brilliantly led this study. Mike and Bob Gibson and Jack Mandel (both faculty in the University of Minnesota system) were deft methodologists, and Bob rapidly generated complex computer-based analyses using a database incorporating data from the finely tuned 16-page study questionnaire and also proprietary tampon fluid capacity and chemical composition data for all brand styles of tampons in the marketplace through early September.[17] This was important because of the perplexing array of products within brand lines labeled as regular, super, and super plus (brand styles). The progression of such terms probably provided many women with relative knowledge about the absorbency of products within brand lines, but consumers had no precise or even relative information regarding absorbency of products across brand lines. For example, one brand's super could be more absorbent than another brand's super plus. The proprietary data were essential to sort this out. With the assistance of legal council, Mike worked with representatives of each of the tampon manufacturers to procure these data, and to their credit, the companies willingly provided it.

Eighty women with TSS with onsets before September 19, 1980, and 160 age- and gender-matched neighborhood controls were randomly selected. Interviews were conducted in person. We found the odds ratio for developing menstrual TSS with any tampon use compared with no tampon use was 18.0 ($P < 0.001$). We were fortunate that there were some non-tampon users in our study. When individual tampon brand use was compared with no tampon use, the brand-specific odds ratios were each significantly associated with TSS and ranged from 5.9 to 27. Similarly, odds ratios for individual brand style use compared with no tampon use were each significantly associated with TSS and ranged from 2.6 to 34.5.[17] In multivariate analysis, tampon fluid capacity (absorbency) and Rely brand tampon use were the only variables that significantly increased the relative risk of TSS; the risk associated with Rely was greater than that predicted by absorbency alone, suggesting that chemical composition of tampons was an important factor. We also found that significant risk factors for TSS recurrence were continued tampon use during menstrual periods after an episode of TSS and not receiving antistaphylococcal antibiotics during an initial episode of TSS. Among women with menstrual TSS, those having both of these risk factors had the greatest risk of recurrence. Those having neither factor had the least risk of recurrence, and those having either factor but not the other had an intermediate risk of recurrence.[18]

IMPACT OF THE CASE CONTROL STUDIES AND CONTROL MEASURES

Each of the studies cited used highly comparable TSS case definitions. Despite divergent methods, the association of menstrual TSS with tampon use was established in six different case control studies by late 1980: the two CDC studies[13,15] and four state-based studies (Wisconsin, Utah, Oregon, and the Tri-State Study).[5,16,17,19,20] The association with Rely use was established in four (CDC-2, Utah, Oregon, Tri-State Study).[16,17,19,20] In a review of these six TSS epidemiologic studies published in 1982, the author, Reuel Stallones, wrote this:[21]

> Early cases were predominantly in menstruating women, and the use of tampons was strongly associated with the onset of illness. Because of widespread publication of this finding, the case-comparison studies had problems due to differential ascertainment and recall bias. However, the number of cases among women was so great and the relation with tampon use so marked that unreasonable assumptions are necessary if the results are to be attributed to these biases. These studies show the power of epidemiologic methods, even given the unfavorable circumstance of an uncommon condition, associated with a common practice.

In October 1980, the Food and Drug Administration published a proposed regulation stipulating that all tampon manufacturers place TSS warnings on their packages.[22] The warnings initially appeared in 1982,[23] but based on data from the Tri-State TSS Study were later enhanced to include information on tampon absorbency as a TSS risk factor, that women use tampons with the minimum absorbency needed to control menstrual flow, and ultimately a scale to indicate the absorbency of the individual units. These warnings are still protecting women.

On December 18, just over 1 year after that initial call regarding three cases in Madison, final expanded reports of the Wisconsin and first CDC case control studies were published in the *New England Journal of Medicine*.[5,13] We included an estimate of TSS rates based on 81 cases reported in Wisconsin during a full year that ended September 30, 1980. Among women of menstrual age (ranging from 12 to 49 years old), TSS incidence rates among women under age 30 years were 3.3-fold greater than among women age 30 years and older. Peak rates of nearly 15 cases per 100,000 menstruating women per year in Wisconsin were noted among women 15 to 19 years old who were regular users of tampons (Figure 6-1).[5] These rates decreased dramatically after September 1980 and during 1981 in Wisconsin and nationwide in response to the clinical

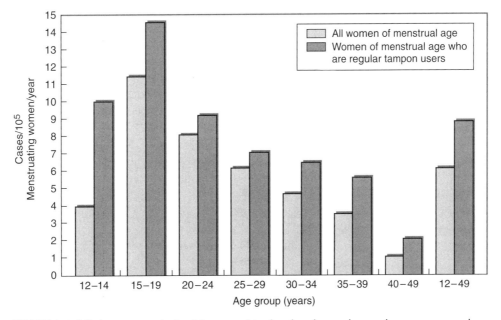

FIGURE 6-1 Minimum crude incidence of toxic-shock syndrome by age group in Wisconsin. From Davis JP, Chesney PJ, Wand PJ, LaVenture M, Investigation and Laboratory Team. Toxic-shock syndrome: Epidemiologic features, recurrence, risk factors and prevention (Fig 2). *N Engl J Med* 1980;303:1429–35, Copyright ©1980 Massachusetts Medical Society. All rights reserved.

management and product-related control measures and recommendations that were disseminated widely and rapidly to a nation captivated by this compelling episode in public health (Figure 6-2).[24,25]

The reported number of TSS cases that occurred in the United States during 1970 through June 15, 1983, was 2,204, among which 2,108 (95.6%) occurred in females and 90% of cases in women had onsets during menses (99% of those women were tampon users). There were over 100 reported deaths, and the case fatality rate decreased from 10% before 1980 to 5% in 1980 and 3% in 1981 and 1982.[24] In Wisconsin during 1972 through 1982, 221 confirmed and 51 probable reported cases of TSS occurred. Among these cases, 5 (1.8%) were fatal.[23]

Within 12 months, much of the TSS unknown had been successfully revealed, and by mid 1981, reports were published of the discovery of the etiologic agent of TSS independently in two laboratories. Merlin Bergdoll at the University of Wisconsin and colleagues isolated and described a new *Staphylococcus* enterotoxin, SEF, produced by isolates from patients with TSS.[26] Similarly, Pat Schlievert at the University of Minnesota and colleagues isolated and described a new pyrogenic exotoxin, PEC.[27] These investigators and others ultimately concurred these moieties were identical, and they renamed the toxin TSST-1.[28]

THE WISCONSIN TSS TEAM: CONTINUING INVESTIGATIONS AND PERSONAL REFLECTION

After these discoveries, the seroepidemiologic features of TSS were rapidly delineated. Merlin and his staff used the purified toxin to develop an assay (radioimmunoassay) for antibody to SEF (TSST-1).[26] The assay was then used to measure the anti-SEF (anti-TSST-1) antibody in the many banked pairs of serum from case patients and sera obtained from various categories of control subjects and from the extensive WSLH general serum bank. Our Wisconsin TSS team, that now also included Jim Vergeront and Susan Stolz, along with Joan, Phil, and Merlin's laboratory colleagues and I, examined SEF-related immune responses. These included the detection and measurement of the presence of antibody in longitudinal specimens obtained from patients with TSS and in sera from controls and the detection and seroprevalence of SEF antibody markers in representative stored sera from different age cohorts ranging from early infancy to old age and in sera collected from young adults in different geographic regions of the United States.[29–31]

I have not focused on nonmenstrual TSS in this chapter, but Art Reingold and colleagues published an early, definitive article on the TSS not associated with menstruation,[30] a condition with a wide range of risk fac-

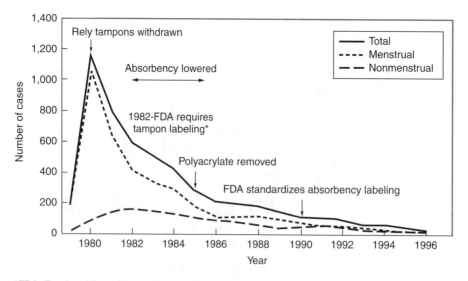

*FDA, Food and Drug Administration; includes definite and probable toxic shock syndrome cases

FIGURE 6-2 Toxic shock syndrome cases, menstrual vs. nonmenstrual, United States by year, 1979–1996. Years of important federal and voluntary measures are indicated [39].

tors that did not decrease substantially in occurrence during the early 1980s.

The intense, sustained investigation of TSS, particularly during December 1979 through December 1980, was exhilarating, challenging, and humbling. It was also exhausting. The number of work hours devoted to our TSS-related studies was immense, and they accrued in parallel to my other duties as state epidemiologist including many investigations of other diseases that were reportable or newly emerging in Wisconsin. I experienced unanticipated intervals of tampon burnout, but I learned more about tampons in 1 year than I ever expected to know during a lifetime. The experience stimulated a sustained TSS-related investigative activity involving our TSS team and clinical and laboratory colleagues that, in addition to continuing to address TSST-1 related immune responses and seroepidemiologic features of TSS, also examined clinical outcomes and sequelae of TSS, epidemiologic trends and TSS surveillance methods, and other issues.[33–38] Most of all, the experience of investigating the many aspects of TSS during the initial year and the years that followed has provided me with a valued network of colleagues for which I am very grateful.

> *I experienced unanticipated intervals of tampon burnout, but I learned more about tampons in 1 year than I ever expected to know during a lifetime.*

REFERENCES

1. Band J, LaVenture M, Davis JP, et al. Epidemic Legionnaire's disease: airborne transmission down a chimney. *JAMA* 1981;245:2404–2407.
2. Dryer RF, Goellner PG, Carney AS. Lyme arthritis in Wisconsin. *JAMA* 1979;241:498–499.
3. Davis JP, Schell WL, Amundson TE, et al. Lyme disease in Wisconsin: epidemiologic, clinical, serologic and entomologic findings. *Yale J Biol Med* 1984;57:685–696.
4. Todd JK, Fishaut M, Kapral F, Welch T. Toxic-shock syndrome associated with phage-group-1 staphylococci. *Lancet* 1978;2:1116–1118.
5. Davis JP, Chesney PJ, Wand PJ, LaVenture M, Investigation and Laboratory Team. Toxic-shock syndrome: epidemiologic features, recurrence, risk factors and prevention. *N Engl J Med* 1980;303:1429–1435.
6. Osterholm MT, Gibson RW, Mandel JS, Davis JP. Tri-State Toxic Shock Syndrome Study: methodologic analysis. *Ann Intern Med* 1982;96(Pt 2):899–902.
7. Wharton M., Chorba TL, Vogt RL, et al. Case definitions for public health surveillance. *MMWR* 1990;39(RR-13):1–43.
8. Toxic-shock syndrome—United States. *MMWR* 1980;29:229–230.
9. Chesney PJ, Davis JP, Purdy WK, Wand PJ, Chesney RW. Clinical manifestations of toxic-shock syndrome. *JAMA* 1981;246:741–748.
10. Gourley GR, Chesney PJ, Davis JP, Odell GR. Acute cholestasis in patients with the toxic-shock syndrome. *Gastroenterology* 1981;81:928–931.
11. Chesney RW, Chesney PJ, Davis JP, Segar WE. Renal manifestations of the staphylococcal toxic-shock syndrome. *Am J Med* 1981;71:583–588.
12. Chesney TW, McCarron DM, Haddad JG, et al. Pathogenic mechanisms of the hypocalcemia of the staphylococcal toxic-shock syndrome. *J Lab Clin Med* 1983;101:576–585.
13. Shands KN, Schmid GP, Dan BB, et al. Toxic-shock syndrome in menstruating women: association with tampon use and *Staphylococcus aureus* and clinical features in 52 cases. *N Engl J Med* 1980;303:1436–1442.
14. Follow-up on toxic-shock syndrome—United States. *MMWR* 1980;29:297–299.
15. Schlech WF III, Shands KN, Reingold AL, et al. Risk factors for development of toxic shock syndrome: association with a tampon brand. *JAMA* 1982;7:835–839.
16. Follow-up on toxic-shock syndrome. *MMWR* 1980;29:441–445.
17. Osterholm MT, Davis JP, Gibson RW, et al. Tri-State Toxic-Shock Syndrome Study. I. Epidemiologic findings. *J Infect Dis* 1982;145:431–440.
18. Davis JP, Osterholm MT, Helms CM, et al. Tri-State Toxic-Shock Syndrome Study. II. Clinical and laboratory findings. *J Infect Dis* 1982;145:441–448.
19. Latham RH, Kehrberg MW, Jacobson JA, Smith CB. Toxic shock syndrome in Utah: a case-control and surveillance study. *Ann Intern Med* 1982;96(Pt 2):906–908.
20. Helgerson SD. Toxic shock syndrome in Oregon: epidemiologic findings. *Ann Intern Med* 1982;96(Pt 2):909–911.
21. Stallones RA. A review of epidemiologic studies of toxic shock syndrome. *Ann Intern Med* 1982;96(Pt 2):917–920.
22. Food and Drug Administration. Update on toxic shock syndrome. *FDA Drug Bull* 1980;10:17–19.
23. Food and Drug Administration. Tampon packages carry TSS information. *FDA Drug Bull* 1982;12:19–20.
24. Update: toxic-shock syndrome—United States. *MMWR* 1983;32:398–400.
25. Toxic-shock syndrome in Wisconsin. *Wisc Epidemiol Bull* 1983;5:1–2, 5.
26. Bergdoll MS, Crass BA, Reiser RF, Robbins RN, Davis JP. A new staphylococcal enterotoxin, enterotoxin F, associated with toxic-shock syndrome Staphylococcus aureus isolates. *Lancet* 1981;1:1017–1021.
27. Schlievert PM, Shands KN, Dan BB, Schmid GP, Nishimura RD. Identification and characterization of exotoxin from *Staphylococcus aureus* associated with toxic shock syndrome. *J Infect Dis* 1981;143:509–516.
28. Bergdoll MS, Schlievert PM. Toxic shock syndrome toxin. *Lancet* 1984;2:691.

29. Vergeront JM, Stolz SJ, Crass BA, Nelson DB, Davis JP, Bergdoll MS. Seroprevalence of antibody to staphylococcal enterotoxin F among Wisconsin residents: implications for toxic-shock syndrome. *J Infect Dis* 1983;148:692–698.
30. Stolz SJ, Davis JP, Vergeront JM, Crass BA, Chesney PJ, Wand PJ, Bergdoll MS. Development of serum antibody to toxic-shock toxin among individuals with toxic-shock syndrome in Wisconsin. *J Infect Dis* 1985;151:883–889.
31. Vergeront JM, Blouse SE, Crass BA, Stolz SJ, Bergdoll MS, Davis JP. Regional differences in the prevalence of serum antibody to toxic-shock toxin (anti-TST). *Twenty-fourth Interscience Conference on Antimicrobial Agents and Chemotherapy*, Washington DC, October 1984; Abst. 610.
32. Reingold AL, Dan BB, Shands KN, Broome CV. Toxic-shock syndrome not associated with menstruation: a review of 54 cases. *Lancet* 1982;2:1–4.
33. Davis JP, Vergeront JM, Amsterdam LE, Hayward J, Stolz-LaVerriere SJ. Long-term effects of toxic shock syndrome in women: sequelae, subsequent pregnancy, menstrual history and long-term trends in catamenial product use. *Rev Infect Dis* 1989;11(Suppl 1):550–551.
34. Vergeront JM, Evenson ML, Crass BA, et al. Recovery of staphylococcal enterotoxin F from the breast milk of a woman with toxic-shock syndrome. *J Infect Dis* 1982;146:456–459.
35. Chesney PJ, Davis JP, Chesney RW. Factors determining severity of the toxic-shock syndrome (TSS). *Pediatr Res* 1981;15:440.
36. Chesney PJ, Davis JP. Toxic shock syndrome. In Feigen RD, Cherry JD, Demmler GJ, Kaplan SL, eds. *Textbook of Pediatric Infectious Diseases*, 5th ed. Philadelphia: Saunders, 2003:836–859.
37. Davis JP, Vergeront JM. The effect of publicity on the reporting of toxic-shock syndrome. *J Infect Dis* 1982;145:449–457.
38. Hayward J, Vergeront JM, Stolz SJ, Bohn MJ, Davis JP. A hospital discharge code review of toxic-shock syndrome in Wisconsin. *Am J Epidemiol* 1986;123:876–883.
39. Hajjeh RA, Reingold A, Weil A, Shutt K, Schuchat A, Perkins BA. Toxic shock syndrome in the United States: surveillance update, 1979–1996. *Emerg Infect Dis* 1999;5:807–810.

LEARNING QUESTIONS

1. Verifying that an outbreak is truly occurring is an early step of outbreak investigation. Investigators often rely on reviewing surveillance data to determine if the number of cases suspected of causing an outbreak is actually greater than that expected. In the case of toxic shock syndrome there was no surveillance system at this time. How did the author attempt to perform this verifying step?
2. The mortality rate for toxic shock syndrome was only 3.2% in Wisconsin but elsewhere it was 25%. What may have accounted for such a large difference in these mortality rates?
3. There are many benefits of outbreak investigation. Make a list of the benefits of the performance of this outbreak investigation.

CHAPTER 7

The Early Days of AIDS in the United States: A Personal Perspective

Harold W. Jaffe, MD, MA, FFPH
United States, 1980s

INTRODUCTION

In the spring of 1981, I was working as an Epidemic Intelligence Service (EIS) officer in the Venereal Disease Control Division at the Centers for Disease Control (CDC) in Atlanta. My stint in EIS was rather atypical in that I had first come to the CDC in 1974, fresh out of internal medicine training. I stayed for 3 years but left when I had the opportunity to do an infectious diseases fellowship. Soon after I returned to the CDC in 1980, the newly elected Reagan Administration decided to reduce the federal workforce, including CDC staff. Fortunately, the EIS was considered, as a training program, exempt from the cuts, and thus, serving in EIS kept me employed!

It was a bit strange to be working on infectious diseases at a time when the public health community seemed to feel that many of the problems posed by infectious diseases had been solved, at least in the developed world. We had vaccines for most of the childhood infections and a broad range of antibiotics available to treat bacterial and even some viral diseases. I recall hearing a lecture by Dr. Robert Petersdorf, a very eminent infectious diseases physician from the University of Washington, in which he argued that the demand for infectious diseases specialists was likely to diminish.

At the same time, however, our group at the CDC was busy studying the newly emerging problem of penicillin-resistant gonorrhea and the increasing rates of syphilis in men who had sex with men (MSM). During my time as an infectious diseases fellow in Chicago, I had "moonlighted" at a sexually transmitted diseases (STD) clinic caring for MSM and had treated many of them for gonorrhea and syphilis. Unfortunately, the era of infectious diseases was not over for them. Thus, when I saw the first report of a strange illness occurring in MSM in Los Angeles, I was more than a little interested.

> *It was a bit strange to be working on infectious diseases at a time when the public health community seemed to feel that many of the problems posed by infectious diseases had been solved, at least in the developed world.*

THE BEGINNING

The report had come to CDC's Division of Parasitic Disease from Dr. Wayne Shandera, an EIS officer assigned to the Los Angeles County Health Department. Wayne had received reports from Dr. Michael Gottlieb, an immunologist at UCLA Hospital, and from several other Los Angeles physicians who had seen young MSM with *Pneumocystis carinii* pneumonia (PCP). These cases were highly unusual because PCP typically occurred in adults with a known cause of immune suppression, such as the receipt of cancer chemotherapy or drugs to prevent rejection of a transplanted organ, but none of these men had these predisposing risk factors.

The first report of these cases, which appeared in the CDC's *Morbidity and Mortality Weekly Report* (*MMWR*) on June 5, 1981,[1] raised a series of questions. First, was this really a new disease, or had similar cases occurred in the past without being reported? Second, were cases being seen elsewhere? Third, were other unusual diseases also occurring in MSM, and fourth, why were the cases occurring in MSM? These questions led to fundamental epidemiologic steps that are essential as one begins to investigate a possible outbreak. Verify whether there really is a new outbreak or an outbreak at all. Determine the extent of the problem by searching for additional cases within and outside of the area of the initial report. More thoroughly examine the problem through case investigation, and consider performing a risk factor analysis to identify whether information can be learned that could create a prevention strategy to decrease the extent of or terminate the outbreak.

To answer the first question, the CDC turned to its Parasitic Disease Drug Service, which supplied American physicians with medications to treat unusual parasitic infections. (At the time, *Pneumocystis carinii*, was considered to be a parasite; more recently, it has been reclassified as a fungal species, *P. jiroveci*) The only drug available to treat PCP in 1981 was pentamidine isethionate. A record review revealed that almost all previous pentamidine requests had been for persons with an obvious cause of immune suppression. Beginning in the second half of 1980, however, a few requests had been received for persons fitting the profile of the Los Angeles cases.[2] Thus, the disease might have begun a bit earlier than 1981, but not much earlier.

The answers to questions two and three came soon after the report from Los Angeles. MSM with PCP were also being seen in San Francisco and New York City. Some of these men were developing other severe infections typically seen only in immunosuppressed persons (called opportunistic infections, or OIs). At a meeting I attended in San Diego soon after publication of the Los Angeles report, I also heard that MSM in San Francisco were developing a very unusual skin cancer, Kaposi's sarcoma (KS), a disease typically seen in older men and organ transplant recipients. I was so worried that I would forget the strange name of the disease that I wrote it on a slip of paper and put it in my wallet so that I could discuss it when I returned to Atlanta. For lack of a better name, we began referring to this new disease as "KS/OI." Why it was occurring in MSM remained a mystery.

EARLY INVESTIGATIONS

Whatever this new disease might be, it did not fit neatly into any of the CDC's organizational units, and thus, a "KS/OI Task Force" was set up under the direction of Dr. James Curran. Because there seemed to be so many aspects to KS/OI, the membership of the Task Force was very diverse and included experts in cancer epidemiology, parasitology, virology, immunology, and STDs. I was asked to join the group because of my experience in working with MSM and was happy to do so. Our initial Task Force meetings included perhaps a dozen people and were mainly brainstorming sessions about what might be going on; however, we all agreed that we needed to begin national surveillance for KS/OI and for that we needed a case definition (Exhibit 7-1). We distributed the case definition to health departments and major teaching hospitals. By the end of August 1981, over 100 cases meeting the definition had been reported. (Subsequently, the CDC began funding health departments, starting with New York City, to establish systematic hospital-based surveillance, a program that remains in place today.)

EXHIBIT 7-1 Case Definition of KS/OI (1981)

- Biopsy-proven KS and/or biopsy- or culture-proven life-threatening opportunistic infections
- Previously healthy persons less than 60 years of age
- Patients excluded with conditions known to cause immunosuppression such as congenital immunodeficiency, lymphoreticular malignancy, and therapy with immunosuppressive agents

> *Physicians seeing cases at one hospital were often unaware that similar patients were being seen at other hospitals in the same city.*

It was apparent, however, that little information sharing about cases was occurring at the local level. Physicians seeing cases at one hospital were often unaware that similar patients were being seen at other hospitals in the same city. In New York City, Dr. David Sencer, the former CDC director and now the New York City Health Commissioner, recognized the problem. To break down these communication barriers, he established monthly meetings at the health department, at which clinicians from all of the major New York City hospitals would come to discuss their cases and hear updates from health department staff.

At this point, we thought it would be important for the physicians on the Task Force to see persons with KS/OI, both to appreciate the clinical presentation of the disease and to start developing an epidemiologic profile of these patients. I was asked to go to San Francisco, and I spent several days talking to patients cared for at University of California, San Francisco. I was struck by how sick these young men were. They had lost large amounts of weight. Those with PCP were on ventilators in intensive care units, and those with KS were covered with purplish lesions (Figure 7-1). In speaking with the men who were able to talk, it became apparent that they were highly sexually active and had used a variety of recreational drugs.

When we gathered again in Atlanta to discuss what we had seen, the profiles of KS/OI patients sounded very similar, whether they were from California or New York. Thus, we again asked ourselves our fourth question, "Why MSM?" Two ideas seemed most plausible. First, we might be dealing with a new STD. Rates of other STDs had been dramatically increasing in MSM, and the men we had interviewed had been very sexually active. The second hypothesis involved an environmental exposure, perhaps to street drugs or an exposure in gay bath houses. I hoped the second hypothesis was right because it would certainly be easier to eliminate something from the environment of MSM than to control a new STD.

Regarding the environmental hypothesis, we were particularly interested in nitrite inhalants or "poppers," whose use to enhance sex was thought to be especially common in MSM. To look at this possibility in more detail, Dr. Bill Darrow, a CDC research sociologist, and I made a visit to the Club Baths, a gay bath house in Atlanta. With the permission of the manager, we interviewed customers about their use of poppers. (We were rather obvious, as we were the only ones wearing clothes!) Although the customers had no particular reason to trust us, most were very willing to sit down and talk for a few minutes. We found out that popper use was almost universal and that poppers could be purchased in bath houses and other gay venues in bottles with names such as "Rush" or "Bolt." In fact, our visit coincided with "Popper Night," with a 50-cent discount offered on each bottle. We subsequently learned that poppers could also be bought in gay bars and bookstores in unlabeled bottles. To find out what was in these bottles, we purchased them in several cities and brought them back to Atlanta for chemical analysis. (My wife was not amused to find them stored in our home refrigerator!) We thought we might find some sort of contaminant, but the bottles contained butyl and isobutyl nitrite, chemicals not associated with immunosuppression.

By the end of the summer of 1981, the Task Force decided to do a case control study of KS/OI. The study would examine a wide range of possible causes but would focus on infectious and environmental risk factors. Because of the sensitive nature of the questions, we decided to conduct all of the interviews in person. The cases would be MSM with PCP and/or KS, but the selection of control patients was more problematic. We thought these persons should be apparently healthy MSM matched to the cases within an age range and by race and city of residence. How should we select them? After much debate within the Task Force, we decided to recruit three MSM control groups and separately analyze our case data in comparison to data from each of

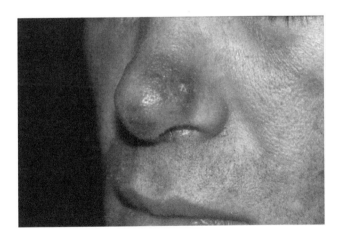

FIGURE 7-1 Kaposis' sarcoma on the nose of a patient with **AIDS**. Courtesy of David Hines, MD, not from the early 1980's.

the control groups: persons attending public STD clinics, persons cared for by private physicians with predominately MSM practices, and friends of cases who had not been their sexual partners. It was very telling that many of the case patients could not name an MSM friend who hadn't been a sex partner.

To do the interviews, we sent teams to Los Angeles, San Francisco, and New York. Being originally from Los Angeles, I was put on the California team. Although the men we interviewed could have had many reasons to distrust us, I was very impressed by how open they were in discussing the most intimate details of their lives. I think this was likely the result of fear in the MSM community, where increasing numbers of men were sick or dying. We did the interviews in our hotel rooms, creating much puzzlement among the desk clerks who must have wondered why all these young men were asking to see us. Taking no particular precautions (we did not wear gloves), we also drew blood from these men in our rooms. In retrospect, we were very foolish, although this was an accepted practice in medical facilities at the time.

The analysis of the case control study indicated that KS/OI was most strongly associated with having a large number of male sex partners.[3] For example, case patients had a median of 61 partners per year as compared with 27 partners for the control patients from STD clinics. This was an especially striking difference given that the STD clinic patients would be expected to be highly sexually active. Although we felt the findings were most consistent with a sexually transmitted cause of KS/OI, we could not entirely exclude the environmental hypothesis because sex and drug use were highly associated in this population.

The epidemiologic proof of a sexually transmitted cause of KS/OI did not come until the spring of 1982. Dr. David Auerbach, the EIS officer who had taken over for Wayne Shandera in Los Angeles, called me to say that he had heard through contacts in the MSM community that some of the men with KS/OI had been sexual partners. He wanted to interview the men to confirm these rumors but had never done this sort of interviewing and needed help. Thus, we sent Bill Darrow to work with him. In just a few days, Darrow and Auerbach were able to confirm the sexual links between these cases. Furthermore, they found that four men with KS/OI in Southern California had sex with a French-Canadian flight attendant who himself had developed KS. This flight attendant, referred to in a published report as Patient O, could also be linked to four other KS/OI patients in New York. As the investigation expanded, a total of 40 patients living in 10 North American cities could be linked by sexual contact.[4] When reported in the popular press, Patient O was described as the "source" of the North American epidemic. Although this was a misinterpretation of the study findings, it did seem likely that a small number of men who were both highly mobile and very sexually active, like Patient O, could have quickly spread the disease among MSM.

AN EXPANDING PROBLEM

By the summer of 1982, more pieces were being added to the KS/OI puzzle. The clinical spectrum of illness began to expand to conditions beyond those initially identified. For example, reports of generalized lymph node enlargements among homosexual men suggested that this condition might be a precursor of KS/OI. Some homosexual men were also reported with unusual forms of non-Hodgkin's lymphoma.

The groups of persons developing KS/OI also expanded beyond the homosexual men initially reported. By June 1982, 13 of the 355 reported KS/OI cases were in women, more than half of whom had used intravenous (IV) drugs. Haitians residing in the United States, particularly in Miami, Florida and Brooklyn, New York, were reported with KS/OI. Almost all of the Haitians were young men; those interviewed all denied homosexual activity. Finally, three heterosexual men with hemophilia A were reported with PCP. All had received Factor VIII concentrate, a blood product used to treat their coagulation disorder.

The early winter of 1982–1983 proved to be a pivotal time in the investigations of what by then was called AIDS (acquired immune deficiency syndrome). The case total in the United States was approaching 800, with a mortality rate of about 40%. Although cases were still concentrated in New York City, San Francisco, Los Angeles, Newark, and Miami, other cities were beginning to report cases. The first key event of this period was the December 10, 1982, *MMWR* publication of a possible case of transfusion-associated AIDS.[5] Dr. Arthur Ammann, a pediatric immunologist at University of California, San Francisco, was caring for a 20-month old infant with unexplained severe immunodeficiency. Although AIDS had not been previously described in children, the features of this child's illness more closely resembled AIDS than other forms of pediatric immunodeficiency. The child had received multiple transfusions shortly after birth to treat erythroblastosis fetalis (a condition that results from a blood group incompatibility between mother and fetus). Investigation of the blood donors by the San Francisco Department of Public Health revealed that 1 of the 19 donors was a man who developed AIDS 9 months after donation. Although initially reported with no known risk factors, subsequent investigation by David Auerbach determined that the donor was a homosexual man.

Only a week later, the *MMWR* reported four other infants with unexplained immunodeficiency.[6] These infants, born in New York City, Newark, and San Francisco, had not received transfusions. Two of the infants had Haitian mothers, whose health status was unknown. The mothers of the other two infants reported IV drug use; one of these mothers died of AIDS, whereas the other had early signs of the disease.

Finally, in early January 1983, the CDC published a report from New York City of two women who had each developed immunodeficiency after repeated sexual contact with a man who had AIDS.[7] One of these men was an IV drug user, whereas the other was bisexual. Neither woman had any other known risk factor for the disease.

Taken together, these three reports plus the "Patient O" investigation strongly suggested an infectious cause of AIDS. Evidence from case ascertainment and analysis of descriptive epidemiologic data supported that the putative agent could be transmitted through sexual contact, either homosexual or heterosexual, from mother to child, and through blood and blood products. Furthermore, the source of transmission could be a person who had not yet developed the disease, implying that the agent could be carried asymptomatically.

In addition to the epidemiologic importance of these reports, they also had a major impact on the media's interest in AIDS and the public perception of the disease. Until this time, the mainstream media paid relatively little attention to AIDS; most of the coverage had been in the gay press. With these new reports, however, AIDS could no longer be regarded as simply "the gay plague." Suddenly, Americans realized that transfusion could put them at risk. My own wife refused to sign a hospital consent form to allow transfusions to be given to her during the birth of our first child unless either she or I agreed that they were absolutely necessary. Infants with the disease, portrayed as "innocent victims," gave special poignancy to the story. I remember seeing camera crews and reporters from all of the major television networks lining up to do interviews with CDC staff to meet the sudden demand for news about AIDS. Although I was glad that the mainstream media was finally paying attention, I wondered why it had taken them so long.

Unfortunately, while the problem was increasing, resources were not. The Task Force continued to operate without a clear organizational home within the CDC. Many of our staff had been "detailed" from other programs. With no specific appropriations forthcoming from Washington, the money to support our work came from funds that had been appropriated for other purposes, particularly STD control.

The lack of interest from the administration was exemplified by an October 1982 press briefing when President Reagan's press secretary, Larry Speakes, was asked whether the President was aware of the growing AIDS epidemic. His first response was "what's AIDS?" When told that it was affecting gay men, Speakes replied, "I don't have it. Do you?"[8] The President himself made no public remarks about AIDS until 1987.

AIDS AND THE BLOOD SUPPLY

The growing concern about the safety of the blood supply gave rise to an important meeting held at the CDC in January 1983. From our perspective at the CDC, the purpose of the meeting with the U.S. Food and Drug Administration, the National Hemophilia Foundation, blood banking organizations, and groups representing MSM was to describe the occurrence of AIDS in transfusion recipients and persons with hemophilia and then discuss potential prevention measures. Prevention options included excluding blood donation from persons known to be at risk for AIDS (such as MSM) or those with laboratory findings known to correlate with AIDS risk (such as a positive hepatitis B antibody test).

As well described by Randy Shilts in his book *And the Band Played On*, the meeting quickly became a contentious debate rather than a constructive discussion.[9] Although the CDC presented a series of cases thought to be AIDS resulting from receipt of blood or blood products, the representatives of the blood banks and hemophilia treatment community said they were not convinced that the disease was AIDS and were unwilling to accept our evidence that the "AIDS agent" was contaminating the blood supply. At one point in the meeting, Dr. Donald Armstrong, Chief of Infectious Diseases at Memorial Sloan-Kettering Cancer Center in NYC, stood up to say that he could hardly believe these comments. In his mind, there was no question that

> *Until this time, the mainstream media paid relatively little attention to AIDS; most of the coverage had been in the gay press*

these were AIDS cases and that something needed to be done, but the other participants simply ignored him.

The other participants also rejected the concept of using a "surrogate," such as the hepatitis B antibody test, to exclude potential donors. In part, this may have represented a legitimate concern about the possibility of creating a blood shortage. In my view, however, much of the discussion simply reflected denial. The blood-banking and hemophilia treatment communities were unwilling to accept the notion that blood and blood products, seen by them as lifesaving, could be transmitting a lethal infection. This decision would later cost millions of dollars in lawsuits. Similar sorts of decisions were made in France in 1985 that resulted in the 1992 imprisonment of officials judged to be responsible.[10]

Needless to say, CDC staff members were very disheartened by the outcome of this meeting. We felt that we had made a convincing case, but the case had been rejected. Fortunately, private discussions held over the next few months proved to be more productive, and in March 1983, the U.S. Public Health Service published the first comprehensive set of recommendations for the prevention of AIDS.[11] The recommendations noted that "available data suggest that the severe disorder of immune regulation underlying AIDS is caused by a transmissible agent." Although no test existed to detect this agent, those at highest risk were noted to be those with symptoms or signs suggestive of AIDS, the sexual partners of AIDS patients, sexually active MSM with multiple partners, Haitian entrants to the United States, past or present IV drugs users, patients with hemophilia, and sexual partners of persons at increased risk for AIDS. The publication then went on to recommend avoiding having sexual contact with persons known or suspected to have AIDS and noted that having multiple sexual partners increased the risk of AIDS. Furthermore, as a "temporary" measure, members of these risk groups were advised not to donate plasma or blood. These recommendations were derived from the epidemiologic data available at the time. In the absence of a screening test for the transmissible agent, this was a rational strategy for decreasing the risk of AIDS transmission though blood and blood products.

Several features of the recommendations might strike contemporary readers as puzzling. First, why not restrict all MSM from blood donation rather than only those with "multiple sexual partners" (a term not further defined)? This recommendation represented a compromise between public health officials, who wanted a wider prohibition, and gay rights advocates, who wanted the prohibition to be as narrow as possible. Because the risk of AIDS correlated with the number of sexual partners, the "multiple partners" language was seen as an acceptable compromise. Second, why were all Haitian Americans excluded from donation when relatively few seemed to be at risk for the disease? Here the problem was that no particular behaviors had been shown to correlate with AIDS risk, and thus, the donation restriction could not be limited to a specific subgroup of Haitians. Undoubtedly, this decision resulted in unwarranted discrimination against Haitians living in the United States. Even in retrospect, however, I think this was the correct public health decision at the time. With the subsequent availability of tests to screen donated blood for HIV, the restriction on Haitians was eventually lifted but remains in effect for MSM and injection drug users.

Putting these controversies aside, I think the most remarkable aspect of the recommendations was that they were essentially correct, even though the cause of AIDS had not yet been discovered. It was not until May 1983 that Luc Montagnier and his associates at the Institute Pasteur in Paris identified a novel retrovirus in the lymph node of a homosexual man.[12] Another year then passed before Robert Gallo and his associates at the U.S. National Institutes of Health could prove that the virus, called HTLV-III by his laboratory, was the cause of AIDS.[13] Thus, the investigations done by the CDC Task Force and many others showed the power of the epidemiologic method to establish the likely transmission routes of a new infectious agent, as well as to develop basic prevention recommendations, before the identity of the agent was known. Furthermore, those investigations helped focus the work of the laboratory scientists who were trying to find the agent.

Unfortunately, the AIDS epidemic did not stop with the identification of the causative agent. Despite the release of the recommendations intended to help prevent further cases of AIDS in the March 1983 *MMWR*, case counts continued to rise. There were many factors that kept these recommendations from being as immediately useful as the removal of the pump handle by John Snow during the 19th century London cholera outbreak. It would be later learned that the virus had a long latency period from infection to AIDS such that these recommendations were too late for many persons who had acquired the virus weeks, months, or years earlier. Much remained and still remains to be learned about how to change human sexual behavior to prevent disease transmission. Almost a million Americans have been reported with AIDS since 1981, and almost 40 million persons are now living with HIV/AIDS worldwide.

CONCLUSIONS

I've often been asked what it was like to be one of the early AIDS investigators. To me, at least, it all began as a medical mystery, just like many other outbreak investigations. I was caught up in being a "medical detective" without much thought of the broader significance of what we were investigating. Perhaps some of my colleagues were astute enough to have seen the future, but I wasn't. As time went on, however, I gradually began to see that what we were studying was something much bigger than I had imagined. Once it was clear that the disease was sexually transmitted, we knew that the disease would not be limited to MSM. After we knew that the agent was in the blood supply, we knew many more people were at risk. The medical mystery would soon become the global pandemic.

ACKNOWLEDGMENT

An adaptation of this chapter was printed in the following: Jaffe HW. The early days of the HIV-AIDS epidemic in the USA. *Nat Immunol* 2008;9:1201–1203.

REFERENCES

1. CDC. *Pneumocystis* pneumonia—Los Angeles. *MMWR* 1981;30:250–252.
2. Centers for Disease Control Task Force on Kaposi's Sarcoma and Opportunistic Infections. Epidemiologic aspects of the current outbreak of Kaposi's sarcoma and opportunistic infections. *N Engl J Med* 1982;306:248–252.
3. Jaffe HW, Choi K, Thomas PA, et al. National case-control study of Kaposi's sarcoma and *Pneumocystis carinii* pneumonia in homosexual men: part 1, epidemiologic results. *Ann Intern Med* 1983;99:145–151.
4. Auerbach DM, Darrow WW, Jaffe HW, Curran JW. Cluster of cases of the acquired immune deficiency syndrome: patients linked by sexual contact. *Am J Med* 1984;76:487–492.
5. CDC. Possible transfusion-associated acquired immune deficiency syndrome (AIDS)—California. *MMWR* 1982;31:652–654.
6. CDC. Unexplained immunodeficiency and opportunistic infections in infants—New York, New Jersey, California. *MMWR* 1982;31:665–667.
7. CDC. Immunodeficiency among female sexual partners of males with acquired immune deficiency syndrome (AIDS). *MMWR* 1983;31:697–698.
8. The White House. Office of the Press Secretary. Press briefing by Larry Speakes, October 15, 1982. http://findarticles.com/p/articles/mi_m0HSW/is_401/ai_n6078340.
9. Shilts R. *And the Band Played on. Politics, People, and the AIDS Epidemic.* New York: St. Martin's Press, 1987.
10. Weiberg PD, Hounshell J, Sherman LA, et al. Legal, financial, and public health consequences of HIV contamination of blood and blood products in the 1980s and 1990s. *Ann Intern Med* 2002;136:312–319.
11. CDC. Prevention of acquired immune deficiency syndrome (AIDS): report of inter-agency recommendations. *MMWR* 1983;32:101–104.
12. Barre-Sinoussi F, Cherman J-C, Rey F, et al. Isolation of a T-lymphotropic retrovirus from a patient at risk for acquired immune deficiency syndrome (AIDS). *Science* 1983;220:868–671.
13. Gallo RC, Salahuddin SZ, Popovic M, et al. Frequent detection and isolation of cytopathic retroviruses (HTLV-III) from patients with AIDS and at risk for AIDS. *Science* 1984;224:500–503.

LEARNING QUESTIONS

1. What were the initial four questions the investigation needed answered early on in the AIDS outbreak and how did they go about answering them?
2. Consider the controversy of the early recommendation that all men who have sex with men refrain from blood donation rather than just men who have sex with men with "multiple sexual partners" (a term left undefined). Do you agree or disagree with this early recommendation in the context of what was and was not understood about AIDS in the early 1980s? If a new condition emerged today (one like AIDS) that appeared to be infectious and could be transferred by blood transfusion but for which no test had yet been created to allow for blood donor screening, and if this condition emerged primarily in a subpopulation and had a 75% 1-year mortality in children with hemophilia, would you support or oppose a policy of excluding that subpopulation from blood donation? Consider the implications of such a policy and consider several different subpopulations.

CHAPTER 8

Verify the Diagnosis: A Pseudo-Outbreak of Amebiasis in Los Angeles County

Frank Sorvillo, PhD

Los Angeles, 1983

INTRODUCTION

Struggling through the laboratory section of Larry Ash's notorious course "Protozoal Diseases of Humans" in the spring of 1978 as part of my master's in public health curriculum at UCLA's School of Public Health, I repeatedly questioned my sanity in taking this six-unit class that had a widespread reputation of brutalizing students. Professor Ash is regarded as one of the leading parasitologists of our era. His discovery of an animal model (the Mongolian jird) for filariasis was considered a major scientific breakthrough that led to numerous significant achievements against a disease that is now considered a target for eradication. Moreover, Ash and his colleague Tom Orihel had produced two highly acclaimed texts, considered the "bibles" of diagnostic parasitology, *Atlas of Human Parasitology* and *Parasites in Human Tissues*.[1,2] They would also go on to produce a series of bench aids for the World Health Organization for use in the diagnosis of parasitic infections. These aids are considered among the most important tools in the recognition and control of parasites of global public health significance. Despite the challenge, Ash's classroom lectures had made the subject of parasitology so captivating that I changed my focus from cardiovascular disease to infectious disease epidemiology. Nevertheless, hours of reviewing hundreds of stained slides, wet mount preparations, and countless baffling artifacts were both exhausting and humbling, and none of us bargained for examining our own stool specimen! The benefits of this torment were realized some time later when, working as an infectious disease epidemiologist with the Acute Communicable Disease Control unit of Los Angeles County's Health Department, I was assigned to the surveillance of parasitic diseases.

Sue Nagamine, the lead secretary for the Acute Communicable Disease Control unit, advised me that an anxious caller from a large, local health maintenance organization (HMO) "needed to speak to someone about parasites." I answered the phone and could quickly sense the obvious concern in the person's voice. It was October 1983 and an outbreak of amebiasis was unfolding in their patient population. Over 30 cases had been diagnosed, and they were anxious for the health department to investigate and find the source.

Amebiasis is caused by the protozoan parasite *Entamoeba hystolytica* and is endemic in most areas of the developing world. Globally, an estimated 50 million cases of amebiasis occur each year, causing approximately 100,000 deaths.[3] Although infection is often asymptomatic, when symptoms do occur, it typically induces diarrhea and dysentery but can cause severe and even life-threatening disease when it becomes invasive and affects tissue of the liver, lungs, or brain. The term histolytica in fact refers to the ability to "lyse tissue," which allows dissemination of the parasite beyond its gastrointestinal niche. Fulminant amebic colitis and cerebral infection, although rare, have a particularly poor prognosis.

Concern about *E. histolytica* had been heightened in the early 1980s with the recognition of very high prevalence rates (20% to 30%) in communities of men who have sex with men. One of the first reports of this phenomenon was Most's classic article entitled "Manhattan: a 'Tropical Isle'" in which he documented the frequent occurrence of pathogenic protozoa among gay men in the New York City area, a phenomenon that typically was seen only in resource-limited areas of the world.[4] Recent immigrants from endemic regions, residents of long-term care facilities, and travelers to developing countries were also known risk groups.[5–7]

The call from the HMO was taken very seriously. We knew that amebiasis could occur in outbreak form with significant accompanying mortality (Table 8-1). A major waterborne epidemic of amebiasis had occurred during the 1933 World's Fair in Chicago, with over 1,400 cases and 98 deaths recorded.[8] Sewage contamination of drinking water led to the outbreak. Other waterborne outbreaks in the United States had been recognized in Chicago and South Bend Indiana.[9,10] Moreover, in 1982, just 1 year prior, Greg Istre, then an Epidemic Intelligence Officer with the Centers for Disease Control assigned to Colorado, had published in the *New England Journal of Medicine* a report of an outbreak of amebiasis linked to "colonic irrigation" exposure.[11] Thirty-six cases were reported with six deaths.

Colonic irrigation, also known euphemistically as "colonic hydrotherapy," is administered through a bizarre, almost medieval contraption that provides a series of enemas over a short period of time. Historically, some proponents of colonic irrigation have contended that many conditions, including everything from impotence to cancer, are caused by fecal impaction of the colon and that these conditions can be cured with colonic irrigation. Practitioners of this procedure include "colon therapists" and naturopaths, as well as some chiropractors. It is a procedure that, regrettably, is often sought by persons who may not have access to conventional medical care for treatment of their ailments or by individuals seeking hope for conditions that may not be curable.

Given the bohemian nature of Los Angeles and its penchant for the unconventional, we were well aware of the procedure. It is not uncommon to find advertisements in various Los Angeles publications trumpeting in large boldface font that "Death Begins in the Colon!" while encouraging people to get their colons "cleansed." Our most bizarre experience with colonic irrigation occurred in the summer of 1988 when a young man in tennis shoes, jeans, and a t-shirt walked into our office carrying a huge contraption that we recognized immediately as a colonic irrigation device. He was a Los Angeles police department vice squad officer, and they had seized the "machine" as part of a raid on what he termed a "bondage and dominance parlor" in the central city area. Anyone entering the establishment had to first submit to a colonic irrigation. Because no police officer would agree to this personal invasion, they were unable to go undercover. The detective had brought the colonic irrigation device to us to see whether we had any information that might be of use for their case against the operation. Because a small amount of cloudy liquid remained in the reservoir (a glass tank capable of holding about 4 to 5 gallons of water), we took several swabs of the liquid for bacterial culture. Our bacteriology laboratory subsequently isolated *Aeromonas hydrophila* as well as several *Pseudomonas* species (which are commonly recovered from water). *A. hydrophila* can cause

TABLE 8-1 Reported Common Source Outbreaks of Amebiasis, United States

Location	Year	No. Cases	No. Deaths	Source
Chicago	1933	1400	98	Water
Chicago	1934	123	Unknown	Water
South Bend	1953	31	4	Water
Colorado	1978–80	36	6	Colonic irrigation device

gastrointestinal illness, and this was the first time that a pathogen had been recovered from one of these devices. Believing that this was important information to share, we documented our findings in a letter format submitted to the *Journal of the American Medical Association*. Wanting a catchy title for this letter, one of the co-authors (Dr. Laurene Mascola, then chief of our unit) suggested that we use "The Holistic Runs." Pleased with this title, we submitted our letter and received an enthusiastic response from the *Journal of the American Medical Association* with one suggestion—that we change the title to "Bondage, Dominance, Irrigation and *Aeromonas hydrophila*: California Dreamin."[12] We had to admit that the *Journal of the American Medical Association* editors had managed to improve substantially what we had thought was a great title.

Given the occurrence of repeated waterborne outbreaks and the colonic irrigation report, clearly the epidemic potential of *E. histolytica* was recognized. Because amebiasis is a fecal–oral transmitted disease, we were concerned that the current outbreak possibly represented the initial cases in a waterborne or foodborne epidemic.

THE INVESTIGATION

Preliminary information indicated that a total of 38 cases of amebiasis had been identified over the 3-month period from August through October. Most of the patients reported acute diarrhea and had improved after treatment with antiprotozoal therapy. Gratefully, none of the cases had died. Based on historic data, the expected number of cases diagnosed at the HMO during this time period was just three (approximately one *E. histolytica* infection per month). We determined that there had been no increase in specimens submitted for "ova and parasite" examination that might explain a jump in cases. Given this information, the number of cases recognized substantially exceeded typical baseline levels and therefore met the criterion of an outbreak.

As often occurs with such circumstances, we initiated several activities concurrently. Two senior epidemiologists, Mike Tormey, a marathon runner who had graduated from that bastion of parasitology, Tulane University, and Marc Strassburg, one of the elite cadre of individuals who had worked on smallpox eradication, provided help (as well as their typical dose of usually valuable criticism). Our preliminary investigation failed to implicate a possible common source of infection. Although this centralized laboratory served several healthcare facilities, there was no clustering of cases from any particular site(s). Moreover, early information indicated that the affected patients were not from recognized risk groups such as recent immigrants or men who have sex with men. At this point, information was not available on possible exposure to colonic irrigation. A review of countywide reported amebiasis cases and a quick survey of other major laboratories and selected physician groups did not reveal an increase in cases beyond that reported by this HMO. Although this information was reassuring, we still had a sizable outbreak yet to resolve.

In his protozoal diseases laboratory section, Larry Ash had drilled into us that *E. histolytica* was a difficult parasite to diagnose. On his dreaded laboratory exams, taken under the duress of 1-minute timed stations, complete with the pressure of a loud timer annoyingly ticking off the seconds, he had always included artifacts or "fake parasites." From this torture we learned that not only could a number of common nonpathogenic protozoa be confused with *E. histolytica* but fecal leukocytes (white blood cells), notably polymorphonuclear neutrophils and macrophages, were routinely mistaken for *E. histolytica* (Table 8-2). Nevertheless, this was a highly respected laboratory that had followed approved procedures for the diagnosis of intestinal protozoa. Their methods were solid. As recommended, permanently stained smears were prepared from polyvinyl alcohol-preserved stool specimens using the Gomori-trichrome staining method. The laboratory had also done well in proficiency testing (independent testing to assure quality control).

Given this information, we were confident in the capability of this laboratory. Nevertheless, infectious disease epidemiologists are indoctrinated that it is essential early in an outbreak investigation to verify or "confirm the diagnosis." Not expecting to find anything irregular,

TABLE 8-2 Artifacts and Organisms that Can Be Mistaken for *E. Histolytica* Infection and Lead to a False-Positive Diagnosis

Artifacts
Polymorphonuclear neutrophils
Macrophages
Epithelial cells

Organisms
Entamoeba coli
Entamoeba hartmanni
Entameoba polecki

we nevertheless went to the HMO facility, where we found a large operation with state-of-the-art equipment. To my relief, we were greeted by a very cooperative laboratory director, a woman with many years of experience in clinical laboratories. We asked whether there had been any recent changes to staff or procedures in the parasitology section. She advised us that there had not been any significant changes of note. A single technician was responsible for reading the parasitology slides and had been employed for the previous 4 years. The established protocol was for all positive findings to be reviewed by a supervisor. The only recent modification was that a new staff member had been assigned to prepare the initial fecal smears. The laboratory director stated that, because of this change, the slides had become "less dense" and were "easier to read." This made sense because organisms can be difficult to see when smears of stool are too thick.

Based on the information provided and our observations of their operation, we had no reason to believe that there may have been a laboratory error and became more concerned that we needed to find a source of the outbreak. In spite of this, just to be thorough, I asked the laboratory director whether I could review the "parasite" logs. In 1983, most logs were large notebooks with entries that were recorded by hand. Going down the list of entries, the benefits of Larry Ash's grueling parasitology course were finally realized. Most of the *E. histolytica*–positive entries had recorded in the comments section that "many white blood cells were observed." Few specimens from other patients had such comments. Because white blood cells are commonly mistaken as amoebae, we now suspected that our epidemic of amebiasis was perhaps not an outbreak at all but rather a pseudo-outbreak caused by false-positive lab findings. The similar appearance of *E. histolytica* and fecal leukocytes is illustrated in Figure 8-1. We asked to take 12 of the positive slides back to the Los Angeles County Public Health Laboratory's Parasitology Section, where Kay Mori, the unit supervisor, reviewed the slides. Kay had decades of experience and, in the early 1980s, was one of the first to recognize the rare protozoan parasite, *Entamoeba polecki*, in Vietnamese immigrants. Each year her lab processed thousands of stool specimens for "ova and parasite" exam. In just a few hours, Kay called to tell us that none of the 12 slides were positive for *E. histolytica* but that frequent leukocytes were observed!

Eventually, 71 slides from the 38 patients were reviewed either by the Public Health Laboratory or UCLA's Clinical Laboratory.[13] A total of 67 (94.5%) specimens from 36 patients were negative for amebiasis; just 4 slides from 2 patients could be confirmed as *E. histolytica* positive. This meant that 95% of the patients were incorrectly diagnosed. Specimens from 34 of the 36 unconfirmed cases were found to have polymorphonuclear neutrophils and/or macrophages. In the remaining two cases, nonpathogenic protozoa were observed. Thinner, "less dense" slides can make the morphology of cells,

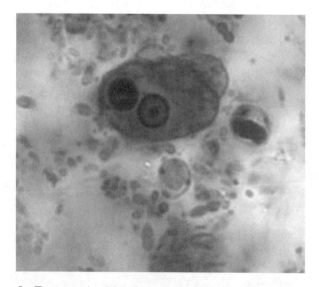

A: Entamoeba histolytica trophozoite

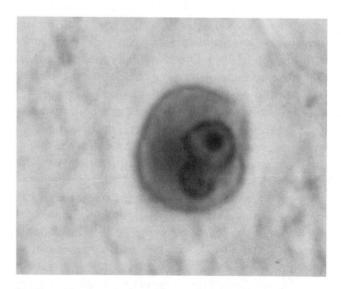

B: Fecal leukocyte

FIGURE 8-1 Comparison of Entamoeba histolytica (trophozoite) and fecal leukocyte from trichrome stained fecal smears under oil immersion. Courtesy of Lawrence R. Ash.

including leukocytes, more defined, and those features of white blood cells that can mimic *E. histolytica* may become more pronounced. The change in procedure by the new technician had resulted in misdiagnosis.

> *It is likely that some of the patients in the pseudo-outbreak mistakenly diagnosed with amebiasis may have actually had bacterial gastroenteritis.*

It is likely that some of the patients in this pseudo-outbreak mistakenly diagnosed with amebiasis may have actually had bacterial gastroenteritis. Such bacterial infections can elicit gastrointestinal inflammation, and the presence of fecal leukocytes is commonly observed in infections such as *Salmonella*, *Campylobacter*, and *Shigella*.[14] Moreover, because these infections are typically self-limited, it could explain the apparent, yet coincidental, response to antiamebic therapy. It is also possible that some patients may have had inflammatory bowel disease, a condition that may mimic amebiasis and one in which white blood cells frequently occur in stool specimens. It was amusing that although the laboratory director informed the patients' physicians of the misdiagnoses, a number of incredulous clinicians called to challenge us stating, "My patients must have had amebiasis because they improved on antiamebic therapy." We listened, politely assuring them of our findings and advising them that the observed patient improvement was simply coincidental.

The microscopic diagnosis of *E. histolytica* can be challenging and requires highly skilled technicians.[1] Krogstad and colleagues investigated seven suspected foci of amebiasis and determined that a number of laboratories had substantially overdiagnosed amebiasis with the principal error found that leukocytes in stools were reported as *E. histolytica*.[15] Two of these laboratories were in community hospitals, and one was in a teaching hospital associated with a medical school and a school of public health. These three laboratories may have mistakenly diagnosed as many as 1,200 cases of amebiasis a year for 20 years. In independent proficiency testing conducted by the Centers for Disease Control using a stool specimen that contained no parasites but had numerous leukocytes, none of 17 reference laboratories reported the presence of parasites; however, 74 of 528 other laboratories (14%) erroneously reported one or more parasites, most commonly *E. histolytica*.[13] Missing the presence of parasites (i.e., false-negative findings), including *E. histolytica*, is another common error, and together, the frequency of underdiagnosis and overdiagnosis speaks to the larger issue of having qualified and quality controlled laboratory personnel in diagnostic laboratories.

DISCUSSION AND CONCLUSION

This pseudo-outbreak of amebiasis underscores the need to verify the diagnosis as one of the initial important steps in outbreak investigations. Failure to do so can waste valuable time and resources, as well as induce unnecessary alarm. Pseudo-outbreaks are not rare. Such events, across a variety of infectious agents and circumstances, have been routinely reported in the biomedical literature and may be more common than appreciated. These apparent outbreaks can be caused by many different factors (Table 8-3). Among the more unusual of such events included a spurious outbreak of gastrointestinal *Pseudomonas aeruginosa* infection that resulted when stool culture samples were taken from feces that had already been excreted in toilets rather than captured in a clean container.[16] An apparent outbreak of pharyngeal gonorrhea was attributed to false-positive test results caused by the presence of commensal oropharyngeal *Neisseria* species.[17] Storing transport media in uncovered bottles under a sink allowed contamination by tap water and led to a pseudo-outbreak of multidrug-resistant *Pseudomonas*.[18] A contaminated ice machine was the source of transient respiratory tract colonization with *Mycobacterium fortuitum*.[19] The following briefly details factors that have been implicated as causes of pseudo-outbreaks and includes accompanying examples.

Improper Specimen Collection Techniques

The pseudo-outbreak of *P. aeruginosa*, referred to previously here, occurred among 10 patients in a hematology unit.[16] Because *P. aeruginosa* is not a recognized cause of diarrheal disease, this was an indication that something might be wrong. In investigating the apparent outbreak, it was observed that nurses obtained specimens for cultures from feces in the toilet. *P. aeruginosa* genetically identical to the "patients'" strain was recovered from toilet water. Pseudomonads are ubiquitous in water sources, including municipal water, and it would be expected to be found in toilet water.

Laboratory Error

A variety of factors can lead to false-positive laboratory findings and the occurrence of pseudo-outbreaks. Such factors include misidentification of nonpathogenic organisms or artifacts (fake parasites) as disease-causing

TABLE 8-3 Factors Implicated in Pseudo-Outbreaks and Examples of Reported Incidents

Cause	Circumstance	Agent	Setting	Number of Cases	Reference Cause
Improper specimen collection techniques	Sampling from feces in toilet	Pseudomonas	Hematology unit	10	16
Laboratory error Misidentification	Commensal organism misidentified	Neisseria Gonorrhoeae	Prostitutes	Unknown	17
Incorrect test cutoff	Antibody testing	Legionella pneumophila	Community-wide	7	20
Inappropriate test performed	Antibody testing	Epstein-Barr virus	College students	285	21
Contaminated equipment	Inadequate disinfection of bronchoscope	Pseudomonas, Serratia	Private hospital	41	22
Contaminated media/reagents	Transport media stored under a sink	Pseudomonas	Infants	16	18
Cross-contamination from control strains	Cross-contamination at a time of processing	Mycobacterium scrofulaceum	Veteran's hospital	3	24
Airborne contamination	Laboratory construction	Aspergillus sydowii	Ophthalmology ward	23	25
Transient colonization	Contaminated ice machine causing respiratory tract colonization	M. fortuitum	Hospital ward for persons with HIV	47	19
Inappropriate testing material	Tuberculosis skin testing	Mycobacterium tuberculosis	Residential facility staff	9	27
Improper reading (e.g., skin test)	Tuberculosis	Mycobacterium tuberculosis	Prison	73	28
Enhanced detection	Expanded culturing by laboratories	Escherichia coli O157:H7	Community-wide New Jersey	46	29
Sporadic cases mistaken for an outbreak	Unrelated cases viewed as cluster	Mycobacterium tuberculosis	Poultry plant workers	4	30
Automated Identification System errors	Software update	Enterococcus durans	Community hospital	29	26
Use of probiotics	Stool cultures taken after probiotic administration	Bacillus cereus	Hospital	3	23
Misinterpretation of testing (low positive predictive value)	Usually antibody testing	Variety of agents	NA	NA	31

NA = not applicable.

agents, as occurred in the amebiasis outbreak detailed here, or the pseudo-outbreak of pharyngeal gonorrhea referred to previously.[17] The use of incorrect test cutoff values as has been reported for Legionnaires' disease,[20] poor laboratory technique, and using the wrong diagnostic test, which has been documented for infectious mononucleosis,[21] can also result in false-positive findings.

Contaminated Equipment

An apparent outbreak of both *P. aeruginosa* and *Seratia marcesans* occurred among 41 hospitalized patients who had undergone bronchoscopic procedures.[22] It was determined that contamination and inadequate disinfection of bronchoscopes were responsible for the pseudo-outbreak.

Contaminated Media or Reagents

The spurious outbreak of multidrug-resistant *Pseudomonas* mentioned previously occurred among 16 infants and was linked to contaminated transport media stored under a sink where a number of bottles were found to be open and without tops.[18] Tap water splashing from the sink was considered the likely mode of contamination.

Use of Probiotic Supplement

An apparent clustering of diarrheal illness thought to be caused by *Bacillus cereus* was linked to the use of probiotic medication.[23] Three patients were given the probiotic supplement after developing diarrhea. Genetically identical *B. cereus* was recovered from the probiotic that had been administered to the patients.

Cross-Contamination from Control Strains

Microbiology laboratories retain reference strains for use as controls to assist in confirming identification of cultured organisms and as a quality control measure to ensure that techniques are reliable. An apparent cluster of three cases of *Mycobacterium scrofulaceum* was linked to cross-contamination of patient specimens with a laboratory reference strain.[24] Because infection with this agent is rare and had not been identified by this laboratory for 10 years, an investigation was initiated. Testing of the patient isolates and reference organism indicated that they were identical.

Airborne Contamination

A pseudo-outbreak of *Aspergillus sydowii* keratitis in 23 patients in an ophthalmology ward and clinic was associated with recent construction and probable airborne contamination of culture media.[25] It was noted that many colonies formed outside of the inoculation zone of the agar plates and that *Aspergillus* was recovered from air sampling in the clinic.

Transient Colonization

As previously discussed, a contaminated ice machine led to transient *M. fortuitum* colonization of 47 HIV-infected patients on a hospital ward.[19] The patients had consumed water with ice from the contaminated machine. After thorough disinfection of the ice machine with vinegar and bleach, no additional cases were observed.

Automated Identification System Errors

The use of automated systems for identification of infectious agents, particularly in large laboratories, has been increasing. An apparent outbreak of 29 cases of *Enterococcus durans* followed an error in the updated system software.[26] Using alternative methods of identification, it was determined that these isolates were likely misidentified.

Improper Testing Material

Nine staff of a residential facility converted to skin-test positive for tuberculosis; however, it was determined that an inappropriate concentration of purified protein derivative (250 tuberculin units) was used for the skin testing. Retesting with the standard 5 tuberculin units yielded no reactions.[27] Improper reading of PPD skin tests can also result in spurious outbreaks.[28]

Enhanced Detection

A community-wide pseudo-outbreak of *E. coli* O157:H7 resulted from expanded culturing of the organism by laboratories. Often, clinical laboratories will not routinely test for pathogens that may be considered rare or less important unless specifically requested by a physician; however, when such agents begin to become more common or well-known, laboratories will increase testing with the result that these agents are more frequently identified. Such enhanced detection of sporadic cases can be mistakenly perceived as an outbreak.[29]

Sporadic Cases Mistaken for an Outbreak

The occurrence of four cases of *M. tuberculosis* in poultry workers initially appeared to be a localized outbreak[30]; however, investigation found that they were unrelated cases that were erroneously viewed as a cluster.

Low Positive Predictive Value

An underappreciated problem is that even highly specific diagnostic assays will result in false-positive findings and subsequent over-diagnosis. For example, a test with 95% specificity will have a 5% level of error. That is, 5 of every 100 noncases will be false positives. In low-prevalence populations, where the large majority of individuals are negative, most of the positives will, in fact, be false positives, and the test will have a low positive predictive value; therefore, in such circumstances, imprudent interpretation of diagnostic test results can lead to the incorrect presumption that an outbreak exists. This phenomenon was encountered in the early years following the discovery of the Lyme disease agent (*Borrelia burgdorferi*), where there was a veritable explosion of testing for this infection using a new serologic test; however, given the protean (many and varied) manifestations of Lyme disease that include dermatologic, arthritic, cardiac and neurologic conditions, huge numbers of patients, many of whom were not even at risk, were now being tested. Moreover, patients with a variety of chronic conditions that were nonresponsive to therapy requested that their physicians test for Lyme disease. During this time, I spoke with many persons who actually desperately wanted to have Lyme disease. Because the infection is treatable with antibiotics, they held the hope that their chronic illness was Lyme disease, which meant that they could be cured with a course of antibiotics. During this period, we began receiving scores of reports of Lyme disease among residents of Los Angeles despite the fact that repeated surveys of local tick populations failed to find the agent. The rapid expansion and national epidemic of Lyme disease was caused, in part, by overdiagnosis through misinterpretation of serologic testing.[31]

> *Epidemiology has been described as "reasoning under uncertainty."*

Epidemiology has been described as "reasoning under uncertainty."[32] Most epidemiologists are either born skeptics or acquire the trait through repeated indoctrination. The saying "believe none of what you hear and half of what you see" could very well have been coined by an epidemiologist. The pseudo-outbreak of amebiasis detailed here should reinforce the admonition to keep an open mind and question everything, even apparent diagnoses from highly regarded sources. It demonstrates that verifying the diagnosis is an essential element of any outbreak investigation.

REFERENCES

1. Ash LR, Orihel TC. *Atlas of Human Parasitology*, 5th ed. Chicago: American Society for Clinical Pathology, 2007.
2. Orihel TC, Ash LR. *Parasites in Human Tissues*. Chicago: American Society for Clinical Pathology, 2007.
3. Petri WA Jr, Haque R, Lyerly D, Vines RR. Estimating the impact of amebiasis on health. *Parasitol Today* 2000;16:320–321.
4. Most H. Manhattan: "a tropical isle." *Am J Trop Med Hyg* 1968;17:333–354.
5. Arfaa F. Intestinal parasites among Indochinese refugees and Mexican immigrants resettled in Contra Costa County, California. *J Fam Pract* 1982;12:223–226.
6. Thacker SB, Simpson S, Gordon TJ, Wolfe M, Kimball AM. Parasitic disease control in a residential facility for the mentally retarded. *Am J Public Health* 1979;69:1279–1281.
7. Steffan R. Epidemiologic studies of travelers' diarrhea, severe gastrointestinal infections, and cholera. *Rev Infect Dis* 1986;8(Suppl 2):S122–S1230.
8. National Institutes of Health. *Epidemic Amebic Dysentery: The Chicago Outbreak of 1933*. National Institutes of Health Bulletin no. 166. Washington, DC: Public Health Service, 1936.
9. LeMaistre CA, Sappenfield R, Culbertson C, et al. Studies of a water-borne outbreak of amebasis, South Bend Indiana. I. Epidemiological aspects. *Am J Hyg* 1956;64:30–45.
10. Hardy AV, Specter BK. The occurrence of infestations with *E. histolytica* associated with water-borne epidemic disease. *Public Health Rep* 1935;50:323–334.
11. Istre GR, Kreiss K, Hopkins RS, et al. An outbreak of amebiasis spread by colonic irrigation at a chiropractic clinic. *N Engl J Med* 1982;307:339–342.
12. Sorvillo FJ, Kilman L, Mascola L. Bondage, dominance, irrigation and *Aeromonas hydrophila*: California dreamin. *JAMA* 1989;261:697–698.
13. Centers for Disease Control and Prevention. Epidemiologic notes and reports, pseudo-outbreak of intestinal amebiasis—California. *MMWR* 1985;34:125–126.
14. Thielman NM, Guerrant RL. Acute infectious diarrhea. *N Engl J Med* 2004;350:38–47.
15. Krogstad DJ, Spencer HC Jr, Healy GR, Gleason NN, Sexton DJ, Herron CA. Amebiasis: epidemiologic studies in the United States, 1971–1974. *Ann Intern Med* 1978;88:89–97.
16. Verweij PE, Biji D, Melchers WJ, et al. Pseudo-outbreak of multiresistant *Pseudomonas aeruginosa* in a hematology unit. *Infect Control Hosp Epidemiol* 1997;18:128–131.
17. Verzijl A, Berretty PJ, Erceg A, et al. A pseudo-outbreak of pharyngeal gonorrhea related to a false-positive PCR-result. *Ned Tijdschr Geneesk* 2007;151:689–691.
18. Heard S, Lawrence S, Holmes B, Costas M. A pseudo-outbreak of *Pseudomonas* on a special care baby unit. *J Hosp Infect* 1990;16:59–65.
19. Gebo KA, Srinivasan A, Perl TM, Ross T, Groth A, Merz WG. Pseudo-outbreak of *Mycobacterium fortuitum* on a human immunodeficiency virus ward: transient respiratory

tract colonization from a contaminated ice machine. *Clin Infect Dis* 2002;25:32–38.
20. Regan CM, Syed Q, Mutton K, Wiratunga K. A pseudo community outbreak of legionnaires' disease on Merseyside: implications for investigation of suspected clusters. *J Epidemiol Community Health* 2000;54:766–769.
21. Centers for Disease Control and Prevention. Pseudo-outbreak of infectious mononucleosis—Puerto Rico, 1990. *MMWR* 1991;20:552–555.
22. Silva CV, Magalhaes VD, Pereira CR, Kawagoe JY, Ikura C, Ganc AJ. Pseudo-outbreak of *Pseudomonas aeruginosa* and *Serratia marcescens* related to bronchoscopes. *Infect Control Hosp Epidemiol* 2003;24:195–197.
23. Kniehl E, Becker A, Forster DH. Pseudo-outbreak of toxigenic *Bacillus cereus* isolated from stools of three patients with diarrhoea after oral administration of a probiotic medication. *J Hosp Infect* 2003;55:33–38.
24. Oda GV, DeVries MM, Yakrus MA. Pseudo-outbreak of *Mycobacterium scrofulaceum* linked to cross-contamination with a laboratory reference strain. *Infect Control Hosp Epidemiol* 2001;22:649–651.
25. Freeman J, Rogers K, Roberts S. Pseudo-outbreak of *Aspergillus* keratitis following construction in an ophthalmology ward. *J Hosp Infect* 2007;67:104–105.
26. Singer DA, Jochimsen EM, Gielerak P, Jarvis W. Pseudo-outbreak of *Enterococcus durans* infections and colonization associated with introduction of an automated identification system software update. *J Clin Microbiol* 1996;34:2685–2687.
27. Grabau JC, Burrows DJ, Kern ML. A pseudo outbreak of purified protein derivative skin-test conversions caused by inappropriate testing materials. *Infect Control Hosp Epidemiol* 1997;18:571–574.
28. Weinbaum CM, Bodner UR, Schulte J, et al. Pseudo-outbreak of tuberculosis infection due to improper skin-test reading. *Clin Infect Dis* 1998;26:1235–1236.
29. Centers for Disease Control and Prevention. Enhanced detection of sporadic *Escherichia coli* O157:H7 infections—New Jersey, July 1994. *MMWR* 1995;44:417–418.
30. Kim DY, Ridzon R, Giles B, Mireles T. Pseudo-outbreak of tuberculosis in poultry plant workers, Sussex County, Delaware. *J Occup Environ Med* 2002;44:1169–1172.
31. Sorvillo FJ, Nahlen B. Lyme disease. *N Engl J Med* 1990;322: 474–475.
32. Greenland S. Probability logic and probabilistic induction. *Epidemiology* 1998;9:322–332.

LEARNING QUESTIONS

1. Summarize the evidence for and against the existence of an outbreak of amebiasis.
2. What are the major factors that have been implicated as causes of pseudo-outbreaks?

CHAPTER 9

Measles Among Religiously Exempt Persons

Charles E. Jennings

Illinois, 1985

During January 1985, I was working for the Illinois Department of Public Health's Immunization Section in Springfield, Illinois. My primary duty was to administer the disease surveillance/outbreak control section for vaccine preventable diseases. Prior to this, I started my career in public health by coordinating the "Swine Flu" efforts for the central and southern areas of Illinois back in 1976. After concern about the "Swine Flu" vaccine being unsafe, with the resulting shut down of the "Swine Flu" program, I continued to work for the Immunization Section by conducting school-based immunization clinics as part of the Centers for Disease Control's (CDC) measles elimination efforts.

On February 13, 1985, I received a report through interstate reporting procedures of a suspected measles case in a Missouri resident who was also one of 714 students at Principia College in Southwestern Illinois.[1] This was an unusual report because measles was uncommon, thanks to the success of the measles vaccine in the United States, and it was a unique population that may have been exposed to measles. Principia College is a college run by Christian Scientists for Christian Scientists. That same day, while I was investigating this report, I received a call from a public school nurse in the area that had heard a rumor of a 17-year-old female that died at a hospital in Alton, Illinois with a suspected rash. Alton, Illinois is a relatively small town, but it was the closest city to Principia College, with medical facilities that serve a wide area of southwestern Illinois. I immediately contacted the hospital, and they confirmed that a 17-year-old female had died of severe dehydration, rash, and a remarkably high temperature of 107°F (41.7°C). I learned that measles was suspected, but no report was made to health authorities, although measles is a class I–reportable illness. In Illinois, our surveillance system mandated that class I–reportable diseases must be reported to health authorities within 24 hours by telephone when there is a suspicion of disease.

After further questioning, I was told that the girl's body was returned to the family for cremation. This was troubling because such an unexplained hospital death should have been referred to the coroner. Fortunately, I contacted the Jersey County coroner and learned that tissue samples had been preserved.

During this very busy day, I received a call from "Cathy" (not her real name) who identified herself as a "nurse" from Principia College. She said that she wanted to comply with the law and to report six students currently in the college sick room with measles. She also said that she had previously reported cases to the Jersey County Health Department but had not received any feedback. I asked how she could confirm measles, and she stated she identified it from a picture in a book. She stated that all cases felt warm and had a rash similar to the picture. Before I could formulate my next questions, she proceeded to explain that as a Christian Scientist nurse she cannot take temperatures or blood pressure measurements or provide any care other than to make the person comfortable, assist with drinking and eating, and guess what something is from text books. I then asked about the 17-year-old female that had died, and she confirmed that she was a student there, including having been in the sick room; however, the family chose to remove her from Christian Science care and seek medical attention. Not liking the way this all sounded and the way the day was going, I consulted with the Jersey County Health Department and left immediately to begin an investigation.

That evening, the Jersey County Health Department Communicable Disease staff and I met to plan our strategy to begin an investigation of this suspected measles outbreak. The items that we discussed included the case definition that we would use in an investigation. The CDC case definition of measles at that time included a fever of 101°F (38.3°C) or greater if measured, a generalized rash lasting 3 or more days, and at least one of the following: cough, coryza (inflammation of mucous membranes, i.e., running nose), conjunctivitis, or photophobia. We decided to modify the case definition for this outbreak because temperatures were not taken; however, a feeling of warmth could be reported. We also discussed how we would approach the investigation the next morning. They further discussed with me their relationship with the college in the past, the people they work with, and about the community of Elsah, Illinois, where the college is located.

Principia College is located high on the bluffs overlooking the Mississippi River on very prime real estate. The college is completely fenced and has only two gates guarded 24 hours a day with tightly controlled access. The village of Elsah, just outside the main gate, is an old rustic sort of town featuring quaint bed and breakfasts, restaurants, and arts and crafts stores. Most residents of the town are closely associated with the college and are either faculty, staff, or former students settling there. The health department said they maintain a good relationship with the college in regards to mandatory food and sanitation inspections and a few communicable diseases in the past.

The Jersey County Health Department admitted that a few rash cases had originally been reported to them by the college, but that they had at this point failed to act on those reports. They would later be penalized during health department accreditation hearings for this lapse. Arrangements were made to meet with the college administration the next morning. Later that first night, I visited the county coroner, who was also a local funeral director, and was given lung tissue, bronchial fluid, and heart blood for shipment to the CDC laboratory. The results that came later from the CDC showed massive Gram-negative bronchial pneumonia with purulent tracheobronchitis and some areas of bronchopneumonia associated with *Staphylococcus* and *Streptococcus*. Measles is often complicated by pneumonias such as these, particularly among adolescents and adults with no prior histories of exposure to circulating measles virus or vaccine.

> *Measles is often complicated by pneumonias such as these, particularly among adolescents and adults with no prior histories of exposure to circulating measles virus or vaccine.*

On February 14, 1985, representatives from the Jersey County Health Department led by Nola Kramer, RN, administrator, and I drove the 20 miles to the campus. This was my first visit to Elsah and the college, and I was very impressed with what I saw. The town of Elsah was like stepping back into time, and I was awed by the beauty of the college campus. Grand old buildings were mixed with modern architecture. They overlooked the Mississippi River and could be seen for miles in all directions. After arriving at the guarded gate, we were told precisely where we needed to go to meet the college administrators and were escorted there by college staff. We were very enthusiastically received and were introduced to the college president, the dean of students, and a representative of the office of information for the Church of Christian Scientist out of Chicago, Illinois.

After all the formalities, I explained what I suspected (measles occurring on campus), what I wanted to do (investigate), and if indeed measles was occurring that we could make efforts to control and contain the disease, including offering clinics for vaccinating students, staff, and families. The college administration stated that they were Christian Scientists and that their religion teaches them to live by the laws of the land but to strive to continue to practice their religion. I stated that I respected their wishes and beliefs but that it was my role to protect the public health of both everyone on the campus and the general public outside the gates of their campus. I requested access to the campus as needed. They arranged for me to visit their "sick room." The sick room on campus is a separate building where students, staff, and families stay when they are sick. This is also where the Christian Scientist "nurses" work from. Here I met "Cathy," who placed the earlier phone call to me. She explained again that as a Christian Scientist nurse she could only observe and view pictures of illness to determine what might be wrong.

To my amazement, there were currently 16 students who had a rash and felt warm in the sick room facility. There was no attempt at isolation of these rash illness cases, and thus, these students in the sick room were sharing common space with other ill students. Being the first part of February, it was my opinion (as I also was responsible for influenza surveillance for the state of Illinois) that influenza was also circulating on campus, as well as in the community and this region of the state. The girl that had died was in the sick room at the same time as others with influenza-like symptoms. If someone who was debilitated with one disease should become infected with another disease, the outcome could be more severe than would normally occur. In fact, the 17-year-old that died was in the sick room with influenza-like illness while incubating measles.

Over the next 6 days my investigation continued. On the second day after arriving at the sick room, the building was surrounded by students singing and praying for those in the sick room. On the same day, the college agreed to close the campus, not allowing people to enter or leave without some proof of previous vaccination. This, I thought at the time, was actually a huge step, as I had been told the day before that as Christian Scientists they do not believe in medical care or immunizations. They did, however, only tell the students that if they had a vaccination record at home they could have someone send it to them, but would not agree to making these records a part of the student's file. We learned later that this "quarantine" of the campus was not enforced to any extent, as sports teams, visiting families, and other groups were allowed to enter and leave the campus freely. Students also knew how to sneak their way off campus through the fence. Serious isolation and quarantine would come later as the outbreak became more serious. Suspected measles cases and those considered susceptible (persons with no history of immunity from past disease or vaccine) need to be isolated from the outbreak for up to 21 days after the onset of rash of the last known case. Measles is a highly communicable virus and is spread by respiratory droplets, so that strict airborne isolation is necessary; however, their restrictions on access did not apply to families of staff attending school at Principia College's grade school and high school across the river in Missouri.

Our access to ill students was limited. Although college officials stated that we could have all of the access we needed, we were always escorted by school officials, and they were always present during any interview. One of my goals was to be able to draw blood for measles specific IgM, for confirmation that measles was occurring. When a student would agree to let me draw blood, he or she eventually would change his or her mind after talking with a school official. I even suggested obtaining throat swabs for viral isolation, as this would be less invasive to the body, but this too was denied. By the third day, school officials were visiting each student before I was allowed to talk to them.

The Christian Scientist nurses were as helpful as possible. They explained to me that if a Christian Scientist is ill, it is because their thoughts and minds are not right with God. While a student is in the sick room, a Christian Scientist reader will come and sit with them for hours reading to them from the bible and from the literature of Mary Baker Eddy,[2] the founder of the Church of Christ, Scientists. They explained that with the girl that died they would read to her and rub her neck to get her to swallow water. When the family decided to put her in the hospital, all Christian Science spiritual assistance stopped. Above the Christian Scientist nurse is the Christian Scientist practitioner (considered the "doctor" of Christian Science). An ill person can hire the practitioner to provide the spiritual care to get the person's mind right with God; however, that spiritual help ends when a person chooses medical care.

The interviews that I conducted with the ill students typically went like this. The school official would introduce me as a new friend here to meet them who would like to talk to them about their being here in the sick room. I would then attempt to do an epi-investigation; however, many factors would hamper the collection of good data. I asked, "How long have you had this rash?" The answer more often than not would be, "What rash?" I came to learn as the investigation progressed that the students would drape towels over their mirrors so that they would not see the rash, as being ill meant that their mind was not right with God. Denial of symptoms seemed to be the norm. If they didn't see it, they didn't have it.

It was also on the third day of investigation that I was told by college officials that a 19-year-old male student had died, but it turned out that he had not been included among the students I had interviewed, which further led me to believe I was not being told everything and/or not being told of all suspected cases. This student who died had been found unresponsive in the bathroom of his dorm, and CPR was attempted to revive him. I immediately asked why CPR was attempted on him when medical care is generally not allowed. I was told that this student, while being read to, went into the bathroom and fell and hit his head, and thus, it was considered an accident and not because of any illness. I was further told that when an accident happens (i.e., a sports injury) that first aid is appropriate. This was confusing to me because the investigation showed this young man to have met the case definition, and an autopsy showed massive Gram-negative bronchopneumonia.

As we attempted to make home visits to interview ill family members, we would see evidence of persons ill in the home (such as bowls out in the open, probably used for vomiting); however, it was believed that ill children were being moved from house to house ahead of our team. We believed this, as not all of the children could be found when visiting homes. Some families would tell us of sick children in other homes, but having to make "appointments" to visit the homes, we would find that the suspected case would be visiting friends or relatives at another location.

At this time, I requested assistance from the CDC and was immediately sent Steven G. F. Wassilak, MD, an Epidemic Intelligence Service officer, to assist in this investigation further. Dr. Wassilak came with a lot of measles experience and was eager to hit the ground running. Steve immediately started analyzing the data and offered suggestions on the investigation. As the investigation continued, three acute-phase IgM measles-specific serum specimens were obtained. The first confirmation of measles came from the sister of the 19-year-old male that died. She was hospitalized with measles and was not a practicing Christian Scientist. The other two confirmed IgMs were from students whose parents agreed to having the blood drawn despite the college administration's wishes.

During our initial discussions with the college administration, they had expressed a desire not to include the news media. I agreed that no information would come from the Illinois Department of Public Health and, should something get out, they would be the ones to handle it; however, in situations like this, the news media is all over it. After the outbreak leaked to someone in the media, it became a full time job just trying to respond to them. My hotel was 12 miles from the campus. On one morning, I actually had two cars and one helicopter follow me to the campus. The news media set up camp outside the gate and helicopters even attempted to land on campus. I encouraged college officials to arrange for a news conference on campus, where they could control what was presented to the media. The college agreed but asked me to take the lead. This was a good opportunity to let the media know what was happening, and I was able to introduce Dr. Wassilak as an expert on measles, which probably helped the media view our work with enhanced credibility and focus on and accept the facts rather than speculation, which could have gone awry given the two deaths. After the news conference was over, the media was satisfied with updates every day, and they left us alone to do our work. The news media seemed to be most happy getting updates on the numbers of cases.

One evening I visited one of the measles cases in the hospital. It was the sister of the 19-year-old that had died. Her father, who was in town to make arrangements for his son's body, was visiting, and we had the opportunity to sit and talk for several hours.

We talked about many things, but I took the opportunity to explain measles and how vaccine can prevent illness. I explained how I needed to get the college to accept vaccine. After he and I shared a tearful 2 hours, he stated that he wished he knew the things we talked about before he lost his son. He asked me whether other parents really knew what was going on, to which I responded that I could not answer that because the college controlled the communication with the parents.

That night I received a phone call at my hotel from the dean of students asking me how quickly I could offer vaccine on campus. He also stated that a 16-year-old female, the daughter of a faculty member, had now died too (another case we knew nothing about!). Without showing just how excited I was, I said we could have a clinic set up by 8:30 a.m. the next day. I learned later that the father to whom I had explained the public health facts about measles, along with many other parents, had put pressure on the college. He had contacted them to allow us to do whatever was necessary to control the outbreak.

At about this same time, I received a call from the Illinois Department of Children and Family Services. They were concerned about a number of complaints that there may be children in this community that were ill and not receiving appropriate health care. They were consulting with me about the possibility of filing child abuse charges against parents and even the college. I approached the college administration to let them know what this state agency wanted to do. I offered that I could encourage the department not to pursue the issue if the college would allow us the opportunity to have all ill persons be examined by a physician of our choice. Dr. Wassilak was chosen to do this, as he had developed a strong relationship with the college administrators; however, the college stipulated that he examine only minor children. One of the minor children that Dr. Wassilak examined, a 12-year-old female, was the sister of the 16-year-old female who had recently died. The parents agreed to allow the ill child to be examined; however, the parents stated that they were only agreeing to the exam because of the agreement we had with the college. They made it very clear that no further medical care was to occur, no matter what Dr. Wassilak determined. While sitting in their home while the exam was being conducted, a little dog was running around the house. The mother of the girl being examined stated that the poor little dog had been sick that day and that they had just taken it to the vet. With a great deal of surprise I had to ask how they were able to seek medical care for the dog but would refuse it for their children. I was told that the dog is not able to think for itself and that it does not have the thought processes that humans do, and thus, they need to make the decision for the dog. Humans are capable of thinking and God has given every person the chance to keep their minds right with God or be punished with an illness.

Because this was my first major outbreak situation in my new role of surveillance/outbreak control, I was fortunate to have had great people to work with. The administrator of the Illinois Immunization Program, Mr. C. Ralph March, and the Division of Disease Control Chief, Byron Francis, MD, were great in allowing me the leeway and the authority that I needed to be able to negotiate and compromise in our effort to contain this outbreak. My immediate boss, Mr. March, and I had an agreement that I should do as I see fit to control the outbreak and that he would do the politics associated with state government. If I made an unpopular decision (politically or medically), he would work to smooth it over. This partnership was important for the eventual containment of this outbreak and demonstrated a trusting administrator–program staff relationship that allowed me to thrive in my job.

By 8:30 a.m. the morning after the college allowed a clinic on campus, staff members from the Illinois Department of Public Health and the Jersey County Health Department were set up and ready to begin vaccinations. I had suggested to college officials earlier that if we could set up a clinic we could use the jet injector device. This is a device that injects vaccines and other injectables directly into the body using hydraulic pressure that pinpoints the stream of vaccine. As there is no needle, I convinced college officials that this method would be less invasive to the body. They requested that this is what they wanted. Another incentive that I offered was that if anyone agreed to vaccination they could immediately have access off campus with no further restrictions. I realized that some who received vaccine could still be incubating disease but that this was a necessary compromise to get the clinic approved. In fact, only one person that received vaccine developed a rash within 7 days of being vaccinated.

That day vaccine was administered to 403 students, staff, and families. One hundred thirty five more were able to prove prior vaccination, and 50 students that declined vaccine were quarantined on campus for up to 21 days after onset of rash of the last case. This quarantine was strictly enforced. An additional 127 persons sought vaccine off campus.

Before it was finally controlled, this outbreak (Figure 9-1) was sustained for six generations of cases with 125 cases among the 714 students and 121 staff and resident family members (an overall attack rate of 15.0%). It was shown that the index case was a student who had traveled to Alaska over the Christmas holidays, returned to the college on the 9th of January, and developed rash on the 11th of January.

There were 11 associated cases. Three died, two students and one 16-year-old child of a staff person residing on campus (case fatality ratio = 2.2%). The case fatality ratio for the United States at that time was < 0.01%. The 11 associated cases were among persons who were not students, faculty, staff or family members and were reported from outside the college and immediate community but had been exposed by students, faculty, or staff.

This outbreak was one of the most important to occur during my career with the Illinois Department of Public Health. I learned many valuable lessons that carried on through many outbreaks of many vaccine preventable diseases. Most of the lessons learned were called on again during April and May of 1994 when another measles outbreak occurred among the same Christian Scientist community.[3] One hundred forty one persons with measles were reported from Illinois and Missouri among the college, an elementary school, and a high school. The same family names were again involved with this outbreak that had been part of the 1985 outbreak. This time I was prepared to handle the college administration. They knew just what we needed, and I

> *This outbreak was one of the most important to occur during my career with the Illinois Department of Public Health.*

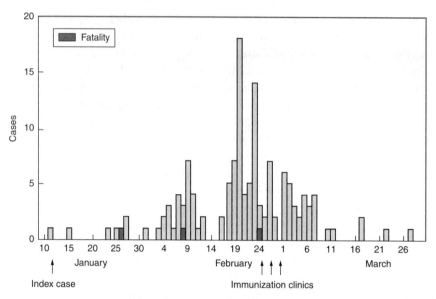

FIGURE 9-1 Measles cases in a Christian Science college in Illinois by date of rash onset, 1985. Novotny T, Jennings C, Doran M, March CR. Measles outbreaks in religious groups exempt from immunization laws. *Public Health Reports* 1988;103:49–54. Republished by permission of the Association of Schools of Public Health, Public Health Reports.[1]

knew what I needed to do. This time I went directly to the parents of the students, as I found that many times perhaps only one parent was Christian Scientist, and found that they were always very cooperative. Most of the families could present immunization records so that I could determine who may be immune. The college was also prepared to enforce strict isolation and quarantine. The college even agreed to allow students to include immunization records as a part of their school records. Following this 1994 outbreak, I do not recall any further outbreaks reported for this community.

During outbreaks, religiously exempt groups (Exhibit 9-1) generally cooperate during health emergencies. Disease-control personnel should learn to understand and develop working relationships with the various leaders of the several diversified groups of people opposed to immunizations. All persons need to be aware of reporting laws and the advantages to early reporting. This will allow disease control per-

> *Disease control personnel must be willing to negotiate and compromise to accomplish the tasks necessary to control and end outbreaks.*

EXHIBIT 9-1 Religious Groups Possibly Opposed to Immunization

- Amish
- Church of Christ in Christian Union
- Church of Christ, Scientist
- Church of the First Born
- Church of God (several types)
- Church of Human Life Sciences
- Church of the Lord Jesus Christ of the Apostolic Faith
- Church of Scientology
- Disciples of Christ
- Divine Science Federation International
- Faith Assembly
- Hare Krishna
- Hutterites
- Kripala Yaga Ashram
- Mennonites
- Netherlands Reform Church
- Rosicrucian Fellowship
- Worldwide Church of God

Source: McLaren N. *A Study of Immunization Attitudes*. Presentation to the Center for Health Promotion and Education, CDC. August 25, 1982.

sonnel to control the disease more rapidly while providing protection to the general public. Disease control personnel must be willing to negotiate and compromise to accomplish the tasks necessary to control and end outbreaks. Sensitivity to the beliefs of these diversified groups needs to be balanced with enforcement of the rules and regulations that are the public health laws of the city, county, or state. It is a difficult and delicate challenge to investigate an outbreak in this setting, but with good communication skills and a good working knowledge of what is required for the control efforts, a successful outcome is ultimately possible.

REFERENCES

1. Novotny T, Jennings C, Doran M, March CR. Measles outbreaks in religious groups exempt from immunization laws. *Public Health Reports* 1988;103:49–54.
2. Eddy MB. *Science and Health with a Key to the Scriptures.* Boston: Christian Science Board of Directors. 1934, Revised 1994.
3. Outbreak of measles among Christian Scientist students—Missouri and Illinois, 1994. *MMWR* 1994;43:463–465.

LEARNING QUESTIONS

1. There were several barriers that the author needed to attempt to overcome as he investigated and attempted to control this measles outbreak. List those barriers and how he dealt with them.
2. The author describes that the media were aggressively pursuing information on this outbreak. What specifically was the media doing to obtain information and how did the author turn this around into a more manageable interaction?

CHAPTER 10

An Outbreak of Fulminant Hepatitis B in a Medical Ward in Israel

Ronald C. Hershow, MD, MPH

Israel, 1986

My path to a public health career in infectious disease epidemiology was a circuitous one. During my internal residency at Washington Hospital Center, in Washington, DC, I was fortunate to do a 2-month elective providing emergency medical care in a Khmer refugee camp in Thailand. While there, I was exposed to the challenges of providing food, shelter, and health care to 140,000 persons who had been displaced by a genocidal Cambodian civil war. This powerful introduction to international health crystallized a desire to expand beyond the primary care focus that had defined me since I had first applied to medical school. Envisioning a possible career in international health, I decided to stay on and do an infectious disease fellowship at Washington Hospital Center. I was first told about the Centers for Disease Control's (CDC) Epidemic Intelligence Service (EIS) by Terry Chorba, a friend from residency who had just begun his EIS fellowship. He enthusiastically described a Cleveland outbreak of Parvovirus B19 that he was investigating. I was hooked. While still an infectious disease fellow, I was accepted to the EIS and subsequently underwent a frenetic week of interviews in Atlanta. I was drawn to the Hepatitis Branch because of a strong mentorship team led by Steve Hadler and James Maynard, the potential for involvement in international investigations, and a diverse group of diseases that exemplified different types of epidemiology. It turned out to be one of the best decisions I ever made.

During my infectious disease fellowship, I had acquired only a rudimentary knowledge of viral hepatitis and had to learn quickly. That early immersion in viral hepatitis was a wonderful period of discovery. I learned just how fascinating my "new" diseases were by delving into their natural history, diagnosis, epidemiology, and prevention. This process affirmed my selection of the Hepatitis Branch in the same way that living in a newly purchased home reveals many unanticipated pleasures. One thing that I came to appreciate was the value of the hepatitis A and hepatitis B serologic assays; in 1986, these had only been available for a few years. For an infectious disease epidemiologist, they are powerful tools, and their development led to an explosive growth in knowledge regarding the epidemiology of these diseases.

Because this chapter concerns a nosocomial outbreak of hepatitis B virus (HBV) infection, I will begin by discussing how HBV serologic tests aid the epidemiologist. In the context of an outbreak, the hepatitis B surface antigen (HBsAg) assay is useful because approximately

30 days after the virus is acquired, the liver begins to manufacture the virus, which spills into the bloodstream and is detectable by this assay; however, among adults, more than 90% of the time, this period of viremia resolves within 6 months as the immune response successfully neutralizes and resolves the infection. Before resolution occurs, most adults will experience a symptomatic acute hepatitis syndrome, with onset generally beginning 60 to 120 days after HBV acquisition, although incubation can range from 45 to 180 days.

Although successful resolution of HBV infection is due to a complicated combination of cellular and humoral responses, the antibody to the HBsAg (anti-HBs) plays a key neutralizing role, and thus, detecting anti-HBs in the blood generally coincides with the resolution of hepatitis B viremia. Soon after anti-HBs titers rise, the HBsAg assay will no longer detect circulating virus; this generally occurs within months of the acquisition event; however, 2% to 6% of acutely infected adults fail to resolve acute infection and progress to chronic infection. For such individuals, the anti-HBs response never develops, and the HBsAg assay remains positive, generally for the rest of that patient's life. Thus, although a positive HBsAg response may signify acute, recently acquired infection, most often it identifies an individual who has developed ongoing, chronic HBV infection.

Fortunately for the epidemiologist, there is a serologic marker that indicates recently acquired infection. In the typical course of an evolving HBV infection, two separate types of antibody appear. One is the already mentioned anti-HBs, but even earlier, the immune system produces antibodies to a core structural element within the HBV, the antibody to the hepatitis B core antigen (anti-HBc). Early on, IgM and IgG anti-HBc are elaborated, but within 6 months of the acquisition event, the IgM class anti-HBc becomes undetectable. In contrast, the IgG anti-HBc generally remains detectable for the rest of the person's life.

> *In the typical course of an evolving HBV infection, two separate types of antibody appear.*

These four assays used in combination provide the epidemiologist with a powerful toolkit. In the context of an epidemic, the IgM anti-HBC (generally used in combination with the HBsAg) provides a way of identifying recently infected individuals. Indeed, HBV viremia may resolve so quickly and subclinical or mild disease presentations are so common that the IgM anti-HBc may be the only way to identify some patients infected during an epidemic. The IgG anti-HBC assay is important to the epidemiologist because it accurately indicates whether a person has ever acquired HBV infection and thus has utility as an epidemiologic tool that allows epidemiologists to measure the seroprevalence of HBV infection in different populations. Such sero-surveys can be used to cross-sectionally map cumulative incidence of HBV infection by country or geographic region, and the assay can be used to screen populations to assess whether given individuals need hepatitis B vaccination. Those with a positive anti-HBc will not require immunization because they have already acquired natural infection and are either naturally immune for life or, less commonly, have developed chronic infection. The anti-HBs are almost as useful to screen populations but will not be positive among those who have gone on to develop chronic infection. Those who have developed chronic infection and are persistently HBsAg positive are at heightened risk of progressing to chronic hepatitis, cirrhosis, and hepatocellular carcinoma, although the majority live out their lives as healthy carriers.

Epidemiologically, the pool of chronically infected persons are of central importance, as they are able to transmit infection to others through sexual contact, through overt parenteral exposure (as occurs when injection drug users share syringe needles), or through less apparent parenteral exposures that occur through contact with blood or blood-derived skin exudates in household settings or during skin-to-skin contact as might occur when children engage in rough play. Skin diseases or lacerations can provide portals of exit or entrance in these situations.

> *Skin diseases or lacerations can provide portals of exit or entrance in these situations.*

Most pertinent to the outbreak described in this chapter is the possible role of patients or providers as sources of HBV-contaminated body fluids in healthcare-related exposures that on occasion result in nosocomial HBV acquisition.

My involvement in this outbreak began with a single phone call. As an EIS Officer, it was my job to answer the phone 2 days a week. A great majority of these calls were routine and could be handled by anyone with a thorough knowledge of "Recommendations for Prevention of Viral Hepatitis,"[1] an incredibly helpful set of recommendations that had been published in the *Morbidity and Mortality Weekly Report* in 1985. In a year of answering questions from concerned individuals, I had heard most of the standard variations. The priest who was worried about offering communion wine to a hepatitis B carrier parishioner for fear that the wine glass would be contaminated, a police cadet who was told that she could not be a police officer because she had tested positive for hepatitis B, and loads of people worried about the safety of immune serum globulin in view of the burgeoning AIDS epidemic. In these examples and on most calls, my job was to reassure that risk was negligible; however, on this particular day in August 1986, a call came in from Haifa, Israel that was of a different sort entirely.

The call was from the Rambam Medical Center in Haifa, Israel, and the facts were as follows. From June 7 to June 26, 1986, four patients were admitted to their Medicine A (or "aleph" in Hebrew) ward with fulminant and ultimately fatal acute hepatitis B. Remarkably, all four patients had been hospitalized on the same medical ward between April 23 and May 8, 1.5 to 2 months before their terminal admission. Recognizing that this cluster of cases probably represented a hospital outbreak, a local investigation ensued that did not identify a cause of the outbreak. As part of this investigation, serologic testing was conducted in late May and early June to identify additional case patients who may not have been ill enough to have been rehospitalized. All living patients who had been on the ward in late April and early May were serologically tested. This revealed a fifth case (IgM anti-HBc positive) who was the only apparent survivor of the outbreak. On August 17, 2 months after the first cluster, a sixth patient was admitted with fulminant hepatitis B. This patient had been previously hospitalized when patients from the first cluster had been present on ward A. Concerned that an ongoing source of virulent hepatitis B had gone unidentified after the first cluster and that a second cluster was about to emerge, hospital officials decided to seek epidemic aid from the CDC. I happened to pick up the phone when they called.

Things developed very quickly from that point. International investigations were often led by senior staff, but fortunately for me, my superiors were all busy with other projects. When I had started in the EIS program, I had selected the Hepatitis Branch in part because of its involvement in international projects; however, an investigation in Israel exceeded my expectations. As a Jew, I had always felt a special connection to Israel and had been there once before. Five years previously, my wife and I had gone to Israel after 6 months volunteering at a mission hospital in Kenya. Even though we had never been there before, our stop in Israel before heading back to the United States felt like an early homecoming. On that first trip, we flew on the Israeli Airline El Al, and I was surprised when my eyes filled with tears as the chant Shalom Aleichem was piped into the airplane before landing. We were welcomed warmly by the people we met, and several even suggested that we might want to consider immigrating to Israel. Although I had always supported Israel in my political views and through donations to charitable causes, those commitments now seemed paltry and effete compared with the daily challenges of the Israelis that we met. I often reflected on that trip and thought that I would like to make some meaningful contribution to Israel; this investigation might provide a chance to do so.

Nonetheless, preparing to depart for an investigation is always hectic. Although I had already been an EIS officer for a year, I had never worked on a hospital outbreak and had to familiarize myself with the ways that the HBV might be acquired in a hospital. In addition, I had to temporarily disentangle myself from all current projects and family commitments. The call had come in just before Labor Day, and my wife's parents were coming for a visit soon. I had even rented a house on a lake in the Smoky Mountains for a late summer getaway. My family enjoyed it without me because in a few days I was on my way to Israel, with a briefcase full of articles hastily copied in the CDC library.

After I boarded the plane, my life simplified, and during the long flight, I was able to review the basic facts of the outbreak and to synthesize what I had learned by reviewing reports of other hospital-based hepatitis B outbreaks. The first cluster of cases with onset dates occurring within a circumscribed 3-week period in June was remarkable in several respects. First, the high mortality rate among cases was extremely unusual, if not unprecedented. Acute hepatitis B generally has a case fatality rate of less than 1%. Even considering that the patients involved in this outbreak were older persons, surveillance data suggested an expected mortality rate of 5%, not the 80% rate that had occurred in the first cluster. Second, assuming that hepatitis B infection was acquired during their earlier admission, the cases had short incubation periods ranging from 1.5 to 2 months, at the lower end of the 1.5- to 6-month textbook description of incubation period for hepatitis B. Third, none of the patients had been exposed to traditional hospital-related sources of hepatitis B infection. Specifically, none had received hemodialysis, blood products, or surgery during the initial hospitalization when HBV infection had likely been acquired.

In pretrip briefings with my mentors (Stephen Hadler, Miriam Alter, and Mark Kane), we identified goals for my investigation. The first centered on confirming that an outbreak had in fact occurred. Laboratory error was ruled out by testing serum specimens from case patients for the serologic marker of acute hepatitis B infection (IgM anti-hepatitis B core antigen positive) in the

CDC viral hepatitis laboratory. Soon after arrival, I also confirmed that the cluster of hepatitis B cases observed on the Medicine A ward exceeded expected Haifa background rates. Indeed, review of district health office surveillance data and laboratory results from the virology laboratory at the Rambam Medical Center revealed that, excluding the ward A cluster, less than 10 cases of acute hepatitis B had been reported in Haifa in the first 8 months of 1986. Furthermore, cluster-associated case patients lacked plausible ways of acquiring infection outside of the hospital. They were older, debilitated patients who tended to live alone so that acquisition by illicit injection drug use or homosexual sex was considered exceedingly unlikely by care providers. Clearly, the tight cluster seen on one ward in Rambam Hospital in June exceeded expected background rates and hospital acquisition seemed virtually certain.

My second goal was to ascertain whether case patients possessed co-factors that might predispose them to fulminant disease and to explore other explanations for the high mortality rate in this outbreak. One hypothesis to explain the high case fatality rate was that case patients may have been co-infected by the hepatitis D (or delta) virus, a highly virulent companion virus that literally parasitizes the HBV that it is dependent on it for its replication and clinical expression; however, all specimens from the six case patients were negative for total delta antibody by a CDC in-house assay that was more sensitive than the commercially available assay that had already been used by the Israelis to investigate this possibility. Furthermore, other than their older, debilitated status, case patients had no specific underlying illnesses or medication exposures that were likely to affect the liver and potentiate the risk of fulminant hepatitis. Ultimately, the reason for the high case fatality in this outbreak remained obscure for many years, but I will return to that issue later.

My preeminent goals while in Israel were to ascertain the mechanism of transmission for the first cluster of five cases in June and to determine whether the sixth case in August was part of a second cluster and, if so, to discover the mechanism of transmission of that second cluster. The first of these goals was daunting because with only five case-patients it would be difficult to identify and statistically link specific hospital exposures with development of hepatitis B infection. In addition, by the time I undertook the investigation, the period of likely acquisition of hepatitis B infection (in late April and early May) was already 4 months in the past. Thus, in attempting to reconstruct hospital exposures, I was almost completely limited to medical record review. I was concerned that medical records might be inadequate to identify important exposures. Furthermore, medical records were in Hebrew, making me totally dependent on the translator who had been assigned to me. Finally, as I got to know my Israeli collaborators, it became increasingly clear that they were extremely competent. The fact that they had conducted an investigation already and failed to identify a cause did not augur well.

> *The fact that they had conducted an investigation already and failed to identify a cause did not augur well.*

In pretrip briefings, my mentors at the CDC had brainstormed with me about possible mechanisms for this outbreak. These included the possibility that there was a HBV-infected staff member who could have transmitted infection to cases through contamination of open wounds or breaks in the skin of case patients. Indeed, there were outbreaks described in the medical literature caused by this mechanism, but they tended to involve transmission from hepatitis B-infected dentists or surgeons to patients during surgical procedures,[2-6] and most often involved practitioners with dermatologic problems affecting their hands (from which plasma derived exudates could contaminate wounds) or technique problems that led to sharp instrument accidents while working in confined operative spaces. In any event, the Israelis had already effectively ruled out this possibility by testing virtually all staff that had been associated with these patients in late April and early May; no hepatitis B carrier or acutely infected staff members were identified.

A second mechanism would implicate patients concurrently on the ward as a potential source of HBV infection. If there was a hepatitis B carrier patient on the unit in late April and early May, body fluids from that patient could infect surrounding patients through a few mechanisms. First, if such patients bled into the environment, patients could be contaminated directly through splashes onto nonintact skin or into the mouth or eyes. Although this seems unlikely, patients with chronic hepatitis B infection can experience catastrophic bleeding from esophageal varices, and bleeding from any site may be exacerbated by coagulation problems caused by advanced liver disease. Blood may contaminate the environment or equipment, and patients may be indirectly exposed to hepatitis B through contact with these sources.

In addition, blood from source patients can occasionally contaminate multidose injectable preparations. For example, Miriam Alter briefed me on a dialysis-related outbreak that she had investigated.[7] This particular dialysis unit was unusual in that dialysis patients were taught to carry out simple nursing functions to facilitate their care. These included going to a common preparation area where several multidose injectable preparations were kept. One of these multidose injectables was a local anesthetic (bupivicaine) that some patients asked dialysis staff to use to anesthetize their skin before the percutaneous insertion of the dialysis canula. Patients were instructed to draw up the anesthetic into a syringe and have it ready for the dialysis technician. In this outbreak, use of bupivicaine was significantly associated with being a case. There were two known HBsAg-positive carriers on this unit who used the bupivicaine. One of them had recently had a minor stroke and had some residual hand weakness and tremors. It is postulated that she jabbed her finger with the syringe needle while attempting to advance it into the rubber stopper of the bupivicaine vial. Instead of discarding the syringe, it is thought that she persisted and readvanced the contaminated needle into the vial, effectively inoculating its contents with her blood. From that point on, other patients who used that vial of local anesthetic were directly injected with hepatitis B-contaminated fluid. In fact, of 11 susceptible patients who had used bupivicaine and received dialysis after the implicated HBsAg carrier, 10 (91%) subsequently seroconverted to HBsAg positive.

Armed with these potential mechanisms, I arrived at Lod Airport and was met by Dr. Edna Ben-Porath, an accomplished virologist who had participated in the Israeli investigation of the first cluster. She drove me to my hotel in Haifa, and I admired the view from the top of Mount Carmel. To be honest, however, as nice as that hotel was, I mainly remember only the bed because from then on I was working the typical 16-hour day of an EIS officer on assignment.

At a meeting the next day, I learned about the basic structure of internal medicine inpatient care at the Rambam Medical Center. The internal medicine inpatient wards at the Rambam were denoted alphabetically, and as mentioned, this outbreak occurred on the Medicine A ward. Inpatient medical wards were staffed continuously by a core group of attending internists who served as faculty for house staff who rotated through that particular medical service. During residency training, house staff members were assigned to one of these teams and remained attached to a given unit throughout their 3-year training period. Attending physicians and residents saw a panel of internal medicine outpatients, and if these patients required hospitalization, they were admitted to ward A. This system differed markedly from the one used by my residency training program. At Washington Hospital center, the medical units were staffed by different attending physicians every month, and I was assigned to month-long rotations on these inpatient units several times a year. I did have a panel of outpatients that I followed, but when these patients required admission, they were assigned sequentially to one of the inpatient units in the order that they were admitted to the medical service. As a result, I rarely cared for my own clinic patients when they were hospitalized. It is interesting to speculate whether this outbreak would even have been detected in my training hospital as patients were not automatically linked to one inpatient unit of the hospital. It was the continuity in staffing of the Medicine A ward and the medical staff's familiarity with their panel of patients that led to the easy recognition of this outbreak when the same group of patients was admitted and then readmitted months later with fulminant hepatitis B.

At that first meeting in the hospital, I was also introduced to Dr. Nahum Egoz, a medical attending on the Medicine D ward who would serve as translator and would slog through medical records with me during many long evenings. Although not part of the Medicine A staff, he was assigned to me in part to insure that he would remain objective and unbiased as we conducted the investigation. We got along extremely well, and I learned much about the Israeli medical system through our acquaintance. Although Nahum maintained a "full-time" position at the Rambam, a public hospital, he also maintained a private medical practice. Attending physicians at the Rambam were generally done with ward rounds by 2 p.m., which left time for this type of dual practice.

I met a number of people who I came to like and admire as the investigation proceeded. Dr. Gideon Alroy was the chief of Medicine A at the Rambam. He was an inspiring, vigorous leader, all the more remarkable because he suffered from end-stage kidney disease and was dependent on peritoneal dialysis administered in his home. Early in my stay, he invited me to dinner at his home (as did Dr. Ben-Porath and many others), and I developed a friendship with his daughter, Tamar, who was an artist. In rare moments, when I had some free time, she was kind enough to show me parts of Haifa. Once she took me to see the first segment of the recently released film "Shoah," a poignant documentary that provides insights into the day to day operation of the Nazi Death Camps by interviewing not only survivors, but also persons who had worked at the death camps or who lived in communities where Jews were being systematically removed. We were riveted for 4 hours, and both of us were speechless after seeing it.

In preliminary discussions, the Israelis had briefed me on the findings of their investigation. Following the June cluster, they had astutely performed serologic testing on all patients who had resided on the Medicine A ward in late April and early May for hepatitis B serologic markers. Their testing window was based on the observation that all four patients with fulminant hepatitis B in June had all been previously together on the unit on only 1 day, April 29th. Around this date, a 1-week interval was constructed. They identified 58 patients who had been on the unit from April 26 through May 2. Of these, five later developed hepatitis B in June. Eighteen died before they could be reached for serological testing. Twenty one were tested and found to be negative for all hepatitis B serological markers. Eleven were tested and had evidence of remote prior hepatitis B infection, and three were chronic hepatitis B carriers who were known by Medicine A clinicians to be positive for HBsAG even before the Israelis conducted this serologic investigation. These results raised some obvious questions. Could one of the four hepatitis B carriers be the source of hepatitis B in this outbreak? In addition, the fact that 18 of the 58 (or 31%) of these patients had died within a few months of their April/May admission seemed to be excessive and raised the possibility that some of these individuals may have been unrecognized victims of the outbreak. Unlike the 5 case patients, these 18 had not been subsequently admitted to ward A, but died elsewhere.

I asked the ministry of health to provide death certificates for these 18 patients to see whether there was any suggestion that they had died a liver-related death. Nahum and I then proceeded to examine the medical records of the five case patients. All case patients were older, but they had little else in common. They had been initially admitted to Medicine A with a variety of apparently unrelated illnesses and had not shared common hospital rooms while in ward A. This lessened the possibility that the outbreak was due to catastrophic bleeding from one of the hepatitis B carrier patients. Indeed, subsequent review of the medical records of the four hepatitis B carrier patients revealed no episodes of bleeding during their residence on ward A. We also noted that all five of the case patients had some form of intravenous access devices in place during their admission. This represented a potential portal of entry for HBV, but without a control group for comparison, it was difficult to say if it was unusual. Thus, we entered the case-control phase of our investigation with a vague hypothesis that having an intravenous access device in place may have played some role in the acquisition of hepatitis B.

Fortunately, we had an obvious source of control patients. The serologic testing that the Israelis had done revealed that 21 patients were negative for hepatitis B serologic markers and therefore susceptible to hepatitis B. Why had these 21 patients avoided infection, whereas 5 unfortunate ward-mates had not? Nahum and I pored over the records of these 21 patients culling out demographic information, bed placement, exposure to medications (particularly injectables), medical examinations patients had undergone, and presence of indwelling intravenous devices. There was only one significant finding: although cases and controls were equally likely to have intravenous devices in place during their hospital stay, the five case patients were more likely to have a heparin lock in place. In fact, from April 26 to May 2, all five cases had had this device at some point compared with only 5 of 21 of susceptible controls (24%) ($P = 0.004$).

I knew a few basic things about heparin locks from my internal medicine residency. A heparin lock is a small tube connected to a catheter that is maintained in a vein to allow convenient venous access. If someone needs periodic but not continuous infusions of a given medication, that medication solution can be run into the heparin lock at scheduled intervals through a needle that is inserted into a rubber port in the barrel of the heparin lock tube.

I was ignorant, however, about how heparin locks were maintained and went back to the ward the next day eager to follow up on this lead. I asked for an interview with the head nurse of the unit. I was careful to begin with some questions about other, unrelated procedures on the ward. Eventually, I asked the critical question, "Could you tell me about the insertion and maintenance of heparin locks on the unit?" The head nurse told me that heparin locks were inserted using aseptic technique, like any other indwelling intravenous catheter. The only difference between the maintenance of an intravenous line and a heparin lock was that the barrel of the heparin lock tube was flushed at regular intervals using heparin solution. This is done so that the blood in the heparin lock barrel will not clot off and eliminate access to the vein.

I probed further and asked whether the heparin flush solution came directly from the pharmacy. The nurse stated that no, in general, the heparin solution was prepared on the unit once a day, usually just after the morning change of shifts. Routinely, at 7 a.m., a nurse would draw up a defined quantity of heparin from a vial and inject it into a rubber-stoppered vial of sterile normal saline. Trying to sound offhand, I asked whether each patient had his or her own designated heparin flush solution vial or whether one vial served as the flush solution for all patients on the ward who needed heparin lock maintenance. She stated that the heparin flush solution was kept at the nurse's station and that nurses would draw up solution as they needed it. All heparin locks on the unit were generally flushed in sequence every 8 hours. I asked whether the same syringe was used to flush multiple heparin locks and received a shocked look. "No, of course not. A new, prepackaged, sterile syringe is used to draw up heparin flush solution, and the same syringe is never inserted into the heparin lock of different patients." Even a fledgling epidemiologist knew enough to be skeptical about that kind of blanket pronouncement.

With further questioning, I established a few other facts. The April 26 to May 2nd interval that we were scrutinizing coincided with Passover, an important Jewish holiday. As a result, ward A staffing was minimal, much as it would have been during the Christmas Holidays in the United States. Although record keeping did not permit the identification of specific persons who had performed the heparin lock flushes during this interval, it was clear that such persons would have been overworked during this time interval. I postulated that under these circumstances a mistake could have been made. If one of the hepatitis B carriers housed on ward A had a heparin lock in place during this interval, an overburdened staff member might have reused a syringe that had been contaminated while flushing that carrier's heparin lock. By readvancing it into the multidose heparin/saline flush solution, the solution itself would have been contaminated. Adding to the plausibility of this mechanism was the fact that additional medical record reviews revealed that of the four hepatitis B carriers on Medicine A in late April and early May, only one was in the hospital on April 29, the day when all five cluster patients had been on the unit on the same day. This carrier individual had a heparin lock in place from April 23 through the morning of May 1. Although there was no way to definitively prove it, I had a highly plausible explanation for the first cluster. This explanation was biologically plausible, consistent with available data, and credible given the tendency for error when staff are rushed or overburdened. With some excitement, I called my supervisor, Steve Hadler, and he agreed that I had identified the probable cause of the outbreak but suggested one additional analysis to bolster my case.

He speculated that the kind of mistake I was hypothesizing would probably be a one-time event because it represented a gross breach of standard practice. As we now knew, the heparin/saline flush solution was changed every 24 hours. Steve therefore suggested that I examine the association between heparin lock placement on each day of the April 26 to May 2 interval (Table 10-1). Of special interest were the data from April 29th, the only day when all five cluster patients were on the unit. On this date, the heparin lock association was nearly perfect. Specifically, four of five cases had a heparin lock on that day compared to none of nine controls.

How could I explain the one patient who did not have a heparin lock in place on the 29th? I carefully reviewed the Medical record again and found that he was admitted to Medicine A from the coronary care unit on the 29th on continuous intravenous therapy. From my own experience as a resident, I knew that when a patient is transferred from one unit to another the patient is jostled and transferred from bed to stretcher and that transient interruptions in intravenous fluid administration may frequently occur. It was possible that while being transported, this case patient's intravenous line clotted off. If so, a staff person on ward A may have flushed the line with the contaminated heparin normal saline solution soon after the patient arrived on ward A. This would be done to salvage the line and avoid the need to reinsert an intravenous line at a different site.

TABLE 10-1 Percentage of Cases and Susceptible Controls With In-Dwelling Heparin-Lock Placement on Medicine A on Consecutive Days in late April and Early May

Date	4/26	4/27	4/28	4/29	4/30	5/1	5/2
% Cases (n)	75 (4)	100 (4)	100 (4)	80 (5)	67 (3)	100 (3)	100 (3)
% Controls (n)	11 (9)	36 (11)	9 (11)	0 (9)	11 (9)	11 (9)	14 (14)
P (Fisher's exact)	.052*	.051*	.004	.005	.127*	.018	.015

*P not significant
n = number of cases or controls present on Medicine A on specific dates.

Statistically, significant associations are demonstrated on other calendar days in the April 26 through May 2 interval, but no other date included all five case patients. Furthermore, it did not surprise me that other days would show an association; a patient who requires a heparin lock on any given day is likely to continue to require it on ensuing days.

Although I remained busy during the following days, it mainly amounted to tying up loose ends. Death certificates from those 18 Medicine A patients who had died after their April/May admission did not reveal any hint of a liver-related cause of death. Furthermore, the hepatitis B serologic testing performed on patients who had been co-residents of the patients who died of fulminant hepatitis in the June cluster on ward A revealed no other patients with evidence of acute hepatitis B. Thus, the sixth case that had occurred in August was an isolated event, not part of a second cluster, and in fact, he did not have a heparin lock in place. He did, however, undergo a bone marrow biopsy during his stay, had a permanent cystostomy in place, and had an indwelling intravenous line for much of his stay. Three of the dying June cluster patients were present on the ward during his admission. All of these patients had marked coagulopathies, and one was noted to have ongoing blood oozing from his intravenous line insertion site. We hypothesized that the sixth case may have acquired hepatitis B through cross-contamination with blood derived from the June cluster hepatitis patients. This blood may have been present in the environment or have been transported to the patient on the hands of staff members and gained entry through breaks in the skin of case 6 provided by indwelling lines and invasive procedures.

After completing the basic investigation, it was time to brief the staff of the Rambam Hospital on my findings and to make recommendations. In that presentation, I reviewed my findings carefully, not only summarizing my positive findings but refuting other potential mechanisms. Further strengthening the case for a common-source, multidose exposure was the tight temporal clustering of the cases and the short incubation periods. The short incubation period favored a high inoculum exposure like that which might result from the direct injection of a contaminated injectable, rather than that which would result if small amounts of infected materials were splashed or rubbed onto an intravenous site.

After completing my presentation, I was taken aback when the chief of staff raised his hand and said that I had left out one important possible explanation for the outbreak—intentional sabotage. He was concerned that a disgruntled or criminal employee had obtained hepatitis B contaminated fluid and intentionally injected it into these patients. I thought about this and asked why a saboteur would inoculate only those with a heparin lock when intravenous lines would provide equivalent ease of access to the blood stream of patients. Without hesitation, he stated that heparin locks have a flat rubberized port, whereas intravenous systems have a rounded rubberized section for introducing needles. With the latter, it is easier to poke yourself, which might have deterred a saboteur. I advanced other arguments against the sabotage theory, pointing to the fact that use of potassium chloride or poisons would be a more typical approach, but these were countered by the assertion that they would have raised greater suspicion of foul play. In the end, I inserted the following sentence into my final report: "The deliberate injection of HBsAG-positive material through the heparin lock cannot be definitively ruled out but accidental inoculation seems far more plausible and has occurred in other outbreaks."[7,8]

It was time to say goodbye. I had acquitted myself well during the investigation and had made a good impression. Before I departed, I was offered a position at the Rambam Hospital and the challenge of developing an infectious disease service there. I seriously considered this offer and even inquired about potential positions for my wife, Judy, who was also a physician. They assured me that something would be arranged. I did not want to leave the EIS program at that point, however, and by the time my tenure in that program ended, the idea had faded in light of family obligations and practical concerns. I said goodbye with sadness, however.

At the end of my stay in Israel, I was told that the outbreak investigation was to be kept strictly confidential. Israeli media had not been informed of the outbreak on Medicine A. Families of the cases would have to be told first and then the decision about publication would be reassessed. I was disappointed in part because it meant that the work might not be published, which affected me personally, but also because the wider world could not benefit from the findings of our investigation.

At the airport, when I was getting ready to board my airplane to return to the United States, I was interviewed by security. They asked me what I had been doing in Israel. I was not prepared for this. As a representative of the U.S. government working for the CDC, I did not want to lie to Israeli security. With some trepidation, I told them that I had been working on a scientific investigation in Haifa with colleagues at the Rambam Hospital. The security agent must have sensed my unease and continued to probe for increasingly specific details of my investigation. Eventually, I divulged that I had been working on an outbreak at the Rambam Hospital. The security official left me alone for a few minutes, and when she came back, I was told I could leave. A few weeks after my return to the United States, I found out that the story had been "leaked" to the Israeli media. I have always wondered if I was that leak. In any event, the outbreak investigation was eventually published.[9]

One last issue remained to be illuminated. There was as yet no explanation for the high mortality rate in this outbreak. At the time I did the investigation, the CDC did not have the capacity to clone and sequence viral DNA from HBV strains that had infected these individuals; however, serum from these individuals was carefully stored in Israel, and 5 years later, Edna Ben-Porath and colleagues at Harvard Medical School were able to do so. Specifically, the presence of HBV was identified by polymerase chain reaction amplification of viral DNA in serum from the hepatitis B carrier patient identified as the likely source of the infecting strain by our investigation, the five patients with fulminant hepatitis B, and five controls with acute, self-limited hepatitis B. The amplified viral HBV DNA samples were then cloned and sequenced. Sequence analysis of viral DNA established that the same HBV mutant with two mutations in the precore region was present in the source patient and the five patients with fulminant hepatic failure, but not in control patients. They concluded that naturally occurring viral mutations in the HBV genome may predispose the infected host to more severe liver injury.[10] This report was gratifying not only because it helped to explain the high case fatality rate in the outbreak, but because it confirmed that we had correctly identified the hepatitis B carrier patient who was the common source for this tragic outbreak.

After this outbreak, I returned to the hepatitis branch and finished up my EIS career. I still consider those 2 years the most exciting professional experience that I have ever had. Toward the end of my tenure in the EIS program, I was offered a few jobs at the CDC that I would have considered the fulfillment of a dream when I first started. There was one position that involved measles control in Africa that was particularly exciting; however, during my EIS years, my son Charlie was born. The measles job would have required at least 4 months of international travel a year, and I chose instead to assume an academic position at University of Illinois at Chicago (UIC). My daughter, Rebecca, was born soon after we arrived in Chicago. The UIC position allowed me to return to the clinical practice of infectious diseases and to garner a joint appointment at UIC's School of Public Health. My background in viral hepatitis proved invaluable. Shortly after my arrival at UIC, the cause of non-A, non-B hepatitis was identified, and the study of hepatitis C virus natural history and epidemiology has been a major focus of my research ever since. Also, because hepatitis B and C share epidemiologic similarities with HIV infection, my training in viral hepatitis proved to be excellent preparation for work that increasingly focused on HIV infection. Shortly after arriving at UIC, I was fortunate to become a co-investigator on the Women and Infants Transmission study. The study of HIV infection as it affects women and substance users has been another important research area for me.

Nonetheless, there have been times that I have wondered about the roads I did not take. Both of my children have graduated from high school now, and as I finish this chapter, I can hear the call of the muezzin from a nearby Mosque. I am in Jakarta, Indonesia launching the first international investigation I have undertaken since I left Israel 22 year ago. I am doing a pilot investigation to identify effective ways to promote successful antiretroviral therapy among injection drug users in Jakarta and Bali. Who knows? Maybe it's time to start planning a sabbatical in Israel.

REFERENCES

1. Centers for Disease Control. Recommendations for prevention of viral hepatitis. *MMWR* 1985;34:313–324, 329–335.
2. Prentice MB, Flower AJ, Morgan GM, et al. Infection with hepatitis B virus after open heart surgery. *BMJ* 1999;304:761–764.
3. Polakoff S. Acute hepatitis B in patients in Britain related to previous operations and dental treatment. *BMJ* 1986;293:33–36.
4. Rimland D, Parkin WE, Miller GB, Schrack WD. Hepatitis B outbreak traced to an oral surgeon. *N Engl J Med* 1977;296:953–958.
5. The Incident Investigations Team and Others. Transmission of hepatitis B to patients from four infected surgeons without hepatitis B e Antigen. *N Engl J Med* 1997;336:178–184.
6. Reitsma AM, Closen ML, Cunningham M, et al. Infected physicians and invasive procedures: safe practice management. *Clin Infect Dis* 2005;40:1665–1672.
7. Alter MJ, Ahtone J, Maynard JE. Hepatitis B virus transmission associated with a multiple-dose vial in a hemodialysis unit. *Ann Intern Med* 1983;99:330–333.
8. CDC. Outbreaks of hepatitis B virus infection among hemodialysis patients: California, Nebraska, and Texas, 1994. *MMWR* 1996;45:285–289.
9. Oren I, Hershow RC, Ben-Porath E, et al. A common source outbreak of fulminant hepatitis B in a medical ward. *Ann Intern Med* 1989;110:691–698.

10. Liang TJ, Hasegawa K, Rimon N, Wands JR, Ben-Porath E. A hepatitis B virus mutant associated with an epidemic of fulminant hepatitis. *N Engl J Med* 1991; 324:1705–1709.

LEARNING QUESTIONS

1. The author recognized several unusual features of this outbreak of hepatitis B virus infection. What were they?

2. What were the possible mechanisms of transmission considered for this outbreak by the CDC staff before sending the author to Israel and what were the strengths and weaknesses of each of these possibilities?

CHAPTER 11

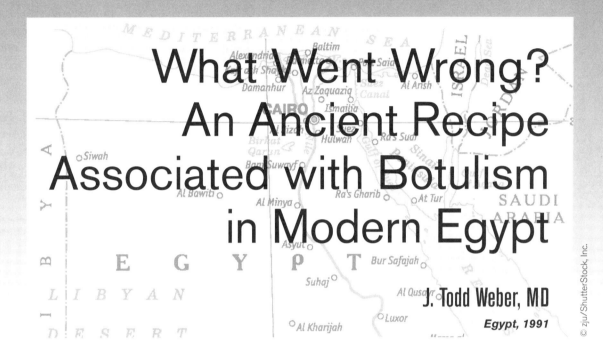

What Went Wrong? An Ancient Recipe Associated with Botulism in Modern Egypt

J. Todd Weber, MD

Egypt, 1991

INTRODUCTION

Terrorism, War, Religious Observance, and a Holiday

On Wednesday, December 21, 1988, Pan Am Flight 103—a Boeing 747-121 named Clipper Maid of the Seas—was destroyed by a bomb. The ruins fell in and around the town of Lockerbie, Scotland. Experts showed that plastic explosive had been detonated in the airplane's cargo hold. The death toll was 270 people from 21 countries. The first leg of Pan Am Flight 103 began as PA 103A from Frankfurt International Airport, West Germany to London Heathrow Airport. An unaccompanied bag had been routed onto Pan Am 103 on an Air Malta flight to Frankfurt and then by flight PA 103A to Heathrow. This unaccompanied bag contained the bomb. The investigation of the bombing went on through 1990, and findings of various groups recommended and led to increased airport security.[1]

The Gulf War began on August 2, 1990, with the invasion of Kuwait by Iraq. Saddam Hussein was known to be developing biological weapons. After defeat by an allied coalition of 34 countries, the war ended on March 3, 1991, when Iraq accepted a ceasefire. Approximately 400 coalition forces died during the war, including 10 from Egypt. The United States estimates that at least 20,000 Iraqis were killed.[2]

In 1991, the month-long Islamic holiday of Ramadan began on March 17 and ended on April 14–15. Ramadan occurs in the ninth month of the Islamic calendar, a lunar calendar, changing dates on the Gregorian calendar each year. In the month of Ramadan, Muslims fast during the day, eating at night and avoiding salty foods. (Because the rules of Ramadan prohibit drinking during the day, foods that make you thirsty are undesirable.) There are exceptions to the requirement of fasting, including for those who are menstruating, pregnant, postpartum, traveling, ill, or in battle—an important point because the Gulf War had only recently ended and coalition troops were still present in the region.

In 1991, the Egyptian Holiday *Sham-el-Nessim* fell on April 8, coincidental with Ramadan. *Sham-el-Nessim* is an annual springtime holiday; it is nonsectarian and is celebrated by Islamic and Coptic Egyptian citizens. It is a public holiday occurring annually on Monday, the day after the Coptic Easter Sunday. Its origin reportedly dates back millennia. The rough translation of *Sham-el-Nessim* is "sniffing the breezes." Typically, families spend the day together outside and share foods traditional to the holiday.

THE OUTBREAK

On the evening of April 9, 1991, the second day of the Centers for Disease Control and Prevention (CDC) Epidemic Intelligence Service (EIS) annual conference in Atlanta, Georgia, I was on call for the Enteric Diseases Branch of the Division of Bacterial and Mycotic Diseases at the CDC. I joined the EIS after training as an internist at New York University in the Bellevue Hospital Center and Tisch Hospital. I received a call at home from an Ohio state health department officer. He needed botulinal antitoxin and knew that the CDC was the only place he could get it. He had received a call from a doctor in his state who was Egyptian and had relatives in Cairo. She told him there were three adults with botulism intoxication in a hospital in Cairo, all on ventilators, and wanted to know how to obtain antitoxin. After consultation with others in the branch, I recommended that this physician contact companies in Europe that produce antitoxin, as shipment from there would be faster.

In the next 24 hours, the CDC received other calls reporting more cases and some deaths. The physician for the U.S. Embassy in Cairo called. He said there were hundreds of Cairo citizens crowding the gates of the embassy and pleading for antitoxin. It was front-page news in the Egyptian newspapers, and the Minister of Health was being called into Parliament to explain what had happened and what was being done. This was the first time botulism had ever been reported in Egypt, and it sounded much larger than a typical botulism outbreak. Antitoxin was ultimately obtained from several European companies and the United States Armed Services. Ban Mishu, the preventive medicine resident in the branch, and I were invited to Cairo to investigate the outbreak. Along with luggage, laptops, printers, and laboratory equipment, we carried with us antitoxin from the CDC's supply. The U.S. Agency for International Development paid for it at the request of their office in Cairo.

The Enteric Diseases Branch (now the Enteric Diseases Epidemiology Branch, Division of Foodborne, Bacterial, and Mycotic Diseases, National Center for Zoonotic, Vector-Borne, and Enteric Diseases, CDC) is available 24 hours a day to provide clinical advice to state health departments and clinicians. The laboratory provides testing for state health departments. The CDC controls most of the supply of antitoxin for the United States and through state health departments supplies it to doctors taking care of suspected cases. (The Alaska Division of Public Health and the California Department of Health Services also maintain supplies of antitoxin for reasons of population size, geography, and incidence of cases.) The CDC maintains control of the supply for two reasons. First, the CDC maintains active surveillance through requests that are received for antitoxin and for laboratory testing. Second, preventive measures may be taken on the basis of the report of a single case of botulism (Exhibit 11-1). This single case may be a sentinel for a larger outbreak, requiring an investigation to prevent further cases from occurring. Such an investigation is usually carried out by the state or local health department. The U.S. Food and Drug Administra-

---

EXHIBIT 11-1 Key Facts About Botulism

Three Main Forms

Foodborne botulism occurs when a person ingests toxin which then leads to illness or death within a few hours to days. Outbreaks of foodborne botulism have potential to be a public health emergency because the contaminated food may be eaten by other people. Symptoms typically begin 18 to 36 hours after eating contaminated food (range 6 hours to 10 days).

Infant botulism occurs when the spores of *C. botulinum* are consumed by infants with subsequent growth of the organism in the gut and toxin is released.

Wound botulism is a rare disease that occurs when *C. botulinum* infects wounds and produces toxin.

Anaerobic conditions promote germination of *C. botulinum* spores and botulinum toxin production.

Among the seven types of botulism toxin designated by the letters A through G, only types A, B, E, and F cause illness in humans.

Classic Symptoms*

- Double vision
- Blurred vision
- Drooping eyelids
- Slurred speech
- Difficulty swallowing
- Dry mouth
- Muscle weakness

Untreated, botulism may progress to cause paralysis of the arms, legs, trunk, and respiratory muscles, leading to death.

---

* Infants with botulism appear lethargic, feed poorly, are constipated, and have a weak cry and poor muscle tone.

Derived from Botulism. Division of Foodborne, Bacterial, and Mycotic Diseases, Centers for Disease Control and Prevention. Retrieved October 21, 2008, from http://www.cdc.gov/nczved/dfbmd/disease_listing/botulism_gi.html

tion is notified of each possible case so that suspect foods may be seized and have their production investigated. Numerous countries have requested the assistance that the CDC provides to states, but the distance to most countries makes timely delivery of antitoxin with an uninterrupted cold chain problematic. Without preservation of the cold chain, the antitoxin, scarce and expensive, can be rendered ineffective. The people in Egypt were not discouraged by this policy, and relatives contacted state health departments and the CDC until the investigation began and the antitoxin was made available from several sources.

American surveillance picked up an Egyptian outbreak. Because there was no botulism expertise in Egypt, the CDC and the U.S. Naval Medical Research Unit 3 (located in Cairo) were asked to assist the Ministry of Health in an investigation in order to prove an association with a vehicle, to assist with management of cases, and to recommend preventive measures. The investigation was supported with resources and logistics by the U.S. Agency for International Development in Egypt. The first stage of the investigation involved finding cases. Suspected cases were reported to the Egyptian Ministry of Health, and all of these were limited to Cairo. The outbreak was well publicized throughout the country, and we spoke with health officials in several other cities to ask whether they were aware of any cases in their districts. They reported none.

THE INVESTIGATION[3]

The Ministry of Health instructed all hospital administrators in Cairo to report cases of suspected botulism based on diagnosis by a physician and then compiled a list of reported patients. We were unable to examine hospital records systematically to determine the completeness of hospital reporting. Investigators examined only those hospital records of patients with botulism-like illness who were interviewed. Patients, family members, and attending physicians were questioned regarding age, gender, religion, date and time of onset of illness, symptoms, date of hospitalization, admission to an intensive care unit, the use of mechanical ventilation, and the type and dose of botulinal antitoxin received. Patients were asked to list all foods eaten during the 72 hours before onset of illness. We defined a case of suspected botulism as illness in a hospitalized patient whose physician suspected botulism and who had at least one of the following symptoms: dyspnea, blurred vision, or ptosis (drooping eyelids).

Ninety-one patients with suspected botulism were reported to the Ministry of Health. Of these 18 (20%) died from the illness. Before discharge from the hospital, 45 of the 73 surviving patients (61%) were interviewed between 14 and 19 April. The age of the patients interviewed ranged from 8 to 85 years, and there was a slight male preponderance (60%).

The onset of illness for 98% of patients interviewed was within 24 hours of April 8th, which was the Egyptian holiday *Sham-el-Nessim*. We made the assumption that the food responsible for the outbreak was served during the traditional meal of *Sham-el-Nessim*, and thus, the mean incubation period was 12.8 hours. This is on the shorter end of the spectrum for botulism, but if our assumption was correct, then it implied there could have been a very high dose of toxin.

Religion was noted for 33 of the patients we interviewed. Remarkably, the vast majority (26 [79%]) were Coptic Christians. Six (18%) were Muslims, and one (3%) was Protestant. This is in stark contrast to the population of Egypt. The *2006 World Factbook* estimates that 7.6 million or 10% of Egyptians are Christian (9% Coptic and 1% other denominations).

After completing interviews with hospitalized patients, we conducted a case-control investigation to prove an association with a vehicle. Five families, found through the hospital case investigation, were chosen, and arrangements were made to interview as many family members as possible who had attended a *Sham-el-Nessim* feast. The case definition required illness in a person during the week following *Sham-el-Nessim* with at least three of these symptoms: blurred vision, dysphagia, dry mouth, dyspnea, and constipation. Controls were other family members who shared the *Sham-el-Nessim* feast and did not meet the case definition. Because a detailed list of foods served could not be generated for each family, open-ended questions were asked about foods eaten during the day of the feast. Some family members had died, and the person who appeared most knowledgeable about what they had eaten was interviewed in their stead. There were 16 cases and 26 controls. Their mean ages and male to female ratios differed.

Five hospitalized patients and their family members were interviewed between 23 and 26 April 1991. The 42 people surveyed ranged in age from 5 to 60 years (median, 25); 20 (48%) were male. Thirty-seven (88%) were Coptic Christians, and 5 (12%) were Muslims. Sixteen (38%) reported symptoms of botulism meeting the case definition. The most frequently reported symptom was dry mouth (81%). Other frequently reported symptoms included blurred vision (69%), dysphagia (69%), weakness (69%), dyspnea (69%), and nausea (59%). Five family case-patients died (31%), all within 1 week after onset of illness.

All 16 of the family case-patients reported eating *faseikh* on *Sham-el-Nessim* compared with 10 (38%) of the 26 controls (odds ratio undefined, $P < 0.001$, lower 95% confidence limit of odds ratio = 6.6). Olive oil and lemon were also associated with illness. Olive oil, lemon, and onions are often put on *faseikh*, however, just before serving. When we asked cases and controls about how much they ate, everyone spontaneously described it in hands: a full hand, half a hand, a finger's worth, and so on. We did our best to represent these in fractions of hands. The mean amount of *faseikh* eaten by cases was 0.70 hands and 0.14 hands for controls ($P < 0.01$).

All five of the families in the case-control investigation purchased *faseikh* from the same store, which was in Shobra, the largest Coptic Christian neighborhood in Cairo. All of the families purchased the *faseikh* between April 7 and 9.

Assuming now that contaminated *faseikh* was responsible for the outbreak, the reason for the Coptic Christian majority among the cases becomes clear because *Sham-el-Nessim* fell during the month of the Islamic holiday Ramadan. *Faseikh* would be avoided by observant Muslims during this time not only because of rules regarding daytime fasting, but because of the very salty nature of *faseikh*, it is a highly undesirable food for the thirst that it might provoke during the day. Coptic Christians are under no such constraint and ate the *faseikh*, causing this group to make up 79% of the hospitalized patients and 88% of the family study case patients, vastly larger than their proportion of the general population. The sole Muslim case in the family case-control investigation was menstruating during *Sham-el-Nessim*. Thus, she was exempt from daytime fasting and ate a bit of *faseikh* as a snack on the day of *Sham-el-Nessim*.[4]

Of the 16 cases found in this investigation, 6 (34%) were not reported to the Ministry of Health. Of the patients who were not reported, three experienced only mild symptoms, and a fourth died at home; these four were never hospitalized and demonstrate the limitations of relying only on hospitals for data on cases that have died. Two other patients died in the hospital but were not reported through ad hoc surveillance. All of these unreported cases were found in families with at least one hospitalized patient. There may well have been families in which all cases died or whose illnesses were mild enough to avoid being hospitalized.

Estimating the actual size of the outbreak is difficult, however, because completeness of hospital reporting was not assessed directly, no population based-survey was conducted, and no records of sale of *faseikh* were available from the implicated shop.

> *Estimating the actual size of the outbreak is difficult, however, because completeness of hospital reporting was not assessed directly, no population based-survey was conducted, and no records of sale of* faseikh *were available from the implicated shop.*

We were told anecdotes that suggest there may have been unreported deaths and cases. In one Coptic Christian neighborhood, we came across a coffin maker. Without saying why we were asking, we asked how business was. He promptly replied that even though his sales were up about three coffins a day because of the increased deaths, he was proud to say that he had not raised his prices. The increased sale accounted for about 40 deaths. We were also told by several residents of the same Christian neighborhood that local shops had run out of mourning clothes because there had been so many families with deaths.

FASEIKH PREPARATION

As Americans have turkey as the traditional dish on Thanksgiving, *faseikh* is the traditional dish served during the feast of *Sham-el-Nessim*. Reportedly, it has been made since the time of the Pharaohs. *Faseikh* is an uneviscerated, salted fish. It is made from grey mullet (*Mugil Cephalus*). The fish are gathered from the Red Sea, several salt water lakes, and fish farms in the Nile delta region near the Mediterranean. Of note, grey mullet are found near the shore. To eat, a grey mullet points its head and mouth down toward the mud and sucks and swallows a mouthful of mud and tiny organisms. It can also filter food particles through its gills, expelling mud and debris and swallowing what it finds edible.[5] If *C. botulinum* spores are present within the unfiltered muck, that the gut or gills of the mullet would be contaminated with them when taken out of the water is conceivable. Although *faseikh* is sold throughout the year, it is especially popular on *Sham-el-Nessim*. It is very soft when it's ready to eat. When it's served, people take a portion and spread it on bread.

To understand better how *faseikh* is made, we spoke with several producers and discussed methods known to the Egyptian Ministry of Health inspectors. Fresh fish are collected and arrive in Cairo within several hours. *Faseikh* shop owners indicated that they refuse fish that arrive on ice as this indicates the fish is not fresh. This is the opposite of what I expected to hear because in the United States chilling fish is the norm to preserve its freshness. Shop owners indicated that they prepare *faseikh* themselves in their own shops or another facility. The fish is placed in large plastic or wooden draining trays that are covered with cotton cloth. We were told that the trays are placed in a dark, cool area for putrefaction, never outdoors or in the sun. One shop owner cautioned that placing the fish in the sun gives the fish a "bitter" taste. The fish are left for several hours to one day until they are optimally "swollen" and soft. If there is *C. botulinum* in the fishes' gut at the time, this creates an environment for it to grow and produce toxin, and this has been shown in the laboratory with other fish spiked with spores. Thus, unfortunately, what is good for *faseikh* is good for the organism that causes botulism. It is no surprise that the Arabic word "*faseikh*," roughly translated into English, means "putrid." The final product smells pretty foul, and I do not recommend keeping it in your hotel refrigerator, as I did.

The fish are then placed in wooden barrels with coarse salt placed between layers. Salt is placed as the lowest and uppermost layers. Approximately 1 kilogram of salt is used for each kilogram of fish. Each barrel holds approximately 20 to 30 kilograms of fish plus salt. No other ingredients, such as oil, spices, or lemon juice, are added.

How quickly the salt penetrates into the bowel of the fish is unclear, and if there is *C. botulinum* there, it may still have time to grow before the salt concentration rises too high. If there is an anaerobic environment created by the barrel or if the shop owner who sold the contaminated fish did something to create one is also unclear, which might have been done by putting on an airtight cover.

The uncovered barrel remains in a dark, cool room for 1 week to 1 year. After several weeks, liquid is drawn from the fish by the salt and accumulated in the barrel; large, flat weights are place on the top layer to prevent upward flotation of the fish.

The Ministry of Health food inspectors described a different *faseikh* preparation method that included placing fish in the sun for 1 day for putrefaction and then placing them in barrels sealed with airtight lids.

We wanted to interview the shop owner, but his shop was closed. Shortly after the outbreak, we were told that the Cairo police arrested him and that he remained in jail. The authorities explained that he was in jail for his own safety because a mob might have attacked him. We were told that he denied ever making *faseikh* in his life, and thus, an interview would probably have been unhelpful.

Human botulism is typically caused by one of the serotypes named A, B, and E. It came as no surprise that this was type E because this type is associated with fish and other marine animals. The majority of Americans' experience with it comes from Alaska. There, type E botulism is associated with fermented fish heads, fish eggs, whale meat, and seal flipper that are prepared by Alaska natives using traditional methods.

> *Human botulism is typically caused by one of the serotypes named A, B, and E.*

During the 20 years before the Egypt outbreak, however, the recipes in Alaska changed for convenience. For example, the traditional method for preparing fermented fish heads involves putting 50 or so salmon heads in a clay pit. This changed to using plastic bags at ambient temperature. These changes undoubtedly create more anaerobic conditions as well as a temperature favorable for growth of *C. botulinum* and toxin production.

Three outbreaks of botulism resulted from kapchunka in the United States between 1981 and 1987, causing 3 deaths and 11 illnesses. Kapchunka, an ethnic food usually produced from whitefish, is also known as "rybetz," "ribeyza," or "rostov." Kapchunka is an uneviscerated, salt-cured, air-dried, whole fish that may or may not be smoked. It is consumed without further preparation, such as cooking. The fish are salt cured under minimum refrigeration conditions for a minimum of 25 days and then air dried at ambient temperature for 3 to 7 days. Kapchunka may be smoked before packing and are commonly stored under refrigeration.

The problems with these products are compounded by the difficulty in attaining sufficient levels of salt in all portions of an uneviscerated fish to inhibit the growth of the *C. botulinum*. Consequently, any fish product (greater than 5 inches long) that is salt cured and then dried, smoked, pickled, or fermented is considered by the U.S. Food and Drug Administration to be a potentially life-threatening health hazard. These products are considered hazardous by U.S. Food and Drug Administration whether stored at ambient temperature, refrigerated, or frozen, or whether packaged in air, vacuum, or modified atmosphere. Toxin may be present in these products even when there are no outward signs of microbiological spoilage or other clear indications to alert the consumer.[6]

Thus, perhaps the jailed *faseikh* producer violated the traditional methods of *faseikh* making. Perhaps, because he expected a large sale for *Sham-el-Nessim*, he put the fish in the sun to speed putrefaction. Perhaps he put in less salt, as a cost-cutting measure. Unfortunately, we just do not know what he did.

LABORATORY FINDINGS

We attempted to obtain serum and stool specimens from all hospitalized patients. The Ministry of Health Central Laboratory obtained partially eaten *faseikh* specimens from affected patients. Whole, uneaten specimens of implicated *faseikh* were obtained from a hospitalized patient. When we completed interviewing this patient, he casually asked whether we wanted some of the fish. Rather surprised, we answered yes, and he got out of bed and removed a plastic bag containing a fish from the locker in his room.

The CDC botulism laboratory received specimens from 32 patients but in such small quantity that direct toxin determination by mouse bioassay was not possible. Twenty-five percent of the specimens had positive cultures for *C. botulinum*, type E. These were from stool and postmortem stomach contents.

Faseikh was tested by the CDC and the Egyptian Ministry of Health central laboratory. The fish were reportedly from the single shop, samples of which were obtained from the patient's hospital locker and the Cairo police. These were all positive. Two specimens were titrated and had 16,000 and 64,000 mouse lethal doses per gram, respectively. One lethal human dose equals 7,000 mouse lethal doses. In other words, there was enough toxin in each gram of edible fish to kill between 2 and 10 people. Fresh mullet caught in the region can weigh approximately 1 kilogram.[7]

> *There was enough toxin in each gram of edible fish to kill between 2 and 10 people.*

We traveled around Cairo and purchased samples nonsystematically from other shops, and none of these was positive for toxin or bacteria.

ANTITOXIN SOURCES AND USE

For ethical reasons, no controlled trial to document the efficacy of botulinal antitoxin has been conducted in humans; however, reports suggest that patients with type A and type E botulism who have received trivalent equine antitoxin early in the course of illness fare better than those who have not.

In response to this outbreak, trivalent botulinal antitoxins had been obtained from commercial sources within and outside Egypt by private physicians and patients' family members. The types of antitoxin used were recorded in patient records as dBIG (F(ab')2 "despeciated" heptavalent botulism immune globulin), French/Pasteur, French/Canadian, German, or a combination thereof.

Subsequent to written entreaty by the Egyptian Ministry of Health, 100 vials of dBIG were provided to the Egyptian government for compassionate use under a U.S. Department of Defense investigational protocol.[8] Available records indicated that no fewer than 54 patients in this group (59%) received botulinal antitoxin of at least one type during their hospital stay. Antitoxin regardless of type was not administered, and data were not collected in a systematic fashion that would allow valid analysis of comparative effectiveness. dBIG appeared to be as safe as commercially available antitoxins under these field conditions.

CONCLUSIONS

This outbreak was associated with *faseikh*, a traditional food, supposedly prepared safely for thousands of years; however, we do not know how this particular batch was made, and therefore, we could not assess the likelihood for recurrence.

This outbreak might have affected even more people had there not been the coincidence of the Muslim and Gregorian calendars that put *Sham-el-Nessim* during the holiday of Ramadan; therefore, Muslims were largely spared because of their holiday requirement of fasting and food preferences. This largely restricted the victims to the Coptic Christian community.

After the investigation was concluded, we recommended that the public be warned that *faseikh* can cause botulism. Given the enormous publicity this outbreak received, however, I am confident most people in Egypt were already aware of this. We also recommended a review of the *faseikh* preparation methods and laboratory studies to reproduce *faseikh* preparation methods using "spiked" fish, fish with a known quantity of spores in them. Only through these kinds of experiments can a safe method for preparation be proved, if it exists.

In 2003, the *Al-Ahram Weekly* (online) reported that 12 people died of *faseikh* poisoning and that authorities impounded approximately 38 tons of spoiled fish and arrested nine Cairo shop-keepers for selling "bad fish." The article suggests that safe *faseikh* can be identified by visual and olfactory inspection (which the U.S. Food and Drug Administration, above, states is not reliable because botulinal toxin is colorless and odorless). Nationwide, centers for the treatment of poisoning announced a 48-hour emergency, and "vaccines" (perhaps antitoxin) to treat botulism were distributed.[9]

An average of 145 cases of botulism are reported to the CDC annually. Approximately 15% are foodborne, 65% are infant botulism, and 20% are wound botulism. Because an outbreak from *faseikh* had never happened in Egypt before, because the Gulf War had only recently ended, and because Saddam Hussein had threatened biological warfare, it was suggested that this was the result of a terrorist act. We found no evidence to support this, however.

> *Because an outbreak from faseikh had never happened in Egypt before, because the Gulf War had only recently ended, and because Saddam Hussein had threatened biological warfare, it was suggested that this was the result of a terrorist act.*

On my return to Atlanta from Cairo, I changed planes in Frankfurt. I was pulled out of the line to enter the plane by airport officials, although I do not remember having identified myself to anyone up to that point. They requested that I accompany them to the tarmac. There I saw my baggage, including the typical large, red Coleman coolers that the CDC uses to transport specimens and laboratory equipment. I was asked to identify all of the cables, electronic equipment, and battery-containing items that were in the coolers. They had a list of suspicious items that I assume were detected through X-ray of the containers. These were systematically identified and shown by me within the specified coolers with several men dressed in white shirts and ties holding clipboards reviewing my activity at a distance. The officials then asked for a remaining cooler to be opened. I did this, and the officials poked their heads in and then practically leaped back in response to the smell of *faseikh*. I was ordered to close it up and to return to the check-in line.

REFERENCES

1. Pan Am Flight 103. Retrieved August 28, 2008, from http://en.wikipedia.org/wiki/Pan_Am_Flight_103.
2. Keaney T, Cohen EA. *Gulf War Air Power Survey*. Washington, DC: United States Department of the Air Force, 1993.
3. Weber JT, Hibbs RG Jr, Darwish A, et al. A massive outbreak of type E botulism associated with traditional salted fish in Cairo. *J Infect Dis* 1993;167:451–454.
4. Weber JT, Hatheway CL, Blake PA, Tauxe RV. Clarification of dietary risk factors and religion in a botulism outbreak. *J Infect Dis* 1993;168:258.
5. Artful Angler. Retrieved October 20, 2008, from http://www.artfulangler.co.uk/fishprofiles/fish_profiles_sea_Mullet.htm.
6. Compliance Policy Guidance for FDA Staff Updated: 2005-11-29 Sec. 540.650 Uneviscerated Fish Products that are Salt-cured, Dried, or Smoked (CPG 7108.17). http://www.fda.gov/ora/compliance_ref/cpg/cpgfod/cpg540-650.htm.
7. El-Gharabawy MM, Assem SS. Spawning induction in the Mediterranean grey mullet. *Afr J Biotechnol* 2006;5:1836–1845. Available online at http://www.academicjournals.org/AJB.
8. Hibbs RG, Weber JT, Corwin A, et al. Experience with the use of an investigational F(ab')2 heptavalent botulism immune globulin of equine origin during an outbreak of type E botulism in Egypt. *Clin Infect Dis* 1996;23:337–340.
9. Fish over reason, Al-Ahram Weekly Online May 1–7, 2003: 636. Retrieved October 20, 2008, from http://weekly.ahram.org.eg/2003/636/eg8.htm.
10. Department of Health and Human Services, Centers for Disease Control and Prevention, Botulism. Retrieved October 20, 2008, from http://www.cdc.gov/nczved/dfbmd/disease_listing/botulism_gi.html#9.

LEARNING QUESTIONS

1. Early in this outbreak the case definition was "illness in a hospitalized patient whose physician suspected botulism and who had at least one of the following symptoms: dyspnea, blurred vision, or ptosis (drooping eyelids)." Describe this definition in terms of its sensitivity versus its specificity for botulism and consider why the investigation used this definition rather than one more specific.
2. Later in the investigation, a case-control study was performed. The earlier case definition was abandoned for a revised case definition. Why was the earlier case definition not used for the case-control study?

CHAPTER 12

Controlling an Outbreak of Shigellosis with a Community-Wide Intervention in Lexington, Kentucky

Janet Mohle-Boetani, MD, MPH

Kentucky, 1991

INTRODUCTION

"There's a large outbreak of shigellosis in Kentucky, and we wondered if you could help out." This was the request to me from Dr. Patricia Griffin of the Enterics Branch in the first week of June 1991. Dr. Griffin was in the middle part of her career as a supervisor in the Enterics Branch for the Centers for Disease Control (CDC). She was known by the EIS officers as a supervisor who paid attention to details in an outbreak investigation. She was also very friendly, and I had often talked with her about interesting outbreaks when I ran into her in the elevator in the CDC building.

I had just about completed my first year of EIS in the Bacterial Meningitis and Special Pathogens Branch and had watched enviously as my colleagues in the Enterics Branch, just down the hall from me, were sent to investigate cholera in South America and botulism in Egypt (Todd Weber). Before joining the EIS, I went to Stanford Medical School, where I developed an interest in epidemiology from our pathology classes and worked on epidemiologic studies of ovarian cancer and breast cancer. In my internal medicine residency at Stanford, I developed an interest in infectious diseases; I thought that the EIS program would be an ideal place to both further explore infectious diseases and expand my skills in epidemiology. In Atlanta, I had worked on engaging and complex projects including a cost-effectiveness analysis of preventive measures for neonatal group B streptococcal disease, but I had yet to be involved with a large epidemic, or even a sizable outbreak. Although Lexington, Kentucky did not seem to be the most exotic location to be sent on an outbreak investigation and shigellosis could not have been a more common disease, the opportunity to work on a large outbreak outside of Atlanta was very appealing to me. I enthusiastically accepted the offer.

After a day spent reading all that I could about shigellosis and its control and packing my bags for an estimated 2-week trip, I boarded a plane for Lexington. I remember immediately being struck by the vast grasslands surrounding the airport. There were horse pastures seemingly everywhere; the health department was in close proximity to a fair ground where horses competed in weekly shows. I arrived at the health department at 9 a.m., and the office was bustling with activity. After being introduced to the Commissioner of Health, Dr. John Poundstone, and a crew of public health nurses, I set to work looking into the statistics that had been gathered on the outbreak.

There were 138 culture-confirmed *Shigella sonnei* infections with onsets from January through May; most of these cases were in persons who attended or worked at child care facilities or elementary schools. The public health nurses had been attempting to control the outbreak using standard public health procedures. Cases were defined as laboratory evidence of infection with *Shigella sonnei*. Cases were reported through standard laboratory surveillance. Each case triggered a public health investigation that included a home visit, collection of stools for *Shigella* culture from close contacts, and instruction in handwashing before meals, after toileting, and after diaper changes.

> *Shigella is a Gram-negative organism that is spread through the fecal–oral route or person to person and causes fever, diarrhea, and stomach cramps about 1 to 2 days after ingestion.*

Shigella is a Gram-negative organism that is spread through the fecal–oral route or person to person and causes fever, diarrhea, and stomach cramps about 1 to 2 days after ingestion. The diarrhea is often bloody, and symptoms usually resolve within 1 week. The organism is carried (by persons who are infected but do not have symptoms) and causes disease in only humans (not in other animals). Because the infectious dose is very low and most infected people are only mildly ill and thus remain in contact with other people, outbreaks are common.

Shigella organisms were discovered more than 100 years ago by Shiga, a Japanese scientist. There are three major species of *Shigella*. *Shigella sonnei* causes two thirds of infections in the United States, and the other third of infections are primarily caused by *Shigella flexnerii*. *Shigella dysenteriae type 1* cause toxic diarrheal epidemics in the developing world.

Public health professionals (primarily public health nurses) also visited all schools and child care centers that were attended by children with culture-confirmed shigellosis. All classmates of culture-confirmed cases were tested for shigellosis. Children in preschool or daycare were excluded while symptomatic (with diarrhea) day care center staff, teachers, and elementary school children were excluded from school or work until they had three consecutive stool cultures negative for *Shigella*.

In March, the health department mailed a notification to the directors of all licensed child care facilities (preschools, day care centers, and family day care homes). The notification included information about the outbreak and advised them to require handwashing on arrival to the facility, after diaper changes, after toileting, and before eating or preparing food.

Despite these meticulous and well-documented investigations, exclusion policies, and notifications, the outbreak persisted and spread throughout the community through the end of May. There was understandable frustration in not being able to control the outbreak, despite following standard public health practices. There was also concern that the outbreak would be exacerbated by summer activities. Because *Shigella* infections are spread person to person and through food handling, shigellosis typically increases in the summer because of increased congregations of people in areas without hygienic facilities (e.g., at camps) or sharing home prepared food items (e.g., weekend picnics). For these reasons, assistance in controlling the outbreak was sought first from the state health department and then from the CDC.

> *Because Shigella infections are spread person to person and through food handling, shigellosis typically increases in the summer because of increased congregations of people in areas without hygienic facilities (e.g., at camps) or sharing home prepared food items (e.g., weekend picnics).*

INITIAL INVESTIGATION AND RECOMMENDATIONS

In the afternoon of my first day, one of the public health nurses took me to a few of the child care facilities that had outbreaks of shigellosis. Despite recent training and written notifications by the public health nurses regarding the need to wash hands, we observed barriers to handwashing in most of the centers we visited. For example, the sinks were too high for children to reach, and no step stools were readily available for the children to get access to the sink after going to the toilet. Also, sinks were not easily accessible to the areas chosen for diaper changing.

After reviewing the data and conducting observations at child care facilities for a few more days, my supervisor in Atlanta, Dr. Griffin, and I developed recommendations for the Lexington Health Department. We recommended promotion of handwashing community wide, surveillance for diarrhea, and rapid diagnosis and treatment of shigellosis. We emphasized handwashing promotion over collection of stool specimens.

I worked diligently on the weekend and called Dr. Griffin at her home to check in on the wording of some of the recommendations. In the middle of one of these very intense conversations, she exclaimed "Wow, he did it!" I asked, "What?" "My son just pooped in his potty chair—his first time!" I found this particularly comical given that we had just been talking about how to phrase our recommendation to wash hands after helping children use the toilet.

An additional recommendation that Dr. Griffin and I developed was that the health department should stop collecting stool specimens from asymptomatic convalescing school children, teachers, and day care staff. We felt that these groups, even though recently infected, would be very unlikely to transmit *Shigella* if they had formed stools and could be relied on to wash their hands after going to the toilet. We also recommended against the practice of testing asymptomatic contacts of persons with shigellosis. We reasoned that the decreased burden of specimen collection, ensuring exclusions from work or school, and following up on multiple stool culture results would permit the public health professionals to focus on handwashing in key locations where people congregated and would permit a proactive rather than reactive approach.

Because we could not be certain that preschool aged children could be expected to wash their hands reliably, we recommended that asymptomatic convalescing preschool aged children be excluded from group child care until two stool cultures were negative for *Shigella*. This recommendation was a policy change from the practice of excluding children from child care facilities only during the time that they had diarrhea. Although we anticipated an increased workload in following these children, we expected that there would be a substantial decrease in workload in following cultures from asymptomatic contacts and from asymptomatic, convalescing, school-aged children and adults.

INITIAL RESPONSE

The Lexington County Health Department responded vigorously to our recommendations. On June 10th, the day after we provided our recommendations, the Commissioner of Health created a Shigella Task Force consisting of health department staff from the clinic, the laboratory, the field service section, the school health section and the environmental health division. The commissioner called a meeting with key leaders in each of these areas and presented our recommendations. I believe the commissioner created the task force to empower the leaders to take responsibility for controlling the outbreak. I credit the commissioner's leadership skills as responsible for the effectiveness of the committee. The leaders decided to implement a community-wide handwashing campaign with monitoring of handwashing at sites controlled by community services considered to be at high risk of transmission. The task force initiated onsite handwashing promotion at day care centers, summer schools, summer camps, and free lunch sites. The handwashing promotion included problem solving at each site to ensure that appropriate handwashing could be accomplished everyday.

> *I believe the commissioner created the task force to empower the leaders to take responsibility for controlling the outbreak.*

In the 3 to 4 days after the creation of the task force, I accompanied public health professionals on several of their site visits to child care facilities, elementary schools, summer camps, and free lunch sites. At each of these sites, I observed the direct advice and problem solving of the public health professionals and recorded and photographed key areas of concern regarding handwashing. For example, we observed and recorded children lining up for free lunches without handwashing and a paucity of handwashing facilities available at summer camps. At child care centers, we observed sinks that were too high for the children to reach to wash their hands. At schools, we observed that no soap was available in some of the bathrooms; this was a safety issue because children would squirt soap on the floor and then slip on the soap. I planned to return to each of these sites in a few weeks to observe changes in the accessibility of soap and water and handwashing practices.

Watching the community join together to implement rapidly community-wide handwashing was one of the most rewarding experiences of my tenure at the CDC. After creating the task force, assistance in handwashing promotion was sought from the community at large. To engage the community, Dr. Poundstone held a press conference and sought cooperation from the media, the Parks and Recreation Office, the Community Services Agency, and the school board. A local television station aired a video several evenings each week that emphasized the prevention of shigellosis through handwashing and taught proper handwashing technique. The Community Services Agency and the Parks and

Recreation provided liquid soap and water to all free lunch sites and summer camps. The school board ensured that all summer students viewed a video on shigellosis and handwashing and that all students would be monitored in handwashing on arrival to school, after using the toilet, and before eating lunch or snacks. I believe that it was Dr. Poundstone's leadership and a strong local public health infrastructure that permitted the rapid implementation of these community-wide preventive actions within a week of my arrival to Lexington.

> *An additional change that was implemented was enhanced surveillance for diarrhea.*

An additional change that was implemented was enhanced surveillance for diarrhea. Child care facilities and elementary summer schools were directed to keep track of illnesses from school or day care and to advise those with diarrhea to seek rapid diagnosis and treatment at the health department clinic. The health department set up a special diarrhea clinic so that persons with diarrhea would not need to wait for an appointment to get tested and treated. All patients were instructed in handwashing in the clinic.

After observing the implementation of the handwashing campaign, I needed to leave Lexington to attend the international conference on AIDS in Florence, Italy. This was a conference that I funded on my own, to present a paper from work I had done during my internal medicine residency. Coincidentally, some of the work that I collaborated on regarding bacillary angiomatosis while I was an EIS officer was also being presented (this is an unusual systemic disease occurring primarily in immunocompromised persons due to infection with the bacteria *Bartonella quintana* or *Bartonella henselae*). As can be imagined, I had a very enjoyable week, both at the conference and traveling in Italy with my boyfriend (now husband) Mark. Mark lived in California while I was in Atlanta, and we very much appreciated any time that we could spend together.

THE SECOND PHASE

The week away was also ideally timed from an investigation standpoint. My departure from Lexington permitted the health department and greater community to implement the handwashing campaign unencumbered by meetings with me. I returned to Lexington just before the 4th of July, and I remember spending a great day with the family of one of the public health nurses; we swam in her backyard swimming pool and ate lots of watermelon. The personal relationships developed in the context of an intense outbreak investigation are a major unspoken reward of field investigations. The public health staff members that I met in Lexington were warm, gracious, and appreciative. Their dedication to public health and collaborative spirit were a large part of the inspiration leading to my decision to pursue a career in public health instead of academic medicine.

After my return to Lexington from Europe, my goals were to (1) observe the implementation of handwashing in a diversity of sites in the community and (2) conduct a study to attempt to determine risk factors for outbreaks of shigellosis in child care facilities. Although many child care facilities had outbreaks, there were several that had no cases or only one case; we wanted to determine whether there were predictors for the spread of shigellosis in child care facilities that could be modified to prevent outbreaks in the future.

My first goal was met through going back to the same sites I had originally visited in the week just before the handwashing campaign. I was elated to see dramatic changes at all of the sites that I visited. For example, at a summer camp where there had been limited access to handwashing facilities, handwashing stations were set up close to the latrines. In the outside picnic area where the children had lunch, two outside sinks were designated as handwashing sinks, and I observed the Parks and Recreation staff requiring children to line up and wash their hands before receiving their lunch. At the camp site, they even incorporated handwashing into one of their routine cheers ("Give me an H, give me an A, give me an N....What's that spell?").

At a free lunch site in the middle of a housing project, soap dispensers were installed in the two outside sinks, and I observed the community service workers monitoring children in washing their hands before providing them with their lunches. At child care centers, I noted the addition of step stools to sinks to ensure that young children could reach the sinks and that nurses had worked with facilities to create diaper changing areas that were close to handwashing facilities (this was particularly challenging at times). I observed elementary schools lining children up to wash their hands before lunch. I documented all of these changes with "after-intervention" photographs. The collection of before and after photos was used to create an instructional video directed to local health departments on controlling a community-wide shigellosis outbreak.

To accomplish the second goal, I worked together with an epidemiologist from the state public health department, Margaret Stapleton, MSPH. My supervisor in Atlanta had also changed. Dr. Griffin was on a summer vacation, and Dr. Paul Blake, the Enterics Branch chief, was filling in. I found it refreshing to have a new supervisor for this phase of the investigation. By this point, I had learned a lot from Dr. Griffin about controlling the outbreak and providing recommendations to a local agency. In this next stage of the investigation, I hoped to do a field analytic study that would provide practical recommendations; I was not disappointed.

On another memorable weekend call, Dr. Blake and I developed a plan for a case-control study. In the information collected by the health department, I had noted that some child care centers had large outbreaks, whereas others had no cases. We wondered whether those centers with no cases were different than those that had large outbreaks. We reasoned that if we could determine factors associated with large outbreaks we could use them in recommendations to prevent outbreaks in the future. We decided to conduct a case-control study in which the "case" was a center with at least three cases of shigellosis among children and a "control" was a center with no cases of shigellosis. Although this method differs from the standard case-control study in which cases are defined as illness in individual people, we felt that the method should work in comparing centers with and without outbreaks.

The health department supplied me with a list of all licensed child care centers and family day care homes in the county as well as basic characteristics of those facilities and the number of culture-confirmed cases of shigellosis identified among children attending each facility. I found that all centers with at least three cases enrolled diapered children and children whose child care fees were paid through a federally funded program (indicating a low socioeconomic level). Because both having children in diapers and low socioeconomic status are known risk factors for outbreaks of shigellosis, we felt we needed to control for these factors. Given the small size of the study (only six "case centers"), we felt the most efficient method of controlling for socioeconomic status was to restrict the control centers to those with diapered children, at least five children who had fees paid by the federally funded program, and no cases of shigellosis. Thirteen centers met the criteria for control centers.

Ms. Stapleton and I collected the information for the case-control study through onsite interviews. First we created a questionnaire addressing policies and procedures and observations. Ms. Stapleton interviewed the directors about practices and policies while I asked the same questions of a staff member who cared for diapered children. We also collected the number of children by age group and the number of toilets used by each age group. Comparing notes with Margaret after our respective interviews was another memorable part of this field investigation. The discordance between the director and staff interviews was notable.

We found an association between having a food preparer (a staff who mixed formula or a cook) who changed diapers and having at least three cases of shigellosis in the facility (100% of case centers vs. 46% of control centers, $P = 0.04$). We found a greater median toddler-to-toilet ratio (the number of 3 year olds per flushable toilet) in the case centers than in the control centers (the ratio was 20 in case centers and 13 in the control centers, $P < 0.05$). We also found an association between the provision of transportation from home to the center and shigellosis (83% of case centers provided transportation vs. 15% of the control centers).

Differences in the response of directors and staff to hygiene questions were identified. Although 42% of staff reported that a cook changed diapers, only 11% of directors reported these combined duties. Directors were also more likely than staff to report that they had policies to prevent diarrhea (89% vs. 32%).

Thus, the case-control study did reveal features of centers amenable to changes that could help to prevent diarrheal outbreaks. Food should be prepared by persons who do not change diapers, if possible. The high toddler-to-toilet ratio found in the case centers could be a reflection of inadequate sinks to permit accessible handwashing. We felt that the finding of transportation associated with the case centers might be a reflection of a tendency to mix different age groups of children, permitting the introduction and spread of communicable diseases such as shigellosis. The discordant answers to questions by staff and directors highlights both (1) the importance of querying staff, in addition to directors, when doing investigations in facilities, and (2) that staff in child care centers may need additional training in infection control.

The second part of my investigation was also rewarding because I was able to observe a rapid decline in the reported cases of shigellosis. The epidemic curve showed an abrupt decrease in cases in the week after community-wide interventions were initiated in mid June (Figure 12-1).[1] Although in June there were 42 cases, in July there were only 10 and subsequently cases were reported at a very low rate, 2 to 14 per month. With the outbreak under control, I spent the last weekend at a horse show and visiting the Appalachian mountains (as suggested by Margaret), where I acquired a woolen

```
January 1991 – the Lexington-Fayette County Health Department receives three reports of
Shigella sonnei infections from the University of Kentucky microbiology laboratory
```

```
January 1 through July 15, 1991 – 186 culture-confirmed S. sonnei infections reported to the
health department
```

```
Investigation identifies that 47% of the initial 111 S. sonnei infections of all ages were
attributed to child day care attendance
```

```
June 1991 – the health department creates a Shigella task force
• Creation of diarrhea clinic to facilitate proper diagnosis and treatment
• Intensification of infection-control training
• Intensification of surveillance for shigellosis
• Encouragement of community-based participation in prevention efforts
• Monitoring of hand washing at day care centers, elementary schools, summer camps,
  and free-lunch sites
```

```
Three weeks after intensive interventions initiated, a substantial decline of culture-confirmed
cases is observed
```

FIGURE 12-1 Timeline of shigellosis outbreak in Lexington-Fayette County, Kentucky, 1991. Data from Kolanz M, Sandifer J, Poundstone J, Stapleton M, Finger R. Shigellosis in child day care centers—Lexington-Fayette County, Kentucky. *MMWR* 1992;41:440–442.

blanket, hand woven by students in Berea College that I use to this day.

CONCLUSION

During this investigation, I learned several lessons. First, some standard public health practices such as stool collection among contacts can divert precious public health resources from health promotion and prevention. Second, community-wide interventions are possible with strong leadership and an effectively functioning health department that is able to collaborate productively with the community at large. Third, the case-control study approach can be used with the facility as the unit (for a case or control) to determine facility characteristics that are associated with disease. Fourth, I learned the rewards of direct field investigation and developed a deep respect for local public health professionals. Finally, I learned that you do not need to be in an exotic location or work on an exotic disease to have a rewarding experience investigating an outbreak. Working on this shigellosis outbreak in Lexington, Kentucky was definitely one of the most gratifying experiences of my EIS career and was a turning point in my decision to work in public health at the local level.

REFERENCES

1. Mohle-Boetani, JC, Stapleton M, Finger R, et al. Community wide shigellosis: control of an outbreak and risk factors in child day-care centers. *Am J Public Health* 1995;85:812–816.

LEARNING QUESTIONS

1. This outbreak illustrates the importance of promoting an effective intervention in a community setting. What did the author and her collaborators do to maximize the success of hand washing promotion?
2. The author refers to finding discordance in her case-control study of day care centers. What discordance was found and how may its recognition have been helpful to the author and the health department?
3. Which steps of outbreak investigation are illustrated in this chapter? Where in the chapter are those steps illustrated?

CHAPTER 13

Pork Tapeworm in an Orthodox Jewish Community: Arriving at a Biologically Plausible Hypothesis

Peter M. Schantz, VMD, PhD, and Mary E. Bartlett, BA

New York, 1990

INTRODUCTION

I had known about neurocysticercosis in veterinary school and experienced it first hand in my first year postveterinary school when I spent a year (1965–1966) as an Academic Fellow at the Department of Parasitology at the Faculty of Medicine, National University of Mexico, Mexico City. It was of special interest to me because it was a cestode (tapeworm) associated with animals.

Neurocysticercosis was usually diagnosed at autopsy at that time, as computerized tomography (CT) and other powerful diagnostic imaging technology were not yet available. I knew that people died from it—seen by pathologists—killed by fatal seizures or by obstruction of flow of cerebrospinal fluid, obstructive hydrocephalus. A tiny minority of people died from the disease—many were asymptomatic.

The adult worm in the human intestine is flat (like all tapeworms), and *Taenia solium* is commonly referred to as the pork tapeworm because of a unique relationship between humans and pigs that allows this particular parasite to thrive. Humans are the only (definitive) host that can harbor the adult tapeworm. When a man or woman eats the meat of an infected pig that is harboring cysticerci (the larval stage tapeworm), the worm develops inside the intestines and attaches itself to the bowel wall. Proglottids (egg-producing factories) are then detached from the tapeworm and released individually or in small "chains" in the feces. The tiny eggs contain tinier larvae, or embryos. If the worm could consciously strategize, it would want its eggs to make their way to another pig so that the larvae can encyst in this human food source and keep the cycle going for its perpetual survival. The likelihood of successful transmission of the tapeworm is favored by the common practice of pigs to eat human feces (coprophagy). The tapeworm has been successful at this for thousands of years (at least). More is presented on the life cycle later; however, it is pretty obvious from this life cycle that persons who eat pork are at potential risk for this disease.

> *Humans are the only (definitive) host that can harbor the adult tapeworm.*

As an anthropology undergraduate major, I had long been fascinated by other cultures and practices. Veterinary medicine too was a passion, and public heath

*Chapter 13 is written from the experiences of Dr. Schantz.

was a means of merging these two interests. Dr. James H. Steele, then Chief Veterinary Officer in the U.S. Public Health Service, spoke to my class in public health at the University of Pennsylvania School of Veterinary Medicine on the role of and opportunities for veterinarians in public health; Jim has been and remains an important mentor to this day.

After postgraduate studies in epidemiology with Professor Calvin Schwabe at the University of California, Davis, I worked in South America with the Pan American Zoonoses Center (PAHO/WHO) in Buenos Aires, Argentina, where I was epidemiologist and head of the zoonosis laboratory. Before the outbreak described here, I had experienced several memorable field investigations at the Centers for Disease Control (CDC) as an Epidemic Intelligence Service (EIS) Officer during 1974 to 1976. I investigated clusters of cases of echinococcosis in the Navajo, Santo Domingo, and Zuni tribes in New Mexico and Arizona. I had been recruited to the CDC by Myron Schultz, MD, DVM (then Director of the Division of Parasitic Diseases).

The CDC was challenged to develop a serodiagnostic assay for neurocysticercosis in response to increasing numbers of clinical calls from physicians all over the country who were newly diagnosing the disease. Because of my prior experience with the disease in Mexico, I assisted in handling the clinical calls at the Division of Parasitic Diseases. At that time (the 1970s), new diagnostics were being developed that would detect cystic lesions in the brain (e.g., CT), which uniquely permitted detection and characterization of intracerebral pathology; however, the intracerebral cysts resembled some other possible pathologic conditions and a specific immunoassay for *Taenia solium* cysticercosis was needed to help confirm the nature and viability of the intracerebral lesions.

My veterinary colleague, Professor John Eckert, Director of the Institute of Parasitic Diseases at the University of Zurich, Switzerland, arranged for his graduate student, Bruno Gottstein, to come to the CDC to acquire experience working in our parasitology program. Under the supervision of Victor Tsang, PhD, Bruno developed an immunoblot assay for serologic diagnosis of *Taenia solium* cysticercosis with high specificity and improved sensitivity. Because cysticercosis is a larval tapeworm cyst disease that localizes in tissues of the brain and muscles, it was difficult to diagnose. The development of an immunoblot assay was an important advance as prior serodiagnostics were nonspecific and had poorly defined sensitivity.

THE INVESTIGATION

Physicians in the United States were not usually familiar with neurocysticercosis because the tapeworm (*Taenia solium*) was not transmitted locally in its life cycle, although cases were seen occasionally in immigrants from Mexico and some other Latin American countries.[1] The development and growing availability of CT scans in the 1980s provided a unique diagnostic technology for detection and characterization of a wide variety of pathological conditions within the central nervous system and other organs. Magnetic resonance imaging further improved technology for brain scanning. After CT and magnetic resonance imaging became widely available for scanning of the brain, together with the immunoblot test, diagnosis of this problem in the United States became more frequent. Most U.S. physicians were not familiar with this disease, and thus, they frequently consulted the CDC for assistance with serologic diagnosis and clinical management decisions when they suspected it. I was the person who most often took those calls because it had become one of my areas of specialization. With rare exceptions, the patients who were subjects of these queries were immigrants from Mexico or other countries where *T. solium* was endemic.

Thus, in 1990, when we started getting calls from physicians in New York City about persons who were not the typical case seen in immigrants, but rather in persons who were born in New York City (and in fact had never traveled outside the United States), I knew we had to look more closely at the situation. Unlike some outbreaks, this one was not explosive. The number of cases was small. There were four persons who were evaluated with recurring seizures.[2] When they received brain imaging, lesions were present that were radiologically consistent with cysticerci; however, what was especially puzzling was the population that this infection was being diagnosed in. These were Orthodox Jewish persons who were 6 to 39 years old. One had been born in Morocco and lived in the United States since 1976, and another had traveled to and spent 1 week in an area where cysticercosis is known to be endemic; however, that travel was 8 years before the onset of his symptoms. It is a religious practice that Orthodox Jews do not eat pork. Thus, this question arose: "How do Orthodox Jewish people get infected with a pork tapeworm?" At this point, we needed to establish a biologically plausible hypothesis to explain what we were observing.

Knowledge of the life cycle of this tapeworm played a fundamental role in considering what questions to

> *Knowledge of the life cycle of this tapeworm played a fundamental role in considering what questions to ask and which answers to dismiss or consider important.*

ask and which answers to dismiss or consider important. Persons who eat cyst-infected pork can become infected with *Taenia solium*, and the tapeworm establishes in their intestines; however, persons who ingest the tapeworm eggs (passed in the stool of persons infected with the tapeworm) become infected with the cystic larval stages of the tapeworm (Figure 13-1). Embryonic larvae (oncospheres) emerge from the tapeworm's eggs, penetrate the intestines, and migrate through the blood stream of the egg ingester and encyst widely in the body. They may encyst in the brain and produce neurologic symptoms, including those observed in the four index cases, such as seizures or aphasia (difficulty using or understanding words). Other neurological changes could occur depending on where in the brain the cyst(s) is/are located.

The unresolved question when facing this group of cases was how did these Orthodox Jews ingest pork tapeworm eggs if they do not eat pork and typically spend much of their time with other Orthodox Jews?

Questioning of their physicians and interviewing family members revealed that a common practice in the community was to hire persons from Mexico as household laborers (domestics) with primary responsibility for food preparation and childcare. Although good hygiene, including rigorous hand washing, would minimize the possibility of exposure of other persons to the tapeworm eggs passed in the stools of infected house maids, such fastidious hygiene was apparently not uniformly practiced in this setting. It can be assumed that the tapeworm-infected domestic servants were having eggs deposited in their perianal area and, at least occasionally, contaminating their hands, which could then have engaged in preparing a salad or other food item for the family that employed them. They also could have had direct hand contact with family members (i.e., childcare) that allowed transfer of the eggs. This tapeworm can live for many months if not many years so the opportunity for someone with *Taenia* infection to infect others may be prolonged. We discovered that there was a clandestine service that organized and facilitated transport of these household laborers from Mexico City to Los Angeles, then to New York City, and probably to other destinations. We did not pursue the details of the labor practices and childcare, as it would have put us in a situation in which the immigrant workers might become reluctant to talk to us. This might threaten the relationship with the local community that employed them and our ability to discern the sources of infection.

For these Mexican women, this clandestine employment was a path out of poverty. They were young, unmarried, and "right off the farm," and you can probably guess what livestock species was present on that farm. In poor areas of rural Mexico, there is often a lack of disposal of human feces in a completely safe and sanitary manner, which gives roaming pigs access and opportunity to ingest tapeworm eggs shed in feces by infected humans.[1] We did not pursue their stories, all of the details of their coming to live and work in New York City, but clearly they were coming from communities where pork tapeworm infection was not rare and pork was a common staple food.

I engaged my colleague in the Division of Parasitic Diseases, EIS Officer Anne Moore, PhD, MD, to followup the outbreak with a serosurvey of the extended families and other members of the involved community.[3] Serologic testing for cysticercosis antibodies was performed to detect people who had been exposed and infected with *T. solium* larva but had not necessarily developed symptoms of the disease. We drew blood on a volunteer basis anonymously. We had good cooperation in no small part because it was a very well-organized community of middle-class families in the New York City boroughs of Brooklyn and Queens. They had an efficient communications network through the temples, and after they were advised of what was happening—that is, people were having seizures—they cooperated because they recognized it to be in their best interest to do so.

Using the enzyme-linked immunoelectrotransfer blot, 17 immediate family members of the cases were tested. Seven persons among 11 tested from families of 2 of the patients were seropositive. Among these 11 family members who went on to also have magnetic resonance imaging, lesions were identified in two of the seropositive family members (both children). They were 6 and 2 years old, respectively. Coincidentally, the day before she was scheduled to have a screening brain magnetic resonance imaging the 6-year-old had a prolonged seizure.

In the past 5 years, each of the four families had employed an average of three housekeepers from Mexico. One of these families had employed at least 10 women; however, it was not possible to identify the particular individuals who were the most likely sources of

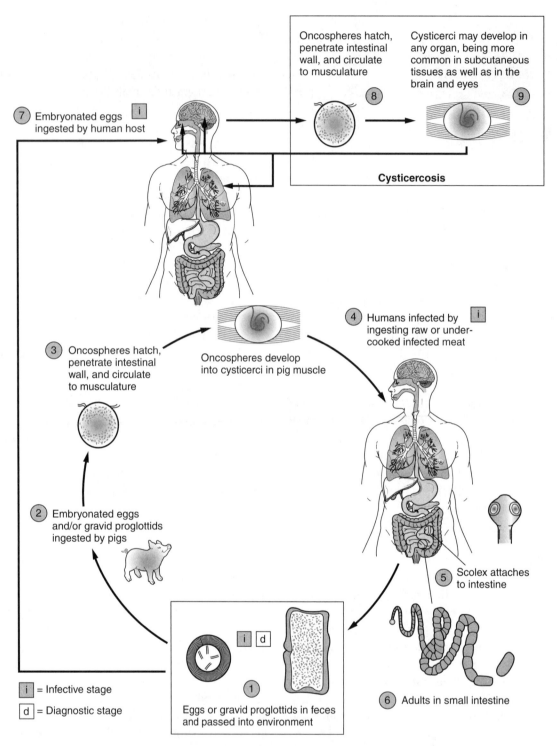

FIGURE 13-1 Cysticercosis. From Centers for Disease Control and Prevention. Cysticercosis. Available at: http://www.dpd.cdc.gov/dpdx/HTML/Cysticercosis.htm. Last accessed October 29, 2008.

the infections because most of these women were not available for testing. In the case of the family of a 16-year-old female patient (in which none of her three immediate family members were seropositive), serum was drawn from one of the housekeepers, and it tested positive for antibodies in the CDC enzyme-linked immunosorbent assay for cysticercosis. Examining her stool revealed *Taenia* sp. eggs. When told of her results, both she and the other housekeeper refused any further interviewing or examination and left the home.[2]

COMMENTS ON THE UNIQUENESS OF THIS OUTBREAK

Taenia solium, the "pork" tapeworm, is not transmitted in its natural life cycle in the United States because swine husbandry practices rarely permit pigs to have access to human feces, a requirement for perpetuation of the life cycle of the tapeworm. Nevertheless, the disease is seen commonly in immigrants, mainly from Mexico and some other countries where the infection is endemic, who acquired their infections in their native homeland but may experience first onset of clinical disease after immigration to the United States. It is the nature of the disease that the larval tapeworm cysts (cysticerci) may exist within the brain for months or years without producing any symptoms of illness. Clinical cases of cysticercosis, larval stage *T. solium* disease, are commonly seen in hospitals and emergency clinics, usually in immigrant patients who were previously unaware of having the infection. These same individuals are also at risk of carrying the "pork tapeworm" (*T. solium*) in their intestines, which they had acquired in their home country through ingestion of uncooked pork containing the cysticerci. This intestinal-stage tapeworm infection is usually without symptoms, although the carriers may be aware of passing tapeworm segments ("proglottids") in the stools. Tapeworm carriers are important to the life cycle and maintenance of the infection if their feces are available to swine, which are the key intermediate hosts for the tapeworm. Coprophagy is a behavior characteristic of swine and allows the transmission of this infection in its human–pig life cycle. Tapeworm carriers are also the source of cysticercosis in humans when humans accidentally ingest food contaminated with feces containing the eggs of the adult tapeworm. The source of the cysticercosis may be the tapeworm carrier himself or herself as a result of direct or indirect fecal contamination.

The cause of the seizures experienced in this community was not apparent until several of the patients had been placed under specialist care with the assistance of the New York City Health Department and the CDC. No one at the local community hospitals had prior experience with this infection and its potential dangers. Surgeons who conducted brain biopsies sent the lesions to pathologists who recognized them as cysticerci (larval stages) of *T. solium*. After the cause and source of the infections were understood, it allowed the investigations to go forward and resulted in development of educational and preventive measures that promptly prevented further transmission.

REFERENCES

1. Despommier DD. Tapeworm infection: the long and the short of it. *N Engl J Med* 1992;327:727–728.
2. Schantz PM, Moore AC, Munoz JL, et al. Neurocysticercosis in an Orthodox Jewish community in New York City. *N Engl J Med* 1992;327:692–695.
3. Moore A, Lutwick LL, Schantz PM, et al. Seroprevalence of cysticercosis in an Orthodox Jewish community. *Am J Trop Med Hyg* 1995;53:439–442.

LEARNING QUESTIONS

1. Referring to the life cycle of the tapeworm, what determines if a human infected with *Taenia solium* will become an egg passer versus potentially have cysts in the brain?
2. Let us say a physician on the Board of Health for New York City learned of this investigation and its outcome and recommended that all Mexican housekeepers should be tested for *T. solium* in their stool. How would you respond to such a policy recommendation?

CHAPTER 14

The Massive Waterborne Outbreak of *Cryptosporidium* Infections, Milwaukee, Wisconsin, 1993

Jeffrey P. Davis, MD
Wisconsin, 1993

INTRODUCTION: APRIL 5, 1993

On Monday morning, April 5, Dr. Gerald Sedmak, a virologist with the City of Milwaukee Health Department (MHD), received calls from individual citizens complaining of gastrointestinal illnesses. Gerry told other MHD staff about these complaints, and in turn, these staff members began an effort to see whether there was an unusual number of individuals with similar gastrointestinal illness—indeed, there were. Kathy Blair, a registered nurse and epidemiologist with the MHD, received calls from the South Milwaukee Health Department, other local agencies, and private citizens regarding widespread occupational and school absenteeism related to diarrheal illness. Gerry, Kathy, and their colleagues could not have known at that time that these were the initial reports of what would unfold as a historically large and unprecedented waterborne outbreak in the United States. Many pharmacies on the south side of Milwaukee had or were nearly sold out of antimotility medications (medication to slow down or stop diarrhea). Additionally, many health care providers were ill and unable to work. Concomitantly, Dr. Steve Gradus, director of the MHD Bureau of Laboratories, and his colleague, Dr. Ajaib Singh, conducted telephone surveys of hospital emergency rooms and laboratories. They learned of an extreme number of weekend visits for diarrhea-related illnesses to emergency departments and increased numbers of requisitions for bacterial culture of stool specimens. The St. Luke's Hospital microbiology laboratory exhausted its supply of media used to isolate enteric bacterial pathogens. Based on this information, MHD officials suspected that the outbreak was predominantly affecting the southern part of Milwaukee and included other municipalities in southern Milwaukee County. Initial newspaper and other media reports circulating on April 5 focused on the unusual number of diarrhea illnesses, the unknown etiology of the illness, and the shortage of antidiarrhea medications. Media interest intensified rapidly.

Kathy called Jim Kazmierczak, DVM, an epidemiologist and colleague in the Bureau of Public Health (BPH), Wisconsin Division of Health (DOH; now named the Wisconsin Division of Public Health), notified him of these events, and inquired whether DOH staff were aware of an unusual occurrence of similar illnesses elsewhere in the state. Up to then we had not been told of similar illnesses elsewhere.

During my initial conversations with Kathy and Jim that morning, we discussed the potential of any one of several etiologic agents to be associated with these events and the need for good laboratory data and illness characterization. Although the agent was not yet known, my initial impression was the illness must be considered to be waterborne until proven otherwise because of the magnitude and widespread occurrence of diarrhea illness. Concomitantly, Drs. Gradus and Singh discovered that most hospital microbiology laboratory staff members were not conducting virus culture of stool specimens and that tests for ova and parasites were infrequently ordered. Accordingly, infection control practitioners were selected to facilitate collection of stool specimens for virus culture at the MHD from the next 10 patients presenting at their facilities with diarrhea illnesses.

Later, we discussed the MHD plan to widely distribute stool kits for virus testing to clinics to test individuals with acute diarrhea illnesses and the results to date of testing for bacterial enteric pathogens at St. Luke's Hospital. We sensed that this was a really big outbreak when we learned that from this one hospital on one weekend about 200 stool specimens were obtained for bacterial culture, and we were confronted with a really big clue when we learned that, despite this high volume of testing, all cultures were negative to date for bacterial enteric pathogens. I suggested testing stool specimens already known to be negative for bacterial enteric pathogens and still remaining at the St. Luke's laboratory for parasitic and protozoan infections at the MHD laboratory. The MHD laboratory was one of two public health laboratories in Wisconsin. The emerging scope and breadth of this outbreak diminished the likelihood that this was a viral illness, and it was important to consider protozoan infections, as they could be associated with large community outbreaks.

Steve arranged for this testing and also requested that microbiology laboratory supervisors begin aggressively testing diarrhea stool specimens for protozoan infections, with specific emphasis on testing for *Cryptosporidium*. Steve also planned to review water treatment records that would be available from the City of Milwaukee Water Works (MWW), the municipal water utility.

Because of the apparent magnitude of the outbreak and implications for residents in multiple jurisdictions, I offered the onsite assistance of DOH staff to join the MHD in the investigation. We would need Tuesday, April 6 to structure a team and plan our activities in Milwaukee and would drive to Milwaukee from Madison early on Wednesday, April 7. The offer of assistance was accepted.

APRIL 6, 1993

On April 6, I spoke with Steve to discuss the findings of his review of the MWW water treatment records. He described some initial resistance to review the records and defense of the quality of Milwaukee's water by the MWW administrators, but he was able to review some recent water treatment records. Generally, during recent weeks, there were increases in coliform counts that were consistent with substantial rainfall at water intake points; however, chlorine levels were high, and *E. coli* counts were within Department of Natural Resources (DNR) recommendations after treatment. Steve also noted spikes in treated water turbidity (one of many measures of water quality) occurred in late March primarily at the South plant, one of the two municipal water treatment facilities operated by the MWW. Turbidity is a technical measure of particles suspended in water. Turbidity can be measured in raw, untreated water and in finished, treated water. Steve was impressed with peaks in turbidity values of treated water on successive days.

While we were discussing these unusual turbidity test results, Steve recalled the Carrollton, Georgia, outbreak of waterborne *Cryptosporidium* infections involving an estimated 13,000 diarrhea illnesses—a lot of illness by any measure.[1] The Carrollton outbreak was associated with a filtered water supply; however, the peak filtered water turbidity was less than 1 nephelometric turbidity unit (NTU). That was surprisingly low. The NTU values in Milwaukee were considerably greater. Based on Steve's preliminary information, the potential that *Cryptosporidium* was the etiologic agent in the Milwaukee outbreak seemed increasingly likely. I requested Steve to arrange a meeting early on April 7 with the MWW directors and an opportunity for our staff to review the water treatment records. This would be our first meeting in Milwaukee after arriving on site.

Typically, notifiable enteric diseases are reported when an etiologic agent is laboratory confirmed, although in Wisconsin outbreaks were to be reported upon suspicion regardless of whether the etiology is known. Also, relatively few individuals with true notifiable infections ever get tested, and diarrhea without laboratory data is not reported by physicians. Thus, several strategic surveillance activities were planned. I contacted Dr. Dennis Juranek, the chief of the Parasitic Diseases Division in the National Center for Infectious Diseases, the Centers for Disease Control and Prevention (CDC). Dennis had extensive experience with waterborne diseases and had directed the CDC's investigation of the Carollton outbreak.[1] We discussed the Carollton outbreak, and Dennis suggested examining illness occurrence in nursing home populations, which were geographically fixed and not likely to obtain their drinking water from other sources or sites.

Later that day Steve set up acid fast smears from three stool specimens known to be bacterial culture negative. The test would determine whether the patients were infected with *Cryptosporidium*. The specimen staining procedure required an overnight interval before the results would be known.

APRIL 7, 1993

While driving to Milwaukee early on April 7 with Mary Proctor, PhD, MPH, and chief of the BPH Communicable Diseases Epidemiology Section, I discussed our prospective and retrospective surveillance needs. We decided it would be valuable to establish immediately a surveillance focus in two settings. Mary would establish and maintain surveillance for diarrhea illness in nursing homes and emergency departments throughout Milwaukee County and its four contiguous counties.

Bill Mac Kenzie, MD, was the CDC Epidemic Intelligence Service (EIS) officer assigned to the DOH who I supervised. Bill, Jim Kazmierczak, Mary and I from the DOH, Steve and Kathy of the MHD, and Wisconsin DNR staff met with MWW officials, and we were briefed on their water treatment methods and distribution system. The DNR had purview over regulation of drinking water utilities.

Drinking water for the City of Milwaukee (1993 population estimate of 630,000) and many of the other 18 municipalities in Milwaukee County was supplied by two MWW treatment plants, one in the northern part of the city (Linnwood Avenue Purification Plant, North Plant) and one in the southern part of the city (Howard Avenue Purification Plant, South Plant). Each plant had a submerged water intake grid in Lake Michigan about 1.25 (North) and 1.44 (South) miles offshore, respectively, where water entered an enormous tunnel and flowed by gravity through additional tunnels until it reached stations to pump water to the respective plants. The North Plant was located just offshore, but the South plant was located 3.5 miles inland from the Lake Michigan south shore (Figure 14-1).

The North Plant was a strikingly beautiful structure situated on a prominence projecting into Lake Michigan that was initially opened in the 1930s, and it could be viewed from the hills overlooking Lake Michigan. I grew up in a village along the north shore in Milwaukee County, passed by the treatment plant many times, and truly appreciated the majesty of this municipal water treatment facility. The same could not be said for the South Plant, built during the 1960s. Nonetheless, both plants housed modern, large treatment facilities.

Treatment capacities of each plant were sufficiently large to supply the entire water district fully. Treated water needs in Milwaukee are great because of its large population and industrial base, which included industries such as brewing that required large volumes of pure water. Should an outage occur in one plant, the distribution infrastructures from each plant were interconnected so that either plant could supply the water needs for the City of Milwaukee and its retail water customers elsewhere in Milwaukee County. With both plants in simultaneous operation, the South Plant predominantly supplies water to the southern portion of the district, and the North Plant predominantly supplies the northern portion. Central Milwaukee was typically supplied by both plants.

At the time of outbreak occurrence, water treatment in both plants followed the same sequence: the intake of raw water, the addition of chlorine as a disinfectant and polyaluminum chloride (PAC) as a coagulant to the raw water followed by rapid mixing, mechanical flocculation to remove solid and particulate material, sedimentation of the flocculent, and rapid filtration. The South Plant had 8 filters, and the North Plant had 16, each of which was enormous. After filtration, the water was pooled in a massive clear well at each plant (35 million gallons at the South Plant) from which it was distributed to customers (Figure 14-2). Parts of the water distribution infrastructure were very old, including large pipes, and MWW staff members were concerned that lead and copper could be leached if the pH of the water was too low. To address

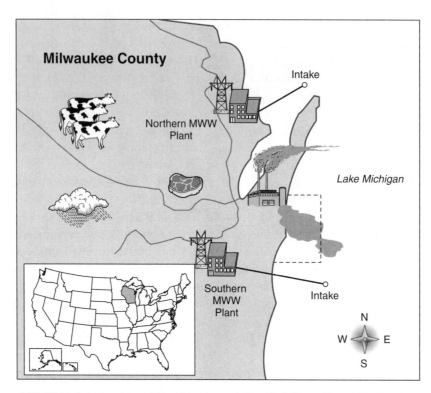

FIGURE 14-1 Location of the North and South Milwaukee Water Works water treatment plants, the water intakes for these plants, the three rivers that flow through Milwaukee County, and the breakfront located in the Lake Michigan harbor.

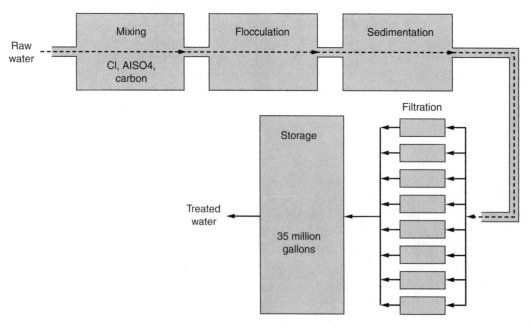

FIGURE 14-2 Schematic of the water treatment process at the South Milwaukee Water Works water treatment plant in March and April, 1993.

this concern, the MWW changed coagulants in late 1992 from the venerable and time tested alum to PAC.

Testing treated water for a variety of water quality indices was required by the DNR and the federal Environmental Protection Agency (EPA) and was done three times each day at each plant before water was released from the clear wells. Tests of water quality included bacteriologic (*E. coli* testing and coliform counts), chemical (residual chlorine, residual fluoride, alkalinity, and pH), and physical (color, threshold odor, raw water temperature, and turbidity) tests. The treated water was then distributed from the clear wells. Treated water leaving the plant was referred to as plant effluent. I do not believe I have ever asked anyone whether they would like a nice tall glass of cold plant effluent.

During March and April 1993, the turbidity of water treated at the South Plant and distributed to customers increased with spikes to historically high values. Early in March, there were no significant increases in finished water turbidity despite turbidity spikes in raw water; however, on March 23, the turbidity of South Plant treated water exceeded 0.4 NTU. This had not occurred in more than 10 years. Furthermore, the peak daily turbidity on March 28 and March 30 reached 1.7 NTU, even though the dosages of PAC were adjusted. When turbidity rises, the concern is that something dirty is getting into the system. The goal is to get it to precipitate out or be filtered out before it gets into someone's nice tall glass of effluent. Chemists at the South Plant aggressively tried to control the turbidity by changing the dosage of coagulant, but PAC was not the coagulant they were used to using, particularly under such extenuating circumstances. Plant staff resumed use of alum instead of PAC on April 2, but a spike in finished water turbidity to 1.5 NTU occurred on April 5.[2,3]

There were substantial differences in daily comparisons of South plant and North Plant finished water turbidity (Figure 14-3); the North Plant treated water turbidity did not exceed 0.45 NTU. The MWW administrators, although mindful that treated water turbidity at the South Plant was unusually high, noted the turbidity results and other water quality measures were in compliance with state and federal regulatory standards. Turbidity related compliance was based on average results over one month. Bill Mac Kenzie and Steve Gradus thought MWW administrators viewed turbidity as less important than other measures of water quality, and more as a measure of clarity. Notably, continually during February through April 1993, samples of treated water for water quality testing obtained from both plants were negative for coliforms. Coliforms are a group of related bacteria whose presence in water may indicate contamination by disease causing microorganisms. Thus, it became strikingly apparent that the likely focus of the outbreak

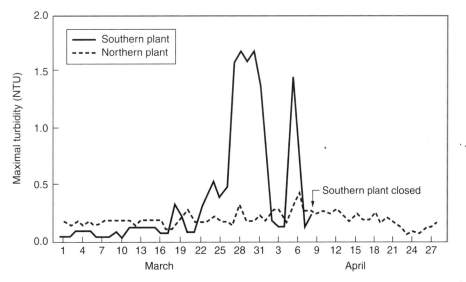

FIGURE 14-3 Maximal Turbidity of Treated Water in the Northern and Southern Water-Treatment Plants of the Milwaukee Water Works from March 1 through April 28, 1993. NTU denotes nephelometric turbidity units. From Mac Kenzie WR, Hoxie NJ, Proctor ME, Gradus MS, Blair KA, Peterson DE, Kazmierczak JJ, Addiss DG, Fox KR, Rose JB, Davis JP. A massive outbreak in Milwaukee of Cryptosporidium infection transmitted through the public water supply. *N Engl J Med* 1994;331:161–67.

was the water treated in and distributed from the South Plant. Using water quality indices, there were clear differences in finished water quality between the North and South Plants during the same time interval. Nonetheless, this did not exonerate treated water from the North Plant.

Later, on April 7, raw and treated water quality records for an interval that exceeded 10 years were available from the MWW. I examined the turbidity data and plotted the monthly peaks in finished water turbidity from each plant for the past 10 years. Indeed, the initial spike in South Plant finished water turbidity of greater than 0.4 NTU represented the first time in more than 10 years that the finished water from this plant exceeded 0.4 NTU. Thus, the three major spikes occurring during March 28 through April 5 were truly historic peaks in turbidity.

After several internal planning meetings early in the afternoon, MHD Commissioner Paul Nannis and I met with the press regarding our initial impressions. I discussed the strong likelihood that this was a waterborne outbreak and that the prime focus of our investigation was the South Plant, but we would also pursue additional hypotheses. I noted that testing of stool specimens for bacterial enteric pathogens was all negative; however, results of testing these negative samples for a variety of other pathogens were pending.

While I met the press, Jim Kazmierczak and Bill Mac Kenzie were meeting with MHD staff when they received a call from Steve Gradus who reported MHD Bureau of Laboratories staff found *Cryptosporidium* oocysts in the three stool samples known to be bacterial enteric pathogen negative that he had set up the day before. In addition, staff from the St. Luke's Hospital laboratory notified Steve that they had detected *Cryptosporidium* oocysts in stools from 4 patients. These stools were obtained from 7 healthy adults who resided in the Southern half of Milwaukee. Steve also received a report of a case of *Cryptosporidium* infection in an older resident of West Allis in southwest Milwaukee County. That laboratory diagnosis was made by an astute microbiologist at West Allis Memorial Hospital who tested the stool specimen for *Cryptosporidium* oocysts even though the test was not specifically ordered. Steve, Bill, and Jim recognized the significance of these laboratory findings. Given our findings and recalling those from the Carrollton outbreak that affected an estimated 13,000 people,[1] these laboratory results from only eight adult individuals were very significant.

After the press session, Paul and I were to meet with Milwaukee Mayor John Norquist to discuss our findings and investigation plans. While walking to the mayor's office, I was met by Bill and Jim and was informed of the eight laboratory-confirmed cases of *Cryptosporidium* infection. They believed *Cryptosporidium* was a highly plausible etiology for this outbreak, and I concurred. Bill raised the issue that a widespread boil-water advisory involving all users of City of Milwaukee municipal water would be needed to prevent additional cases.

The meeting with the mayor involved a substantial number of MDH, MWW, DNR, mayor's administration officials, and our DOH team. The water treatment and quality data and state and federal water related regulations were discussed in detail with the mayor. Based on preliminary findings and illness characteristics, an outbreak of this nature that was so widespread would be considered as waterborne unless proven otherwise. We discussed the likelihood that this large waterborne outbreak was caused by *Cryptosporidium* infection based on laboratory data that we had just become aware of. We informed the mayor of our investigation plans to consider all possible sources of these infections.

The discussion ultimately focused on what could and should be done to control the outbreak. A variety of approaches were discussed, including disinfection and a boil-water advisory. *Cryptosporidium* was a highly chlorine-resistant protozoan, thus disinfection would not be effective. To be clear, chlorine will kill *Cryptosporidium*; however, the concentration needed would be great, and treating water with a concentration of chlorine that can quickly kill *Cryptosporidium* would make the water unsafe to drink or bathe in for too long of an interval and at great expense given the magnitude of the water supply. The pros and cons of a boil-water advisory were considered. Although *Cryptosporidium* oocysts were heat sensitive and inactivated with boiling, the downside involved the need to boil all water treated in MWW plants to be used for eating and drinking, the personal injury risks associated with boiling water and with consuming recently boiled water, and the bump in energy use that would be associated with a prolonged advisory. The educational needs to conduct this activity effectively would be enormous. Plus, all of these considerations were based on limited and newly available information. Ultimately, the mayor focused his attention on a soft drink can that I brought to the meeting and asked me, "Would you drink a glass of water here, right now?" I replied, "No." Mayor Norquist then stated, "That's it. We need to go public with what our suspicions are."[4] Clearly, if I would not drink the water, he would not let Milwaukee residents and visitors drink it unless it was safe to do so.

With no pun intended, this was a watershed moment. The mayor would invoke a boil-water order, and his staff notified the media of a press conference that evening. Precision was needed to provide clear instructions to all users of the water. The implications of this massive boil-water advisory were enormous. Municipal staff members would need to answer many questions. That evening during the press conference, the mayor told all city residents and all users of MWW water to boil their drinking water for 5 minutes and discard all ice.

Because of the need to obtain critical water samples to document any presence of *Cryptosporidium* in water from each of the implicated treatment plants, systematic sample collections were planned for April 8, and the South Plant would be closed for an undetermined interval beginning on April 9. From April 8 throughout this undetermined interval, all drinking water in Milwaukee would be supplied by the North Plant.

This was an enormous news story with national and international implications. The local media gave this virtually unprecedented coverage. The two major (and competing) Milwaukee newspapers collaborated in publishing a special issue in Spanish. Plans for daily media updates were announced. A half-page ad for an over-the-counter antimotility medication appeared, but now that a boil-water order was invoked, what would be needed to lift it? It was my responsibility to answer that question, but there were so many questions to answer and avenues to explore to describe fully the scope and all aspects of this outbreak, to generate and test hypotheses regarding how it occurred and why it was so large, and to determine whether measures were to be effective in controlling it.

THE OUTBREAK AND THE OUTBREAK INVESTIGATION

This is what was known about *Cryptosporidium* before April, 1993:

We needed to learn quickly what was known about *Cryptosporidium*, particularly regarding its associations with waterborne disease outbreaks. At the time of this outbreak, relatively few public health officials had much knowledge of this protozoan parasite and its associated illnesses, nor was it well known as a pathogen by those charged with keeping local supplies of drinking water safe.

Although initially detected in animals in 1907 and for years thought not to affect humans, *Cryptosporidium* was first reported as a human pathogen in separate case reports of enterocolitis in immune competent[5-7] and compromised[8,9] patients. *Cryptosporidium* became a prominent pathogen when it was recognized in 1981–1982 as an AIDS-defining illness and opportunistic infection. The initial report in 1984 of a waterborne disease outbreak of cryptosporidiosis was associated with an artesian well in San Antonio, Texas. During 1986 to 1992, waterborne *Cryptosporidium* infections were associated with surface water exposure in New Mexico (1986), post-treatment contamination of drinking water in Aryshire, UK (1988), and filtered water supplies in Carrollton, Georgia (surface, 1987), Swindon and Oxfordshire, UK (1989), the Isle of Thanet, UK (1991), and most recently in Jackson County, Oregon.[10-14] The outbreak that was most similar to ours was the one in Carrollton.

Early Logistics

It was rapidly apparent this outbreak investigation would require work well beyond even the larger outbreaks I had focused on during my tenure as a state epidemiologist. Each of the outbreak's many facets would need a person in charge. Information by necessity would flow in one direction, but nominally, and those providing data needed to understand this; however, information would be continually shared with those who needed to know. Thus, organization and appropriate use of human resources were critical elements of this investigation. As the state epidemiologist and the state's leader of this multijurisdictional outbreak investigation, my time was focused on generating hypotheses, overseeing the generation of outbreak related data and information, communicating important findings, whether positive or negative, and assuring that all aspects of the investigation were proceeding in a timely, efficient way. My time would not be well spent working out the logistics of having enough staff available to conduct certain aspects of the investigation, although it was important for me to request and obtain the resources when needed. Ivan Imm, BPH Director, and John Chapin, DOH Deputy Administrator, were masterful in generating the personnel and supply resources needed and would

> *It was rapidly apparent this outbreak investigation would require work well beyond even the larger outbreaks I had focused on during my tenure as a state epidemiologist.*

remain on site for nearly 2 weeks to run interference. We had a large room in the Milwaukee Municipal Building for our investigation with dedicated phones, computer resources, and even a new fax machine needed on short notice for our surveillance activities that was purchased by the State Health Officer, Ann Haney. Several additional venues were established for activities requiring phone banks and dedicated teams could be rapidly deployed for survey purposes. Ultimately, nine teams, each of which focused on separate investigation components and all of which involved public health personnel, were created during the early phase of the outbreak investigation and were staffed by various combinations of City of Milwaukee and DOH personnel (Exhibit 14-1).

Early on we needed an experienced investigator to join our investigation and focus on special laboratory and surveillance projects. I had worked with David Addiss, MD, since 1985 when he began his 2-year term as an EIS officer assigned to our health department, and I was his field supervisor. We collaborated on many investigations since then. Dave was working as a medical epidemiologist in the Parasitic Diseases Division at the CDC and was extremely familiar with systems in Wisconsin. I invited Dave to join our investigation in Milwaukee, and fortunately, this was possible.

Review of MWW Data

Raw Water Source

The Milwaukee watershed includes three rivers that flow through Milwaukee County: the Milwaukee, Menomonee, and Kinnikinnick Rivers. Environmental

---

EXHIBIT 14-1 Investigation of the Massive Waterborne Outbreak of *Cryptosporidium* Infections: Epidemiologic and Laboratory Studies Initiated and Health Education and Logistic Functions (Selected)

Studies to define the outbreak
- Laboratory confirmed case surveillance: determine outbreak trends, characterize the illness in healthy populations and in immunocompromised and other special populations, and establish case definition, collection, and storage of serologic and other specimens for future studies
- Emergency room log database and case surveillance
- Nursing home database and surveillance
- Random digit dialing (RDD) surveys:
  - RDD 1: description of clinical disease, risk factors for acquiring *Cryptosporidium* infection in the community, early estimate of magnitude
  - RDD 2: description of trends, age and zip code-specific attack rates, epidemic curve, estimates of outbreak magnitude, use of clinical services, hospitalization, economic impact, secondary transmission
  - RDD 3 and 4: survey to assess morbidity before and after reopening the South Plant
- Single day (short duration) of exposure database and surveillance: determine when problems with water treatment began, specific days that water was contaminated, incubation period calculations, quantify occurrence of secondary transmission
- Immunocompromised, AIDS/HIV assess multiple risk factors, natural history, prevention measures—large ill and well cohorts
- Surveillance in child care and daycare settings
- Satellite outbreak investigations in communities outside of greater Milwaukee areas

Environmental Studies
- MWW: plant protocols and engineering reviews, water quality data reviews
- River and estuaries data: cooperative study to monitor the Milwaukee River watershed and subwatershed, the sewage treatment plant influent and effluent, beach sites and MSS treatment plant influents and effluents. Five samplings at 21 sites through Spring 1994
- Efficacy of point of use filters in an outbreak setting
- Meteorological data analysis
- Laboratory testing of stored ice for *Cryptosporidium* and additional environmental testing

City of Milwaukee government activities (selected)
- Press-related coordination and releases, risk communication, phone banks coordination, fact sheets development, and translations and other health education related functions
- Quality assurance and inspections
- All agencies availability (24/7) and interagency coordination and committees
- Infection control and coordination with all health related facilities

sources of *Cryptosporidium* oocysts that could impact on these rivers and associated watersheds could have been agricultural, industrial (meat packing), and wildlife related. The three rivers converge a short distance before emptying into Lake Michigan within a harbor area protected by a large breakfront (see Figure 14-1). There are three major gaps in the breakfront, including a large central gap allowing boat access and egress, and smaller north and south fair weather gaps. The ambient current in the harbor and within the breakfront was southerly. The flow of water from within the breakfront through the south fair weather gap created a plume that was typically directly toward the raw water intake grid for the South Plant, which was located 7,600 feet offshore at the bottom of Lake Michigan under 50 feet of water.

The central sewage treatment plant operated by the Milwaukee Metropolitan Sewage District is located at the point where the river, created by the confluence of the three rivers, empties into Lake Michigan, and the effluent from the sewage treatment plant empties into the harbor within the confines of the breakfront.

Laboratory-Based Active Surveillance and Testing[2,15]

Steve transmitted information on *Cryptosporidium* detection to the directors of 14 clinical microbiology laboratories throughout the five county greater Milwaukee area and established laboratory-based surveillance with data to be reported to him. Compared with the usual parasitic testing of stool specimens, an additional flocculation step and special staining of the pellet with Kinyoun acid fast stain was needed to detect *Cryptosporidium* oocysts, and although it was the gold standard for testing at the time, the test was insensitive. This test was used in 13 of the laboratories. Because of the nature of the test, relatively few tests of stool for *Cryptosporidium* were requested before the occurrence of this outbreak, and these were primarily for testing patients with AIDS who had diarrhea, particularly chronic diarrhea.

Preoutbreak (prepublicity) baseline *Cryptosporidium*-related data were generated by retrospectively examining results of testing during March 1 through April 6 and were then compared with results of prospective testing during April 8 through April 16. During March 1–April 6, among 42 stool specimens submitted for *Cryptosporidium* testing, 12 (29%) were positive. This compares to 331 of 1009 specimens (33%) tested during April 8 to April 16. Of note, other pathogens accounted for only a very small proportion of the *Cryptosporidium* test-negative illnesses, and the percentage of specimens *Cryptosporidium* test positive (39%) during the Carrollton outbreak was similar. The similarity in the proportion of test positive principally among immunocompromised individuals with persistent diarrhea prior to the outbreak (29%) and among principally previously healthy persons of all ages in a wide range of demographic settings (33%) was striking and perplexing.

One question to be answered prospectively was the efficacy of *Cryptosporidium*-related laboratory tests that were or would be in development. To address this, Dave Addiss and a microbiologist from the CDC worked with Steve and other MHD laboratory staff members to obtain and archive stool and serum specimens for current and future testing.

Clinical Characteristics of Illness and Generation of a Case Definition[2]

The magnitude of this outbreak provided an opportunity to examine the clinical spectrum of illness among many individuals with laboratory-confirmed or clinically defined infections. Early in our investigation, we examined clinical signs and symptoms of illness and illness onset data among those with laboratory-confirmed *Cryptosporidium* infection to generate a reliable clinical case definition. We observed a virtual 100% occurrence of watery diarrhea among these individuals. Onset data suggested this outbreak emerged after March 1, 1993. We determined the illness onset interval of March 1 to April 9 would be inclusive of outbreak-related exposure until the South Plant was closed.

Although we recognized many thousands of cases likely occurred through May 15, the MHD received reports of 739 individuals with laboratory-confirmed *Cryptosporidium* infections; a more workable sample of 312 of these patients was selected, and extensive interviews were completed on 285, which was nearly a 40% sample and highly adequate for our purposes. This would be our study cohort with laboratory-confirmed infection. To understand the occurrence of illness in the community, we conducted the first of our four random digit dialed phoned surveys during April 9 to 12 to help describe clinical and other features of outbreak-related infections and generate a cohort of members with clinically defined illness to compare to the cohort with laboratory-confirmed illnesses. This first random digit dialed phoned survey (RDD 1) was administered by the DOH Sexually Transmitted Disease program staff who had substantial interviewing skills and by public health nurses, including an energetic group of retired public health nurses in southeastern Wisconsin who were a great resource and donated much time. The retired nurses, all of whom had long public health careers, literally stepped forward and asked us if they could be of service. Among 482 adult Milwaukee city residents, 42% had illness meeting the clinical case definition of cryptosporidiosis, and 6% of those individuals were hospitalized for their illnesses. We recognized the laboratory-confirmed illness cohort were ill enough to seek medical care and have their physicians order appropriate stool exams; indeed, 17% were immunocompromised, and 46% were hospitalized.

We found the cohorts to be similar in mean age, gender distribution, dates of illness onset, and in occurrence of abdominal cramps, fatigue, and muscle aches (Table 14-1). As anticipated, because the case group was comprised of patients ill enough to have consulted physicians and then be tested, those with laboratory-confirmed illness had diarrhea of longer duration (9 vs. 3 days), more frequent stools (median maximum of 12 vs. 5 stools

TABLE 14-1 Clinical Characteristics of Case Patients with Laboratory-Confirmed Cryptosporidium Infection and Survey Respondents with Clinical Infection

Characteristic	Laboratory-Confirmed Infection (n = 285)	Clinical Infection* (n = 201)	P value[†]
Symptoms—number of patients of respondents (%)			
Diarrhea	285 (100)	201 (100)	NA
Watery diarrhea	265 (93)	201 (100)	NA
Abdominal cramps	238 (84)	168 (84)	0.9
Fatigue	247 (87)	145 (72)	< 0.001
Loss of Appetite	230 (81)	147 (73)	0.03
Nausea	199 (70)	119 (59)	0.01
Fever	162 (57)	72 (36)	< 0.001
Chills	65 (64)[‡]	91 (45)	0.04
Sweats	55 (54)[‡]	83 (41)	0.04
Muscle or joint aches	152 (53)	100 (50)	0.6
Headache	53 (52)[‡]	122 (61)	0.2
Vomiting	136 (48)	37 (18)	< 0.001
Cough	68 (24)	56 (28)	0.3
Sore throat	48 (17)	35 (17)	0.7
Mean duration of diarrhea (days)	12	4.5	0.001[§]
Mean maximum number of stools/day	19	7.7	0.001[§]
Mean maximum temperature (°C)	38.3	38.1	0.09[§]
Mean duration of vomiting (days)	2.9	2.0	0.07[§]
Mean maximum number of vomiting episodes/day	3.9	2.6	0.36[§]

* The criterion for clinical infection was the reported presence of watery diarrhea.
[†] Unless otherwise noted, Yates' correction has been applied to P values. NA denotes not applicable.
[‡] Data are from 101 case patients interviewed during phase 1 of the study.
[§] By Kruskal-Wallis test.
From Mac Kenzie WR, Hoxie NJ, Proctor ME, et al. A massive outbreak in Milwaukee of Cryptosporidium infection transmitted through the public water supply (Table 1). N Engl J Med 1994;331:161–167.

daily), and higher rates of vomiting (48% vs. 18%) and fever (57% vs. 36%). Nonetheless, those with clinically defined illness were also quite ill.

Nursing Home Surveillance[2,3,15]

To determine whether and for how long gastrointestinal illness was associated with drinking water supplied by the South Plant, Mary Proctor established the aforementioned retrospective and prospective surveillance system for diarrhea illness among residents of representative samples of northern Milwaukee and southern Milwaukee nursing homes. Nursing home residents are relatively nonmobile (fixed populations) among whom information on diarrhea is collected routinely by nursing home staff. With their limited possibilities of exposures outside of their nursing homes, they represented an ideal human population to study. We defined diarrhea as three or more loose stools in a 24-hour period. Among residents of the nine nursing homes in northern Milwaukee, the prevalence of diarrhea remained less than 2% during March and April. In stark contrast, the prevalence of diarrhea among residents of six of the seven southern Milwaukee nursing homes increased to 16% during the first week of April and remained high until 2 weeks after the boil water advisory was issued (Figure 14-4c). Mary was particularly excited when she noted that the one nursing home in southern Milwaukee that did not observe an increase had a private well, and the prevalence of diarrhea among residents at that home remained less than 2%... serendipity at its finest. Furthermore, of stool samples prospectively collected from 69 southern Milwaukee nursing home residents with diarrhea (during April), 51% were positive for *Cryptosporidium* compared with none among samples from 12 northern Milwaukee nursing home residents with diarrhea. Clearly, if there were any doubts about the early association of illness with the South Plant, these data dispelled them.

Emergency Department Surveillance

While classically emergency department surveillance is useful during outbreak investigations, this was of greatest value to us only during the early phase of our investigation to facilitate case finding, clinical characterization, and case definition generation. To monitor the course and impact of the outbreak, other more focused surveillance activities proved to be superior.

Estimation of Magnitude of the Outbreak[2]

Because the outbreak magnitude was so large that it precluded any reasonable estimate through standard illness reporting means, we planned to generate this estimate by conducting the second of our RDDs (RDD 2). Bill Mac Kenzie, working closely with Neil Hoxie of the DOH, was the lead on this critical component of our outbreak investigation. With objectives of estimating the magnitude of the outbreak and its temporal and geographic impact, a questionnaire was created for use by telephone surveyors, and sample selection was conducted using computer-generated, random telephone numbers for the greater Milwaukee area. The survey was written by the University of Wisconsin Survey Research Institute (SRI) based on a set of key data needed by the DOH. DOH and SRI staff generated the final instrument. SRI staff members were finely honed to conduct these types of surveys and conducted all of the calls and completed all forms and data entry. Based on RDD 1 data, watery diarrhea with onset between March 1 and April 28 was used as a reliable definition of cryptosporidiosis. The survey included questions about watery diarrhea occurrence and frequency, other signs and symptoms, illness duration, health care visits, hospital stays, mortality, and demographic features. The survey sample included households in Milwaukee County and the four counties contiguous to Milwaukee County; the five-county greater Milwaukee area population was an estimated 1.61 million people. During April 28 through May 2, among the 840 households contacted, 613 (73%) participated representing 1662 household members from Milwaukee and the four surrounding counties. Household-related information was provided by interviewing the most knowledgeable adult member. The sample distribution was similar to the five county population distribution based on 1990 census data.

The clinical definition of cryptosporidiosis was watery diarrhea, but the time frame of onset was March 1 through April 28 to assess the impact of the boil-water order and other recommended control measures. Among the 1662 household member sample, 436 (26%) had illness meeting the definition of clinical cryptosporidiosis. These data were excellent for generating an epidemic curve to examine outbreak trends (Figure

CHAPTER 14 ■ The Massive Waterborne Outbreak of *Cryptosporidium* Infections, Milwaukee, Wisconsin, 1993

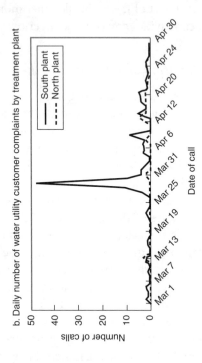

a. Daily maximum water treatment plant effluent turbidity by treatment plant

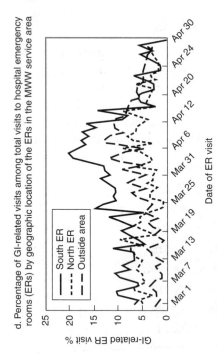

b. Daily number of water utility customer complaints by treatment plant

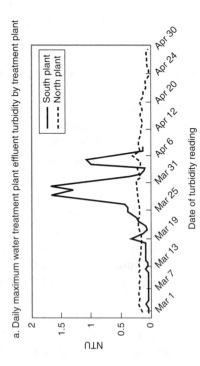

c. Daily nursing home (NH) diarrhea prevalence rates per 100 residents by geographic location of nursing home in the MWW service area

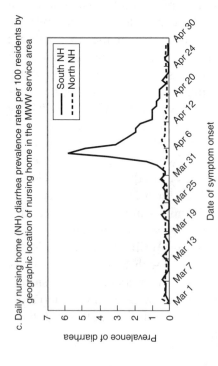

d. Percentage of GI-related visits among total visits to hospital emergency rooms (ERs) by geographic location of the ERs in the MWW service area

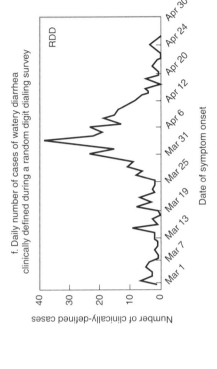

f. Daily number of cases of watery diarrhea clinically defined during a random digit dialing survey

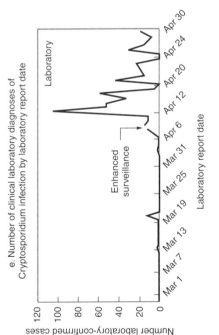

e. Number of clinical laboratory diagnoses of Cryptosporidium infection by laboratory report date

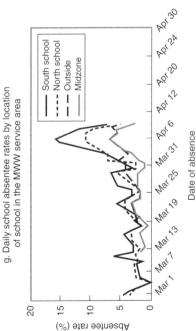

g. Daily school absentee rates by location of school in the MWW service area

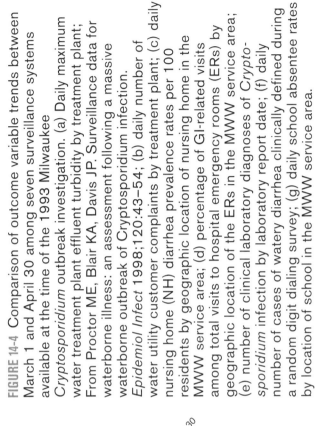

FIGURE 14-4 Comparison of outcome variable trends between March 1 and April 30 among seven surveillance systems available at the time of the 1993 Milwaukee *Cryptosporidium* outbreak investigation. (a) Daily maximum water treatment plant effluent turbidity by treatment plant; From Proctor ME, Blair KA, Davis JP. Surveillance data for waterborne illness: an assessment following a massive waterborne outbreak of Cryptosporidium infection. *Epidemiol Infect* 1998;120:43–54; (b) daily number of water utility customer complaints by treatment plant; (c) daily nursing home (NH) diarrhea prevalence rates per 100 residents by geographic location of nursing home in the MWW service area; (d) percentage of GI-related visits among total visits to hospital emergency rooms (ERs) by geographic location of the ERs in the MWW service area; (e) number of clinical laboratory diagnoses of *Cryptosporidium* infection by laboratory report date; (f) daily number of cases of watery diarrhea clinically defined during a random digit dialing survey; (g) daily school absentee rates by location of school in the MWW service area.

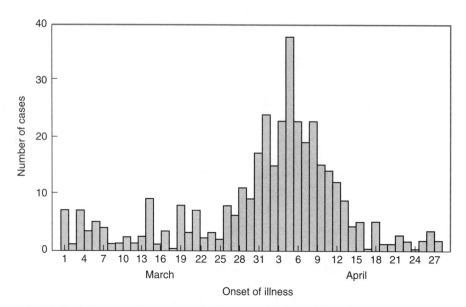

FIGURE 14-5 Reported Date of the Onset of Watery Diarrhea During the Period from March 1 through April 28, 1993, in 436 Cases of Infection Identified by a Random-Digit Telephone Survey of the Greater Milwaukee Area. Reprinted with permission from Mac Kenzie WR, Hoxie NJ, Proctor ME, Gradus MS, Blair KA, Peterson DE, Kazmierczak JJ, Addiss DG, Fox KR, Rose JB, Davis JP. A massive outbreak in Milwaukee of Cryptosporidium infection transmitted through the public water supply. *N Engl J Med* 1994;331:161–167.

14-5). The occurrence of watery diarrhea began with a small increase in morbidity beginning about March 18 followed by a larger increase in the five-county area beginning about March 24, a peak during April 1–April 7 with a distinct mode on April 4 followed by a rather sudden decrease in morbidity on April 13. This observed decrease in morbidity provided strong evidence that the boil-water order was effective.

Among participants residing within the MWW service area in Milwaukee County, the attack rate of watery diarrhea was greatest (52%) among residents in southern Milwaukee, lowest (26%) among residents of northern Milwaukee, and intermediate (35%) in the mid-zone region in which water could be supplied by either the South or North Plants. The attack rate among participants residing outside the MWW service area was 15%; however, among residents who lived outside the MWW service area but worked within southern Milwaukee, the attack rate was 39%.

To digress momentarily, it is logical to wonder why there was such a big difference in attack rates among residents in southern Milwaukee households (52%) and residents of the southern Milwaukee nursing homes (16%), who are typically thought of as being more vulnerable. We observed attack rates in this outbreak to be age dependent, and the older population had the lowest attack rates. This is likely associated with prior immunity. There were similar outbreaks during the 1930s, each involving tens of thousands of people prior to the construction of the north plant, and I suspect that individuals who lived in Milwaukee at that time were more likely to be immune.

By projecting the overall attack rate (26%) onto the five-county population (1.61 million), we estimated that during March 1 through April 28, the number of persons with watery diarrhea who resided in this area was 419,000. Subsequently, in another RDD survey (RDD 3), a background rate of watery diarrhea among residents in this area was estimated to be 0.5% per month. Application of these background data resulted in a final estimate of 403,000 residents of the five county area with watery diarrhea attributed to this truly massive outbreak. The RDD 2 data were used to estimate health care seeking and occupational impacts. Among the 436 household participants with watery diarrhea, 50 (11%) saw health care providers (estimated 44,000 persons seen as outpatients) for their illnesses, and 5 (1%) were hospitalized (estimated 4,400 persons hospitalized). Furthermore, for each case individual, the mean days of reported lost productivity (work or school) was 1.8 days, which projected to an estimated 725,000 days lost productivity attributed to this outbreak.[2,16]

These were astounding numbers. The outbreak was the largest waterborne outbreak documented in the United States, and perhaps in the developed world!

Using these data as the estimates of morbidity, several years later after appropriate hospital-, workplace-, insurance-, and government-related records were reviewed, estimates of the fiscal impact of this outbreak were generated.[16]

Cases in Visitors to Milwaukee[17]

While most BPH communicable disease epidemiologists were involved in the onsite investigation, one, Wendy Schell, remained in Madison. In addition to memoranda circulated widely to physicians, public health officials, and infection control practitioners throughout Wisconsin, on the day after the announcement of the boil water advisory, I generated a memo. This memo included information regarding the occurrence of the large waterborne outbreak, descriptive epidemiologic data, and data pertaining to the *Cryptosporidium* etiology and the boil water advisory. Wendy distributed this memo nationwide to all state and territorial epidemiologists with instructions for the reporting of cases. These memoranda were used to establish regional and national surveillance for confirmed and suspected cases of *Cryptosporidium* infection among individuals residing outside of the five-county greater Milwaukee area. This surveillance activity was very fruitful. Numerous reports of cases were received from state and local departments, and after regional and national press coverage of the outbreak and related events, the DOH received numerous self-reports of illness from individuals who resided outside the five-county region but visited Milwaukee and subsequently became ill.

As questions and hypotheses mounted, we recognized that residents of the greater Milwaukee area had too many opportunities to become infected to be helpful in addressing some of them; however, interviewing individuals with short term visits to Milwaukee would be key to determining the incubation period, how long *Cryptosporidium* was present in the water supply, and the extent of secondary transmission in households.[17]

> *Interviewing individuals with short term visits to Milwaukee would be key to determining the incubation period, how long* Cryptosporidium *was present in the water supply, and the extent of secondary transmission in households.*

During April 12 through May 20, out of region participants with suspected or confirmed *Cryptosporidium* infections were interviewed by phone using a standardized questionnaire focusing on demographic features, illness characteristics, length and site of stay, and water consumption; 130 of those interviewed had laboratory or clinically confirmed cryptosporidiosis, and 94 case individuals had brief (<48 hours) visits to the MWW service area. We had a unique opportunity to measure the interval during which *Cryptosporidium* was present in the water by noting the dates of the brief visits of these 94 case individuals. Among those with these brief visits, particularly the 63 with visits of 24 hours or less, we determined the incubation period by examining the intervals between dates of illness onset and dates of arrival to Milwaukee. The median incubation period was 7 days (range, 1–14 days). Among those with brief exposures, the earliest date of exposure was March 24, and the last date of exposure (with one exception) was April 5. The peak days of exposure were March 27 and 28, and based on arrival date information, *Cryptosporidium* was present in the municipal water supply continuously and daily during March 24 through April 5. Because of the brief durations of exposure, including several strikingly brief airport layovers, we could quantify consumption of tap water and beverages containing tap water while in the MWW service area. The median amount consumed was 16 ounces, and 23% of brief exposure participants drank 8 ounces or less.[17]

Important clinical observations among this cohort included the low (5%) risk of secondary transmission within households where the index case patient was an adult; however, cryptosporidiosis during this outbreak appeared more severe when compared with cases described in previous case series reports. The recurrence of watery diarrhea after apparent recovery from clinical illness was a frequent event among short-term visitors to Milwaukee with laboratory-confirmed infections (39%) as well as in Milwaukee County residents with clinical infections (21%) and contributed a significant proportion of cases of postoutbreak diarrhea in the community.[17] The significance of this observation among the short-term visitors was that it excluded re-infection with *Cryptosporidium* as a cause of recurrence.

Response to Questions from Business

The boil-water order affected many businesses in Milwaukee County. Because of the importance of beer (as an industry and as a beverage to be depended on more often than usual in the days to come), one early concern involved the cold-filtered brewing process used by a major Milwaukee brewing company; however, this company pasteurized its water before it was used in the brewing process, and its filters were sufficiently small to remove *Cryptosporidium* oocysts effectively. Before and during the outbreak, this brewing company donated a very large volume of pasteurized, purified water for individuals who were immunocompromised and needed a reliable source of pure drinking water.

Many questions came from food processors and the health care industry. The only food-related industries with prevailing concerns were those that prepared food that was not to be heated to an adequate temperature to kill *Cryptosporidium* oocysts. Regional and nationwide recalls (all voluntary) of many of these types of products, such as prepared salads and dips, were needed and we depended on the Food and Drug Administration and U.S. Department of Agriculture to help with these actions.

Studies of Special Populations

Impact on Children and in Childcare Settings[18,19]

We were very cognizant of the importance of the observation of widespread school absenteeism in the recognition of this outbreak. Although much effort was focused on understanding the occurrence of illness in fixed populations, we needed to understand the impact of *Cryptosporidium* infection on children, particularly because of hygienic issues that may contribute to transmission in households, day care facilities and other settings, but also to determine the extent of asymptomatic infection and persistent shedding of *Cryptosporidium* in this population. To address these issues, two very specific Epidemic Aid investigations were generated with Dave Addiss serving as the CDC supervisor; Ralph Cordell focused on the impact of *Cryptosporidium* infections in child day care settings,[18] and Helen Cicirello focused on broader impacts among children.[19]

Ralph coordinated the screening of 129 diapered attendees of 11 day care centers in metropolitan Milwaukee and found 35 (27%) with *Cryptosporidium* oocysts in their stool, 10 of whom did not have diarrhea during the outbreak. Thus, at least in this very young population, asymptomatic or minimally symptomatic *Cryptosporidium* infection appeared to be somewhat frequent.[18] There was no systematic assessment of asymptomatic shedding of *Cryptosporidium* among those without diarrhea.

Helen coordinated a study of the clinical, laboratory, and epidemiologic features of outbreak-associated cryptosporidiosis among children who sought medical care at the Wisconsin Children's Hospital during the outbreak. As with other diarrhea illnesses for which multiple stool examinations increases the opportunity to make a diagnosis, those children who had laboratory-confirmed *Cryptosporidium* infections had stools specimens submitted more frequently and later in their illnesses than those with stool exams that were negative.[19]

HIV Infection[20]

In outbreak settings, it was not known whether *Cryptosporidium*-related diarrhea illness attack rates were greater in HIV-infected persons than in the general population. There was great concern among the public health community and the HIV/AIDS advocacy community regarding the impact of this outbreak on those with HIV-infection and what could be done to prevent *Cryptosporidium* infections from occurring. Chronic diarrhea caused by *Cryptosporidium* is an AIDS-defining condition, and the massive exposure to *Cryptosporidium* among the HIV-infected community in Milwaukee could result in many new AIDS cases with substantial suffering because of the lack of an effective treatment. This outbreak occurrence provided an opportunity to survey a large community of HIV-infected individuals exposed to a point source of *Cryptosporidium* contaminated water to examine epidemiologic features and severity of clinical illness.

A group headed by Holly Frisby, DVM, an epidemiologist in the DOH AIDS/HIV Program, conducted a case control study incorporating a randomized sample of 263 among 703 HIV case-management clients in the five-county greater Milwaukee and one age- and gender-matched control selected from the general population using RDD methods. To facilitate participation and assure patient confidentiality, case patients were known only to their case managers. Case and control survey questions were similar. The survey participation among the sample of HIV-infected individuals was high (82%). During this outbreak, the attack rate of watery diarrhea among HIV-infected persons (32%) was less than among matched controls (51%); however, although HIV-infected individuals were not more likely to experience symptomatic *Cryptosporidium* infection than persons in the general population, once infected with *Cryptosporidium*, the duration and severity of illness were greater in HIV-infected individuals, particularly among those with CD4+ T-lymphocytes < 200 per mL.[20]

Mortality[21]

The media focused on severe and ultimately fatal *Cryptosporidium* infections in several individuals with previously diagnosed AIDS. During the first several weeks of our investigation, we were not aware of any deaths attributable to this outbreak that involved individuals who were not immunocompromise or had some other serious underlying illness. We realized measurement of mortality attributed to this outbreak must be deferred because of delays inherent in obtaining accurate mortality data. When final state mortality data were available for 1993–1994, we were able to measure this. I was continually concerned regarding the arbitrary and unfortunate number of 100 deaths attributed to the outbreak and circulated in the media, as there were no data to support this, and we would be the ones to provide an accurate assessment. Our approach was to assess death certificate data that specifically indicated cryptosporidiosis as a cause of death that could conclusively be attributed to the outbreak, and to measure the AIDS-related mortality during the first 6 months after the outbreak (the near term observed mortality that likely would be acutely associated with the outbreak) and compare that with expected AIDS-related mortality during this interval and to the AIDS-related expected mortality during the subsequent 6 months. We observed greater than expected AIDS-related mortality during the first 6-month interval and less than expected AIDS-related mortality during the subsequent 6-month interval. Thus, in addition to death certificate data (50 outbreak attributable deaths, 86% among persons with AIDS), we were able to measure premature mortality attributable to this outbreak among persons with AIDS with no death certificate mention of cryptosporidiosis (19 deaths).[21] The "official" outbreak-related attributable mortality was 69 deaths, of which 93% occurred in persons with AIDS.

> The "official" outbreak-related attributable mortality was 69 deaths, of which 93% occurred in persons with AIDS.

Detection of Cryptosporidium in the Water Supply

Another of our objectives was to demonstrate *Cryptosporidium* in water or other material sampled during the actual outbreak interval. Our first lead was a company that manufactured very fine absolute pore-size filters. For many days in a row, their test filters were discolored by an apparent water impurity. Fortunately, the filters were dated and saved by the company and available to us.

Perhaps the most fortuitous opportunity involved a call from an ice manufacturing company to Greg Carmichael, a quality assurance officer who worked for the City of Milwaukee. The company, located near the South Plant, manufactured large (50 gallon) blocks of ice for sculpture. During March 25 through April 9, impurities in the ice spoiled its color and clarity; however, representative blocks were saved! A tremendous opportunity existed, and we generated a plan to use these slabs. Under Dave's supervision, each block of ice would be melted separately, and the resulting water would be divided into two aliquots, one of which would be filtered using a standard, nominal spun polypropylene cartridge filter, which was notoriously unwieldy to use and assay and crude in accuracy of results. The other aliquot would be filtered using a large (11.5 inch) Millipore membrane filter with a 0.45-micron fixed pore size that was suspected to be superior. Unfortunately, despite these elegant plans, there was confusion within the company, and all but the blocks of ice made on March 25 and April 9 were discarded. Nonetheless, the manufacturing dates of the remaining blocks were well timed for our purposes, and the study was completed according to plan.[2] Dave reported that the concentration of *Cryptosporidium* oocysts in ice produced March 25 and April 9 and filtered using the membrane filter was 13.2 and 6.7 oocysts per 100 liters compared with 2.6 and 0.7 oocysts per 100 liters, respectively, using the spun cartridge filter. Regardless of the filter used, *Cryptosporidium* was confirmed to be present in each block at substantial concentrations even though freezing reduces the recovery of oocysts. The March 25 data were notable as the peak turbidity of South plant water that day was 0.5 NTU, which was substantially less than the NTU peak days later when the measurable concentration of oocysts would be projected to be considerably higher. As expected, the submicron membrane filter was functionally far superior to the standard spun cartridge filter.

Investigation of the Milwaukee Water Works South Plant

During my first conversation with Dennis Juranek of the CDC regarding the outbreak, he provided me with the names of raw water and drinking water experts: Walt Jakubowski (EPA, Cincinnati), Stig Regli (EPA, Washington, DC), Joan Rose (University of South Florida), Mark LeChevalier (American Water Works Association [AWWA]), and others. I called each of these individuals shortly after my initial review of the finished water quality and the invoking of the boil-water order. One aspect of the conversation with Walt was the need to conduct an in-plant inspection of both of the MWW plants by an EPA engineer who was expert in all aspects of the drinking water treatment process. Walt mentioned that Kim Fox would be particularly skilled to conduct this aspect of the investigation. Kim and an EPA colleague Darren Lytle arrived in Milwaukee on April 12 and began their investigation by reviewing detailed operational and water-quality data from both plants followed by in-depth onsite inspections of the South and North plants and extensive interviewing of plant and other MWW personnel. In the report of this investigation, Kim noted that the South Plant received a highly variable quality of raw water from Lake Michigan (the influent) for processing and noted that during March 18–April 9, 1993, the raw water turbidity levels ranged from 1.5 to 44 NTU (usually 3 to 4 NTU in prior months), and raw water coliform concentrations were also quite variable. Specific deficiencies that may have contributed either to a delay in recognition of a problem or the inability to bring finished water turbidity to plant baseline values included the lack of historical use records for the coagulant used (PAC was used only since September, 1992). Also, the residence time for the water in the plant was relatively short, and the time required to see a result in treated water quality after chemical adjustment was relatively long. These factors contributed to difficulty in optimizing the coagulant dose. In addition, the finished water turbidity was measured in the clearwell rather than as the water left each filter. The clearwell was the massive receptacle where water from all the filters was pooled before it was released as effluent from the treatment plant. Also, although the filters were frequently backwashed to remove impurities and maintain optimal filtering capability, the backwash water was recycled through the plant instead of being discarded.

Comparison of the Efficacy of Different Surveillance Methods Used in this Outbreak Investigation[15]

The availability of a rich array of surveillance data from seven categories of data source provided us with an opportunity to compare the efficacies of using each category of surveillance data during this waterborne outbreak investigation. We found that surveillance systems that could be easily linked with laboratory data were flexible in adding new variables, and those that demonstrated low baseline variability were most useful. Notably, geographically fixed nursing home residents served as an ideal population with nonconfounded exposures; however, the signals that were most timely (i.e., the shortest interval needed to learn about the peak) were consumer complaints to the South Plant utility (the best) and aberrant and peak finished water turbidity (Figure 14-4). Although not indicators of disease, these signals can be effectively used in stimulating heightened surveillance for human illness and generating timely messages to the public and persons at greater risk of water related illness and help reduce potential outbreak-related morbidity. This would be particularly helpful to implement in communities with populations greater than 100,000 with water supplies derived from surface water.

Unusual Clusters and Anecdotes

There were several unusual clusters. The Finals (Frozen Four) of the NCAA hockey tournament were held in Milwaukee April 1–3. We conducted a follow-up with cooperation from respective state epidemiologists to determine whether diarrhea illnesses occurred in any team or entourage members. Indeed, cases occurred among members or associates of three teams, but not among the team from the University of Maine that brought its own bottled water supply as a standard practice, and they won the NCAA championship. Bottled water generally should not be viewed as a panacea, but it sure was healthful in this instance. A large number of individuals with watery diarrhea illness were seen in the clinic facility at the speedway in North Wilkesboro, NC during a NASCAR event. All ill individuals had attended the funeral of the beloved NASCAR driver and Milwaukee resident Allen Kulwicki (killed in a crash of a private airplane) in Milwaukee 1 week previously. An outbreak of *Cryptosporidium* infections investigated in Michigan occurred among a Coast Guard crew on a boat that had its potable water supply tank filled in Milwaukee.

Professional sports were not spared. Several Milwaukee professional athletes became ill, and there were concerns raised among teams that had recently traveled or would be traveling to Milwaukee. The largest event of concern for which numerous special precautions were taken was the Milwaukee Brewers home season opening game that occurred before the boil-water advisory was lifted. Of course, the beer was safe to drink.

Invoking and Lifting the Boil-Water Advisory

When boil-water advisories are enacted, it is important to envision the terms and conditions needed to discontinue (lift) them. After becoming familiar with water testing processes and having numerous phone conversations with experts at the AWWA, EPA, CDC, the Wisconsin DNR, and in academia, I began the process of generating a Delphi survey that involved the repeated interviewing of these experts regarding what they felt the standard should be for lifting the boil-water order. The South Plant was closed, and thus, all of our attention was on the North Plant. We needed to demonstrate that the North Plant water was safe. This would involve repeated measurement of *Cryptosporidium* oocysts in samples of North Plant effluent water and representative samples of water obtained from distal sites in the municipal water distribution system. Also, spun cartridge filters, the standard at that time, would be used to filter samples of finished water and would then be tested for the presence of *Cryptosporidium* oocysts. The filters were sent to the AWWA laboratory in Belleville, Illinois. Mark LeChevallier and his colleagues in Belleville provided exceptional expertise and service during this outbreak.

After several rounds of calls, the Delphi process ultimately focused on the demonstration of less than one *Cryptosporidium* oocyst per 100 liters of filtered water at each of the sampling sites (one central and four distal) and in two consecutive samples at each of the central and distal sites. The samples would involve 12-hour collections at each site. With shipping, the cycle to process each filter took 2 to 3 days. I realized that it would probably take a minimum of 5 days to have the data needed to lift the advisory, and one sample from any site with results that exceeded the threshold could add another 3 days to the process. Sometimes my patience in waiting for test results wore rather thin.

Finally, the boil-water advisory was lifted on the evening of April 14 after receipt late on April 14 of the results of processing samples collected during the third round on April 13. The city was served exclusively by the North Plant until June, when the water filters replacement and refurbishing was completed at the South Plant.

Additional Investigations and Studies

Protection from Point-of-Use Filters[22]

During a press conference in the early phases of the outbreak, I requested that individuals who had point-of-use (filters that were installed in homes or workplace settings) water filters installed in their homes before the outbreak contact us because we were interested in evaluating whether they were effective in preventing diarrhea illness during this outbreak. The response to this request was overwhelming, and many individuals volunteered to actually donate their filter if needed. Bob Pond, an Atlanta-based EIS officer, joined Dave Addiss and me in Milwaukee to conduct this evaluation. We surveyed 155 filter owners and 99 completed the self-administered questionnaire. Among residents and users of water in the southern or central Milwaukee, we found users of submicron (pore size less than one micron) point-of-use filters during the outbreak were significantly less likely to experience watery diarrhea than those who consumed unfiltered tap water in a public building and those who had home water filters with pore sizes greater than 1 micron. Being conservative in interpreting our data, we concluded that (even in these extraordinarily adverse field conditions) submicron point-of-use water filters may reduce the risk of waterborne cryptosporidiosis.[22]

Postoutbreak Transmission of Cryptosporidium[23]

Surveillance for new infections was sustained for many months. Postoutbreak secondary transmission of *Cryptosporidium* was expected to occur; however, of great concern was the potential of sustained waterborne transmission of *Cryptosporidium* that could be occurring with clinical muting of symptomatic illness related to the widespread emerging immunity to *Cryptosporidium*. In a follow-up investigation of 33 individuals with onsets of laboratory-confirmed *Cryptosporidium* infection during May 1 to June 23 and neighborhood and household control subjects, we found waterborne transmission was not associated with these late illnesses. Risk factors for postoutbreak illness included immune compromise and living in a household with one or more children less than 5 years old suggesting person-to-person transmission. Despite biases introduced by the greater likelihood that immune-compromised individuals would be tested during the postoutbreak period, this study provided reassurance that new *Cryptosporidium* infections were not occurring as a result of drinking MWW water.[23]

Swimming Pool-Related Outbreaks

We were mindful that chains of transmission could be sustained as *Cryptosporidium* can be transmitted from person to person or an infected individual can contaminate a new, more limited water supply. Shortly after the Milwaukee outbreak and throughout the summer of 1993, outbreaks of *Cryptosporidium* infection among users of public or hotel pools were reported from several counties.[24,25] The earliest such outbreak north of Milwaukee could be directly attributed to the Milwaukee outbreak; however, the phenomenon continued through the summer as additional pools in Wisconsin and elsewhere were seeded with the chlorine-resistant *Cryptosporidium* oocysts and pool users became infected and then contributors to multiple generations of illness. The optimal concentration of chlorine in swimming pools was not sufficiently high to kill the oocysts before an unsuspecting swimmer ingested a small volume of pool water.

Genotyping

Speciation and further characterization of the outbreak strain of *Cryptosporidium* were another objective of this investigation. To accomplish this, three volunteers who had been ill during the outbreak and had laboratory-confirmed infections were recruited to donate large volumes of stool. To our disappointment, after shipment to and maintenance of these specimens at a CDC laboratory, the *Cryptosporidium* in these specimens became nonviable. These specimens still proved useful because they were ultimately (more than a year later) used to test the *Cryptosporidium parvum* DNA to determine genotype of the strains. An important goal of the genotyping was to determine the source of the *Cryptosporidium*. Although limited, genotype information provides clues regarding whether the source strain was human or bovine. In Milwaukee, the source strain was suggested to be human based on the genotype testing[26]; however, I believe the extremely small number of specimens from the Milwaukee outbreak used in the genotype investigation and perhaps the sources of stool specimens tested make these observations more conjectural. The suggestion of a human source is supported by the limited data available, but I do not believe that it is proven. It is conceivable that multiple genotypes were circulating.

Serologic Studies

We were very interested in the prospect of testing banked sera from ill and well individuals during this outbreak to assess immune responses when a reliable assay became available at some unspecified time in the future. More than 5 years after the outbreak, plasma samples obtained from 553 Milwaukee children aged 6 months to 12 years old who were being tested for lead exposure during the time of the outbreak were tested at CDC laboratories for *Cryptosporidium* antibodies[27] using an enzyme-linked immunosorbent assay to detect IgG to two immunodominant antigens of *C. parvum*. Samples were obtained during five distinct periods in a 5-week interval between March 1993 and May 1993. Each child was bled once, but the prevalence of antibody among children bled during each distinct period could be measured. Data were also available to compare antibody prevalence by region of residence in Milwaukee. The prevalence of antibodies increased from about 16% to 85% during the 5-week interval among children from southern Milwaukee ZIP codes and from about 21% to 45% during the 5-week interval among children from northern Milwaukee ZIP codes. Median antibody reactivity was also substantially greater among the children from southern ZIP codes compared with northern ZIP codes. In addition to corroborating our earlier epidemiologic observations, these data suggest that *C. parvum* infection was more widespread than initially measured based on our RDD studies.[27] Because the samples were obtained without accompanying clinical information, it is not known what the proportions were of subclinical or asymptomatic infection.[27]

Theories on Why This Massive Outbreak Occurred: A Perfect Storm[2,3]

Outbreaks of great magnitude are generally not easily explained, nor was this one; however, a confluence of likely contributing factors and events during March and April 1993 was exceptionally compelling and provided unique opportunities to dramatically amplify case occurrence.

The South Plant Intake Grid Location and Unusual Weather Conditions

The placement of the South Plant intake grid was unfortunate at best. As previously noted, the three rivers flowing through Milwaukee County join together to flow into a bay and harbor along the Lake Michigan shore. This harbor is protected by a large breakfront. The breakfront has three large outer gaps through which water can flow in and out of the harbor. As previously noted, the ambient current in the harbor contained within the large breakfront was southerly. Water flowing out the south fair weather gap typically flowed directly toward the South Plant intake grid. During and after rainy and other high-flow periods when increases in runoff and storm sewer overflow in the rivers are noted, the discharges of dirt and particulate matter into the harbor can be striking (Figure 14-6). This was occurring during a prolonged, intense high flow period compounded by unusual weather conditions:

- There was a high snow pack during the winter that melted rapidly while the frost line was still high. The runoff was excessive, and its impact was likely compounded by runoff manure spread onto

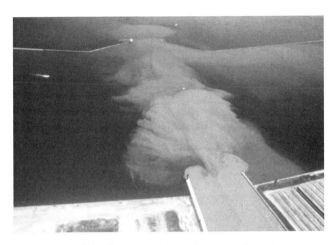

FIGURE 14-6 Discharge of run-off and related materials from the Milwaukee River into the Lake Michigan Harbor during or following a period of high flow, Milwaukee, Wisconsin, 1993.

the snow by farm workers intent on getting rid of it and concurrently enriching their fields.
- There was record setting rainfall in March and early April that contributed to runoff within the river watersheds. Within the City of Milwaukee, this rainfall contributed to widespread storm sewer overflows resulting in vast volumes of sewage that could be disinfected but otherwise bypassed treatment in the Milwaukee Metropolitan Sewage District facility before it drained into the bay that was protected by the breakfront.
- The wind conditions and direction were highly unusual. There was a prolonged period of northeasterly winds occurring in late March and early April. During this time, there was likely accentuation of the southerly flow of water within the breakfront with more flow of water in the bay out the south fair weather gap, which likely amplified plumes flowing directly toward the South Plant intake grid. Prevailing winds in other directions would have facilitated their dispersal.
- These conditions would have enhanced the transport of *Cryptosporidium* oocysts toward the South Plant water intake.

Cross Connection Between a Sanitary Sewer and a Storm Sewer

In early March 1993, during the construction of soccer fields near the Menomonee River and close to downtown Milwaukee, a linkage of a storm sewer draining the fields with a central main sewer was being created when a large volume of impacted contents was noted in the main sewer. The contents included animal material, particularly animal intestines. In addition, there were many rubber rings that were used to prevent spillage of enteric contents when bovines were slaughtered and eviscerated. Further investigation by local officials resulted in the detection of a cross connection between an abattoir kill floor sanitary sewer and the storm sewer. After elimination of this cross connection and correction of sewage flow, the storm sewer was cleaned during a multiple week process. The cross connection was estimated to have existed for years. Material from the abattoir kill floor that impacted in the storm sewer or flowed directly to the river via the cross connection would now travel through the sanitary sewer and be treated at the sewage treatment plant or be disinfected and bypass treatment during periods of high flow (heavy rains). It is not known whether *Cryptosporidium* oocysts were released directly through the storm sewer into the Menomonee River during or preceding these events or whether a bolus of oocysts properly flowing through the sanitary sewer during cleanup procedures may have bypassed sewage treatment during a period of high flow.

Change in Coagulant

The change in coagulant routinely used in both the North and South Plants 6 months before the outbreak and the difficulty in coagulant dosing during a period of abnormal turbidity to bring the turbidity under control were factors. Furthermore, the Milwaukee Water Works interpretation of finished water turbidity as an aesthetic indicator may have contributed to late recognition of the difficulties (or later recognition of the importance of the difficulties) they were having with water treatment. The occurrence of this outbreak provided a focus on the importance of turbidity as a water quality indicator.

Human Amplification

The amplification of the burden of *Cryptosporidium* oocysts among residents of the greater Milwaukee area was a critical factor. In humans, the infectious dose of *C. parvum* that can result in illness is small. Among healthy adult volunteers with no serologic evidence of past infection with *C. parvum*, the median infectious dose has been determined to be 132 oocysts[28]; however, billions of oocysts are excreted each day in the stools of symptomatic individuals, and excretion of oocysts typically continues for several weeks after symptoms resolve. Shedding can be more prolonged in those who are immunocompromised. Additionally, the oocysts can remain infective in moist environments for 2 to 6 months. Thus, the opportunity for infection in this outbreak was extraordinarily, perhaps incomprehensibly, high. This was compounded by the aforementioned rainy, high-flow conditions when storm sewers typically overflowed and, other than disinfection, most sewage was not treated before discharge into the harbor. This all contributed to a sustained vicious cycle of oocyst and illness amplification.

Limited Testing Prior to Outbreak Recognition

There was some delay in recognition of this outbreak. Based on the sporadic occurrences of diarrhea illnesses weeks prior to the outbreak peak, the outbreak probably began in early March but was initially recognized on April 5. This delay can in part be explained by understanding that testing stool specimens for *Cryptosporidium* was not commonplace in medical practice at the time of this outbreak. Typically, testing for *Cryptosporidium* infection was requested in individuals with HIV infection who were experiencing diarrhea. The number of tests requested per month was relatively small, and most healthcare providers would not readily have suspected this diagnosis in healthy patients with brief or even prolonged diarrhea disease. If they requested obtaining a stool specimen to test for parasites, *Cryptosporidium* was not a pathogen routinely looked for. Tests for *Cryptosporidium* required an additional requisition. Indeed, a major factor in the limited number of test requisitions was the complexity caused by the additional pelleting and staining procedures and the attendant greater expense of testing. These factors may have contributed to this insufficient testing demand with consequent delay in ascertainment of an outbreak.

POLICY IMPACTS AND INFRASTRUCTURE IMPROVEMENTS

Standards

The massive Milwaukee cryptosporidiosis outbreak was historic. It is the largest known outbreak of waterborne disease ever documented in the United States and possibly in the developed world. The magnitude of this outbreak coupled with the direct association of illness with a municipal water treatment plant that was operating within existing state and federal regulatory standards at that time had an immediate powerful impact that focused widespread public concern on the quality of drinking water, underscored the need to have far more stringent regulatory standards, and raised awareness of cryptosporidiosis as a diarrheal illness. A specific need to create specific regulatory standards for *Cryptosporidium* in drinking water was apparent.

The Milwaukee Water Works expeditiously adopted standards and quality indices that were maximally stringent and far more stringent than state or federal standards. Wisconsin state standards were also strengthened and clarified. The antiquated and confusing use of monthly or other interval averages in turbidity as a threshold standard was eliminated.

The EPA was in the process of generating and releasing its Information Collection Rule, which provided water treatment facilities with a list of laboratory tests and measures that would be needed to ultimately generate a final set of standards. The occurrence of this massive outbreak in the midst of this process had bearing on the content of the Information Collection Rule.

Infrastructure Improvements

Virtually immediately after the boil-water order was invoked and with the assistance of many experts, officials began planning to make extensive changes to the Milwaukee water treatment infrastructure. Nearer term improvements included the revision of filters and filter beds (removal of all media, sandblasting all filter beds, structural changes, installation of new media) and installation of particle counters and automatic alarms for each filter (when very low threshold turbidity or particle counts are exceeded, there is automatic filter shutdown and diversion of affected water so that it did not enter the clear well). Longer term projects that took several years to complete included the construction of ozonation facilities at each treatment plant. Because *Cryptosporidium* oocysts are highly chlorine resistant, standard disinfection procedures are not sufficient to inactivate them. Ozonation as an adjunct to disinfection is effective because it inactivates oocysts by disrupting their cell walls and it is effective in disrupting other microorganisms found in raw water. The North and South Plants are now state of the art facilities and have been visited by utility related personnel from many states and countries.

CONCLUDING REFLECTIONS

The Milwaukee outbreak, the results of our collective investigations, and the local and state responses were of great interest to drinking water related regulators, utility (public and private) administrators, and municipalities throughout the United States, Canada, Europe, Japan, Australia, and elsewhere. Although fear of such a large outbreak is a great motivator, the significant and tangible improvements in water treatment authorized by the City of Milwaukee administration has had substantial impact on voluntary and required improvements in water processing and in water quality in communities in many states and countries. The transparency of these processes has improved as have communications between the water treatment and public health communities. These efforts were certainly apparent throughout Wisconsin when communities recognized that Lake Michigan turbidity events were not limited to Milwaukee (Wisconsin DPH, unpublished data). Clearly, we learned the importance of the need for improved surveillance for infections that may result from waterborne pathogens and for aberrations in water quality. This requires cooperation, coordination, and communication among public health agency and water utility staffs.

The high level of civic resolve to focus on solutions to rapidly control this massive outbreak and prevent even teeny ones from occurring in the future was extraordinary. As a native of Milwaukee County, I was deeply moved and very proud of this enormous yet efficient effort. Our team was very impressed with the exceptional cooperation received from local government, businesses large and small, and private citizens. We could not have accomplished as much as we did without the degree of cooperation and collaboration that we experienced. As expected, the greater Milwaukee community did this with a great sense of humor, at times magnificently sharp and self-deprecating, and civic pride. In one photograph featured in the newspaper at that time, an illuminated sign from a pharmacy-food mart says simply, "We have Immodium AD. Open Easter." In another photo of a man walking to the front of a bar, the sign overhead says simply, "Mexican vacation? Why bother. Stay here."

Without question, application of the lessons learned from this outbreak has had a sustained impact on preventing subsequent outbreaks in the United States and other developed countries.

REFERENCES

1. Hayes EB, Matte TD, O'Brien TR, et al. Large community outbreak of cryptosporidiosis due to contamination of a filtered public water supply. *N Engl J Med* 1989;320:1372–1376.
2. Mac Kenzie WR, Hoxie NJ, Proctor ME, et al. A massive outbreak in Milwaukee of Cryptosporidium infection transmitted through the public water supply. *N Engl J Med* 1994;331:161–167.
3. Addiss DG, Mac Kenzie WR, Hoxie NJ, et al. Epidemiologic features and implications of the Milwaukee cryptosporidiosis outbreak. In Betts WB, Casemore D, Fricker C, Smith H, Watkins J, eds. *Protozoan Parasites and Water*. Cambridge, England: The Royal Society of Chemistry, 1995:19–25.
4. Marchione M. Detective story: Skill, luck come to fore. *Milwaukee J* 1993;April 11:1, 12.
5. Nime FA, Burek JD, Page DL, Holscher MA, Yardley JH. Acute enterocolitis in a human being infected with the protozoan *Cryptosporidium*. *Gastroenterology* 1976;70:592–598.
6. Jokipii L, Jokipii AMM. Timing of symptoms and oocyst excretion in human cryptosporidiosis. *N Engl J Med* 1986;315:1643–1647.
7. Wolfson JS, Richter JM, Waldron MA, Weber DJ, McCarthy DM, Hopkins CC, Cryptosporidiosis in immunocompetent patients. *N Engl J Med* 1985;312:1278–1282.
8. Meisel JL, Perera DR, Meligro C, Rubin CE. Overwhelming watery diarrhea associated with cryptosporidium in an immunosuppressed patient. *Gastroenterology* 1976;70:1156–1160.
9. Current WL, Reese NC, Ernst JV, Bailey WS, Heyman MB, Weinstein WM. Human cryptosporidiosis in immunocompetent and immunodeficient persons: studies of an outbreak and experimental transmission. *N Engl J Med* 1983;308:1252–1257.
10. D'Antonio RG, Winn RE, Taylor JP, et al. A waterborne outbreak of cryptosporidiosis in normal hosts. *Ann Intern Med* 1985;103:886–888.
11. Gallagher MM, Herndon JL, Nims IJ, Sterling CR, Grabowski DJ, Hull HF. Cryptosporidiosis and surface water. *Am J Public Health* 1989;79:39–42.
12. Richardson AJ, Frankenberg RA, Buck AC, et al. An outbreak of waterborne cryptosporidiosis in Swindon and Oxfordshire. *Epidemiol Infect* 1991;107:485–495.
13. Joseph C, Hamilton G, O'Connor M, et al. Cryptosporidiosis in the Isle of Thanet: an outbreak associated with local drinking water. *Epidemiol Infect* 1991;107:509–519.
14. Leland D, McAnulty J, Keene W, Sterens G. A cryptosporidiosis outbreak in a filtered-water supply. *J Am Water Works Assoc* 1993;85:34–42.
15. Proctor ME, Blair KA, Davis JP. Surveillance data for waterborne illness: an assessment following a massive waterborne outbreak of Cryptosporidium infection. *Epidemiol Infect* 1998;20:43–54.
16. Corso PS, Kramer MH, Blair KA, Addiss DG, Davis JP, Haddix AC. The cost of illness associated with the massive waterborne outbreak of Cryptosporidium infections in 1993 in Milwaukee, Wisconsin. *Emerg Infect Dis* 2003;9:426–431.
17. Mac Kenzie WR, Schell WL, Blair KA, et al. Massive outbreak of waterborne Cryptosporidium infection in Milwaukee, Wisconsin: Recurrence of illness and risk of secondary transmission. *Clin Infect Dis* 1995;21:57–62.
18. Cordell RL, Thor PM, Addiss DG, et al. Impact of a massive waterborne cryptosporidiosis outbreak on child care facilities in Metropolitan Milwaukee, Wisconsin. *Pediatr Infect Dis J* 1997;16:639–644.
19. Cicirello HG, Kehl KS, Addiss DG, et al. Cryptosporidiosis in children during a massive waterborne outbreak,

Milwaukee, Wisconsin: clinical, laboratory, and epidemiologic findings. *Epidemiol Infect* 1997; 119:53–60.
20. Frisby HR, Addiss DG, Reiser WJ, et al. Clinical and epidemiologic features of a massive waterborne outbreak of cryptosporidiosis among persons with human immunodeficiency virus (HIV) infection. *J Acq Immun Defic Syndr Hum Retrovirol* 1997;16:367–373.
21. Hoxie NJ, Davis JP, Vergeront JM, Nashold RD, Blair KA. Cryptosporidiosis-associated mortality following a massive waterborne outbreak in Milwaukee, Wisconsin. *Am J Public Health* 1997;87:2032–2038.
22. Addiss DG, Pond RS, Remshak M, Juranek D, Stokes S, Davis JP. Reduction of risk of watery diarrhea with point-of-use water filters during a massive outbreak of waterborne Cryptosporidium infection in Milwaukee, 1993. *Am J Trop Med Hyg* 1996;54:549–553.
23. Osewe P, Addiss DG, Blair KA, Hightower A, Kamb ML, Davis JP. Cryptosporidiosis in Wisconsin: a case-control study of post-outbreak transmission. *Epidemiol Infect* 1996; 117:297–304.
24. Mac Kenzie WR, Kazmierczak JJ, Davis JP. Cryptosporidiosis associated with a resort swimming pool. *Epidemiol Infect* 1995; 115:545–553.
25. Cryptosporidium infections associated with swimming pools—Dane County, Wisconsin, 1993. *MMWR* 1994;43: 561–563.
26. Sulaiman IM, Xiao L, Yang C, et al. Differentiating human from animal solates of Cryptosporidium parvum. *Emerg Infect Dis* 1998;4:681–685.
27. McDonald AC, Mac Kenzie WR, Addiss DG, et al. Cryptosporidium parvum-specific antibody responses among children residing in Milwaukee during the 1993 waterborne outbreak. *J Infect Dis* 2001;183:1373–1379.
28. Du Pont HL, Chappell, Sterling CR, Okhuysen PC, Rose JB, Jakubowski. The infectivity of Cryptosporidium parvum in healthy volunteers. *N Engl J Med* 1995;332:855–859.

LEARNING QUESTIONS

1. Early on in this investigation, it was clear that there was an emerging public health problem because the health department was receiving calls from several sources. So if they already knew they had a problem, then how did performing active surveillance by calling emergency departments and laboratories around the region to determine diarrhea-related illness numbers help the health department investigators?
2. A suggestion from an expert at the CDC allowed the health department investigators to have greater confidence that this was an outbreak from municipal drinking water rather than from any other source of water. What was that suggestion and the rationale behind it?
3. An early problem was the lack of any surveillance system for cryptosporidiosis or diarrheal disease (as a syndrome). Where did the health department set up diarrheal disease surveillance and why in these specific places?
4. What were the three environmental sources that were suspected of possibly being the source of *Cryptosporidium* into the three rivers that flow into Lake Michigan?

CHAPTER 15

A Community Outbreak of Hepatitis A Involving Cooperation Between Public Health, the Media, and Law Enforcement, Iowa, 1997

Patricia Quinlisk, MD, MPH; Yvan Hutin, MD;
Ken Carter; Tom Carney; and Kevin Teale

Iowa, 1997

INTRODUCTION

When an outbreak of hepatitis A occurred in Iowa during 1996 and 1997, Yvan Hutin was an Epidemic Intelligence Service (EIS) officer with the Centers for Disease Control and Prevention (CDC). Patricia Quinlisk was the state epidemiologist in Iowa. Ken Carter was the state's director of the Division of Narcotics Enforcement. Kevin Teale was the communications director for the state health department, and Tom Carney was a reporter for the Des Moines Register. In this chapter, they share the actions they took, while shedding light on their unique perspectives and how they interacted with each other while they were trying to understand and control an outbreak of hepatitis A in methamphetamine users. Although several counties were involved in the 1997 hepatitis A epidemic, the chapter focuses on Polk County, where Des Moines, the capital, is located (Figure 15-1).

Hepatitis A is a virus that can cause no symptoms at all or it may lead to jaundice, severe fatigue, tea colored urine, loss of appetite, diarrhea, and rarely death.[1] The virus is excreted in the feces, and is spread from one person to another via fecal contamination of water or food from unwashed hands. It is found in humans worldwide, but it is especially common where sanitation is poor. Where it is most common, outbreaks are less likely to occur because sporadic human-to-human transmission can maintain a relatively high level of exposure among the population. As a result, most of the population would be immune because long-term immunity occurs after infection, and much of the transmission occurs in a developing country during childhood. Many studies have shown that the seroprevalence of hepatitis A increases with increasing age, indicating that the longer one lives in an endemic region, the greater the likelihood one will become exposed and subsequently infected.

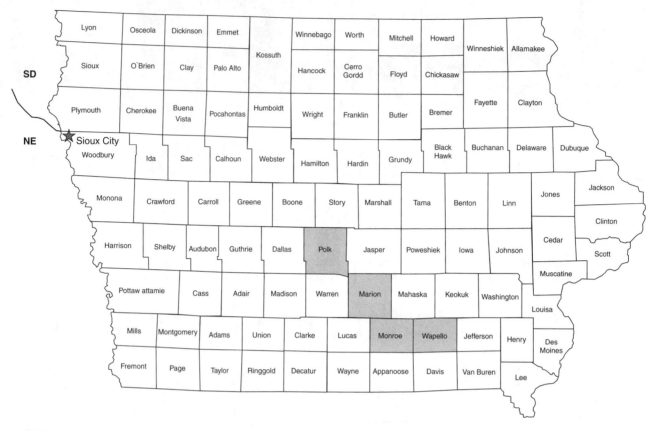

FIGURE 15-1 Iowa and Neighboring States were Involved in this Hepatitis A Outbreak.

Sanitary conditions, in a developed country like the United States, minimize the risk of person to person and waterborne transmission of hepatitis A; however, American child care centers are often foci of spread because of attendance by diapered children who easily spread diseases via feces. Food-borne outbreaks occur sporadically but are not a major source of transmission. As recently as 2006, the Advisory Committee on Immunization Practices recommended that all children should receive hepatitis A vaccine at age 1 year. In addition, the hepatitis A vaccine has been administered to many U.S. citizens because of compliance with a variety of public health recommendations, including efforts to immunize groups where the epidemiology has demonstrated increased risk of either being exposed to the disease or of developing complications if disease occurs, such as travelers, men who have sex with men, persons with clotting-factor disorders, persons working with nonhuman primates, and users of injection and noninjection drugs.

Health departments determine when a hepatitis A exposure has occurred (such as when a restaurant food handler works while infectious and may have exposed hundreds of customers). Then, applying knowledge of the relatively long incubation period for hepatitis A (ranging from 15 to 50 days), the health department determines who can still be protected with immune globulin (IG) (i.e., up until what date could those who were exposed be offered IG as an effective disease prevention measure). The usual time from exposure until it is too late to give IG is 14 days.[2]

Drug use is not the first risk factor one might think of when considering hepatitis A. In fact, when considering drugs, especially injection drugs, one is much more likely to think of hepatitis B or hepatitis C because they are transmitted primarily via blood and blood products. Activities like sharing needles or other blood-contaminated drug paraphernalia fit nicely into the understanding of transmission of hepatitis B and C. Thus, an outbreak of hepatitis A among methamphetamine users is unique.

> *Drug use is not the first risk factor one might think of when considering hepatitis A.*

An infectious disease outbreak involving collaboration with the media and law enforcement without a bioterrorism angle is even more unique. This investigation also demonstrates how the incubation period of an infectious disease can influence policy decision. This investigation also illustrates that health departments must sometimes act based on their interest in protecting the public even though they cannot predict with certainty what would happen if they did not act.

Many features of outbreak investigation are nicely displayed in the presentation of this outbreak: (1) the importance of good communication, (2) coordination between involved governmental entities, (3) community involvement in controlling an epidemic, and (4) the use of an epidemiologic study's findings to intervene and control an outbreak. The health department was challenged with a hard to reach population (drug users), a disease with prevention activities that need to be performed within a specific time frame to be effective (such as administration of vaccine and IG), information that needed to be handled very delicately to keep a clear message, and intense media and public interest.

The voices in the chapter include the following:

CDC: Yvan Hutin, EIS officer, CDC
Narcotics: Ken Carter, director, Division of Narcotics Enforcement, Department of Public Safety
Newspaper: Tom Carney, Science Writer, *Des Moines Register*
Press Liaison: Kevin Teale, Communications Director, Iowa Department of Public Health (IDPH)
State Epidemiologist: Patricia Quinlisk, State Epidemiologist, IDPH

State Epidemiologist: Historically, Iowa has had relatively low rates of hepatitis A, punctuated by occasional small outbreaks[3]; however, in the first few months of 1996, hepatitis A began to increase in the "Siouxland" area (around Sioux City, Iowa, including parts of Nebraska and South Dakota), resulting in a community-wide outbreak that lasted about 1 year. A case-control study was performed during that time in collaboration with the local Siouxland District Health Department, the IDPH, and the federal CDC. This study identified three population groups at increased risk for hepatitis A; those who injected methamphetamine, those who used emergency rooms more than other health care facilities, and those who participated in the WIC (Women, Infants, and Children) program. Prevention and control interventions were expanded, and by the end of 1996, this community outbreak had essentially ended.[4]

Hepatitis A is a reportable disease in the state of Iowa. Thus, health care professionals, including laboratorians, are required to report any disease that the Iowa Board of Health determines to be significant because of public health importance, like hepatitis A. Usually diseases are made reportable if they can spread from one person to another (or from an animal to a human) and/or when public health intervention will modify the transmission or course of disease.

> *Usually diseases are made reportable if they can spread from one person to another (or from an animal to a human) and/or when public health intervention will modify the transmission or course of disease.*

Press Liaison: For at least 3 years prior to 1996, no public health announcements concerning hepatitis A had occurred. Then, in February of 1996, media coverage about the outbreak in the Siouxland area began. At the same time, both the *Sioux City Journal* (the local paper) and the *Des Moines Register* (located in central Iowa, but with statewide readership) did stories about the sharp increase in the number of cases. Although the *Sioux City Journal* article stressed prevention, the *Register* article focused on the possibility that the outbreak might have been tied to drug use. Siouxland health officials expressed concerns that the mention of a drug connection might hamper efforts to control the outbreak.

When press releases or information are released about a health concern, the media often asks many questions. With the exception of large media markets that may have trained health reporters, most news items are handled by general assignment reporters who do not have a background in health or science. Additionally, reporters are trained to produce stories with a reading level of third or fourth grade. It is sometimes difficult to work in the basic facts of a health concern (who, what, when, where, and why) and also work in medical information in a simple form. A delicate balance needs to be struck between keeping the media message uncomplicated and not missing important facts for simplicity's sake.

Also, the number of questions asked or the time spent by a reporter with informants may not be an indication of how large a story will be published or the placement (front page or back page) of the story. The same story may get very different placement in different outlets on the same day

> *The number of questions asked or the time spent by a reporter with informants may not be an indication of how large a story will be published or the placement (front page or back page) of the story.*

because of other stories that the media outlet may be working on.

Sometimes public health officials will ask that key information or issues be contained in a story to address a specific concern, but we really have to rely on the media's cooperation for this to happen. That is why it is important to establish good relationships between the public health community and media outlets before a crisis situation erupts. We are fortunate in Iowa to have a media that understands health issues and very often will oblige our requests.

CDC: In recent outbreaks in the Midwest and the Northwest, a high proportion of the case patients with hepatitis A had reported use of illicit drugs, mostly injected drugs such as methamphetamine. Attempts had been made to determine why these drug users were at increased risk for hepatitis A, but the reason(s) continued to be unclear. These previous investigations had attempted to determine the risk factors for acquiring hepatitis A, but this had necessitated interviewing drug users, who were understandably reluctant to tell "the government" about their drug habits; however, Iowans are notorious for being cooperative, and thus, it was thought that a study there might be successful.

Narcotics: The Iowa Division of Narcotics Enforcement's (DNE) primary responsibility is to be the lead agency, by Chapter 80 of the Code of Iowa, in the investigation of major drug organizations, both within Iowa and in areas that have direct ties to Iowa. This mission is carried out within DNE through specialized enforcement, to include general narcotics, financial conspiracy, diversion, clandestine laboratories, marijuana eradication, and gang-related investigations.

Methamphetamine (or "meth") use had dramatically increased in Iowa in the 3 years before 1997. Although only two clandestine meth laboratories had been seized in 1994 (neither in Polk County), by 1997, 63 laboratories were seized, 28 of which were in Polk County. Additionally, in 1994, only 26 people had been arrested in Iowa related to methamphetamine or amphetamine, but by 1997, 234 were arrested. Finally, in 1994, only 11,433 grams of methamphetamine or amphetamine were seized, but during 1997, 52,472 grams were seized.

Meth is a central nervous system stimulant and allows users to go for days without sleep or food. When users are "coming off" the drug, acute paranoia and violent behavior are quite common. This is when child or spousal abuse occurs and when behavior can be very unpredictable and explosive.

In Iowa, about 85% of meth comes from Mexico or the United States–Mexico border area; however, the number of meth laboratories in Iowa was exploding. With information about how to manufacture meth readily available (e.g., on the web), people are setting up "laboratories" (i.e., manufacturing facilities) in homes, hotel rooms, and farm outbuildings. Meth is produced from commonly available materials such as anhydrous ammonia (a farm fertilizer) and sinus/cold medication that was available over the counter at that time. Combining these components can be dangerous; for the short term, they can explode, but for long term, they can be carcinogenic.

> *Meth is a central nervous system stimulant and allows users to go for days without sleep or food.*

State Epidemiologist: In early 1997, a truck stop food handler developed hepatitis A and was reported to us by the laboratory that did the serologic test. There was potential for the spread of the virus to the public. We found that his exposure to hepatitis A may have been linked to use of drugs that had been obtained in the Des Moines area. He prepared foods in such a way that he could have contaminated ready to serve foods with his hands that were carrying specks of feces laden with hepatitis A virus. Because the only tool the health department has to prevent disease in those who might have been exposed to hepatitis A via eating this contaminated food is by "going public," we put out a press release recommending those who had eaten at the truck stop to get IG shots. We also announced where the shots were available and clinics were opened at the local health departments.

The potential for spread of the hepatitis A virus to the public from an infectious food handler has four main components. We determine: (1) whether the food handler had diarrhea while handling the food (high risk for transmission since the virus is found in feces), (2) whether the food handler neglected to wash his/her hands after using the restroom (increased risk for transmission even if no diarrhea), (3) what foods the food handler handled (wet, rough, uncooked foods, such as salads, are highest risk; foods cooked thoroughly after handling are no risk), and (4) how many times a patron might have been exposed (increased "dosage" or amount of exposure to contaminated food may increase the risk of becoming ill).

In situations like this, we have to weigh the restaurant's need to be protected from bad publicity against the public's need to be able to protect themselves from disease. If there is a possibility of disease transmission, we feel that the public's needs far outweigh the restaurant's concerns; therefore, we put out a press release to notify those who may have been exposed to hepatitis A. We do try to minimize the damage to the restaurant, however, by stating that remedial steps have been taken, that it is safe to eat there now (if this is true), and how well they are cooperating. We do not release the food handler's name, as no purpose would be served by doing so.

Newspaper: The readers of the *Des Moines Register* became better acquainted with hepatitis A in February of 1997, when the state health department announced that a food handler at a truck stop had potentially exposed the public to hepatitis A. This was worrisome because the truck stop was located on Interstate 80, near the intersection with Interstate 29, one of the major crossroads of mid-America. The location raised the possibility that the disease could have been spread all over the Midwest, or even all over the country.

At this point, we published a straightforward news story about a food-borne illness. Although the story was important because of the potential for the spread of infection, we were simply following our most basic mission of publishing news reports on occurrences around the state. One of the criteria news organizations have for determining what constitutes "news" is impact. We consistently ask ourselves what has the greatest impact on the greatest number of people. This story had potential for great impact.

State Epidemiologist: After alerting the public to the potential exposure to hepatitis A at the truck stop, public health clinics provided several hundred people in Iowa and neighboring states with IG shots to prevent the disease. Luckily, no further cases of hepatitis A were reported related to this incident.

There are three main ways to prevent hepatitis A. The first and most obvious is to prevent exposure by not having ill persons handle anyone else's food, and for everyone to wash his or her hands, especially after going to the bathroom and before preparing food. The next method is to vaccinate a person who is at high risk of being exposed to hepatitis A. Before Iowa's epidemics, travelers to developing countries were the most commonly vaccinated Iowans. Today, many states require hepatitis A vaccination before school entry. The last method, and the only one that can be used after an exposure has occurred, is to give an injection of IG as soon as possible (usually within 14 days of the exposure because IG probably does not provide much protection if given more than 14 days after exposure). IG is a blood product that contains preformed antibodies to hepatitis A. Because antibodies are proteins (formed by the blood donor's immune system), they are eventually degraded by the receiver's metabolic system; thus, protection only lasts a few months. In contrast, vaccines stimulate the receiver's own immune system, thus that person is protected for a long time, perhaps even for the rest of their life.

In March of 1997, routine public health surveillance demonstrated that the number of hepatitis A cases was increasing in Polk County (Des Moines is in Polk County and has a population of about 400,000 in the metro area). In 1996, only between zero to three cases had been reported per month in the county; however, in March of 1997, 12 cases were reported, and that was obviously more than expected.

Meetings were held between the Polk County Health Department and the IDPH to determine appropriate actions. There was concern that this was the beginning of a community-wide outbreak. We suspected that drug use might be a risk factor (because of what had happened in the Siouxland area), and we thus began discussing community interventions, such as education of jailed persons (many of whom use drugs), persons attending substance abuse treatment centers, and a media campaign targeted at young adults. Also, we gave a "heads up" to restaurants and day care centers (since hepatitis A can be spread easily in these settings). In addition, in April, public health and substance abuse professionals in Iowa discussed two very important issues: the increase in hepatitis A cases possibly associated with substance abuse, and potential strategies to address the current situation. We reviewed what had been tried in the Siouxland area and what had worked, and the kind of general strategies that are usually done when hepatitis A begins to spread in a community.

On April 1, however, before these measures could be implemented to any great extent, the great nationwide 1997 "hepatitis A in frozen strawberries" situation began.[5] Frozen strawberries that had potentially been contaminated with hepatitis A virus had been distributed to schools around the country, including Iowa, via the U.S. Department of Agriculture surplus food program (Exhibit 15-1). These berries were incorrectly labeled as grown in the United States when they were actually from Mexico. Thus, children at many of Iowa's schools had potentially been exposed to hepatitis A. Although the schools had received the strawberries in

EXHIBIT 15-1 Headline

Hepatitis Prognosis: No Cause For Alarm
This headline was published by *USA Today* on April 3, 1997.

January, after discussion with the Iowa Department of Education it was believed that the majority of the strawberries had either not been served until recently in celebration of the spring holidays (i.e., on the Friday before Easter or before spring break starts), or were still in the school's freezers.

A "quick and dirty" epidemiologic investigation was performed. "Quick and dirty" refers to a type of preliminary survey that is usually done by interviewing those who have become ill or who have been exposed. It is "quick" because it can be completed in a few hours and "dirty" because open-ended questions are asked and sometimes opinions are elicited. The data obtained in this way are not considered "clean" or "precise." The main benefit of this method is that information is quickly obtained that can be used to form an emergency response or to provide guidance for designing a more precise and scientific survey or study. This type of study can also be used for hypothesis generation.

If the "quick and dirty" investigation had supported a hypothesis that students and teachers were getting hepatitis A from strawberry exposure, then to protect those who had been exposed, but not yet ill, IG shots would have been given to stop the development of disease. This would have been an important public health intervention. The risk from an intramuscular injection of IG (a sterile preparation of antibodies made from human plasma) is minimal. Usually soreness at the site of the injection is all that is noted among recipients, with rare exception.

The "quick and dirty" epidemiologic investigation led to a very quick but formal survey of all schools that had received the strawberries. This survey found that only a few students or teachers in Iowa schools had any illnesses consistent with hepatitis A after eating the strawberries, and thus, we conducted emergency hepatitis A testing of the ill people to determine whether they had had hepatitis A. These laboratory tests showed no sign of recent hepatitis A infection. Thus, it was highly unlikely that the lots of strawberries distributed in Iowa were contaminated with the hepatitis A virus; therefore, the decision was made *not* to give any IG to any Iowa students or teachers, as we felt the risk from getting IG shots (i.e., soreness) was greater than the risk of getting hepatitis A from eating the strawberries.

Iowa's recommendation was in contrast to the CDC's recommendations that were released that same day, which said that all school children and school staff who had eaten any of the strawberries should be given an injection of IG. We quickly discussed with the experts at the Hepatitis Branch of the CDC the fact that we were not going to follow their recommendations and the rationale for our course of action. They understood our position and agreed that we had sufficient proof that the specific lots of frozen strawberries served in Iowa were not contaminated. Thus, Iowa was the only state in the United States that did not provide IG to its students and teachers. The remaining frozen strawberries were destroyed just in case.

In the end, no cases of hepatitis A associated with these strawberries occurred in Iowa; however, there was major media attention on this situation, both nationally and in Iowa, that continued to increase the public's awareness of hepatitis A.

Newspaper: In the "contaminated strawberries" story, the epidemiologists at the state health department reported that no students or school staff who had consumed the strawberries had become ill. Thus, the strawberries in Iowa were most likely not contaminated, and the IG shots were not needed. We reported that the risks from the shots were probably greater than the risk of getting hepatitis A from the strawberries. Apart from the news value, the *Register's* story presumably helped to calm the fears of parents, students, and staff members about their risks of infection and the usefulness of the shots in this situation.

My principal interest was in reporting the news in as comprehensive a way as possible, helping readers understand the situation, and providing information on what action, if any, they should take. In this case, getting the IG shots was not among actions recommended by the state epidemiologist—who for me, my newspaper, and readers was the principal authority on the issue.

State Epidemiologist: This incident was a good example of the immense help the media can offer by immediately distributing information in situations that are rapidly evolving. There is no other way the health department can quickly educate large segments of the population. These articles really helped to answer questions from people all around the state and to help explain why IG shots were not being recommended or offered.

After all of the press attention to the Iowa truck stop situation where IG was given and all the front page articles in national papers, like the *USA Today*, about schools being given IG, we had started to create the impression in the public's mind that IG is always the answer to potential exposures to hepatitis A. These media stories helped the health department to explain why the shots were not recommended in this situation, where the risk of disease was so low.

In dealing with the media, having your SOCO in mind is very helpful. A SOCO is your "single overriding communication objective," that is, what exactly is the main point you want to get across to the reporter and therefore to the public. In this situation, my SOCO was "shots aren't needed because the risk of getting hepatitis from the strawberries in Iowa was nil." Everything else was extraneous.

Press Liaison: We worked with the media to insure that the correct information was available to the public. Although the "SOCO" was relatively simple, the reasoning behind it was not.

Relationships with the media must be a constant part of the work of public health. In times of a health crisis, there is no other realistic way to get information out to a large number of people without the cooperation of the media. That means responding to all media inquires in a timely, factual manner, no matter how obscure the request may be or how busy we are. Working with the media in a noncrisis situation promotes good relationships and allows the health community to practice delivering a concise, uncomplicated message about health issues, while "educating" the media about science and public health.

Newspaper: A few days after the strawberry story, I noticed a full-page advertisement in the *Register* by a pharmaceutical company. The ad urged readers to see their doctors and "ask about getting vaccinated against hepatitis A." Because at this time the vaccine was considered useful only prior to exposure (see note at end of the chapter), it was therefore too late to be used to prevent illness in those who had eaten strawberries, even if their strawberries were contaminated with hepatitis A. I contacted a family practitioner, who stated that the vaccine was good but would not be useful for people concerned about the strawberries. We then ran an editorial about this situation; we felt that a vaccine manufacturer had used the public's concerns to promote the use of a vaccine that was not appropriate.

Having educated myself and readers about the hepatitis A vaccine, I was surprised by the ad and wondered whether I had misunderstood the vaccine's usefulness in this situation or whether the pharmaceutical company was being overzealous in promotion of its product. Either way, it was new information on the "contaminated strawberries" story and needed to be checked out and reported. I presented the case by the pharmaceutical company and response from the health department, and—to expand the scope of authority in this case—I referred to a family practitioner who had some familiarity with the vaccine. Believing that the pharmaceutical company was presenting false information, I informed our editorial department, whose staff did its own research and wrote an editorial trying to clarify the issues (even though the pharmaceutical company had paid a great deal of money to place a full-page ad in our newspaper).

State Epidemiologist: A few days before Memorial Day weekend (May 24–26, 1997), concerns about a hepatitis A epidemic exponentially increased when the salad maker at a busy, landmark Des Moines restaurant was diagnosed with hepatitis A. Unfortunately, misleading information was given to the emergency room personnel where he had sought medical care and been tested for hepatitis A, resulting in a delay in the public health officials locating and interviewing him (and finding out that he was a food handler!). It was then realized that he had potentially exposed thousands of people to hepatitis A. The amount of time since the last day of this exposure to the public was determined, but because it was more than 14 days, it was too late to give IG to the exposed persons (and prevent them from becoming ill). Thus, at this point, there was major concern that these exposed persons would develop hepatitis A and potentially transmit it to others before realizing the cause of their illness.

A person with hepatitis A becomes infectious about 1 week before symptoms begin and can remain infectious for a week or two after symptoms start. Those with diarrhea are more likely to spread the disease because their hands can become so contaminated with fecal material (and therefore hepatitis A viruses) that washing may not clean them completely; however, anyone with hepatitis A who does not wash their hands after using the bathroom can spread this disease, regardless of the symptoms they have at the time.

When a food handler at a restaurant gets hepatitis A, it can become a public health disaster if appropriate control measures are not undertaken. In our outbreak,

> *A person with hepatitis A becomes infectious about 1 week before symptoms begin and can remain infectious for a week or two after symptoms start.*

the control measure was to educate the public with a very unusual message: People eating at this landmark restaurant had been exposed, but it was too late to prevent them from becoming ill; however, we explained that if they took appropriate precautions, they could prevent spreading it to their family and friends.

Press Liaison: One of the difficulties with the possible outbreak from this restaurant was that our normal hepatitis A message had to be changed. Instead of a simple message of "get IG," the message here was complicated: "It is too late to protect the customers at this restaurant. But if those people become ill, they need to know what action to take to protect their family and friends." A substantial amount of media attention began after the press release with its complex message. The media stories after this ranged from a theme of "if it can happen here, it can happen anywhere," to the historical link to drug use, to the training sessions planned by the county health department for day-care centers and restaurants. We were fortunate to have the full cooperation of the landmark restaurant's owner, when we went public with the news of this possible exposure of the dining public.

Newspaper: At the press conference announcing that consumers had been exposed at the restaurant, the restaurant owner showed obvious signs of stress about what this announcement would do to his business, but it was obvious that the health officials considered this a serious threat to the public health, warranting the risk to a prominent business and business owner.

The landmark restaurant's owner was unusually frank, saying that the salad maker had told him that he had been hospitalized simply for an "infected liver." Despite comments by the health officials that such an infection didn't mean the restaurant had bad sanitary conditions, his business plummeted. In a Memorial Day interview at his home, he said his business, in the days since the press conference, had been only about 10% of normal. "I'm a victim," he said. "I tried to do right to protect my customers. I'm sure I'm a laughingstock among restauranteurs." Since this episode, the owner has been seen by the community as very responsible and is praised for his action; however, he did suffer a temporary decline in business because of his forthrightness.

Once again, the *Register* provided information to readers about how hepatitis A is transmitted. It published the recommendations that these restaurant goers be especially careful when handling food and to wash their hands often. "Wash, wash, wash," Dr. Julius Connor, medical director of the Polk County Health Department, was quoted as saying. It was apparent that health officials were beginning to worry about the increasing number of cases. Up to that point in 1997, 36 cases had been reported in Polk county, compared with only three during the same period of the previous year, and over 50% of cases in 1997 were occurring in people between the ages of 25 and 44 years, a very different age group than in the past when child care centers were the focal points of transmission.

I was pleasantly surprised that public health officials had named the restaurant, not because I was interested in jeopardizing the restaurant's business, but because that famous name was a major part of the story. Here is where the interests of the media and those of public health officials sometimes part. The reporter considers those familiar names to be part of the public record and by law available to the public—no matter the consequences to the restaurant or the impact on other restaurants that come forward with such information. I was interested in presenting as much accurate information as possible, acting on the traditional press value that information is power. Public health officials often want to protect the identities of sources of outbreaks to help assure their cooperation in future outbreaks. (In my opinion, this position is not supported by Iowa law, which calls for openness unless some specific Iowa law precludes it.) Nonetheless, in this case, there was no conflict, and the interest of the press and public health officials coincided.

State Epidemiologist: Over the Memorial Day weekend, the Polk County Health Department established a hot line number for people to call if they had questions about hepatitis A. Between Friday evening and Tuesday, they reported receiving about 240 calls. The hotline continued service until late June 1997. As the outbreak continued, the hotline number was widely published, and the county health department became a reliable source of quality information.

Getting out the correct information during times of crisis can sometimes be as important as other interventions. If a community is left without information, rumors can get started, often complicating the situation, and public health officials end up spending more time trying to correct false information than they would have if they had been proactive. (You may hear the voice of experience here!) Thus, I have come to the belief the more information given the better, and at times, I probably release more information than needed. I also believe in being "up front" with the media. If I get asked something that I know the answer to, but don't want to release, I say just that. I have found that this is better than trying to evade the question.

Some information, however, is considered confidential, such as an individual's medical information (i.e., the name of the people who have hepatitis A) and, at least under Iowa law, entities (i.e., restaurant names) associated with outbreaks. We do not violate this confidentiality unless it is necessary to protect the public's health.

Narcotics: The DNE initial exposure to the hepatitis outbreak resulted from the press conference concerning the people who may have been exposed at the restaurant. The Polk County Health Department discussed with the DNE the possible connection between the use, distribution, and manufacture of methamphetamine and the outbreak of hepatitis A in Polk County. After the phone conversation, DNE was invited to attend a meeting at the Polk County Health Department a couple days before Memorial Day 1997. The Coordinator of the Governor's Alliance on Substance Abuse also attended this meeting. The meeting discussed the increasing number of hepatitis A cases and the increasing number of illegal methamphetamine laboratories being seized in the central Iowa area. Information was also shared about the manufacturing procedures to help officials understand how meth was made, thus allowing them to determine whether and at what point hepatitis A could contaminate the product. At this meeting, several participants expressed concern over law enforcement being involved as a potential barrier to those that might seek treatment or prophylaxis for hepatitis A.

At this point, we were not interested in obtaining information about individuals with hepatitis A who might have used meth. Also, we understood the need for public health intervention in this group to stop the spread of hepatitis A. Our concern about the health risks to our narcotics agents was also discussed, and determinations were made of actions that could be taken to lower their risk.

The potential for meth to become contaminated with feces via dirty hands is quite extensive. For example, after drying the meth crystals, it is crumbled by hand prior to weighing and packaging it for sale; however, meth is quite acidic, and thus, the virus may not be able to survive on the meth crystals for long. As another interesting tidbit, meth is often colored by the "manufacturer" with food coloring for marketing purposes—that is, a user might prefer "purple" meth over "brown" meth.

State Epidemiologist: As we started to address the drug user link to disease, we were very concerned about the drug-using community having confidence in the health department's code of confidentiality. If we needed to do public health interventions in this community, we would need their cooperation, which we felt we would not get if they did not trust us. Thus, we were careful to maintain a distance from law enforcement, while accepting their assistance. The narcotics enforcement people understood our concerns and always acted professionally.

Outbreaks can make for strange bedfellows, and this can be one of the more interesting aspects of investigating outbreaks. I must admit that I never thought I would learn how to make methamphetamine, but the narcotics agents spent an afternoon teaching us not only how meth was made but how it was used so that we could understand how someone using meth might become infected with the hepatitis A virus.

Press Liaison: One media complication surrounding the situation at the restaurant was that a food handler came forward and declared that he was the one with hepatitis A, but that he was not a drug user. Even though this man had "gone public" about his identity, because of the state health departments policy on medical confidentiality (and the state law), we could not, and never will, confirm or deny if this man was the restaurant worker with hepatitis A.

The issue of confidentiality overshadows media/public health relations. Media outlets want to personalize a story as much as possible, while breeches of confidence can undermine the ability of public health workers to investigate health issues. It is difficult to draft a black and white rule for confidentiality, other than to say that no personal identifying information should be released without the consent of the patient except in extreme situations. Sometimes the best action is to have the patient go directly to the media if they are interested in being identified publicly, thus taking the health department and our concerns of confidentiality "out of the loop."

Other information release "rules" vary based on the situation (see http://www.idph.state.ia.us/adper/common/pdf/cade/disclosure_reportable_diseases.pdf). Describing a patient as being an 11-year-old Hispanic male is obviously of less concern in a Southern California county than it is in a rural Iowa county (where there may only be one 11-year-old Hispanic male, thus allowing the individual to be identified). The decision to name a restaurant that has a worker who may have spread hepatitis A infection is driven by the need to communicate information about an ongoing health risk to a specific population where there is no other way of identifying that population. In the case of a food borne outbreak at a private gathering where a complete guest list was maintained, there may not be a need to communicate news of the outbreak to the general public, as we would already know who was potentially exposed. In other situations, such as a follow-up to an industrial injury, it may not be necessary to identify the specific location or business involved, if the circumstances that lead to the risk have been eliminated. One option that can be tried, if time and circumstances permit, is to have the public health community act as a go-between to approach the patient or institution to see whether they are willing to "go public," and then give them the reporter's phone number that they can then call. The primary reason for doing so is to educate, in the hope that this prevents others from going through the same experience.

Newspaper: On May 29, 1997, we ran a front-page story "Ex-worker at *landmark restaurant* is Sorry for Health Risk." In this article, the food handler with hepatitis A identified himself and was quoted as saying, "I would never have knowingly hurt anyone. I probably have infected someone or their family or their loved one or their significant other. That hurts me, and I can't say sorry enough. It's not like I'm some drug addict or street junkie." He admitted that he told hospital officials that he was not working at the time but said that he had given them a series of addresses where he had been staying. He said that he had decided to come forward, even though his name had not been made public, because of a man's kindness at the unemployment office. "When I went in, he asked me my last employer, I said *landmark restaurant.* Then he asked me my last position. I said a salad bar worker. The man just looked at me and I hung my head. He told me 'you don't have to hang your head.'" At the end of the article, we quoted him as stating, "I'm a victim too." In this article, a manager at the restaurant stated that they "are the ones who forced him to go to the doctors. We wouldn't let him work until he did."

A companion article in the same issue had the headline of "Doctors to Dine at *landmark restaurant* to Assure Public of Safety" for a story on local doctors having dinner at the restaurant to demonstrate their support and confidence in the safety of the restaurant's food. The food worker's public apology and the visit of local doctors to the restaurant were both important follow-up pieces in the hepatitis A story. It added more "human" elements to a story that was becoming as much about the effects disease has on patients, their families, and society as about the epidemiology.

THE FIELD EPIDEMIOLOGIC INVESTIGATION BEGINS: LATE MAY 1997

State Epidemiologist: We realized that we had an opportunity to study the modes of transmission of hepatitis A. We called the CDC and asked for an "Epi-Aid."

Epi-Aids are called when a state has a health event occurring that has (or may have) national impact and when the state needs assistance in order to investigate it fully. Because the CDC has investigators looking for events to investigate, expert consultants available, and laboratories with the capacity to perform large numbers of tests, we felt that Iowans would be best served by collaboration between the state health department, the local health departments, and the CDC. Together we might not only be able to stop the outbreak, but also be able to learn something that could prevent or help control future outbreaks.

We were particularly concerned about the link between the spread of hepatitis A to methamphetamine use for several reasons. Iowa had recently experienced a community-wide outbreak of hepatitis A in Siouxland and the epidemiological investigation revealed a statistically significant correlation to drug use. Also, by this time we had two recent case reports of hepatitis A in restaurant workers that may have been using drugs obtained in the Des Moines area. In addition, nationally, methamphetamine use was being linked to hepatitis A transmission.

CDC: In May of 1997, when this request came in, I was at the end of my first year as an EIS officer working in the Hepatitis Branch of the CDC. EIS is described as a "unique 2-year post graduate program of service and on-the-job training for health professionals interested in the practice of epidemiology." One of the core functions is to help in epidemiologic investigations, and in this capacity, I had already been to Iowa once.

The previous fall (of 1996), during the outbreak of hepatitis A in Siouxland, I had investigated the causes. In that outbreak, a high proportion of cases had reported injection drug use, particularly methamphetamine. A case-control study had been done in Sioux City, Iowa to identify what population group could be identified at highest risk and targeted for intervention.[4]

Even after the study, the methods of hepatitis A transmission among illicit drug users remained unclear. The Siouxland study had been started after the outbreak had been occurring in that greater community for several months. This meant that the outbreak had expanded by then and new subpopulations were involved that had different modes of transmission than had originally occurred. Therefore, when the central Iowa outbreak first started, it was recognized that this was a great chance to study transmission of the virus in its early phases and perhaps better determine the primary and initial routes of transmission.

State Epidemiologist: When we were told that Dr. Yvan Hutin would be sent as the CDC primary investigator, we were thrilled. We knew Yvan quite well from the Sioux City outbreak and were very impressed by his abilities. Thus, we were in good spirits as we geared up for the intensive investigation. We also used the arrival of the two CDC investigators (Dr. Hutin and Dr. Keith Sabin) to generate more publicity that might help continue the effort to educate the public. We felt that the more the community knew about the situation, the better chance public health had in getting it under control. With diseases like hepatitis A, it is the community that has to take definitive action (such as good hand washing and seeing a physician for diagnostic evaluation early in the course of illness). Public health's responsibility is to make that action as easy as possible for the public to achieve.

Newspaper: On June 3, Iowa's health officials announced that they had asked federal investigators to help unravel the mystery of the hepatitis A outbreak in central Iowa. When interviewed about the arrival of the CDC's investigator, the state epidemiologist replied, "We said, 'Great, we'd like to have some help.'" The CDC spokesperson said that their investigators typically work alongside the state epidemiologists and state health care providers to help identify a source.

We reported that it was not clear yet what was causing the increase of hepatitis A cases in Iowa, but that hand washing was critical, particularly after using the bathroom, after changing an infant's diaper, and before preparing food. We also reminded people to go immediately to a doctor if they had been exposed to hepatitis A and to go to a doctor if they were having symptoms of hepatitis A, because as the state epidemiologist said, "If you already have hepatitis A, there's not much we can do for you, but there are things we can do at that point to protect your family and friends." By this time, our goal at the newspaper was to provide any new information about what had become an ongoing story.

State Epidemiologist: After the CDC investigators arrived in Iowa, we met with them and the local health department's epidemiologists to discuss the outbreak, interventions, and investigations. At this meeting, it was decided that one of the most critical items was to determine the way that hepatitis was being transmitted; therefore, between June and July of 1997, a case-control study was conducted to identify specific modes of hepatitis A transmission among persons using methamphetamine. The first step was to identify all persons reported with hepatitis A having onset dates between April 1 and July 24, 1997, the dates from when the outbreak started and when the study needed to end. Then, in early June, a pilot study involving 13 of the people with hepatitis A, also known as case-patients, was performed to help generate hypotheses about potential modes of transmission. Pilot studies are often done to test the feasibility of the study design, including the patient questionnaire, and for a quick check of the hypotheses. If you have time, performing a pilot study can be indispensable for fine-tuning your investigation.

Narcotics: On June 4, 1997, the DNE was contacted by the CDC to notify us that they had an individual en route to Polk County per the request of IDPH. On June 12, personnel from CDC, IDPH, and the Polk County Department of Health met at the DNE headquarters in Des Moines for further information on the increasing number of clandestine meth labs and how this substance was illicitly produced. This allowed the epidemiologists more insights into the possible points during production and distribution of meth that contamination with hepatitis A virus could occur.

From information gathered by us at this meeting, it was decided that hepatitis A shots would be provided to all members of the DNE because of the high potential of coming in contact with law violators who were infectious with hepatitis A. Divisional agents have a large number of undercover investigators who have contact with potential and known methamphetamine distributors. During the months of June and July, all DNE Special Agents received the first of the two doses in the hepatitis vaccine series.

CDC: In the pilot study, the 13 case-patients were asked both open-ended and close-ended questions about meth use, practices associated with meth usage, paraphernalia use, and injection practices. Open-ended questions have no set answers, such as "What did you do last night?" Close-ended questions, however, such as "Did you eat the

> *Open-ended questions have no set answers.*

> *Close-ended questions have limited answers (i.e., yes or no).*

potato salad last night?" have limited answers (i.e., yes or no). This information was used to generate an appropriate questionnaire. Of the 13 case-patients, 10 identified using the emergency room as their primary health care source. This was important because the emergency room had been found to be an important source of health care for the hepatitis A cases in the Sioux City outbreak, and it provided a contact point for case ascertainment (finding people that have or had hepatitis A) and for possible intervention.

We then put together our primary team of investigators consisting of two CDC investigators and two epidemiology students (doing rotations at the state and Polk County health departments). With additional assistance from other professionals at the health departments, we began our main study. Then we had to find people who were like the case-patients except that they were not ill with hepatitis A. These would serve as our control patients.

Because the pilot study identified the emergency room as the primary source of health care for the meth users, controls were recruited prospectively from patients seeking medical care at two emergency rooms in the area (in Polk and Wapello counties) and at a clinic associated with the public hospital in Polk County. During the study period, the triage nurse in each facility asked all patients between 15 and 45 years of age about methamphetamine use in the last 12 months. Patients who admitted to use during this time period were recruited as controls.

We did have exclusion criteria for controls. Each was asked to give a blood sample for hepatitis A testing, and if found positive for IgM (evidence of acute disease), they were excluded from the study. Potential controls who could not or would not be tested were also excluded.

The investigation team trained interviewers, from both the state and local health departments, to administer the questionnaires to study participants, collecting data on demographic characteristics, living conditions, use of social and public assistance services, exposure to day care centers, contact with a hepatitis A case, international travel, sexual activity, history of substance abuse, behaviors associated with methamphetamine used during the 2 to 6 weeks before illness, quantity and routes of administration of each type of meth used, paraphernalia use, and injection practices.

If the persons who design the questionnaire are using others to administer it, it is important to train the interviewers. This ensures consistency in asking questions and in recording answers. It can be surprising how many ways someone can answer even simple questions such as this: "Did you eat the potato salad?"

There were 95 case patients with onset dates after April 1, 1997; of these, 75 were interviewed. Of the remainder, 19 could not be located; only one refused to participate (and she suggested that the interviewer return when she was feeling better).

When performing studies like this, when the CDC investigators take the lead role, it is critical to have the support of state and local public health personnel. In this situation, both the state and local health departments provided logistic and personnel support, which allowed the study to be so successful. Also, it is the local health department people who knew the community partners that became involved in the study. For example, in this study, the local health department personnel helped us to contact and coordinate with the hospitals and emergency rooms to help us identify potential cases of hepatitis A and vaccinate those at high risk.

State Epidemiologist: We had a running joke in the office about how cooperative Iowans were, even the illicit drug users. In the study, 75 out of the 76 hepatitis A cases (99%) contacted agreed to participate in the study. It was my understanding that a similar study had been tried in other parts of the country with little success, because the drug users were unwilling to cooperate, to the point of meeting interviewers at the door with guns!

I'm happy to report that none of our interviewers felt unsafe while doing this study, although this was a concern when the investigation began, especially because some of the interviewers were young female students, inexperienced in public health interventions or working with this population; however, the drug users were willing to tell interviewers about their health and drug use. The only piece of information that we were not able to get was from whom they bought their drugs. It would have been nice to trace back the drugs to the production point to evaluate potential "bad batches" and types of potential contamination, but it was not absolutely necessary for the investigation.

While the CDC study was getting started, the health departments stepped up efforts to control the outbreak. In general, a two-pronged approach was used: to try to prevent disease in the groups at highest risk for becoming infected (e.g., those using meth) and to prevent transmission from groups at highest risk for spreading the virus (primarily food handlers and those associated with day care centers). Thus, in June, both on weekdays and on weekends, the local and state health department personnel provided seminars for restaurants, other food serving establishments, and day care centers, with instruction on how to reduce their risk of transmitting hepatitis A. Food establishments are at high risk because of the potential for exposing large numbers of people via contaminated food or, in the case of day care centers, because their children are often in diapers, allowing for fecal contamination of the environment with easy spread to other children.

These seminars were very well attended. In fact, some national chain restaurants sent managers from regional offices to attend. There was also extensive media coverage of the seminars, reinforcing for the public what needed to be done to decrease the transmission of the virus (Exhibit 15-2). Also, many handouts, such as brochures and fact sheets, were either developed or modified for distribution to the public, parents, day care center employees, and food handlers.

Newspaper: On June 4, we ran a story on the "prevention" seminars being offered to child care providers and restaurant workers in Des Moines. In this story, we reported on the briefing that had occurred that day, and we helped advertise the sites and times of future briefings. The article focused on children and child-care facilities, and why they were of such concern, that is, that children often had no symptoms but still spread the disease, that children in diapers and those still being potty trained can spread the disease more easily than others, and why hand washing was so important. The side bar to this article listed pertinent facts on hepatitis A. Providing information about the response, including prevention seminars, was considered part of our mission to keep our readers informed about the outbreak.

Narcotics: After discussions about the potential for methamphetamine to transmit the hepatitis A virus, we were asked whether it might be possible to obtain some meth, confiscated in a raid or arrest, for testing for the virus. Thus, the Division of Narcotics Enforcement attempted to obtain samples during the execution of search warrants on clandestine meth laboratory sites. Coordination was accomplished with the United States Attorney's office in Des Moines to permit the DNE to immediately release evidentiary samples to the IDPH for analysis. Appropriate storage containers and packing materials were also purchased to preserve any samples for future analysis. Unfortunately, with the exception of one laboratory site, syringes possibly containing meth were not located. The one syringe that was obtained was not fit for analysis because of improper storage.

State Epidemiologist: We appreciated the narcotics staff's willingness to go to such lengths to help us obtain some drug samples for hepatitis A virus testing. It was not easy for them to get permission to give us illegal drugs for testing. If we had been able to obtain some and test it, it would have allowed us to "close the circle" of the outbreak. Unfortunately, this was not possible in this situation.

The preliminary public health surveillance information suggested that injecting drug users and men who have sex with men were the groups at highest risk for developing hepatitis A in central Iowa, and because the Advisory Committee of Immunization Practices (the committee that recommends how vaccines should be used in the United States) already recommended hepatitis A vaccination for these risk groups, it was decided in early June (before the study was started) to go ahead with a vaccination campaign. It was estimated that over 3,000 people would need to be vaccinated and that approximately 5,000 doses of vaccine would be needed. Although two doses of vaccine are recommended for full protection, from experience we only expected about 50% to return for the second dose of vaccine 6 months later.

Several barriers existed to a successful vaccination campaign: (1) difficulty in getting the vaccine to a

---

EXHIBIT 15-2 Headline

Huge Hepatitis Outbreak Feared

"We are asking for your help and cooperation so that we don't end up with hundreds, if not thousands, of people infected in Polk County."

    Dr. Patricia Quinlisk, addressing restaurant owners

This was quoted in the *Des Moines Register*.

population that may not want to be identified (e.g., running an ad in the newspaper asking all illicit drug users to come to the health department on Thursday for shots would probably not work), (2) most of the population that needed the vaccine would not have the resources or perhaps the willingness to pay for a $50+ per dose vaccine, (3) the hepatitis A vaccine requires two doses over a 6-month period for full protection, and (4) the health departments did not have money in their budgets to pay for the amount of vaccine needed.

One of these barriers was addressed politically. On June 12, 1997, after discussions with the state health department and the CDC, U.S. Senator Tom Harkin (D-Iowa) announced that the CDC had agreed to provide Iowa with a "significant amount" of vaccine. He stated in his press release, "I am grateful to the CDC for their prompt and dedicated assistance to our state in dealing with this public health problem."

Newspaper: Out of our Washington bureau, we ran an article that the CDC would pay for 5,000 doses of hepatitis A vaccine to head off the outbreak in Iowa. We also reported that the CDC had committed about $160,000 to the vaccine effort and had sent two investigators to Iowa in the wake of reports of 140 cases of hepatitis A in the state since January. In addition, the CDC action was important because of the potential for a community-wide outbreak to develop involving hundreds of thousands of people.

We wanted to provide information on the outbreak from any and every source, and a reporter in our Washington bureau had an angle—the activities of the CDC in the outbreak—that I didn't hear about in Des Moines.

CDC/State Epidemiologist: Now that we had the vaccine, we needed to decide how best to get it to those at highest risk. It was decided to focus on the four counties in central Iowa with the highest rates of hepatitis A—Marion, Monroe, Polk and Wapello—and to use various access points, such as health departments, emergency rooms, jails, drug treatment centers, sexually transmitted disease clinics, malls, churches, and HIV screening sites. We also ran a clinic in the lobby of the local gambling casino in the middle of the night on the advice of the Narcotics Enforcement people that this was a good place and time to find meth users.

Believe it or not, there are a few places to go in Des Moines in the middle of the night if you are unable to sleep. The local casino is open all night long and with meth being a stimulant drug, it makes sense one might find some meth users in this environment late at night. We ended up vaccinating quite a few people there.

A variety of techniques were used to get the word out to those who needed to be vaccinated (or possibly be given IG because of a recent exposure), including health department personnel speaking about the issue whenever possible. Pamphlets were widely distributed in places where drug users and/or men who have sex with men might congregate, such as gay bars and drug treatment centers. Educational cards were given to those diagnosed with hepatitis A to distribute to their drug sharing partners, friends, and families who they might have exposed to hepatitis A. These cards could then be presented at a vaccination site, at which time they could be vaccinated without having to answer any questions. This was done to encourage anyone who might be in a risk group for hepatitis A or may have been exposed to the case patient to be vaccinated and/or be given IG.

In mid June, the state health department developed a "Recommended Protocol for Hepatitis A Vaccination Programs for Targeted Populations." It addressed issues such as administration costs, standing orders for vaccination, informed consent, vaccine ordering and handling, and patient recall (for the second dose). This packet also contained a sample letter for ordering the vaccine, a consent form, a fact sheet for the patient, and a report form to send back to IDPH on the number of doses of vaccine administered by month. This was distributed to all appropriate local health departments and vaccination sites.

Developing clear guidance, including the protocol and forms, was an important coordinating function for the state health department to perform, especially when multiple jurisdictions and agencies get involved as happened here. It helped to organize the vaccination efforts, ensured consistency in procedures across the counties, and helped to track efforts. Consistency is especially important because different protocols in different counties can cause the public to become concerned. "What does that county know that my county doesn't know?" Inconsistency can undermine the credibility of a health department's efforts and interfere with control of an outbreak.

Even with all of the efforts everyone was making in June, we knew that it would be several months before we would know whether the rates of hepatitis A were decreasing since the incubation period—time from exposure to the virus to the onset of symptoms—can be up to 6 weeks. Throughout this time we remained very concerned that it would spread to the general population.

Newspaper: On June 9, 1997, we reported that the Blood Center of Central Iowa had sent letters to 5,300 blood donors asking whether they ate a meal at the landmark restaurant between April 21 and May 5, when they might have been exposed to hepatitis A. If they had, they were asked to contact the blood center. The center would then destroy the donated blood to reduce any risk of transmitting hepatitis A to blood recipients. Our report also noted that all persons attempting to donate blood were being deferred from donating if they had been exposed to hepatitis A at the restaurant.

Once again, our intent was to provide any new information about the continuing story.

State Epidemiologist: Although much of our communication efforts were aimed at a general audience, in early June, we were pretty confident that illicit drug users were one of the major, if not *the* major group, spreading the disease. We were hesitant to go public with this information at the time for several reasons: (1) During the Sioux City outbreak the previous year, the drug use connection had been made public, but local public health officials felt this had made their jobs more difficult and had possibly stopped some people from being diagnosed. (2) We were doing a study to determine the modes of transmission, and thus, we wanted to be able to document this connection and determine some way of addressing this issue before making it public, and (3) we were not absolutely confident that drug use was the real risk factor. Thus, when we went public with the vaccination clinics, we recommended it for all the high-risk groups identified in the national recommendations (for hepatitis A vaccine use), which included drug users.

The public health departments, however, had already began a targeted education program for drug (primarily methamphetamine) users and men who have sex with men, as these two groups appeared to be at highest risk, but may not be getting information through regular channels, such as the media. Thus, pamphlets with target population specific information were also handed out at drug treatment centers, gay bars, sexually transmitted disease clinics, and so forth.

Newspaper: On June 23rd, we reported the opening of free hepatitis A vaccination clinics. We also reported that the shots were being recommended for (1) anyone who has injected illicit drugs or used meth in the last year, (2) men who are having sex with men, (3) friends and families of these two risk groups, (4) friends and family members of those who have hepatitis A, (5) persons with chronic liver disease, and (6) persons with blood-clotting disorders. To encourage acceptance, it was reported that those seeking vaccination would not be asked about lifestyles or drug use.

The article also reported concerns about the outbreak spreading to the general community, and that if it did it would be almost impossible to stop. If a community outbreak did occur, health officials stated that it could take up to 2 years and hundreds, if not thousands, of cases before it ended.

We wanted to report the latest development in this story and without overstating it; we wanted to inform readers about the risks of the outbreak spreading to the general population. To convey these risks, we depended on the state epidemiologist, who helped us put it all in perspective.

State Epidemiologist: We had watched the reports of cases of hepatitis A carefully for any cases reporting exposure to the landmark restaurant. By the beginning of July it became apparent that this had not occurred. In the end, there were no cases of hepatitis A that we could directly link to exposure to food at this restaurant.

Even though there was no spread, we were comfortable with our actions the month before (going public about the potential transmission of the virus from the food handler and the subsequent outbreak that could occur). It would be great if we could predict the future, but this is obviously not possible. Thus, we prepare for the worst and hope for the best.

Newspaper: On July 3, we reported "Hepatitis Epidemic Apparently Avoided," but that central Iowans weren't in the clear yet. Health officials reported that there had not been a community-wide outbreak from the food handler at the landmark restaurant with hepatitis A and attributed part of this to the "incredible" public response to the warnings and recommendations.

It was reported that most cases were occurring in 23 to 38 year old adults, although health officials declined to speculate why the disease was prevalent in that age group. Dr. Connor, the Polk County medical director, was quoted as stating that the health officials hadn't determined how the virus had been spreading in Polk County, but that it had been decided to recommend the vaccine to high-risk groups.

On July 10, an article titled "Hepatitis A Still Rising Among the Young" was published. It reported that health officials were increasingly concerned about the continuing rise in the number of cases. A possible second case of hepatitis A in a Polk County food handler was also noted.

We were still interested at this point in continuing to inform the public about developments, being careful to make distinctions in the July 3 and July 10 stories to avoid the perception of a contradiction. The epidemic had *not* spread to the general population on the one hand; on the other, the incidence of the disease were still rising among the young. Our thinking in this and other health messages, such as the results of current research, was that we would present information as clearly and succinctly as possible, having confidence that the majority of readers would get the true picture.

CDC: By late July, the investigation of the modes of transmission had definitively identified that the groups at increased risk included meth users and injecting drug users. The case control study found that, among meth users, having used meth with someone who had hepatitis A and injecting meth with a syringe were the two factors statistically associated with getting hepatitis A. Not all the meth users who got hepatitis A reported injecting the drugs, indicating that at least some fecal–oral transmission probably occurred. Among injectors, only half reported sharing needles. Sharing paraphernalia such as spoons, cotton (for filtering the drug solution), and cups was common among the injectors, even if they did not share needles. We concluded that the injecting paraphenalia was probably becoming contaminated by handling during use and then shared with others, infecting them. We termed this mode of transmission "fecal–percutaneous."

> *We concluded that the injecting paraphenalia was probably becoming contaminated by handling during use and then shared with others, infecting them.*

State Epidemiologist: Yvan Hutin, Dr. Julius Connor, and I had a press conference to announce these results on July 23. We were concerned that the general public hearing these results might do a couple of things, such as "blame" the outbreak on the drug users and think themselves safe and thus relax precautions such as careful hand washing. We stressed that those at risk were victims of this disease and should not be blamed and that there could still be a community-wide outbreak if everyone didn't continue to do their bit. The importance of those at risk getting vaccinated was reinforced as a public health intervention. It was announced that more vaccine clinics would be held at health departments, emergency rooms, substance abuse treatment centers, and sexually transmitted disease clinics. Polk County Health Department helped staff some of these clinics.

There was a lot of discussion about how to encourage drug users to come in for vaccinations—for example, how to allow a person to remain anonymous, how to use those that came in for vaccination to encourage their families and fellow drug users to come in, how to overcome the distrust of government agencies that many drug users have, and whether or not we should use this opportunity to address other health risks in this group of people (i.e. HIV and hepatitis B and C). It was decided that hepatitis A prevention was our first priority, and if there was time and opportunity for other issues, they could be addressed.

At the press conference, it was emphasized that those using drugs should stop. If they were going to continue to use drugs, they needed to wash their hands prior to drug use and not share drug paraphernalia, and if a drug user's drug-sharing partner develops hepatitis A, the user should get an IG shot immediately.

There was also concern about how we would be able to deliver the second dose of the two-dose hepatitis A vaccine 6 months after the first. It was felt that we were morally obligated to try to encourage those that obtained the first dose to get the second. Usually, the vaccinee would be contacted and reminded by a "reminder postcard" or a phone call; however, many of these vaccinees might be reluctant to give identifying information about themselves, and we had promised that the vaccine could be obtained anonymously. Thus, we ended up explaining about the need for a second dose and offered to remind them if they would leave us a way in which to contact them.

Narcotics: On July 24, the drug czar of Iowa publicly applauded the decision by health officials to seek out meth users for hepatitis A vaccinations. He stated that he hoped the attention would heighten public awareness about the serious consequences of the drug's increased prevalence in Iowa. "It should open some eyes," he said, to the dangers associated with using meth. "…It's going to spread to the community beyond the drug users and spread in the family to the younger, innocent family members."

State Epidemiologist: By July 29, Polk County Health Department alone had vaccinated over 1,200 people. The clinics were so successful, partially because of all of the publicity the outbreak was receiving, that they were extended. In late July, other counties in central Iowa, such as Wapello, had started vaccination campaigns also. By August 9, over 1,540 doses had been given in Polk County alone.

Unfortunately, but not unexpected because of the lengthy incubation period, the number of cases continued to rise. For the month of July, Polk County reported 79 cases (compared with 9 in the same time period the year before), and Wapallo County reported 45 (compared with 1 the year before).

Because of the epidemic, Polk County Health Department found themselves in need of extra staff. This resulted in the Polk County Board of Supervisors appropriating funds to hire more nurses and program aids to assist in this effort (Exhibit 15-3). This action allowed Polk County Health Department to continue to address the problem aggressively and fully implement the interventions needed to stop the outbreak.

> *This action allowed Polk County Health Department to continue to address the problem aggressively and fully implement the interventions needed to stop the outbreak.*

CDC: By the end of July, our study was coming to an end in Iowa, although some laboratory results and quite a bit of analysis still needed to be done. This part of the study would be completed after my return to the CDC.[6]

We concluded that methamphetamine users in Iowa, especially injecting drug users, were at increased risk for hepatitis A. Hepatitis A was being transmitted from person to person through multiple routes among drug users, including sharing of drug paraphernalia. Also, a common source cluster of cases associated with a contaminated batch of "brown" methamphetamine may have occurred.

The benefits of our investigation included that it provided scientific data on the modes of hepatitis A transmission among drug users and that it provided information to support nationwide recommendations on vaccine use and prevention of hepatitis A transmission.

Narcotics: During the outbreak period, I constantly updated my colleagues at the division, as well as the four other states in the Midwest High Intensity Drug Trafficking Area (Midwest HIDTA), which combats the continuing rise of methamphetamine use. None of the other states reported outbreaks of hepatitis A in their areas. In mid January 1998, divisional agents received their second hepatitis A shots.

Newspaper: As a journalist, my role in all of this was to report what I heard and saw from health officials and other sources and develop any other related stories that would help readers understand the subject and the players. Fortunately for the public, other journalists, and myself, there are good relationships between the media and those at the state and local health departments. As the state epidemiologist was once quoted as saying, "Getting information to the public is a huge piece of the job, and we couldn't do it without the media."

State Epidemiologist: As steps were taken to control the outbreak, the CDC investigation was completed, and the media attention dissipated, we watched the case numbers carefully. By early fall, they began to decline, and although the numbers briefly increased again later, the outbreak was over by the spring of 1998.

In 1997, 1,574 doses of hepatitis A vaccine were given in Polk County. Of these, 78 were given anonymously. The rest provided names and addresses to facilitate sending second dose reminders, of which 1,496 were sent. Just over 250 of these reminders were returned by the post office for reasons that included insufficient address or resident no longer at that address. Although no response was received from 720 people, 492 persons did return to the local health department to receive the second dose of hepatitis A vaccine.

The fact that so many people gave their names and addresses to the local health department for the second shot reminder demonstrates the confidence that the people in these risk groups (e.g., the drug users) had in public health to keep this information confidential. It says a lot about how comfortable this community felt in working with the local public health workers, especially the nurses.

In the end, a lot of resources were used to investigate and control this outbreak, but hepatitis A never expanded to a community-wide outbreak. We felt we had been successful.

EXHIBIT 15-3 Headline

Hepatitis Outbreak Spreads

Cases in August were the highest in Polk County this year, and the county health chief should seek help.

This was quoted from the *Des Moines Register*.

CONCLUSION

Epidemic investigations are never done in isolation. As you can see by the previously mentioned example, many people, organizations, and the public participate in stopping an outbreak. By definition, epidemics occur in a community or a portion of a community, and ultimately, it is the community's actions that contain or stop an outbreak. Public health's main role is to determine the cause(s) of the outbreak and then to assist the community in implementing the actions that would be most effective in halting the epidemic. If the community is not behind the public health efforts, it is unlikely that the epidemic will be controlled.

REFERENCES

1. Heymann DL. Viral hepatitis A. In Heymann DL, ed. *Control of Communicable Diseases Manual*, 18th ed. Washington, D.C. American Public Health Association, 2004:247–253.
2. Centers for Disease Control and Prevention. Prevention of hepatitis A through active or passive immunization. *MMWR Morb Mortal Wkly Rep* 2006;55:1–23.
3. Iowa Department of Public Health. Reportable Diseases by Year. 1930 to Present. Retrieved April 20, 2007, from http://www.idph.state.ia.us/adper/common/pdf/cade/decades.pdf.
4. Hutin YJF, Bell BP, Marshall KLE, et al. Identifying target groups for a potential vaccination program during a hepatitis A community-wide outbreak. *Am J Public Health* 1999;89:918–921.
5. Centers for Disease Control and Prevention. Hepatitis A associated with consumption of frozen strawberries—Michigan, March 1997. *MMWR Morb Mortal Wkly Rep* 1997;46:288.
6. Hutin YJF, Sabin KM, Hutwagner LC, et al. Multiple modes of hepatitis A virus transmission among methamphetamine users. *Am J Epidemiol* 2000;152:186–192.

Note: In 2007, the Advisory Committee on Immunization Practices (ACIP) revised the national guidelines to include the use of hepatitis A vaccine postexposure. See http://www.cdc.gov/mmwr/preview/mmwrhtml/mm5641a3.htm/.

LEARNING QUESTIONS

1. The authors explain that they needed to have a hepatitis A vaccination campaign that emphasized immunizing methamphetamine users. What were the barriers they recognized and how did they deal with them?
2. A food handler at a landmark restaurant was implicated as potentially having spread hepatitis A virus to many persons who ate at the restaurant. Why was this restaurant not closed down and what was done to try to prevent possible restaurant-associated hepatitis A transmission?

CHAPTER 16

Tracking a Syphilis Outbreak Through Cyberspace

Jeffrey D. Klausner, MD, MPH
San Francisco, CA, 1999

INTRODUCTION

It was April 1999. I was less than a year into my new job as deputy health officer and director of the Sexually Transmitted Disease (STD) Prevention Section in San Francisco. At that time, the section had about 70 staff members, operated the municipal STD clinic, and conducted surveillance, epidemiology, disease intervention, and sexual health education and promotion with a budget of about $4 million. Whenever I mention my job title, folks always comment how tough it must be to have such a role in San Francisco. It seems that "Baghdad by the Bay" continues to have a reputation of unbridled sexual expression, resulting in the unmanageable consequences of the spread of sexually transmitted infections. Trying to control such diseases in San Francisco must be a Sisyphean task, they think.

Fortunately, I was well trained. I attended Cornell University for my undergraduate and medical school education, completed an internship and residency in internal medicine at Bellevue Hospital in New York City, and received a Master of Public Health degree from Harvard University. After all that, I became a member of the Centers for Disease Control and Prevention's (CDC) Epidemic Intelligence Service, the nation's premier investigators of disease outbreaks, and was posted in the local health department in San Francisco. Finally, I completed a fellowship in infectious diseases at the University of Washington in Seattle to be certain that I would be able to get a great job in public health.

In this new position as a public health official—my first "real job"—having finished 12 years of postgraduate education, I was seriously concerned that I would lose touch with patients and the care of sick individuals. To reduce that likelihood, I volunteered weekly at the San Francisco municipal STD clinic every Monday morning. It was a great way to start the week, meeting men and women who have waited all weekend for the STD clinic to open and get treated for the various bumps, sores, ulcers, and discharges emanating from their genitalia.

One Monday morning in the spring of 1999, I was interviewing a new patient at the STD clinic about his sexual behavior. When asked how many new sex partners he had in the past 6 months, he said 14. When asked how many new sex partners he had in the past 2 months, he said 14. Nonplussed, I asked him what happened 2 months ago. He paused, smiled and replied, "I got online."

I was curious and allowed my training as a CDC investigator to manifest itself and asked the patient to tell me more. The story he related I will never forget. That story has become the foundation for an entire new field in sexual and reproductive health promotion and disease control—using the Internet to promote healthful behaviors, conduct disease investigations and partner notification, and offer screening and treatment for STDs.

Bill (whose name has been changed) told me that he went every day to America Online (AOL) to a specific chatroom named "SFM4M." In that chatroom, men looked for an immediate "hookup" (an in-person sexual encounter). When I looked at the screen for this chatroom, it showed that all the city sites were full—each had a capacity of 23 members at a single time. AOL members initiated a conversation through "instant messaging" and gave their "stats" such as age, hair and eye color, height, weight, and chest, arm, and penis size or provided a link to a webpage with photographs and additional specifics such as preferred sexual activity or meeting place.

Bill described how he—a self-described HIV-positive, balding, overweight man in his late 40s who had been finding it difficult to meet new sex partners lately—could now go online, meet a potential new sex partner in just a few minutes, and speak to them on the telephone. If he liked their voice, he would invite them to his house. Peering through his living room window, he'd check them out and decide whether to let them in. Once inside his home, often verbal communication stopped, and he and his new partner had sex. Whether they had sex again or not was of little interest to him. He was just amazed at how easy and quick it was to find a new partner. Bill said that on some occasions hookups could be initiated and realized in less than 15 minutes. He seemed quite pleased with his recent discovery. I, however, felt much different. My emotions shifted from cool clinical detachment to an acute sense of epidemiologic foreboding.

THE OUTBREAK

In the summer of 1999, the CDC launched the fourth effort in the history of the United States to eliminate syphilis. Syphilis cases were approaching an all time low, and Congress had allocated $30 million a year in new funding to help the CDC reach that goal. Locally, we formed a syphilis elimination team with health department staff members, including the syphilis disease control investigators and representatives from a variety of community-based organizations. We drafted an outbreak response plan and met biweekly to review and improve current syphilis control efforts. In addition, I personally reviewed each and every new case to assure adequate treatment and to try to identify additional opportunities for the interruption of disease transmission.

Before the AIDS epidemic, syphilis was common in San Francisco, in particular among gay men and other men who have sex with men. Case counts hovered at about 2,000 cases a year in the 1970s, making San Francisco the nation's leader in new cases of syphilis. With the advent of the AIDS epidemic and the profound fear surrounding that untreatable and deadly disease, sexual behavior changed dramatically, and the number of cases of syphilis in San Francisco dropped substantially from over 2,200 cases in the early 1980s to a few dozen by the late 1990s. More importantly, there were only eight cases in gay men and other men who have sex with men in 1998, the lowest number ever recorded in San Francisco. It was perfect timing to eliminate syphilis. All of the conditions required for potential disease eradication were in place—only human-to-human transmission, low case counts, an easy and accurate test, and highly effective treatment that both prevented and cured infection. In the spring and summer of 1999, we were hypervigilant trying to detect the early signs of an outbreak—an increase in the number of cases over the expected rate. We performed a team review of every new case and carefully tried to rule out any evidence of sustained person-to-person transmission. Because the number of baseline cases was so few, any cluster of cases could be considered a potential outbreak.

> *All of the conditions required for potential disease eradication were in place—only human-to-human transmission, low case counts, an easy and accurate test, and highly effective treatment that both prevented and cured infection.*

Upon hearing Bill's story, I requested the syphilis team to inquire about Internet use and subsequent sex partnering or "hookups" among new cases of syphilis. I asked them to ask new syphilis cases who had used the Internet to meet sex partners what specific Internet sites they used and where they met—at someone's house, public space, or bar. In July, just 1 month later, we had two cases that reported meeting partners on AOL at SFM4M. One patient had met partners at that site only.

Bingo! To identify additional cases, the investigators went back and reinterviewed persons with prior cases of syphilis infection acquired in the past year reported to the health department in 1999. The investigators found that all but one new syphilis case who used the Internet to find sex partners used AOL and the specific AOL chatroom SFM4M. I asked the disease-control investigators to collect "handles" or the screen names that AOL members use when they log in and use the chatrooms. I thought that we might be able to link cases through their screen names, as many case patients did not know the names or have other personal identifying information about their partners.

Based on our initial investigation of syphilis cases in gay men and other men who have sex with men in San Francisco, we were able to create a sexual network of interconnected cases. Figure 16-1 shows that network, the early cases, and subsequent secondary cases. That one AOL chatroom linked all of the cases.[1] We defined cases as "early-stage syphilis among gay men reported to the San Francisco Department of Public Health in July and August 1999." (Early syphilis is defined as a patient who has acquired syphilis in the past year.) Examining the sexual network demonstrated that the cases were all linked through the use of the chatroom and revealed the increased number of sex partners reported by some cases. One case reported 47 partners in the past 6 months. A moderate proportion (42%) of the contacts identified by the case patients had confirmed clinical evaluations (Figure 16-1). Overall, however, that moderate proportion of contacts receiving evaluation would make syphilis control in this population very difficult.

From case identification and confirmation of the outbreak, we had to move to a very important stage of our outbreak investigation—public health response. That was going to be tricky, as this was completely new territory, uncharted by prior epidemiologists and unknown to the CDC. This was cyberspace. We needed to act in parallel to warn users of the chatroom of their increased risk and determine the extent of their risk. I knew that the network diagram would be insufficient evidence for some, in particular for some fringe but outspoken gay men who were concerned at that time that the health department was falsely reporting increases in STDs in gay men and other men who have sex with men in its efforts to stigmatize gay sex further. (By 2001, my family and I received death threats that resulted in felony charges and prolonged jail time for two renegade gay male activists— but that is another story for another time.)[2] In addition, we needed very strong evidence because a multina-

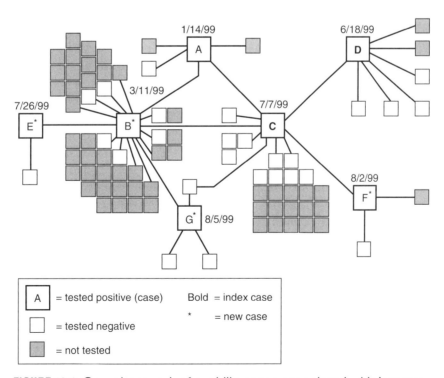

FIGURE 16-1 Sexual network of syphilis cases associated with Internet use, San Francisco, 1999. Adapted from Klausner JD, Wolf W, Fischer-Ponce L, Zolt I, Katz MH. Tracing a syphilis outbreak through cyberspace. *JAMA* 2000; 284:447–9. Copyright © 2000 American Medical Association. All rights reserved.

tional corporation such as AOL could try to refute the potential damaging association of syphilis and chatroom use. A nay sayer would argue that the frequency of Internet sex partnering is very common such that seven syphilis cases from one chatroom would not be beyond what might be expected.

Fortunately, after that discussion with Bill in April, I had immediately thought of the need to understand more about the use of the Internet and its role in sexual health at the population level. I collaborated with a PhD candidate at the University of California–Berkeley, Andrea Kim, who was looking for additional projects related to her thesis about the epidemiology of sexually transmitted diseases. We initiated a voluntary confidential survey of gay men and other men who have sex with men attending the municipal STD clinic to learn about the characteristics of men who used the Internet and measured the frequency of Internet use to find sex partners. Those survey results were linked to each participating patient's STD testing results, and I could easily identify a control population—a group of somewhat similar patients who were tested for syphilis and who were uninfected.[3] I then could do a case-control study and compare the frequency of recent Internet use (the exposure) among those control patients from the survey with the frequency of recent Internet use among case patients. For the case-control study, I defined case patients as San Francisco residents with reported early syphilis infection (syphilis acquired in the prior year) from July to August 1999. I chose early syphilis as the disease classification because early syphilis is recently acquired—persons are infected by definition in the past 12 months—and did not include patients with late syphilis or syphilis of unknown duration to reduce misclassification. In addition, I restricted the case population to gay men and other men who have sex with men to match the surveyed population of control patients.

Using standard epidemiologic analytic techniques, I made a 2 × 2 contingency table comparing the frequency of exposure in case-patients: 4 of 6 (67%) used the Internet to meet sex partners versus 6 of 32 (19%) who used the Internet to meet sex partners among control patients. The odds ratio or measure of association between the odds of being a syphilis case and recent use of the Internet to meet sex partners was 8.7. That value was statistically significant ($P = 0.03$) and thus was very unlikely to be due to chance. In other words, syphilis cases were nearly nine times more likely to have used the Internet to find a new sex partner than patients without syphilis. I had the evidence I needed. The evidence was irrefutable in the court of epidemiology.

Because of the strong and significant association between men using the Internet to meet sex partners and the fact that five of the six cases reported using the AOL chatroom SFM4M, my next steps were to inform AOL and alert the community and medical providers in San Francisco. As part of our outbreak response plan, we had a list of contact information for key community leaders, community-based organizations, local newspapers, and medical care providers, including those who took care of patients with HIV-infection and dermatologists—skin specialists who often see patients with diseases such as syphilis. We sent out a letter through the mail and facsimile stating that we had identified an increase in the number of syphilis cases in gay men and other men who have sex with men that were linked to meeting in a chatroom, AOL SFM4M. We informed readers of the basic signs and symptoms of syphilis and provided treatment and management recommendations and a link to our website (www.sfcityclinic.org) with more information.

Reaching someone at AOL who would collaborate in our investigation and public health response was a significant challenge. How many of us have tried to reach an Internet service provider and were successful in speaking with a live person? I was no different and had no special access. I went to the AOL website and tried to identify the location of the corporate headquarters (Virginia) and attempted to call someone who would work with me to inform AOL members and handle the gathering media storm. Realizing that this was as much about public relations as anything else, I asked to speak with someone in public relations who might provide some assistance. My main aim, initially, in working with AOL was to gather additional locating information for cases of which I only had screen names. AOL certainly had personal and contact information such as name, home address, electronic mail, and various telephone numbers, including likely cellular telephone number. With that information, I could have the investigators contact AOL SFM4M users, directly notify them of their potential exposure, and encourage them to get tested and treated for a possible exposure to syphilis.

Because the incubation of syphilis is on average 3 weeks, if a person is given preventive treatment after exposure with injectable penicillin, the syphilis infection can be aborted. Fortunately, the same dose of penicillin

> *Syphilis cases were nearly nine times more likely to have used the Internet to find a new sex partner than patients without syphilis.*

used for preventive treatment is used for the treatment of early syphilis; therefore, even if treatment is delayed in exposed patients, it is still adequate.

My second aim was to convince AOL to work toward proactively preventing future outbreaks of STDs associated with its members meeting sex partners in chatrooms. I suggested they post advertisements in the chatroom about the syphilis increase, promote regular STD and HIV testing, provide links to further information about safer sex practices, and create a chatroom environment that was conducive to healthful sexual encounters.

Reaching anyone within AOL who would collaborate with me proved very difficult, however. No one would return my calls. Because the headquarters of AOL was in Virginia, I contacted the Virginia Department of Health and asked them to help me. Although not definitely obstructive, the state epidemiologist in Virginia at the time did not agree with me about the urgency to contact AOL. He had spoken to others at the CDC who seemed to agree and were reluctant to exercise their public health authority in the response to the outbreak. I do not think that they appreciated my unique perspective here in San Francisco where Internet partnering was rapidly increasing and the Internet was becoming a very popular place to meet sex partners. Over time, my concern was validated, and Internet sites have become the most commonly cited place where new cases of syphilis in California report meeting sex partners (Figure 16-2). Finally, as the news of the outbreak began to be covered in the media, I did reach an AOL public relations executive, Peter (whose name has been changed).

The power of the media is an important lesson that I have learned in public health.

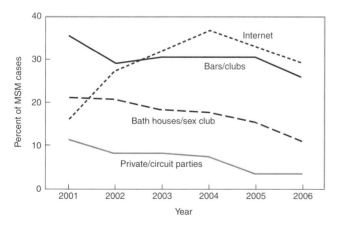

FIGURE 16-2 Percent of Interviewed Gay Male Primary and Secondary Syphilis Cases.

The power of the media is an important lesson that I have learned in public health. When the media calls a company or institution, someone has to comment, and the person making those comments is often a senior executive within the company. After that person's name is associated with the issue in public, that person owns, at least partly owns, the problem; however, Peter was not willing to facilitate my getting further contact information on AOL members who used the SFM4M chatroom. Members' information was private. I became frustrated but soon obtained a lucky break.

Through a personal contact in San Francisco—a friend's sister worked at AOL corporate headquarters—I learned the name of an AOL corporate attorney in Virginia. I sent her e-mail, facsimiles, and certified letters by the U.S. postal service making sure that she was aware—and there was ample documentation of my communications—of the serious nature of the current situation. Through other contacts, I learned that a former high-level gay male governmental official in the Clinton Administration was now working as a senior executive for AOL-Time Warner in New York City—the parent corporation of AOL—and thinking that he might be sympathetic to such issues in gay men's health sought his advice and cooperation. With the continued pressure that I applied, I was ultimately and officially informed that such personal contact information of AOL members could only be released on Federal subpoena or in the case of an imminent grave danger—such as homicide or suicide. I could not justify that syphilis infection posed an immediate and life-threatening danger (with the advent of penicillin and other antibiotics, death due to syphilis infection had become rare in the latter half of the 20th century, and I had never seen a patient die of syphilis infection). A Federal subpoena seemed possible but would take a long time and be expensive and not by any means a guaranteed success.

Of course, I had informed my colleagues at the CDC at the Division of STD Prevention and even further up the hierarchy to include the Director of the National Center for STD, HIV, and TB Prevention. Again, I sent e-mails and facsimiles and mailed letters to the CDC. Although personally sympathetic, various persons at the CDC felt it could not directly intervene with AOL, did not want to make a "federal case" out of it, and would leave things to me in San Francisco. It seemed to me that leaders at the CDC failed to recognize the significance of the outbreak as a harbinger of much larger things to come.

Fortunately, the public relations executive from AOL, in his never ending quest to get rid of me and delegate what only could be a massive headache and public relations disaster for him, put me in touch with Ted (name has been changed), the Chief Executive Officer of PlanetOut, an online community for gay, bisexual, lesbian, and transgender persons headquartered in my hometown in San Francisco. The PlanetOut website offered a range of services, including travel, news, weather, and an online community and was partly owned or supported at that time by AOL. Ted was what I needed. He was a tall, gregarious man with the "can do" "24/7" attitude working in the midst of the 20th century Internet gold rush of 1999, building his great profit machine in cyberspace. Media attention was what he needed and wanted most. Ted detailed a dozen of his staff—various programmers, writers, and marketing personnel—to go online to AOL SFM4M for 2 continuous weeks and inform users about the syphilis outbreak, offer syphilis education, and encourage users to get tested. Because of the privacy concerns of both of the companies, we do not have data about the number or frequency of users who were informed, got tested, or received preventive therapy. Based on chatroom usage patterns, we estimated that thousands were made aware of the outbreak and learned about syphilis, and many of those sought medical care. To evaluate those prevention efforts, we polled a sample of users of SFM4M about the appropriateness of the information campaign. The online survey revealed that 25 of 35 respondents (71%) thought that the awareness campaign on the Internet was useful and appropriate.

To enhance community awareness further and further persuade AOL into being more cooperative, the San Francisco Department of Public Health issued a press release in August of 1999 identifying the direct link between use of the AOL chatroom to meet sex partners and the increase in syphilis cases. In that press release, we also highlighted the lack of willingness of AOL to inform its members but the welcome assistance of staff from PlanetOut. I felt that shaming AOL in view of the general public might prompt them into action. Using the media to confront corporations is a potentially useful but dangerous tactic. No one likes to be embarrassed in the media, particularly public companies. It is a tactic, however, that I have witnessed to be very effective in certain areas of AIDS activism. It is necessary to avoid hyperbole and let the reader or viewer draw his or her own conclusions. Because the media is neutral and is primarily interested in selling newspapers or advertising time, the media does not really care whether the story is about an overzealous local government or an uncaring corporation. The media will go where the most provocative story is. In my case, because my main goal was to raise awareness about the outbreak, any local media I could generate would be beneficial. National media would not help local persons at risk for syphilis but could sway AOL into action. At the minimum, the CDC could not deny its awareness of the situation and might also be pushed into action.

Steve Case, the founder of AOL, had attributed the rapid and sustained success of AOL to its use by the gay community. In public comments, Mr. Case stated that the gay community's use of features like electronic mail, chatrooms, and instant messages unique to AOL at the time was key to AOL's success. He went on to thank the gay community for their early support and allegiance to AOL. "The gay community was a godsend for the company," wrote *Wall Street Journal* technology reporter Kara Swisher in her book *AOL.com: How Steve Case Beat Bill Gates, Nailed the Netheads, and Made Millions in the War for the Web*.[4] "AOL offered a 'live and let live' online space and gays responded by generating huge amounts of revenue for the company." Steve Case said, "Thank God for the gays and lesbians," according to Swisher, noting that use of the online service by gays was particularly heavy in sexually themed chat rooms.

Privacy concerns among Internet users became an issue of national debate. Many national newspapers, including a lead front-page article in the *New York Times* ("Privacy Questions Raised in Cases of Syphilis Linked to Chat Room"),[5] reported on the varied opinions of privacy experts and public health advocates regarding an individual's right to privacy and the government's mandate to protect public health.

In addition to collaborating with Ted at PlanetOut to conduct specific awareness to the potentially exposed population identified through our outbreak investigation, we developed new protocols for public health disease control investigators on how to use the Internet to conduct online partner notification.[6] It is hard to believe that in 1999 many county and state health departments in the United States did not have Internet access or use electronic mail. For those that did, some could not access Internet sites on the World Wide Web outside of their own local network. Many localities had administrative policies specifically stating that personnel could not access the World Wide Web and used firewalls and other techniques to block staff from such use.

By late Fall 1999, the number of new syphilis cases who reported meeting sex partners on AOL SFM4M declined. Unfortunately, that was not the end of increases in syphilis among gay men and other men who have sex with men in the United States. Over the next several years, San Francisco experienced an increase in syphilis from that low in 1998 of 8 cases in gay men and other men who have sex with men to over 550 cases by 2004. Other cities such as Seattle, Los Angeles, San Diego, Chicago, Houston, Atlanta, Miami, Fort Lauderdale, and New York have experienced similar increases. In many cities, those increases continue today. Similar increases have been seen internationally in major cities of Australia, Canada, and Western Europe. The use of the Internet by gay men and other men who have sex with men to meet sex partners has helped to let the syphilis "genie" out of the bottle.

Currently, asking whether new cases of syphilis have met recent partners on the Internet is a routine component of syphilis surveillance. In California, the frequency of meeting partners on the Internet among syphilis cases increased from about 10% in 2000 to over 40% in 2005, making it more common than traditional sites such as bars/clubs, sex clubs, or parks (Figure 16-1). The Internet has become the bathhouse of the 21st century.

> *Chatrooms have given way to entire Internet sites that exist for the expressed purpose of linking sex partners.*

Chatrooms have given way to entire Internet sites that exist for the expressed purpose of linking sex partners. Persons can post photos, maintain a record of prior contacts, and search and sort by a variety of sexual preferences. Sites such as Manhunt and Adam4adam have replaced AOL as the most frequently reported venue for new syphilis cases to report meeting sex partners. Sites such as Craigslist that have city-specific sites like CraigslistSF.org allow for persons traveling to certain cities to identify and plan sexual encounters in advance. To its credit, Craigslist has allowed its site to host online sexual health message boards and provides a routine warning to users of categories such as "men seeking men" about the increases in syphilis transmission associated with meeting partners online.

IMPLICATIONS

Recognizing that the Internet has become the most common venue for gay men and other men who have sex with men at risk for sexually transmitted diseases, including HIV infection, required me to develop a new approach to sexual health promotion and disease prevention. With the additional resources for syphilis control made available in San Francisco by the CDC's effort for national syphilis elimination and the requirement that a proportion of those funds be directly allocated to community-based organizations, I helped stimulate the creation of a new organization called Internet Sexuality Information Services, Inc. (www.ISIS-Inc.org). ISIS-Inc. provides a variety of Internet-based prevention services targeting gay men and other men who have sex with men. Originally focused on men in San Francisco, now ISIS-Inc. works with health departments and community-based organizations worldwide. Innovations developed by Deb Levine, the founder of ISIS-Inc. and I include an online syphilis testing program (STDTest.org) where the public can complete their own syphilis test requisition form, print it out, and bring it to a private laboratory for a free syphilis test. Test results are available securely online. The health department contacts all testers with syphilis and assures timely and adequate treatment. Currently, about 10 to 20 persons a week use the testing service, and the rate of syphilis positivity is about 5% (much higher than any other screening program in San Francisco).[7]

Another innovation includes a site called inSPOT.org, which allows cases of STDs (any STD including HIV infection) to notify a recent sex partner either anonymously or confidentially of exposure to that infection through an electronic postcard with embedded links to more information about the disease, referral information for testing. In the specific case of chlamydia and gonorrhea, inSPOT.org provides access to a free online prescription for treatment. Partners can print out the prescription and take it to a local pharmacy in San Francisco. This augmented peer-to-peer effort for partner notification empowers the user and the community and allows those who wish to take personal responsibility for partner notification an easy opportunity to conduct this important task. Anywhere from 10 to 100 notifications are made monthly in San Francisco, with the highest number of notifications occurring for cases of chlamydia and gonorrhea.

Further Internet-based prevention efforts include banner advertising on major websites named by recent cases of syphilis or HIV infection. These advertisements promote testing or other websites with information about STDs and safer sex practices. By monitoring the frequency of the display of these banner advertisements and the number of click-throughs to the site advertised, one can calculate the cost to the health department per click-through. We have measured a range of costs from less than 5 cents to over $10 per click-through, depending on the site and advertisement. "Ask Dr. K" at AskDrK.org (I am "Dr. K") is a website with honest and evidence-based answers to common questions about sex, sexual health, and sexually transmitted diseases. Although it has limited promotion, over 100 new questions are submitted each week. Frequently asked questions are posted to provide readers with ready and searchable answers.[8]

Other researchers and health officials have also developed Internet-based prevention interventions. Basic services like websites allow users to access sexual health information and clinic operating hours and see sites like Californiamen.net where users can download an electronic black book to record contact information of recent sexual encounters and follow the personal blogs of newly identified HIV-infected men. In 2007, the CDC funded the first Internet-based prevention research center at the Denver Department of Public Health, whose mission is to evaluate and promote effective Internet-based interventions. Scientists at the University of Washington in Seattle have developed and evaluated computer-based personal risk-reduction interventions. If adopted, promoted, and scaled to Internet users at risk for STDs and HIV infection, this intervention has the potential to have a profound impact on sexual risk behavior.[9]

Finally, Internet sex partnering sites run by health organizations that serve to facilitate both sex partnering and safer sex are in development. The move from the old model of bathhouses of the 1970s to 1980s that had no focus on sexual health to the new model of current bathhouses that supply safer sex materials (condoms, lubrication, educational pamphlets) enforce no sex without condom policies, restrict substance use on site, and make STD or HIV screening available is similarly and rapidly occurring on the Internet in its own context. Such sites have online health educators, links to information about sexual health, STDs and HIV infection, links to sites with testing information, and policies mitigating substance use and trafficking of illicit drugs such as methamphetamine.

Perhaps the most exciting aspects of Internet-based sexual or reproductive health promotion and disease prevention are its widespread availability, ease of use, and broad applicability to a range of health issues, in particular those health disparities affected by access to health care. In its first few months of operations, an online service in San Francisco for increased access to Plan B, the age-restricted over-the-counter medication for emergency contraception, has rapidly become a common site for adolescents—those under age 18 years of age who have limited access to Plan B—to obtain information and a free prescription, which they can use at any pharmacy in San Francisco.

CONCLUSIONS

What my patient relayed to me that Monday morning in the spring of 1999 set the stage for the identification and control of the first infectious disease outbreak associated with the use of the Internet to meet sex partners. Furthermore, with broad training in medicine, infectious diseases, and public health, as well as the availability of flexible resources and a highly supportive department director, I was able learn from the outbreak and stimulate the creation of a new field of health promotion and disease prevention. I am often asked to lecture in the United States and across the globe (e.g., Canada, England, Germany, Peru, Brazil, India) about the Internet, the outbreak of syphilis, and disease prevention. People seem fascinated by the combination of technology and sex. To update the old adage "sex sells," today I would say "sex and the Internet" sells. Every new successful technological advance—printing press, photography, telephone, cinema, television, and the Internet—seems to have one thing in common: its ability to enhance life's sexual experiences.

Actively investigating outbreaks, including incorporating and even acquiring new knowledge during fieldwork, is what the term in the CDC's Epidemic Intelligence Service "shoe leather epidemiology" is all about. It is where the rubber meets the road. I hope this brief description of my experience in tracking a syphilis outbreak in cyberspace will allow future practitioners and policy makers to apply similar lessons in public health and observational epidemiology to improve the community's health and the conditions in which we all live.

REFERENCES

1. Klausner JD, Wolf W, Fischer-Ponce L, Zolt I, Katz MH. Tracing a syphilis outbreak through cyberspace. *JAMA* 2000; 284:447–449.
2. Winter G. San Francisco AIDS debate leads to criminal charges. *New York Times*, December 24, 2001:A10.
3. Kim AA, Kent C, McFarland W, Klausner JD. Cruising on the internet highway. *J AIDS* 2001;28:89–93.
4. Swisher K. *AOL.com: How Steve Case Beat Bill Gates, Nailed the Netheads, and Made Millions in the War for the Web*. New York: Random House, 1998.
5. Nieves E. Privacy questions raised in cases of syphilis linked to chat room. *The New York Times*, August 25, 1999:A1.
6. Kent CK, Wolf W, Nieri G, Wong W, Klausner JD, Peterman TA. Internet use and early syphilis infection among men who have sex with men—San Francisco, California, 1999—2003. *Morb Mortal Wkly Rep* 2003;52:1229–1232.

7. Levine DK, Scott KC, Klausner JD. Online syphilis testing—confidential and convenient. *Sex Transm Dis* 2005;32:139–141.
8. Klausner JD, Levine DK, Kent CK. Internet-based site-specific interventions for syphilis prevention among gay and bisexual men. *AIDS Care* 2004;16:964–970.
9. Mackenzie SL, Kurth AE, Spielberg F, Severynen A, Malotte CK, St Lawrence J. Patient and staff perspectives on the use of a computer counseling tool for HIV and sexually transmitted infection risk reduction. *J Adolesc Health* 2007;40:572.e9–16.

LEARNING QUESTIONS

1. The author refers to conditions that are required for potentially eradicating an infectious disease. What are those conditions?
2. Enhancing community awareness about syphilis was an important part of the author's attempt to mitigate this outbreak. How did he go about doing this?

CHAPTER 17

Eschar: The Story of the New York City Department of Health 2001 Anthrax Investigation

Don Weiss MD, MPH and Marci Layton, MD

New York, NY, 2001

INTRODUCTION

Definition:

Eschar (es´kär)

[Greek eschara, a fireplace, a scab caused by burning]. A dark scab, coagulated crust or slough resulting from the destruction of living tissue following a burn, the bite of a mite or as a result of anthrax infection (adapted from the Oxford English Dictionary).

(The term anthrax is used here to describe clinical disease caused by infection with *Bacillus anthracis*. The terms *Bacillus anthracis* and *B. anthracis* are used when referring to the bacterium).

Late on the afternoon of October 4, 2001, Marci Layton, Assistant Commissioner of the Bureau of Communicable Disease, New York City Department of Health (DOH) called us into her cramped office. She would not call it cramped, but if more than three people met with her at the same time, one had to squeeze into a chair wedged between the bookshelf and the table. I moved to that seat in anticipation of Joel Ackelsberg and Annie Fine joining Sharon Balter, Mike Phillips, and myself. Joel, Annie, Sharon, and I were the bureau's core of medical epidemiologists, and Mike was our first-year Epidemic Intelligence Service (EIS) officer. Marci, as assistant commissioner, ran the operation. Sharon and I and a legion of others who certainly would not fit into Marci's office had just spent the weeks following the destruction of the World Trade Center (WTC) towers setting up a new disease surveillance system in New York City. This system was implemented to bolster detection of unusual disease events, specifically bioterrorism, and relied on placing an EIS Officer in each of 15 sentinel emergency departments. We worked 12- to 18-hour days, doing everything from playing den mother to the 40 EIS officers to investigating unusual clustering of patients with febrile and other illnesses.

Just a few days before the meeting in Marci's office, we had returned to our 125 Worth Street offices. The damage at the WTC had affected the local power grid and phone service in the area, and this, along with the pungent air, forced a 2.5-week relocation uptown. Although power was restored, most phone service remained out. My cluttered cubicle looked as foreign to me as a time capsule opened after 50 years of internment. The Centers for Disease Control (CDC) wanted their EIS officers back, and thus, our task was to convert the mostly manual system to an exclusively electronic one, all while trying to get back to our usual and long-neglected tasks such as investigating cases of typhoid fever, meningococcal disease, and West Nile virus. Thus, we exhaled deeply as we moved into Marci's office and prepared for the news.

A high-level epidemiologist in the CDC's bioterrorism response program, stationed in New York City since 9/11, had pulled Marci aside to tell her that the Florida Health Department and the CDC were about to announce a case of inhalational anthrax in a 63-year-old man who worked as a photo editor. His disease onset was September 30; he had evidence of meningitis as well as mediastinitis and was doing poorly. The investigation was examining possible natural exposures, as the individual was reportedly an avid outdoorsman who had taken a recent fishing trip to North Carolina. In the initial public comment about the case, Secretary of Health and Human Services, Tommy Thompson, offered the conjecture that the patient acquired anthrax from drinking spring water contaminated by a dead animal carcass. We are, by nature and experience, a skeptical lot. Although we all immediately considered this bioterrorism until proven otherwise, a photo editor and the Florida location seemed an unlikely choice of a terrorist. There was a rumor about an airport near the patient's home that may have been used as a training location for the 9/11 hijackers. Rather than indulge in debate, our oft and wanton pastime, we began constructing a plan for enhanced surveillance for inhalational anthrax in New York City. Over the next 2 days we made what would become the first of several rounds of active surveillance calls. Concerned that there might be an undiagnosed anthrax case, we called every hospital and laboratory operating in New York City to inquire about possible anthrax and to remind the medical community to report suspect cases.

> *The disease anthrax is caused by infection with the spore-forming bacterium* Bacillus anthracis.

The disease anthrax is caused by infection with the spore-forming bacterium *Bacillus anthracis*. Named for the coal-black scab (eschar), which forms at the site of skin invasion, it is mostly a disease of animals but has plagued humans since antiquity. It can be found worldwide and persists in soil in the dormant spore form. Several clinical syndromes are recognized and differ by the route of entry into the human body. Cutaneous anthrax occurs when *B. anthracis* enters through a breach in the skin's protective barrier. A pimple forms which progresses to an ulcer and heals with the characteristic black scab. Cutaneous infections mostly remain limited to the skin and area lymph glands; however, bloodborne infection can occur. Although the mildest form, untreated cutaneous anthrax may kill up to one fifth of its victims. Gastrointestinal anthrax occurs when the bacteria are ingested. This form usually occurs by consumption of contaminated meat from animals that died of anthrax. After a period of abdominal pain, fever, and vomiting, bloody diarrhea and sepsis may ensue, claiming half of those infected. Inhalational or pulmonary anthrax occurs when spores are inhaled. The most serious form of anthrax, it is fortunately rare and in the modern era has mostly occurred in workers exposed to aerosols generated during the commercial processing of animal hair and hides. An infection in the lung's lymph nodes and surrounding tissue, known as mediastinitis, is the major clinical finding. The bacteria then enter the blood where released *B. anthracis* toxins cause a rapid collapse of the circulatory system. Once in the blood stream, *B. anthracis* can travel to other locations, causing multiorgan failure and meningitis. Death is the usual outcome in inhalational anthrax cases. The vast majority of anthrax cases are the cutaneous form and the disease is quite rare in the United States.

> *The vast majority of anthrax cases are the cutaneous form and the disease is quite rare in the United States.*

THE OUTBREAK AND INVESTIGATION

I could not help thinking, as we organized staff to make the enhanced surveillance calls, that we had only just returned to our offices and had begun reconstituting routine surveillance activities. One thing we did not do very well during 9/11 was involve enough of the DOH workforce. Now we needed to get people back to work. Resuming normalcy was one way to try and put the horror of September behind us. Thus, while getting staff involved in making the calls to hospitals and labs was not exactly their normal activities, it did bring them into the investigation. We targeted emergency departments, intensive care units, infectious disease department chair persons, infection control practitioners, and laboratorians. We told them what we knew of the Florida case and asked them to be particularly observant. Should a previously well person come in with sepsis, respiratory failure, or meningitis, he or she should keep anthrax in their differential diagnosis. Should a Gram-positive rod appear in a culture broth, do not discount it as a contaminant; instead, look into it further, and above all, call us. They could expect a medical alert from Marci soon explaining all of this in detail. We also conducted retrospective surveillance asking clinicians whether they had seen any patients going back to September 11 that fit the symptoms of inhalational, meningeal, or gastrointestinal anthrax. Four to five calls to 70-plus hospitals and labs kept staff occupied. I figured typhoid fever could and would have to wait a bit longer. To handle incoming calls after hours, we divided up the city giving the Poison Control Center, which received after-hours calls from clinicians, our cell phone numbers. Marci took all calls from Manhattan hospitals. Sharon got Queens. Annie took Brooklyn, and I took the Bronx and Staten Island. It was not long before our phones began ringing at all hours.

Meanwhile, Marci prepared a medical alert. The medical alert system was her own creation and had served DOH well during the West Nile virus outbreak of 1999. At the time, it was relatively low-tech, blast faxes sent to hospitals and laboratories with information, instructions, and specific requests for assistance. Hospital-based health care providers had come to expect these alerts and trusted that if there was something going on the DOH would communicate it to them in all due haste.

What several of us did not know at the time was that Joel had evaluated a white powder threat letter and suspicious cutaneous anthrax case on October 1. As our bioterrorism readiness coordinator and intra-agency liaison, he regularly responded to such incidents, a dozen or more since joining the department the previous summer. All of the incidents had turned out to be hoaxes. The woman in question was Tom Brokaw's assistant at NBC News, and she noticed on September 25 a flesh-colored bump about the size of a pea just below her left collar bone and rimmed by scant erythema (redness). Over the next few days, it enlarged and became a fluid-filled vesicle. The surrounding skin became more inflamed and swollen, resembling an oblong cigarette burn. The weekend passed fitfully for her; she experienced headache and malaise, and after repeated urgings from her husband to see a doctor, she began taking left-over antibiotic that she had at home. That Monday, October 1, the erythema increased, and the normal contour of her collarbone was obscured by the swelling. She showed it to the physician at NBC. Recalling the unusual threat letter containing powder that spilled on her chest the previous week, she raised the possibility of anthrax.

When Joel heard her story, he followed the protocol he had written. The FBI retrieved the threat letter and powder, which were tested at the New York City Public Health Laboratory (PHL). The powder was negative for *B. anthracis* by direct fluorescent antibody and culture. Direct fluorescent antibody is a staining technique in which antibodies specific to the *B. anthracis* cell wall are linked to a chemical that glows when exposed to a certain wavelength of light. It is an extremely powerful tool for identifying *B. anthracis*, as it can be used on powders as well as clinical specimens. A routine swab of the wound for bacterial culture was negative, not surprising because the patient had been on antibiotics. Based on these results and that she was improving on treatment, there appeared little reason to perform a biopsy, the excision of a small amount of wound tissue to examine for *B. anthracis*. The patient's unusual skin lesion was attributed to the bite of a Brown Recluse spider that had ventured far from its normal range. NBC, as we were soon to learn, received these types of letters quite frequently.

We followed the Florida investigation like football fans watching the OJ Simpson trial, hoping it was not so. Secretary of Health and Human Services Thompson was again speaking publicly, emphasizing the isolated nature of the case. We remained dubious. The Florida patient died the next day, October 5. Investigations in North Carolina and the patient's office had not turned up any clues. The EIS officers, now stationed in 12 New York City hospitals, kept looking for unusual cases, and we triaged calls from worried clinicians seeing patients who were ill and bore some distant connection to Florida. By October 7, the CDC and the FBI knew that the Florida case was bioterrorism. People in Florida likely knew as well because the FBI had sealed off the America Media Inc. (AMI) building, where the patient had worked, as a crime scene. The next morning the rest of the country found out that environmental samples taken at AMI, from the work space of the Florida case, were positive for *B. anthracis* and that a second AMI worker had inhalational anthrax.

October 8 was Columbus Day, a holiday, although most of us worked anyway. Marci spent the morning evaluating a smallpox case that wasn't and the afternoon through evening at another white-powder incident at a British Company in midtown Manhattan. The rest of us were busy fielding an increase in anthrax calls from worried New Yorkers and the physicians caring for them that had been provoked by the breaking news from Florida. It was nearly 10:00 p.m. when Marci returned to an empty DOH building. Her momentary peace was interrupted by a call from the FBI agent who was with her at the white-powder hoax earlier that afternoon. The incident was not why he was calling. The sick NBC employee called him. She was following the news closely, and she wondered whether her unusual skin lesions could be anthrax after all. Marci called the NBC employee and the woman described to her in chronological detail the progression of her skin infection and then e-mailed Marci links to web images of cutaneous anthrax that looked like her own lesion. Over the next 24 hours she was seen by an infectious disease specialist who felt certain this was cutaneous anthrax and then by a dermatologist who concurred. Sharon met her at the dermatologist's office where a biopsy of her lesion and a blood sample for *B. anthracis* antibodies were obtained. Sharon next called the CDC to ask that they test the tissue and blood. The emergency response center at the CDC informed her that they were swamped with the Florida investigation and suggested that she try the New York State lab. This did not sit well with Marci, who out of experience, or perhaps premonition, knew that this was an important sample that needed to go directly to the CDC. Although the New York State Wadsworth Center was a very good laboratory, they lacked the experience with *B. anthracis* and would not be able to perform immunohistochemical staining (IHC) on the skin biopsy sample. IHC is a tissue-staining technique that uses antibodies specific to what you are looking for, in this case the anthrax bacillus. The antibodies are linked to a molecule that produces a color reaction, thereby highlighting the presence of the organism. Marci made a call to a high-level official at the CDC who she knew from her many interactions with them, from the 1996 Cyclospora in raspberries outbreak to initial U.S. outbreak of West Nile virus in 1999. He agreed to test the clinical specimens as well as the September 25 threat letter. Both were immediately flown to the CDC in Atlanta, GA by a special courier, who happened to be the same CDC staffer who first informed Marci of the Florida anthrax case. The specimens arrived contemporaneously with a power outage at the CDC, which postponed testing until October 11. While awaiting the results, we stayed busy with phone calls and preparing for the worst case scenario.

One of the things that worked well during our response to 9/11 was computer and network access. Within hours of our relocation to the PHL back on September 12, 2001, the information technology team had us up and running. Their support throughout the anthrax investigation was to prove invaluable. Thus, when I arrived at my cubicle on October 9, I was unprepared to see the "blue screen of death," a well known sign of serious computer trouble. Perhaps it was an omen of what was to come because that very evening I found myself on Staten Island sorting through trash outside a suspect case's home, looking for a threat letter with powder reportedly postmarked from Florida (Figure 17-1). The recipient and his family had vague medical complaints but were not seriously ill. My rumpled appearance and odd questions about tape and excessive postage on envelopes, possible signs of tainted letters, must have made me seem like Detective Columbo. The next day, October 10, I recorded in my notebook a heightened sense of anxiety at work. More calls were coming in from community physicians. The chief of staff's assistant stopped by to inquire about a rumor that the FBI had some tests results. This I could not confirm, and when I approached Marci, even she was uncharacteristically terse.

Another young woman, who regularly opened mail at NBC for Tom Brokaw and worked closely with his assistant, was herself ill in late September 2001. For her, it began with throat soreness, swollen glands, and a few papules on her face. She too experienced fever and fatigue and saw her doctor on the same day as her coworker, October 1. After a few days recuperating at home, she returned to work just as the news about the Florida inhalational anthrax case was breaking. She began to put it together. Brokaw, on learning of another of his staff with a suspicious skin lesion, arranged to have her seen by the same infectious disease specialist who had seen his assistant. On October 10, Sharon spoke with the doctor and then the young woman. Sharon learned that among the many "critic" letters there were actually two recent ones that had contained powder. The letter that arrived on September 25 and had tested negative for *B. anthracis* bore an uncanny similarity in penmanship in the eyes of NBC staff to the letter that had

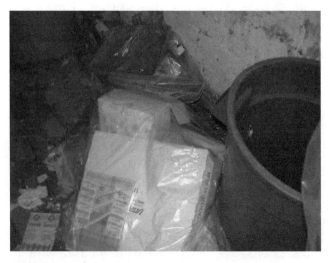

FIGURE 17-1 Sifting through trash for a threat letter on Staten Island. Courtesy of Don Weiss.

arrived a week earlier around September 18. The first letter arrived a week after the WTC attacks and contained a crushed brownish material. Written on the enclosed note was, "Death to Israel, Allah is God." The powder she had discarded, but the letter was kept. When the second letter arrived, this time with a finer, white powder, security came to take it and instructed staff not to open these types of letters anymore. In retrospect, we might have decided to send in a team of moon-suited investigators to search for the September 18 letter. This would have most certainly disrupted operations at NBC and caused alarm among their staff and a nationwide media stir. We had no evidence yet of anthrax in New York City, and it seemed prudent not to move to this step before we had proof based on laboratory confirmation of human illness or environmental contamination.

Results from the CDC on the skin biopsy from Tom Brokaw's assistant, as well as retesting of the envelope, came near midnight on October 11. The September 25 NBC letter (the second one received) had again tested negative. Polymerase chain reaction (PCR) testing on the skin biopsy was also negative for *B. anthracis*. PCR is an extremely powerful laboratory method that can detect small quantities of DNA specific to a particular organism, in this case *B. anthracis*. I think the building breathed a sigh of relief; otherwise, I do not think Marci would have left work at all that night. What remained were the IHC and antibody results. Although some of us slept uneasily at best, senior epidemiologists and laboratorians at the CDC met in the early morning hours and agonized over apparently conflicting results. Although PCR on the letter and biopsy were negative, the immunohistochemical stain of the biopsy was positive for *B. anthracis*. This stain targets specific proteins in the *B. anthracis* capsule, and it was "lighting up" under a microscope. Sherif Zaki, a seasoned CDC pathologist, read the slide and was convinced that it was real. The implications of anthrax from a mailed letter were staggering, and the CDC deliberated as dawn approached. The final test for antibodies in her blood sample would not be ready for several more hours. Just before 3:00 a.m., CDC Director Jeffrey Copeland awoke Marci to tell her the news; they were considering this positive for *B. anthracis*. Marci next switched on the phone tree that jolted the rest of us out of our fitful slumbers. Anthrax was here, in New York City. Report for work at 6:00 a.m. Among the thoughts running through my mind was a line from the Robin Williams movie *Good Morning Vietnam*. Williams as disc jockey Adrian Cronauer crows on the radio, "It's oh-six hundred hours," and then pointedly adds that the "oh" stands for, "Oh my f-ing God its early."

In as much as Cronauer's expletive was more a comment on the Vietnam war than the early hour of reveille, our churning stomachs cared less about the hour of our congress than its topic.

October 12 was the beginning of a massive public health mobilization and multipronged investigation that was to last through Thanksgiving. In addition to the cutaneous anthrax case at NBC, we would hear about other highly concerning cases at three more major media corporations as well as letters, illnesses, and environmental contaminations requiring investigation. Over the ensuing 3 weeks, we performed an average of three concurrent investigations each day and as many as six on some days (Figure 17-2). The following pages describe the major investigations in the order in which we learned of them. Details for each investigation are given as they unfolded over several days. The chronology of the story then returns to October 12 to follow the thread of the next investigation. Unspoken, yet never far from the minds of all involved in the investigation, and likely the entire city, was the apprehension about inhalational anthrax. If cutaneous anthrax was in New York City, could inhalational be far behind?

A team was dispatched to NBC to interview workers in the same office as the index case. A point of distribution (POD) clinic was rapidly mobilized to dispense prophylactic antibiotics. A multiagency environmental assessment team was formed to create a *Bacillus anthracis* sampling plan. Mike and Marci went to 30 Rockefeller Plaza (the location of NBC offices), whereas Sharon stayed at our office to handle the deluge of provider calls. A medical alert was quickly drafted and distributed (Exhibit 17-1). It announced the case at NBC and added the clinical and diagnostic findings of cutaneous anthrax to the previously distributed descriptions of pulmonary and meningeal anthrax sent after 9/11 and again on October 5. The alert reassured the medical community (and indirectly the public) that both traditional and syndromic surveillance systems had not uncovered any suspicious inhalational anthrax cases.

After the first case was verified, we actively sought out additional cases through interviews of co-workers and review of worksite employee health records. Surveillance was established for those currently ill, anyone whose illness in the past month met the case definition, and for future cases. At sites where threat letters were found, tracking the letter's path allowed us to focus the epidemiologic and environmental investigations on individuals at highest risk.

My assignment on October 12 was a stomach tossing, lights and sirens ride in an unmarked police car to

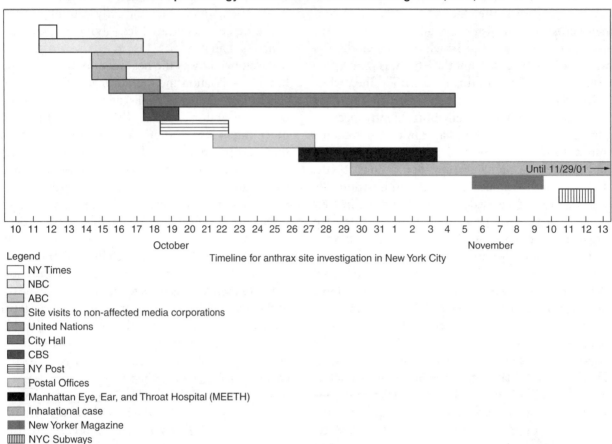

FIGURE 17-2 Timeline of anthrax investigations.

the *New York Times* building, where a journalist had just opened a threat letter filled with powder. The target was a former Middle East correspondent who had recently written extensively on the risk of bioterrorism. She sliced open the letter at her desk in a large open room filled with work stations. Removing the single sheet, the pure white powder fell into her lap and onto the floor. The letter advised her to "go away for the next 4 weeks" and "watch the Sears tower come down." Witnesses described the powder as flour or talc-like with both a perfume and acrid odor. It turned out to be a hoax, but not before a long and tortuous journey to get the powder tested that involved the *New York Times* flying the specimen to the Massachusetts State laboratory in its own private jet. The journalist never did get her favorite sweater returned, which was submitted for testing.

At NBC, while Mayor Rudy Giuliani and Health Commissioner Neal Cohen announced the first anthrax case to the city from a hastily convened press conference, epidemiologists and law enforcement, alerted to the possibility of a second threat letter, began the search in parallel. When notes were compared, we learned the path that mail took through NBC. It was believed to have arrived on September 19 and was promptly x-rayed, as was the procedure for all mail. It was next taken to the 2nd-floor mailroom, where it was sorted into a pile destined for the 3rd, 4th, and 6th floors. It was further sorted to the 3rd-floor Nightly News offices, where it was given to a page, the woman Sharon had interviewed a few days earlier with suspicious skin lesions. She opened it just outside of the office of the first case, getting some of the crushed brown substance on her hands. The powder was dumped in the trash, the odd letter receiving no more notice than its mention of "Death to Israel," and "Allah is God." The envelope and letter were paper-clipped and given to Brokaw's assistant. It was then placed in a gray interoffice envelope and set aside, on her desk, next to the printer and forgotten. On October 9, NBC security came and retrieved the gray envelope along with a stack of unopened, suspicious letters, placing them all in an ordinary plastic shopping bag. The bag was next brought to the 16th floor and left on a chair. Security moved the let-

> **EXHIBIT 17-1** Medical Alert Announcing the First Cutaneous Anthrax Case in New York City
>
> The City of New York
>
> DEPARTMENT OF HEALTH
>
> October 12, 2001
>
> ALERT #8: 1–Case of cutaneous anthrax in an employee at 30 Rockefeller Center possibly exposed to a contaminated envelope.
>
> [Correction: Prior communication that you may have received was inaccurate; at this time, NYC DOH is recommending prophylaxis and routine anthrax testing for *only* those who were on the 3rd floor of 30 Rockefeller Center on September 18th and 25th.]
>
> The New York City Department of Health
>
> - Requests Immediate Reporting of any Suspected Cases of Cutaneous, Pulmonary, Gastrointestinal, or Central Nervous System Anthrax (see Appendix I)
> - Strongly Recommends Against Prescribing Prophylactic Antibiotics for anyone who was NOT on the 3rd floor of 30 Rockefeller Center on September 18th and 25th.
> - Encourages Healthcare Providers to Remain Alert and Immediately Report any Unusual Disease Manifestations and Clusters
>
> Please Share this Alert with All Medical, Pediatric, Nursing, Laboratory, Radiology, and Pharmacy Staff in Your Hospital
>
> TO: Emergency Medicine Directors, Infection Control Practitioners and Infectious Disease Physicians, Laboratory Directors and Others on the NYCDOH Broadcast Alert System
>
> FROM: Marcelle Layton, MD, Assistant Commissioner
>
> Communicable Disease Program
>
> Case of cutaneous anthrax in New York City: On October 12, the New York City Department of Health was notified by the CDC that a specimen from a skin lesion was positive for *B. anthracis* by immunohistochemical stain. The patient is also serology positive.
>
> Source: City of New York Department of Health.

ter over the next several days to different offices, eventually returning it to the mailroom where the plan was to x-ray it again. Knowing the exact trail and possible contact with other mail would become important not only to make sense of the subsequent environmental findings but to understand transmission dynamics of the cases yet to come.

Thus, two threat letters with powder arrived at NBC in September 2001. One postmarked September 18 and the other September 25. The letter of the 25 had already been tested and was negative at both the PHL and the CDC. The letter postmarked September 18 was located on the afternoon of October 12 in the 2nd-floor NBC mailroom and taken into evidence by a New York City Police Department detective and FBI agent. It was couriered to the PHL, where lab technologist Marie Wong was assigned to process the specimen. Inside a large, clear plastic Ziploc bag she found the folded gray interoffice envelope that contained the mailing envelope. A smaller Ziploc bag, also inside the larger one, contained the letter opened flat so that it could be read through the bag. Marie had been the laboratorian who tested the previous NBC letter (postmarked September 25), which contained a copious amount of powder that was not *B. anthracis*. This letter looked different.

Taking the specimens into the biosafety hood for testing, she observed that the mailing envelope that had contained the threatening letter had very little powder. First, she delicately dug into each corner with a spatula, returning nothing. She slanted the envelope and tapped. Still nothing. Pausing for a moment, she noted that the handwritten address was slanted and looked like a child's writing. Peeling back the wrapper of a sterile swab, she applied a few drops of sterile saline and gently worked it into each corner of the envelope. When she pulled it out, stuck to the fuzzy tip were brown and black specks along with some sparkling white crystals. Pretty crystals, she thought. She prepared a wet mount and peered down into the microscope. She saw many large, oval structures lying on top of each other, packed like sardines. The entire slide was filled with them. Uh-oh, she thought, these look like spores. She called over two of her colleagues. They were not sure but knew additional testing would answer the question. Marie promptly proceeded to set up the tests that within hours would confirm her initial observations that this was really *B. anthracis*.

Although the various law enforcement teams that routinely respond to powder threat incidents are usually exceptionally scrupulous about donning personal protective equipment and sealing off areas before entering a possible "hot zone," the chaos of that day, and perhaps concern over alarming NBC staff, disrupted standard operating procedures. The NBC letter had been stored in an ordinary, open plastic shopping bag and was transferred to the sealed plastic bag in open air. The gray interoffice envelope, which had for days contained the letter, was moved about without consideration that it too might be contaminated. Before testing occurred, the letter was photocopied down the hall from the bioterrorism lab, spreading *B. anthracis* spores throughout the copy room as well as the lab. This led to three PHL laboratorians and the detective courier testing positive on nasal or facial swabs. There may have been others contaminated by aerosolized spores, including myself, as the letter and bag made their way from NBC to the PHL, but no others were tested. I was in hallway outside the laboratory that evening to interview the detective and lab staff on what had transpired. The New York City bioterrorism lab was shut down because of *B. anthracis* spore contamination, just as the first batch of what would eventually number over 3,000 samples were arriving. While the PHL was prepared to respond to a bioterrorism event, consisting of one or a few samples, protocols and staffing were not designed to handle the daily influx of hundreds of environmental samples and nasal swabs from the media investigations, clinical specimens from hospitals, and items submitted from an increasingly unnerved general public. The loss of the primary laboratory served only to hasten the saturation point of laboratory capacity. What ensued has been termed "white powder hysteria" that not only affected New York City and the rest of the United States, but spread throughout the world. Anthrax scares disrupted government offices in Canada, England, France, Germany, and Australia in the week after the announcement of the NBC case. Powders closed newspaper offices, grounded planes, held people in quarantine for hours, and caused stocks to tumble.

Another of my assignments, along with our public health veterinarian Bryan Cherry and recent EIS alumnus Denis Nash, was to assist at the PHL with a specimen accession and result tracking system for environmental samples. The pressure for rapid reporting of results came from all sides—the mayor, the health commissioner, the CDC, media moguls, and the public. Their urgency clashed with antiquated laboratory information management systems. After the bioterrorism lab was closed, another lab was quickly outfitted, but the backlog of samples was immense. Some samples were shipped to other state laboratories whose own capacity was severely challenged by their own powder incidents. Although necessary, the use of these reference labs further compounded the problem of tracking results. Help also came in the form of laboratory teams from the CDC and the Department of Defense, but even with the extra hands there was really no keeping up with the influx of specimens, some of which were rather unusual.

The public was seeing threatening white powders where before they had seen ordinary items of their daily routines. Items such as parmesan cheese, Little Debbie Devil Creams, Apple Jacks, onion powder, and 40 fifty-dollar bills coated with a white substance were viewed with new suspicion and submitted for testing. Each panicked public call required the police or other law enforcement officers to evaluate, package, and transport the item(s) for testing. One prankster placed a small pile of talcum or the like on a sheet of toilet tissue in a common bathroom stall and then rolled it up so that the next patron got a very different puff than the one they had expected. Items clogged the storage area at the PHL and overflowed to the loading dock. Some items, like a sofa from Tom Brokaw's office, couldn't fit in the lab safety hood and presented additional challenges. PHL, CDC, and Department of Defense laboratory staff divided into teams and worked in shifts, 24 hours a day just to keep up, despite the implementation of a protocol to prioritize which specimens needed to be tested.

Specimens from a patient with a clinically worrisome illness consistent with any form of anthrax were given the highest priority. Incidents in which there was documented dispersal of powder with a possible risk to many came next, and the third level was for letters or packages in which law enforcement had determined a credible threat existed. Credible threats were those that appeared similar to letters already found, with one or more of the following characteristics: a threat letter mentioning anthrax or referencing 9/11; no return address, suspicious postmark, or handwriting; common word misspelling; excessive postage or securing materials such as tape; noticeable bulk; marked as "personal" or "confidential"; or sent to a high profile person such as Tom Brokaw. Other items were either not tested or testing was postponed. One FBI agent, who through his integrity and open communication had already earned the respect and admiration of many involved in the investigation, practically lived at the PHL triaging the incoming samples.

> *Specimens from a patient with a clinically worrisome illness consistent with any form of anthrax were given the highest priority.*

Returning to the swirl of events on October 12, an interminably long day for those of us in the field and certainly equally exhausting for those left back at the home base to receive phone calls, we learned of other suspicious cutaneous cases at ABC, CBS, and the New York Post. These new reports fit the profile of a clinically compatible skin infection in a person who handled mail for a high-level media employee. In order to handle multiple investigations the DOH re-activated its Incident Command System, which had precious few days to recover from responding to the World Trade Center attack. The Incident Command System was developed in order to coordinate the multiagency response to large forest fires and relied on a military-style structure of responsibility and reporting. An associate commissioner or comparable level staff was assigned to each media site to function as the direct link to the health department. His or her job was to oversee the teams dispatched to conduct epidemiology interviews, perform environmental sampling, assess risk exposure and distribute prophylactic antibiotics at point of distribution (POD) centers, and provide education about anthrax.

In the beginning, what we knew about anthrax all came from textbooks and expert consultants who like us had never dealt with a bioterrorism attack. Educational sessions at the media sites in the early days of the outbreak were daunting. Dr. Isaac Weisfuse, then associate commissioner for disease control and site liaison to NBC, faced an anxious and agitated crowd of investigative reporters on that first day, October 12. Because of concerns of spore dissemination, the air conditioning system had been shut off. For what seemed like hours, they pummeled him with tough, unanswerable questions. The implacable Dr. Weisfuse realized the right thing to do was to acknowledge that we simply did not know all the answers, rather than reassure the public based on insufficient data. The critical decisions of risk communication that emerged that day and over the course of the outbreak were deftly managed by the DOH communications director, Sandy Mullin. For Dr. Weisfuse, however, the temperature in the room was not the only thing broiling that afternoon.

The environmental investigation was complicated by the absence of existing protocols for *B. anthracis* environmental testing. What is the normal background rate of *B. anthracis* spores? What is the threshold limit that poses no human health threat? Conventional wisdom held that once spores fell to the ground, they would remain, pinned in place by electrostatic forces. Was this really true? If spores were tracked elsewhere, was there any risk to human health? Environmental testing occurred

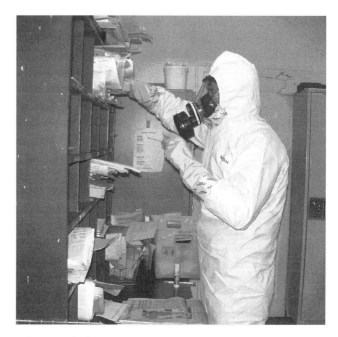

FIGURE 17-3 Swabbing mailboxes for *Bacillus anthracis* spores at a media site. Courtesy of Don Weiss.

at all media sites in which a clinical case was detected as well as media sites without cases in order to detect exposure before disease occurred (Figure 17-3). The role of nasal swab testing for *B. anthracis* spores was purely to learn the location and expanse of exposure, not for individual patient treatment decisions; nevertheless, employees at the involved media sites, who learned of the swab test, had come to expect their noses to be swabbed and treatment decisions based on the results. We were in uncharted waters—icebergs seemed to be everywhere and safe port invisible beyond the horizon.

The next media site investigated was ABC. The call also came in on October 12 about a 7-month-old boy who was hospitalized with a skin infection. He attended a seemingly innocuous workplace birthday party, held on September 28 at ABC's upper west side studio, with his mother, a producer at ABC World News Tonight. The next day he developed a weepy, silver-dollar size sore above his left elbow that oozed yellowish fluid through his shirt. The child appeared unfazed and the sore was initially regarded as an insect bite. The next day his pediatrician decided to treat the sore as cellulitis, a skin infection, and prescribed an oral antibiotic. The infant did not tolerate the medication and was hospitalized on October 1. The wound continued to progress through stages: becoming purple with significant erythema and arm swelling and then ulcerating and finally forming a black eschar on the same day the Florida inhalational anthrax case was announced. Despite other complications, the child was well on the way to recovery when the news of the NBC cutaneous case first broke. The patient's mother immediately reminded physicians of her occupation and the call was made to the DOH initiating the investigation that confirmed the child as another victim in the evolving outbreak of cutaneous anthrax. The site investigation at ABC officially began on October 15, a day after the child's diagnosis was confirmed at the CDC. Although no specific threat letter could be recalled by staff or was ever found, *B. anthracis* spores were detected in the mailroom and staff mail slots.

Sharon Balter had just joined the DOH 2 months before the attack at the WTC and the subsequent anthrax outbreak. Fortified by her experiences as an EIS Officer and CDC epidemiologist, she possessed the requisite sense of humor and ability to take adversity in stride to do well at the DOH. She took to her position with the bureau like a duck to water, which was a good thing, not only because she was the head of our Waterborne Disease Program but because she was one of the few left in the office when yet another call came in late on October 12. The particulars were eerily familiar—this time the sick woman was the personal assistant to CBS anchorman Dan Rather, and as part of her job, she opened from 2,000 to 4,000 letters a day. She first noted two small red dots on her left cheek on October 1. These were accompanied by swelling that began beneath her eye and spread across her face. She was nauseated and light headed. By October 4 she was convinced this was a reaction to an insect bite, something she had experienced before in her life. Her physician prescribed antibiotics. After a few more rough days of feeling light headed, the swelling began to subside, and she was feeling better. A co-worker of the CBS case, on hearing the news about the NBC situation, decided to reach out to the DOH through a mutual friend who was a medical epidemiologist with the bureau. Sharon was tasked to make the initial call to the patient and arranged to meet the woman at her doctor's office. Both patient and doctor were quite skeptical that this was anthrax. Sharon took a digital picture (Figure 17-4), and despite her urging, diagnostic testing did not occur at that visit. Sharon arranged to meet the patient again, after the unfolding events convinced the woman that she should be tested. At Dan Rather's office on October 16, Sharon drew more blood to check for *B. anthracis* antibodies (the initial sample had clotted). A day later at the patient's dermatologist office a skin biopsy was performed. Both the biopsy and blood test confirmed her as the fourth cutaneous anthrax case in New York City. The investigation at CBS began on October 18, and with both the

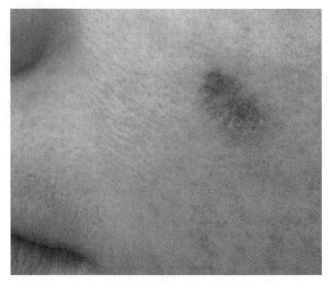

FIGURE 17-4 Cutaneous anthrax, 16 days after onset.
Courtesy of Sharon Balter.

NBC and ABC investigations already underway, the resources of the DOH were severely stretched. Experiences from the first two investigations, however, proved valuable as the CBS investigation proceeded quickly. No one recalled a threat letter with powder and none was found. CBS president, Andrew Hayward, Dan Rather, and DOH staff did much to put the risk of disease into perspective for the CBS employees. Many had been overseas in war-torn nations. What was a little cutaneous anthrax compared to a Scud missile? Rather himself refused to take antibiotics despite spores being found on a desk he used. It was reassuring that in the 2-plus weeks since the patient's onset there had not been any further cases of any form of anthrax at CBS. As a result, many fewer employees had their noses swabbed, and none was put on long-term prophylactic antibiotics.

Before the sun had the chance to set on October 12 we were to hear about one more case. At yet another media organization, an editorial assistant at the New York Post had a suspicious blister on her middle finger. She first noted pus draining near the second joint of her right middle finger while at a friend's wedding on September 22. Her onset date, if confirmed, would make her the earliest case, the true index case of the outbreak. The progression was much as the preceding cases with swelling, ulcer formation, and the characteristic black eschar. She too received antibiotics with the addition of a surgical procedure to remove necrotic tissue and radiographs to exclude bone infection. A hospital guard noted the upward position of her bandaged right middle finger as she exited the emergency department and inquired whether it was a statement meant for

Osama Bin Laden. A photograph of the same image was later published on the tabloid's front page above the exclamation, "Anthrax this!"

As the editorial assistant her job included opening mail. She explained that she opened several weird letters a day but none with powder stuck in her mind. She placed these letters in a box beneath her desk and thought that they had been thrown out by the time we interviewed her on October 12. She too heard the news about the NBC case on October 12 prompting her to contact us and arrange a visit to an infectious disease specialist. As her infection was well along in the healing process, the biopsy did not find evidence of anthrax; however, her blood showed specific antibodies. This was evidence that she had fought off *B. anthracis*, not something a New York City newspaper woman should have coursing through her blood stream, unless her previous assignment was embedded with a troupe of African animal hide traders (naturally occurring anthrax has historically been associated with the handling of animal hides).

Fortunately, staff members at the New York Post were already suspicious about their worker's finger infection after hearing about the anthrax letter received by Tom Brokaw. Thus, they rounded up all the letters from the desks of editors into several U.S. Postal Service containers. The letters were reviewed to assure that no important correspondence was included, and the pile was transferred to a green garbage bag, which ended up at the bottom of the freight elevator. The FBI and New York City Police Department eventually located and searched the bag of letters on October 19, finding one letter with the recognizable child-like, hand-written address and bearing a Trenton, NJ postmark. The letter had not been opened, perhaps explaining why the editorial assistant did not recall it and tested positive for *B. anthracis*. It contained the identical five-line, three-words-per-line, 15-word message as did the NBC letter (Figure 17-5). *B. anthracis* spores were found in the mailroom and on desks of editorial staffers at the New York Post.

By the end of the third week of October, it appeared as though the outbreak might be drawing to a close. The media investigations at NBC, ABC, and CBS were in the environmental remediation stage, and the epidemiology component was winding down. Although two additional cutaneous anthrax cases subsequently came to light, they were both tied to the same exposure, the positive letter at the New York Post. The sixth New York City case occurred in a 34-year-old New York Post mailroom worker, perhaps out of carelessness, and the seventh case in a 38-year-old editor out of curiosity, as they sorted through

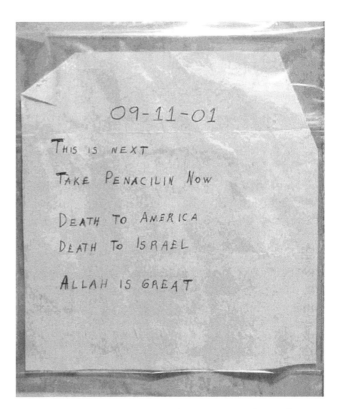

FIGURE 17-5 Image of the anthrax contaminated letter sent to NBC anchor Tom Brokaw. Image by FBI.

the boxes of suspicious mail after it was known that a tainted letter may lie therein. Both likely handled the letter postmarked September 18 from Trenton, NJ.

While we were immersed in prophylaxing hundreds of individuals in the face of cutaneous anthrax, another serious situation was unfolding in nearby states. Postal workers from New Jersey and Washington, DC mail distribution centers were in the initial throes of inhalational anthrax. It was on the afternoon of October 22 that I first heard the news that four postal workers from the same facility had inhalational anthrax; two were already dead. Within 40 minutes I was in a car headed uptown to the James A. Farley Post Office in Manhattan. In the car with me were two CDC physician epidemiologists, the double cell-phone toting Stephanie Factor, and the taciturn yet meticulous Tom Matte. Our tasks were to trace the path of the NBC and New York Post letters through the New York City mail grid, learn how mail was handled and where there were potential risks for spore exposure, and double check that no New York City postal workers were ill with symptoms of any form of anthrax. The James A. Farley building is the width of two city blocks and sits majestically on 8th Avenue across from Madison Square Garden and Pennsylvania station. Its familiar façade, inscription, and Corinthian Colonnade are as familiar to New Yorkers as the Statue of Liberty or Empire State Building. Whenever I think of the place, I can not help seeing its immense stone blocks glimmering in a fusillade of snow with legions of "couriers" trudging great sacks of mail to and fro. In an elegant, richly wood-paneled conference room with enveloping chairs, we learned that mail entering the city first arrives at the Morgan Processing and Distribution Center (P&DC) stretching from 28th to 30th streets between 9th and 10th Avenues. After leaving the Morgan P&DC, mail headed to both NBC and the New York Post passed through a secondary post office, the Times Square post office. Mail to ABC passed through Ansonia post office and mail to CBS through the Radio City post office. On October 21, a contractor had done swab samples along the path the letters passed in the Morgan facility, and these were being processed at a commercial laboratory.

Next, we walked down the block to the workhorse of the New York City Postal Service, the equally immense, but minimally adorned Morgan P&DC. On the third floor we met the stalwart of the Morgan facility, the delivery bar code sorter machine. Mail from all over the country arrives by truck and is unloaded and placed in carts that transport it to conveyer belts that bring it up to the Area Distribution Center. Here the crates of mail for all the New York City zip codes are unloaded and wheeled to rows and rows of bar code sorter machines. One postal worker grabs a yard-width stack of mail and places it in a spring-loaded bin, jogging it to level the letter bottoms. The end holder snaps into place and guides the letters into the machine, which sucks each letter along a lengthy line of rollers, squeezing through a reader that picks up the bar code that had been imprinted by the originating post office. The letters are then expelled into bins, sequentially separating the letters into zip codes and then postal routes. Although the line of rollers was covered, dust and bits of letters could be seen above, behind, and all around the machine. Hanging from the ceiling was a compressed-air hose that was used to unclog the sorter machines by blowing out the dust at 70 lbs/in^2. A large fan stood nearby; it was evidently hot work. We could see lots of places where a letter carrying *B. anthracis* spores might release some of its contents. As we stood in the cavernous floor, looking at row after row of delivery bar code sorter machines an alarm went off. We followed our guide towards the stairs where a worker hurried over with news. A plastic bag filled with white powder had just been found near the time clock, on top of a wooden shelf. Hazmat was on the way; we would have to evacuate the floor.

Back at our offices, staff members were again busy making calls. With the news breaking of postal workers in the District of Columbia and New Jersey ill with inhalational anthrax, we again called hospital emergency departments, intensive care units, and infection control practitioners. In addition to wanting to hear about previously well individuals with either sepsis, respiratory failure, or meningitis and clinical presentations that could be any of the various forms of anthrax, we now asked specifically about postal workers. The newly reported inhalational cases began their illnesses with vague, influenza-like symptoms of fever, chills, malaise and dry cough. Thus, we broadened our inquiry to include postal workers with any influenza or respiratory complaints. As influenza season was approaching, we began including in our medical alerts community influenza surveillance data, which at this point of the season was fortunately rare. To assist clinicians further in differentiating influenza from more worrisome illness in individuals at higher risk for inhalational anthrax as discovered in our epidemiology investigation, a guidance document on how to discriminate influenza from possible inhalational anthrax was also distributed.

It came as little surprise that several of the delivery bar code sorter machines from the third floor of the Morgan P&DC tested positive for *B. anthracis* spores because all of the contaminated mail with New York City destinations passed thorough this facility. The initial testing by the contractor was confirmed by samples taken by a National Institute of Occupational Safety and Health (NIOSH)/CDC team. What did seem unusual was that of the several "downstream" post offices of Rockefeller, Times Square, Radio City, and Ansonia, the intermediate recipients of actual and hypothesized letters to NBC, New York Post, CBS, and ABC, none was positive for *B. anthracis* on initial and repeat testing. Furthermore, nearly 300 nasal swabs of postal workers from these locations were also negative. There were no cases of anthrax, cutaneous or inhalational, in any New York City postal worker. Curiously, contamination could be found at Trenton, the letters' entrance into the mail system, at its next step, Morgan P&DC and at the destination sites. Perhaps there was something about the handling process at the *B. anthracis* negative facilities that differed, the absence of delivery bar code sorter machines to aerosolize spores, or perhaps we just did not look hard enough. This is one of the many questions in the 2001 anthrax outbreak that remains unanswered.

The massive effort to administer prophylaxis to postal workers in New York City was performed by the

CDC (as federal employees). From October 24 to 27, over 7,000 postal workers were given a 10-day supply of antibiotics at a POD held at the James A. Farley Building while awaiting the results of environmental testing. A second POD was held from November 2 to 6 for individuals who did not attend the first POD and to distribute the remainder of the recommended 60-day course to workers exposed to the positive sorter machines. Over 4,000 postal workers were seen at the second POD.

By the third week of October, the U.S. outbreak had expanded to include 20 cases of anthrax from an intentional act of bioterrorism, with 7 cases in NYC and 13 other cases in residents of five states (Florida, Maryland, New Jersey, Pennsylvania, and Virginia) plus Washington, DC. Eleven were the milder, cutaneous form, and nine the more deadly inhalational type. Three had died, all from inhalational anthrax. Those who died were the photography editor exposed at the AMI building in Boca Raton, Florida and two postal workers from the Brentwood P&DC in Washington, DC. The presumed exposure for all of the cases was letters or packages laced with powdered *B. anthracis* spores. Some received or handled the tainted mail, whereas others breathed in the spores as they were aerosolized by mail sorting machines or the compressed air used to clean them. The simultaneous criminal investigation paralleled and intersected the public health one, until the two investigations eventually merged with the report on October 28 of an anthrax case of a different ilk.

Among the abundant facts and skills learned in medical training is microscopy. Pioneered by Van Leeuwenhoek in the late 1600s, the microscope is perhaps the oldest medical instrument still in use today. I remember fondly closing the door to the emergency department mini-laboratory during residency training in order to secure a few moments away from the chaos beyond. There, with the simple implements of glass slides, stains, and a trusty, if not rusty, Zeiss microscope, one could spend a few minutes in diagnostic bliss. Just after 6:00 p.m. on October 29, I found myself once again staring down the barrel of a microscope. The cell walls of certain bacteria absorbed the dye crystal violet and appeared purple-blue. I was seeing blue. Bacteria come in various shapes, sizes, and arrangements. Most are either rods (oval) or cocci (round) and can appear in pairs, clusters, or chains. Large rods in short chains were on the slide before me. The hospital microbiology laboratory director had stayed late just to be there when I arrived, and he could not help from beaming at his staff's diagnostic acumen, despite its ominous implication. Was I looking at *B. anthracis*? The slide had been prepared from a culture of blood taken less than 18 hours earlier, unusually fast growth, but consistent with *B. anthracis*. I asked whether it was nonhemolytic and nonmotile, as these are discriminating characteristics of *B. anthracis*. It was nonhemolytic; however, motility testing was not yet complete. There was still a chance this was not anthrax after all. Before taking the culture to the PHL for confirmation, I was escorted to the intensive care unit to see the patient. She was on a ventilator and was heavily sedated; there would be no interview. I was shown the computerized tomography scan and saw the enlarged mediastinal nodes, a telltale feature of inhalational anthrax. No one in the intensive care unit seemed to believe it, yet none doubted what they were seeing.

> No one in the intensive care unit seemed to believe it, yet none doubted what they were seeing.

The unfortunate source of that blood was a 61-year-old woman originally from Vietnam. Kathy Nguyen had come to America in 1976 as a refugee seeking a better life. She had worked for the last 12 years in the stockroom of a local specialty hospital, the Manhattan Eye, Ear, and Throat Hospital (MEETH). The hospital provided mostly outpatient services and same-day surgical procedures with few inpatient beds. She was well liked by all who knew her but precious few details were known of her life outside of work. Her illness began a few days earlier, on October 26, with muscle soreness, weakness, cough, and shortness of breath that progressively worsened. When she coughed, her phlegm was tinged pink. After 2 days at home without improvement, she arrived at the hospital at 11:00 a.m. breathing fast and shallow, signs of respiratory distress. Her oxygen test was low, and there was no fever. Kathy Nguyen told doctors that it hurt right below her breastbone and that she needed three pillows in order to sleep (three pillow orthopnea is a cardinal sign of heart failure). With a past medical history of hypertension, orthopnea, and a physical examination suggesting lung congestion, her initial diagnosis was pulmonary edema caused by heart failure (a noninfectious condition). The chest radiograph was consistent with this diagnosis showing bilateral pleural effusions (a collection of fluid in the spaces surrounding the lungs). Nothing in her initial laboratory tests indicated another diagnosis, but as a routine, a culture of her blood was taken. Treatment for pulmonary edema proved ineffective, and an echocardiogram of her heart failed to establish a cardiac cause for her respiratory distress. She remained without fever, but her pulse was increasing while her blood pressure fell. Her doctors had to look elsewhere to explain her rapidly deteriorating condition. The emergency department physician received his daily call from Dr. Michael Tapper, an infectious disease specialist and hospital epidemiologist. Since 9/11, Dr. Tapper made a practice of calling the emergency department at least once a day to learn about potentially worrisome cases. He was told about Kathy's illness and came down and saw a suggestion of mediastinal widening on the chest x-ray. He brought it to the radiologist, who concurred. Dr. Tapper instructed the emergency department physicians to begin antibiotics immediately to cover for the possibility of anthrax. Next, he dialed Dr. Layton to report his concerns. The computerized tomography scan of the chest done later that night revealed the enlarged chest cavity lymph nodes and blood, both ominous evidence of hemorrhagic mediastinitis, a hallmark of inhalational anthrax. Early the next afternoon the Gram-positive rods were visible in Kathy Nguyen's blood that prompted my trip to the lab.

A team was quickly mobilized and dispatched to MEETH to begin the investigation. When Joel and Sharon arrived, they were met outside the hospital by the New York City Police Department chief of counterterrorism. All around them were police and emergency vehicles. Specially trained officers had donned their Tyvek protective suits, whereas others stood before the hospital entrance, not allowing anyone to leave or enter. New Yorkers cruised by on their hurried Monday afternoon commute home unconcerned with the goings on at the hospital. The chief was concerned for his officers' safety and explained that his men were not going into the building until the DOH could assure them that it was safe to enter. Joel explained to the chief, in a calm, pedantic monologue, that he could not give him that assurance. For all he knew, there could be a dissemination device inside. An impasse arose. The chief was known for his passionate if not zealous approach to his work. He grew visibly impatient, and the fire in his eyes caused Joel to wonder whether the chief was not considering throwing him in jail for his honest yet blunt assessment. Sharon, out of exhaustion, frustration, or both announced, "If there is anthrax in there, we'll just take antibiotics," and marched in. The New York City Police Department eventually followed, but the FBI set up across the street to conduct interviews. The scene typified both the difficulty in making decisions in the absence of precedent and scientific data, as well as the conflicting needs of public health and law enforcement; however,

in contrast to this auspicious beginning, the New York City inhalational anthrax case investigation enjoyed the greatest integration of public health and law enforcement of any of the anthrax investigations. Joel would later remark, "It was like I was embedded within NYPD."

The first phase of the investigation focused on the hospital basement stockroom where the patient had worked. When I arrived near midnight that first evening, a POD was being set up, and the hospital staff members that had been forced to remain were clearly anxious and eager to leave. The few inpatients the hospital had were transferred and visitors prohibited. That night and into the next day, over 200 employees were interviewed and given antibiotics pending the results of environmental testing. Few of the patient's co-workers knew her regular routine. Her tasks did not include processing incoming mail, and none of the MEETH employees had seen or heard of any suspicious mail arriving at the hospital. A nurse recalled that sometime in the last week the patient had come to her requesting to have her eyes flushed, remarking about the dust down in the basement. It might have been on October 25. That would have been one day before onset, and if it occurred in the hospital, there should be a trail of spores. Hospital staff members that worked in the mailroom, stockroom, and basement were tested by nasal swab, and all were negative. On three separate occasions, the CDC, NIOSH, the FBI, and the New York City Police Department donned their protective gear and took environmental samples: first from the basement, the location of the stockroom and mailroom, then from multiple locations in the hospital, and then again from the basement. Items from the patient's locker were checked twice, the second time using a method to enhance the recovery of *B. anthracis* spores. All tests were negative. Surveillance of MEETH workers turned up several with recent respiratory and skin infections, but none with anthrax. The 1,500 patients and visitors to MEETH over the preceding weeks who had been started on antibiotics at the POD were instructed to stop. Kathy Nguyen became the fourth fatal victim of the intentional anthrax attack on October 31, 2001.

Ms. Nguyen had lived for more than 15 years in a largely Hispanic neighborhood located near the elevated subway in the Southeast Bronx. She lived alone and had infrequent visitors. Efforts to locate relatives were unsuccessful. She was described by neighbors and co-workers as friendly and generous, often buying gifts for others. She was reserved in social interactions and was said to have distrusted banks, choosing to pay her rent using postal money orders. She was reported to have enjoyed shopping. Her one bedroom apartment was neat and uncluttered, suggesting frugality. In her home the FBI took the lead on sampling. Greeting cards, her comb and brush, the television screen, a fluorescent light, a letter opener, her address book, towels, shoes, hats, her cell phone, receipts, and even her Chapstick lip balm were tested. When these results were negative, sampling expanded to other parts of her building—her mailbox and the elevator. Swabs of the mail found in her apartment were examined for *B. anthracis* spores, as were the local post offices serving her home and work. No spores were found. Items, such as her clothes, were vacuumed with a high-efficiency particulate air filter to trap items as small as 1 micron. This too failed to find any spores. Her neighbors were interviewed to learn information about her life that could lead to *B. anthracis* exposure and to search for possible cases. The DOH held a meeting for tenants with Spanish interpreters to answer questions and explain the investigation. One woman was identified with a suspicious skin lesion that tested negative for *B. anthracis*.

With nothing uncovered from the most likely locations, on November 3, the investigation turned toward more remote exposure possibilities. By using her New York City subway fare card (Metro card), credit card statements, receipts, and accounts from her co-workers, Kathy Nguyen's schedule in the weeks preceding her death was reconstructed. Each swipe of her credit card-purchased Metro card recorded the date, time, and station of entry. The sum of her electronic footprints still did not provide a comprehensive timeline of her activities, however; in the absence of a case interview, it was our best lead toward identifying possible exposures to *B. anthracis* spores.

Epidemiologists, using shopping receipts as guides, visited stores she frequented with her picture hoping to extract snapshots of her life to piece together how she encountered *B. anthracis*. She was said to have attended church, although the exact one was uncertain. EIS officers visited churches near her home and place of work, speaking to priests and parishioners, some who recalled her, most who did not. No leads were produced. Along the route she would have walked from the train station to her apartment were several stores and businesses. Other than clerks in the nearby laundromat and grocery stores, none knew her. The check cashing office in the neighborhood had a file for Ms. Nguyen, but it did not indicate any activity in several years. No receipts were found for postal money orders to trace back to a contaminated post office. On the off chance that her exposure could have been along this route, store owners and staff were asked about recent illnesses; none was reported. Teams visited Macy's Department Store in the Bronx and various businesses in Chinatown, two locations she was known to frequent. Still, no leads were uncovered.

What remained was the unthinkable and the possibility was approached delicately. Kathy Nguyen took the subway nearly every day. Could she have been exposed on the platform or the train? The implication threatened to raise the anxiety level in New York City to a new fever pitch and extend anthrax surveillance indefinitely. Before the results on her home and work came back, a plan to test the New York City subway was drafted. Critical to the plan was consideration of how to respond to a positive finding. With over 4 million riders daily, any interruption in service would have major ramifications for people and business in the greater metropolitan New York area. The goal was simply to try and identify where Kathy Nguyen might have been exposed to *B. anthracis*, not to evaluate risk posed by riding the subway. It was reasoned that because there was only a single case among millions of riders and several weeks had passed without any other anthrax cases not directly connected to mail, a positive finding would represent little risk to the public health. Surveillance of Metropolitan Transportation Authority workers, which began shortly after the 9/11 attacks, had not identified any worrisome cases either that supported this response plan. Five stations used by Kathy Nguyen and four control stations whose trains did not intersect with the target stations were tested. Within the station, areas presumed to retain dust particles or be a possible risk area were tested. It was decided that in the absence of any evidence of disease, spores found in a station used as a control location represented very little risk to public health. Positive findings at a station visited by Kathy Nguyen would result in thorough cleaning. Such a finding did not indicate the need for nasal swabs of Metropolitan Transportation Authority workers or riders, nor would antibiotic prophylaxis be warranted.

> *Surveillance of Metropolitan Transportation Authority workers, which began shortly after the 9/11 attacks, had not identified any worrisome cases either that supported this response plan.*

When the results from the subway testing came back in early November, the Mayor and Health Commissioner discussed them at a press conference. Commissioner of Health Dr. Neal Cohen remarked straight faced that although no *B. anthracis* was found in the New York City subway system, "We can now conclude that the New York City subways are not a sterile environment." Injecting humor into what had otherwise been a dire conversation was much needed and a skillful use of risk communication. It helped to place in perspective both the results and massive effort put forth by the DOH, the New York City Department of Environmental Protection, the federal Environmental Protection Agency, the CDC, NIOSH, the New York City Police Department, and the FBI to find how Kathy Nguyen was exposed to B. anthracis. When the leading hypothesis became cross-contamination of mail, I believe it was the open and communicative handling of the investigation that facilitated the public's acceptance of this theory. The truth remains that there were very few alternative hypotheses, and cross-contamination was the least improbable.

The final case in the multistate anthrax outbreak occurred in a 94-year-old Connecticut woman whose activities were quite limited. As with the Kathy Nguyen investigation, no B. anthracis spores were found anywhere that she had been in the immediate period before her illness, but unlike the NYC case investigation, spores were detected at the local post office that processed her mail. It was determined that a letter postmarked in Trenton, that passed through the delivery bar code sorter machine shortly after a known-to-be tainted letter, traveled through the Wallington Distribution Center in Connecticut and was delivered to a home in a neighboring town. That letter was found and tested positive for B. anthracis. No illness was associated with the letter, but it added much needed credibility to the prevailing cross-contamination theory.

> *If you hang around public health bioterrorism experts long enough, you will invariably hear them all say something like this: "It isn't a question if another bioterrorism event will occur, it is when."*

If you hang around public health bioterrorism experts long enough, you will invariably hear them all say something like this: "It isn't a question if another bioterrorism event will occur, it is when." For those of us on the ground in state and local health departments, the question is really how? Despite the numerous hoax letters that preceded the actual tainted ones, we did not expect B. anthracis spores to be mailed because it was not believed to be an efficient method of dissemination. The letters sent to television icons and U.S. Senators dispelled this notion. We did not consider that an ordinary sealed envelope, squeezed through the high-speed postal machinery, could spread spores. No one expected that letters, whose paths merely crossed with contaminated letters that became contaminated by passing through sorting machines after the tainted anthrax letters, would be able to cause inhalational disease. Evidence from the outbreak suggests that the minimum infective dose for inhalational anthrax is much lower than conventional wisdom held in 2001, perhaps as low as a few spores adhering to the surface of an envelope. We did not expect cutaneous cases either. The ability to make or acquire weapons-grade B. anthracis spores was believed to be nearly impossible for all but the most accomplished bioweapons scientist. These former truths guided our initial approach to the investigation. Although much was learned during the anthrax investigation, we likely will not know the "how" in advance of another bioterrorism attack. This continues to be the crucial public health task upon which disease mitigation depends.

CONCLUSIONS

Doctors are trained to think of common ailments first when evaluating a patient's symptoms, not the rare ones. More than a few medical students have been admonished by the adage, "When you hear hoof beats, think horses, not zebras." In 1999, when West Nile virus made its first western hemisphere appearance in New York City, it was initially believed to be an outbreak of St. Louis encephalitis. The bird die-offs that preceded the outbreak were not thought to be linked to human illness; we were wrong on both counts. In public health, we have now come to replace the old adage with a new one: "Expect the unexpected." The anthrax ordeal lasted just over 2 months and resulted in 22 cases nationally, small when compared with such public health enemies as lung cancer or AIDS. More than 12 work sites, 8 confirmed cases, and well over a hundred suspect case reports were investigated in New York City (Figure 17-2). The anthrax mail attack was unprecedented, malignant, and shocked the nation. Although this chapter ends here, the story does not. Health departments across the country continue to plan and drill for the next act of bioterrorism. The criminal case remains unsolved, the FBI investigation open, and the perpetrator at large.

ACKNOWLEDGMENTS

The following current and former DOH staff graciously agreed to be interviewed for the project. They provided valuable recollections and insights from their experiences as part of the 2001 Anthrax Investigation team: Polly Thomas, Susan Blank, Hadi Maki, Andrew Tucker, Annie Fine, Sarah Perl, Tom Matte, Ben Mojica, John Kornblum, Laura Mascuch, Isaac Weisfuse, Sheila Palevsky, Jeannine Pru'dhomme, Sally Beatrice, Marie Wong, Denis Nash, Joel Ackelsberg, Marci Layton, Sharon Balter, Michael Phillips, Andrew Goodman, and Adam Karpati.

EDITOR'S NOTE

Since this chapter was written, a sad and remarkable story has emerged that may have identified who is responsible for these anthrax cases in the United States in 2001. According to an article in *The New York Times* published January 3, 2009, Bruce Ivins, PhD, a scientist who worked for many years at an Army laboratory at Fort Detrick, had become the prime suspect in the FBI investigation. He had worked to develop an anthrax vaccine and was considered an expert on the organism. According to the article, "Dr. Ivins had the equipment and expertise to make the powder in his laboratory." Scientists have even discovered evidence that "the chemical signature" of the water used to grow the anthrax was like the water near Fort Detrick. Also of concern, Dr. Ivins "had worked unusually late hours in his laboratory for several nights before each of the anthrax mailings." And there was more evidence as well although it was circumstantial. Dr. Ivins had written e-mails that admitted to serious mental health problems and he committed suicide in July 2008. The FBI has closed its investigation with Dr. Ivins as the likely source of the 22 anthrax cases (including the ones described in this chapter in New York City). However, neither direct evidence nor a confession had been found leaving the situation still controversial.
(See http://www.nytimes.com/2009/01/04/us/04anthrax.html?_r=1)

LEARNING QUESTIONS

1. Case ascertainment was critical in the anthrax investigation. What was done to increase the likelihood that cases would be recognized?
2. The investigation of inhalational anthrax in Kathy Nguyen was a thorough attempt to try to identify how she was exposed. List each of the possible exposures considered and how the investigators attempted to evaluate those exposures.

CHAPTER 18

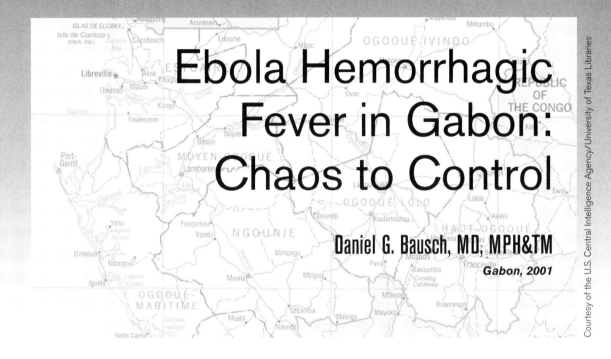

Ebola Hemorrhagic Fever in Gabon: Chaos to Control

Daniel G. Bausch, MD, MPH&TM

Gabon, 2001

INTRODUCTION

The Usual Inconvenient Beginning

Damn...did I screw up. I would have bet you a million dollars that that kid did not have Ebola. Not fun—this feeling of incompetence. What am I doing here in Gabon making misdiagnoses? It was the usual inconvenient beginning: December 12, 2001. Christmas was approaching, and I had long-made plans to visit my fiancée in Switzerland for the holidays and then to help her move to London to begin the tropical medicine program at the London School. I am in some routine meeting in Atlanta when Tom Ksiazek, chief of the Special Pathogens Branch of the Centers for Disease Control and Prevention (CDC), sticks his head in and points to me—"Can I see you for a minute?" Tom is not known for being the chatty touchy-feely type, so I knew he was not calling me out to wish me a Merry Christmas. In fact, before I even got out of the door, I knew that the holiday was gone—no Christmas in Switzerland, no visit with fiancée, no move to London. No, my Christmas would be spent attending to an Ebola outbreak in Gabon and the Republic of the Congo. By the way, for anyone aspiring to this kind of work, sudden calls to Ebola outbreaks that ruin your Christmas plans seem dramatic and exciting only once.

Why not just refuse? All of these plans that you have had for so long are ruined in just a second. It is not so much pressure from your boss or even machismo. It is more black and white; you are either in the outbreak business and attend to it when it happens (damn it), or you are not (although there are limits, as evidenced by my staying home to watch my son be born instead of heading to Angola for the 2005 epidemic of Marburg hemorrhagic fever).

Why me? I would like to think that it had something to do with my experience and expertise—an infectious disease doctor with degrees in public health and tropical medicine, having been at the CDC since 1996 and with experience in outbreak responses and control efforts for a number of different hemorrhagic fevers—Ebola and Marburg in Uganda and the Democratic Republic of the Congo, Lassa fever and yellow fever in various spots in West Africa, and dengue in El Salvador. True, all of that helps, but all of the medical training and field experience were more prerequisites than a deciding factor. In reality, I knew that there was an equally important reason, one that (fortunately) comes up frequently: I speak French—a lucky break brought about by required classes in junior high (in which I started out doing quite poorly), my parents' foresight in enrolling me in a summer exchange program in France as a teenager, and later on, a succession of fortunate professional opportunities. Thus, here is the first lesson for would-be international virus hunters: Leave the advanced molecular biology and volunteering at the hospital alone for a minute and learn a language. French is great for sub-Saharan Africa, but others will work too. It does not matter; pick an area of the world and a corresponding language that interests you, and sign up for conversational classes on Thursday nights at your local community college.

I never planned on a career in viral hemorrhagic fevers. In fact, after finishing my infectious disease fellowship and Master's of Public Health degree at Tulane University in New Orleans, I turned down a spot in the CDC's Epidemic Intelligence Service to take a position directing a community education and training project with a tiny nongovernmental organization (NGO) working in the Central America country of El Salvador—a place in which I had been very involved since medical school. The position entailed training community health workers and doing some clinical work in the rural area of Suchitoto half the week and, as a visiting professor, teaching infectious diseases to medical students and residents at the Universidad Nacional de El Salvador in the capital the other half. The person who learned the most, however, was me. The major lesson was that, although I did and still do support it philosophically as an appropriate health care delivery strategy, I was not cut out for being the primary implementer of a community-based health care project.

After an often frustrating year and a half in El Salvador learning what I was not good at, I was ready to explore new opportunities elsewhere and mentioned this in a phone call to Barney Cline, one of my professors from Tulane and a key mentor and friend over the years. As it happened, C.J. Peters, then the chief of the CDC Special Pathogens Branch and a friend of Barney's, was coming to lecture at Tulane the following week. Barney offered to inquire with C.J. regarding possible opportunities with the CDC. I knew a little bit about C.J.: he lectured to our public health class at Tulane, and by chance (or was it fate?), I had recently read Richard Preston's *The Hot Zone*, which chronicles C.J.'s tussle with Ebola in a monkey facility in Reston, Virginia. Although I had never envisioned myself as anything close to a "virus hunter," I was intrigued enough to listen to any ideas he might have.

C.J. and Barney called me the next week. The initial discussion centered on the possibility of working with the CDC to analyze data collected on a disease called hemorrhagic fever with renal syndrome dating back to the Korean War. As this entailed primarily sitting in front of a computer in Atlanta, I was not too enthusiastic. We were just about to end the conversation when C.J. asked, "You don't speak French by chance?" Thus, the door opened to head up another project that C.J. had in mind: to establish a field station for research on Lassa fever in Guinea, a French-speaking country on the coast of West Africa. A year or so later I joined the CDC and started learning about and working on the viral hemorrhagic fevers.

EBOLA OUTBREAK RESPONSES

In the absence of effective vaccines and therapeutics, the response to Ebola outbreaks has relied almost solely on the classic measures of communicable disease control: case isolation and contact tracing.

> *In the absence of effective vaccines and therapeutics, the response to Ebola outbreaks has relied almost solely on the classic measures of communicable disease control: case isolation and contact tracing.*

An outbreak team is assembled, almost always consisting of personnel from the Ministry of Health of the involved country and local health care workers in the area of the outbreak, assisted by a diverse group of international partners from groups such as the World Health Organization (WHO, usually the coordinating body), the CDC, the National Institute for Communicable Diseases in South Africa, Health Canada, and Médecins Sans Frontières (MSF) and other NGOs.

The group is usually divided into teams, including the epidemiologists who work on case identification, contact tracing, and keeping the primary database; clinicians who establish and maintain isolation wards and treat patients; water-sanitation experts who are responsible for important aspects of the physical maintenance of the isolation wards; laboratory personnel who perform diagnostic testing, establishing field laboratories when necessary; community health workers who deal with social mobilization and prevention campaigns; and zoologists and ecologists who seek to identify the Ebola virus reservoir. Depending on the outbreak and the needs, I might be involved to some degree in virtually all these activities, although my primary roles, including in Gabon, were usually as part of the clinical and epidemiology teams, always with an eye for collecting useful research data in the course of these activities.

Excluding a few laboratory infections, human infection with Ebola virus has been exclusively noted in sub-Saharan Africa (Figure 18-1). Gabon and the neighboring Republic of the Congo were and are hotspots. This is not by chance. Being two of the few countries with large tracts of rainforest still intact, the critter that carries Ebola virus (a bat?) still has a habitat. Consequently, humans in the region are also bound to stumble into an Ebola virus now and then. At the CDC we were honestly not overly enthused about participating in Ebola response operations in Gabon and Congo. First, with their sparse populations, the number of cases was usually few and dispersed in remote, hard-to-reach areas, not easily amenable to control efforts or scientific study. Second, being former French colonies, the conventional wisdom is that this region is "French turf," where participation of the CDC (who sometimes carried a reputation, rightly or wrongly, of barging in and taking over) was less than enthusiastically welcomed; however, this particular time, rumor had it that Senator Kennedy heard that there was an Ebola outbreak in Gabon and wanted to know what the CDC was doing about it. So there was to be no Christmas in Switzerland for me. I was going to Gabon.

OUTBREAK RECOGNITION AND LABORATORY CONFIRMATION

Recent reports had trickled in of cases of a febrile illness, often associated with bleeding, some of them in health care workers, in Gabon's remote Ogooué Ivindo Province, a heavily forested region bordering Congo (Figures 18-1 and 18-2). As Ebola had been seen in Ogooué Ivindo before, this was the diagnosis until proven otherwise. In fact, the diagnosis of Ebola was not in doubt. A Gabonese research center, the Centre International de Recherches Medicales de Franceville (CIRMF), had already made the laboratory diagnosis. Furthermore, it had been confirmed at the South Africa National Institute for Communicable Diseases by my old friend and internationally renowned virologist and zoologist Bob Swanepoel, who simply ran the best and most reliable laboratory in the world. If Bob said that it was Ebola, it was Ebola.

Unlike many other types of outbreaks, by the time outbreak investigations and control efforts for the filoviruses (Ebola and Marburg) are initiated, laboratory confirmation of the pathogen has almost always

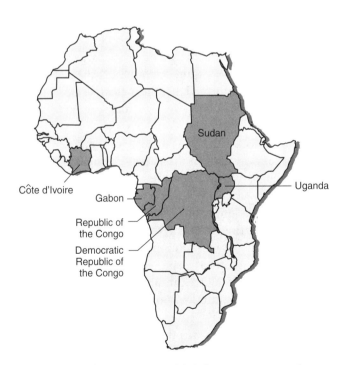

FIGURE 18-1 Countries in which human cases of Ebola hemorrhagic fever have been confirmed, excluding imported cases and laboratory infections.

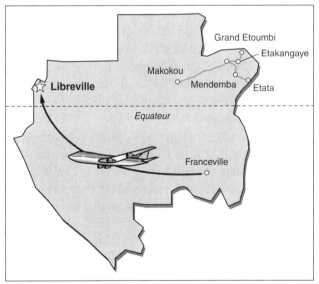

FIGURE 18-2 Geographic distribution of cases of Ebola hemorrhagic fever in Gabon, October 2001–March 2002. Nkoghe D, Formenty P, Leroy EM, Nnegue S, Edou SY, Ba JI, et al. Multiple Ebola virus haemorrhagic fever outbreaks in Gabon, from October 2001 to April 2002. *Bull Soc Pathol Exot* 2005;98(3):224–9.

already occurred.[1] In fact, the unclenching of the entire outbreak response process usually depends on it. Recognizing the severe consequences of both false positives and negatives, a battery of diagnostic tests is usually performed, including the enzyme-linked immunosorbent assay (ELISA), polymerase chain reaction (PCR), and virus isolation; however, there are only a few laboratories in the world where these tests are performed and, paradoxically, very few in sub-Saharan Africa where Ebola is endemic. In contrast to popular belief, this is much less related to the danger of performing the assays (ELISA and PCR can be safely performed using inactivated antigens and samples) than to the unavailability of reagents. There are no commercially available assays for the filoviruses, and existing "in-house" tests rely on the production of antigen derived through the culture of live virus in a high-containment laboratory followed by inactivation, safety testing, and optimization of the assay—a laborious and expensive process that few countries and laboratories have the will and the means to undertake.

The benefit of having a laboratory-confirmed diagnosis before you go has obvious advantages; the considerable resources, both human and financial, required to mount an outbreak response in remote areas of sub-Saharan Africa are not wasted. The wheels are set in motion only when we know that something bad is truly going on; however, the price of this approach is that the response is delayed. In most filovirus outbreaks, transmission smolders at a low level for weeks or even months until a blood sample from a suspected case finally gets drawn and sent, often with the aid of an international NGO working in the area, to one of the few laboratories in the world where filovirus diagnostics are performed. The need to build public health and diagnostic capacity in the endemic area for diseases such as Ebola would later become a major factor in the direction of my career, but that is another story (discussed later here).

In a strange sense, having laboratory confirmation of one of the most lethal pathogens in the world makes things, well…more comforting. When you know what you are dealing with, you know the drill—the mode of transmission, the precautions to take in the field and laboratory. I appreciated this a few years later when SARS cropped up and I headed off to Vietnam with just a description of a syndrome, but no pathogen, no mode of transmission, and no concrete guidelines for what safety and control measures were effective. How do you protect yourself with that uncertainty? What advice do you give to others in your role as a public health expert and consultant?

THE INITIAL ASSESSMENT

Getting back to Gabon—okay, it is Ebola. I will go. I will do my thing. Anyway, the word from the ground, perhaps reflecting wishful thinking as much as any scientific evidence, was that this was a small outbreak, likely to be rapidly controlled, so maybe I would even be in Switzerland for New Year's.

The beginning is always easy. You show up in some capitol city in the tropics, in this case, Libreville. Somebody meets you at the airport (in this case, Ray Arthur, who was secunded from the CDC to the WHO and who was often my contact for these outbreaks), takes you to a hotel that is well above the means of 99% of the African population, and then you go to dinner on the same scale. Over lobster and the Gabonese *Regab* beer, Ray and I discussed the situation. It is interesting, almost fun. You feel important. The next day you meet with the national and local authorities and the WHO country office. Still interesting. Still feeling important.

Next day. Time to hit the field! A small plane was chartered for us. We would fly first to Makokou, site of previous Ebola outbreaks and where a suspected case had been recently reported (Figure 18-2). It was only supposed to be a quick evaluation stop before heading on to Mekembo, epicenter for the outbreak. Ray and I showed up at the small hospital in Makokou in the mid afternoon, the peak of the dry season heat, when most sane people are lying as low and still as possible in the shadiest spot that they can find. The place looked deserted, but we managed to drum up a nurse in charge and introduced ourselves. We inquired about the suspected case of Ebola and were informed that the patient, herself a nurse at Makokou, was holding her own and seemed to be responding to antimalarials. Good news, but I nevertheless thought it was worth taking a quick look at her.

The nurse led us to the patient, being cared for in one of the hospital's small three-bed wards. This being sub-Saharan Africa, I did not expect the patient to be in a negative-pressure room, of which there are precious few on the continent. Furthermore, even if you had one, it would be an extra precaution; although we would certainly use this with a suspected case of Ebola in the United States, it is not technically required, given the lack of evidence of natural airborne transmission of the filoviruses.

Of more concern was the absence of personal protective equipment (i.e., gloves, gowns, and masks) necessary to maintain barrier nursing precautions. I was not worried for my own safety during the brief visit with the patient. I knew that Ebola virus was spread by direct

> *Of more concern was the absence of personal protective equipment (i.e., gloves, gowns, and masks) necessary to maintain barrier nursing precautions.*

contact with blood and bodily fluids.[2,3] I could therefore safely see and speak with, but not examine, the patient as long as I kept out of respiratory droplet range (that is, where droplets the patient might cough up could reach me—about a meter), keeping my arms folded across my chest to not inadvertently touch anything; however, as daily patient management could not be conducted in this way, there were worrying implications for possible exposure to the hospital staff.

The patient, a woman in her early 20s, was quite sick, but there was nothing particularly remarkable from a medical standpoint—fever, headache, malaise, nausea, and vomiting. No bleeding. It could have been a million things, but there was one more unusual and identifying sign—that subtle rash on her face. I had seen a lot of cases of Ebola during an outbreak in Uganda a few years back[4] and knew that making the diagnosis on clinical grounds was extremely difficult, especially in the early phases of the disease. In contrast to much of the popular press, the infected person's eyeballs do not melt, and the liver does not turn to mush. In reality, even if you are the best doctor in the world, distinguishing a case of Ebola from all the malaria, typhoid fever, and host of other febrile illnesses in the region (which do not take a vacation just because there might be an Ebola outbreak) is usually difficult, if not impossible; however, I knew that a measles-like skin rash is sometimes seen on the face and trunk. The rash does not occur in everybody (maybe only approximately 20%) and is usually very fleeting. Its absence does not exclude Ebola, but if you see it, the patient probably has the disease. In other words, it is a specific but not very sensitive sign.

Thus, despite the nurse's diagnosis of malaria, her rash made me suspicious of Ebola. Then there was the other clue—the patient was a health care worker. Tragically, the major clue to almost every outbreak of viral hemorrhagic fever I have investigated has been the death of one or more health care workers. Death of a health care worker should always raise the red flag of possible nosocomial, or health care-associated, transmission, especially if there are clusters. Nosocomial transmission lies behind virtually all large filovirus outbreaks. Health care workers in resource-poor settings without consistent supplies of personal protective equipment, clean syringes, and disinfectant (materials usually taken for granted in the United States) are particularly vulnerable. This really hits home when almost every scientific paper you publish is dedicated to someone "who died investigating the outbreak and disease reported in this manuscript."

When you see health care worker involvement, you have to go back to the hospital records and talk with the doctors and nurses. If a hemorrhagic fever virus is circulating, you will very often find that the health care worker treated a patient with a similar syndrome just a week or so ago. The important point is to make sure that the exposure was within the 3-week maximum incubation period for Ebola, in which case, again, nosocomial transmission should be considered, if not assumed. Indeed, the sick nurse in Makokou had cared for a sick child about 10 days ago—a child brought in from Mekembo.

While Ray and I and the nurse were seeing the patient, another barely noticeable event occurred that was a harbinger of things to come. Although to maintain strict infection control we should not lay a hand on anything, doctors and nurses often can not help themselves from somewhat haphazardly touching things when they are at the patient's bedside. Even if not indicated at that particular moment, we have to check something—the chart, the IV site, the patient's conjunctiva, the turgor of the skin. I suppose that it is the professional equivalent of caring mothers fluffing the pillows when a child is home sick—it does not do anything, but it makes her feel better. While seeing the patient, I noticed that the nurse raised his ungloved hand to adjust the patient's IV drip. There was no visible blood anywhere, and the nurse considered the patient to have malaria (which is not generally directly communicable); however, this would prove tragically prophetic for subsequent events in Makokou.

I stayed on in Makokou for a few days, mostly working with local physicians, Julien Mayoun, chief of the Medical Service at Makokou Regional Hospital, and Prosper Abessolo Mengue, regional health director for Ogooué Ivindo, as well as members of the MSF-Belgian team, Catherine Bachy and Christian Katzer, to assist Makokou hospital in setting up an isolation ward. There was considerable debate, mostly out of fear and politics, as to where the ward should be placed. Sadly, the sick nurse I saw the first day died; however, there were no new cases, and I was starting to think that the stateside predictions of a small outbreak with rapid resolution might be true (Switzerland, here I come?), although I knew that things were still more active around Mekembo.

In fact, Makokou being quiet, the plan was for me to move over to Mekembo to lend a hand. On the day before my departure, a mother brought her teenage boy to Makokou Hospital. I did not consider his story to be suggestive of Ebola at all—low grade fever, no systemic symptoms. True, he had unexplained bleeding, but it was mild and localized to an area around his upper right molars, where he also had pain. I suspected that his problem was primarily dental, perhaps a periapical abscess, the bleeding probably brought on by the mother's constant jamming of her bare fingers into the boy's mouth to show us where the problem was.

ISOLATION WARDS AND INFECTION CONTROL

> *In contrast to what's often portrayed in the popular press, "space suits" or respirators are not necessary, although these may be required for laboratory manipulation of Ebola virus, where virus culture and techniques such as centrifugation have the potential for significant amplification and dissemination.*

The principles of an isolation ward are relatively simple—a "souped up" version of barrier nursing precautions, including masks, gowns, double gloves, head covering, and foot protection, are employed, designed to protect against direct contact and respiratory droplets. In contrast to what is often portrayed in the popular press, "space suits" or respirators are not necessary, although these may be required for laboratory manipulation of Ebola virus, where virus culture and techniques such as centrifugation have the potential for significant amplification and dissemination.

Even under the best of circumstances, admission to an isolation ward is a harrowing experience. Sick patients, some of whom may never have been admitted to a hospital, suddenly find themselves surrounded by strangely clad and unrecognizable health care workers, often foreign, in a potentially frightening atmosphere of sterility. Access to one's family is, of course, limited (usually to a single patient attendant, who is also required to wear protective material and not allowed to touch their family member). Perhaps the most daunting aspect of the whole affair is the prospect of dying and being buried by the isolation ward staff without the funeral rituals often so integral to African culture. To this highly charged environment must frequently be added the vestiges of colonial era suspicion of foreigners and present-day frictions between ethnic groups.

Furthermore, because the case-fatality rates for the filoviruses are so high (often approaching 90%), it unfortunately stands to reason that most patients admitted to an isolation ward with confirmed filovirus infection die. This often gives an appearance of causality to the local population—that is, *if* you go into the isolation ward you will surely die. No matter what, *avoid this*. Certainly with this fear in mind, the mother was adamant that her son's problem was not Ebola but a "normal disease." Given the very atypical clinical presentation, I was inclined to agree with her. The pressure to not isolate patients also comes sometimes from the political sector; in the worst case scenario, establishing isolation wards and isolating patients can be interpreted as the signal to the community that a terrible disease is circulating in the village, with the implicit, if not explicit message, of *do not come here*. This obviously can have catastrophic consequences to the local economy.

With the presentation seeming so inconsistent with Ebola, I discounted the kid as a real case. Nevertheless, because his fever and unexplained bleeding technically met the case definition (discussed later here), I hedged my bets and took blood to send to CIRMF for testing, to receive the results in a week or so. Partly because of the atypical presentation, but also, it must be said, influenced by the family and political pressure to not isolate patients, I did not place the boy in isolation and did not think much more about it. Believing Makokou to be pretty well tucked in, the next day I moved on to Mekembo, a 3-hour drive during which (and I am not making this up) our Toyota Land Cruiser, traveling at a swift pace through a deep stretch of bamboo forest, suddenly and sadly collided with a big leopard crossing the road, the wild-eyed cat bounding into the forest, likely to die, I surmised. I elected not to get out of the car to test this hypothesis.

In Mekembo, a larger team of expatriates and Gabonese, maybe 25 altogether, was already hard at work, including Mary Reynolds, the CDC Epidemic Intelligence Officer sent to work with me. The number of cases was still small, and there were only one or two in the isolation ward; however, there was nevertheless plenty to do tracing contacts, collecting specimens, and working on coordinating prevention efforts. I reviewed the isolation ward briefly and, finding little to do there, joined the epidemiologists in the field activities.

THE CASE DEFINITION AND DESCRIPTIVE EPIDEMIOLOGY

One of the earliest and most important steps in any outbreak investigation is to make a case definition. In most previous outbreaks of Ebola, previous contact with a suspected or confirmed case was the biggest risk factor.[2,3,5] Nosocomial risk factors (i.e., being a health care worker or recently being admitted to a health care center) were especially pertinent.[6] Consequently, determination of possible previous contact with an infected human constituted a major part of the standard case definitions and reporting forms developed by the WHO. These WHO standards were the ones we were using at the beginning of the outbreak in Gabon (Table 18-1) and most of us on the response team had used these case definitions before and felt pretty comfortable with them.

There was, however, the usual difficulty of sensitivity versus specificity. To not miss a case, you could consider everybody with fever to have Ebola. The rookie usually feels most comfortable with this strategy, which is indeed prudent in outbreak settings where missing a single case can have disastrous consequences; however, the problem with this approach is that you will soon fill up your isolation ward with a whole bunch of people who indeed do *not* have Ebola and not have enough room for those who *do*. Furthermore, although infection control guidelines are put in place to prevent it,[7,8] there is still a chance that a patient who does not have Ebola might contract it in an isolation ward. Thus, difficult as it is (and it is *very* difficult), you have to find some balance, to give up some sensitivity for specificity. We add on various signs and symptoms commonly seen in Ebola to try to increase the specificity but, because the early clinical presentation is so similar to most other systemic febrile diseases, they do not help much (Table 18-1).

After some weeks into the outbreak in Gabon, we began to realize that there were some twists on the epidemiology compared with previous epidemics.[1,5] There were a few nosocomial cases, but the numbers were not large. Instead, clusters were noticed in families, sometimes with incubation periods between cases too short to be consistent with human-to-human spread. Furthermore, the initial cases were predominantly male and often members of the same hunting party.

Hunting is the major source of food and protein in inland Gabon, and the killing of a broad array of wild game, including nonhuman primates such as gorillas and chimps, is common (although not necessarily always legal). Like their human cousins, nonhuman primates are susceptible to Ebola virus, rapidly developing severe and usually fatal disease (a fact that excludes them from consideration as the natural reservoir). In fact, over the past decade Ebola has posed a major challenge to the survival of great apes in West Africa, even threatening extinction.[9] Nonhuman primates and perhaps other wild animals are also capable of transmitting Ebola virus to humans who come in contact with them during the course of their illness, usually through hunting.[10,11] An epidemiologic pattern distinct from the nosocomially fueled course seen in most previous outbreaks began to emerge in Gabon; small hunting parties of around five males would head into the forest for expeditions of days to weeks. While there, they would get infected with Ebola virus, perhaps through direct contact with the still unknown primary reservoir or, probably more frequently, through hunting Ebola-infected wild animals (and, logically, the gorilla or chimp suffering from Ebola would be the easier one to catch). Members of the hunting party probably most frequently get infected when they butcher the animal shortly after

TABLE 18-1 Definitions for a Suspected Case of Ebola Hemorrhagic Fever Employed in the Outbreak Response in Gabon and the Republic of the Congo, 2001–2002

Original Case Definition

- Fever and contact with a case of Ebola hemorrhagic fever
- Fever and unexplained bleeding of any kind
- Unexplained death in a person having presented with an acute onset of fever
- Fever and three or more of the following symptoms: headache, vomiting, anorexia, diarrhea, weakness or severe fatigue, abdominal pain, body aches or joint pains, difficulty swallowing, difficulty breathing, and hiccups

Revised Case Definition

- Fever and contact with a case of Ebola hemorrhagic fever
- Fever and unexplained bleeding of any kind
- Unexplained death in a person having presented with an acute onset of fever; fever in a hunter having entered into the forest or other person having contact with wild animals, living or dead, in the 3 weeks before onset of illness
- New onset of fever within 3 weeks of having been hospitalized in Ogooué Ivindo Province
- For patients who do *not* meet any of these criteria: acute febrile illness that persists despite at least 48 hours of appropriate antimalarial and/or antibiotic therapy

killing it. Although the hunting party may come home with infected meat, Ebola virus is sensitive to heat and unlikely to last very long in the hot tropical environment. Refrigeration is rarely possible in these areas, and the virus will certainly be inactivated on cooking.

The bigger danger to the family members at home is not the meat, but rather the hunters incubating Ebola virus. In fact, hunters were the index cases of all the chains of transmission except one in Gabon. After a few days at home, one or more members of the hunting party fall sick. The females, traditionally the care takers of sick persons in the household, now become the at-risk group, exposed to infected blood or bodily fluids as they care for their male family members, damping away blood from the mouth or cleaning up after and emptying plastic pails of Ebola-contaminated feces or vomit. In turn, the women fall sick. Still another wave of infection occurs when remaining females in the household take care of their sick mother, daughter, or sister. Over a few weeks, a small cluster can be recognized, males early and females later. This distinct epidemiology relative to other Ebola outbreaks was reflected in the gender ratio of cases. Because of the predominance of female caretakers in the home, most Ebola outbreaks are skewed toward females[1,6]; however, in Gabon, the majority (52%) of the cases were males, reflecting the fact that hunting is almost an exclusively male activity.[5] Recognizing the key role played by hunters in the epidemic in Gabon, we added elements of hunting, forest entry, and exposure to wild animals to our case definition, allowing us to increase the specificity (Table 18-1). We also narrowed the case definition for nosocomial cases by adding a geographic restriction—Ogooué Ivindo Province, where, at that point at least, all the cases had been seen.

THE SCREW UP AND NOSOCOMIAL TRANSMISSION

A few days after my arrival in Mekembo, the results of a batch of samples sent to CIRMF for Ebola testing came back. That kid with the periapical abscess had Ebola! How could this be? How could I have missed this diagnosis? I was shocked and devastated, consumed by guilt and self-doubt. Not having placed the patient in isolation, I wondered how many cases of secondary transmission there would be. How many people might die because of my blunder? I and a small team rushed back to Makokou to address this new crisis and, despite the mother's continued vigorous protest, isolate the boy.

As it turned out, the boy got rapidly better and went home. None of his family members, other contacts, or the health care workers that cared for him got sick, but I passed some nervous days waiting to see what would happen. To their credit, rather than finger pointing, the outbreak team supported and encouraged me. Two members of the MSF team, Christian Katzer and Isabelle Delbeke, were especially kind to me during that time, for which I will always be grateful. Two take home points here are these: (1) Avoid equivocation and half-way measures, which just confuse everybody (including yourself). Decide whether the patient fits the case definition that you have set, and if so, implement your full control strategy as planned. (2) Appreciate the potential for diverse clinical pathogenesis and presentation, especially of diseases that have not been extensively studied. The interaction between virus and innate and adaptive immune responses is complex and can likely result in a spectrum of clinical presentations.

To this day, I think that there was something strange about that case. If this was Ebola, how could the mother, with so much direct exposure to the boy's blood, possibly have escaped infection? Did she carry some gene that rendered her immune, like the gene for Duffy antigen that confers protection from infection with *Plasmodium vivax* malaria? Perhaps, although unrecognized, she had previously had Ebola herself and survived and was now immune? Seroprevalence studies suggest that circulation of Ebola virus in eastern Gabon is not rare,[10,12,13] and mild and asymptomatic Ebola has been described.[14–16] I will never be able to explain it (and could not get blood from the mother to test for evidence of previous infection) and still wonder whether maybe the laboratory result was a false positive (although subsequent tests confirmed it). This is, of course, irrelevant now—probably just still hoping to cover for my mistake.

Events such as this boy's case should be a signal to us, stimulating the scientific side of our brains to develop and test hypotheses to understand better the disease and how to control it. Especially with diseases such as the viral hemorrhagic fevers, where the remote and sporadic nature of the diseases usually make prospective study difficult,[17] outbreaks need to be looked at as not only public health responses, but our chance to learn about what is going on. Public health comes first, but scientifically and ethically sound research, with the appropriate safeguards and approvals from the patients and institutional review boards, is an essential part of most outbreak response efforts and indeed is in the best interest of public health. There have been organizations and persons who have opposed this, sometimes with a "damn it—we're trying to save lives here while you're just interested in your data and publishing papers" attitude. I notice that these are often the same people that call to ask you questions such as "how long does the virus last in the blood?" and are disappointed if there is no definitive answer. No blood collected—no research, no answer.

Although the boy, his mother, and those treating him dodged the bullet, it was becoming clear that others exposed at the hospital in Makokou were not so fortunate and that the lack of barrier nursing and infection control practices that I had noticed the first day was, unfortunately, having an effect after all; the two other patients that shared a room with the nurse I had seen the first day, considered at the time to have malaria, had fallen ill with febrile illnesses, eventually fatal, after returning home from the hospital. Both were subsequently confirmed as cases of Ebola. There were numerous other nosocomial infections of Ebola in Makokou Regional Hospital. The only thing that perhaps prevented a major nosocomial outbreak was that, as word slipped out into the community of a dangerous disease contracted at the hospital, visits and admissions to the hospital drastically tailed off.

FRICTION IN THE COMMUNITY

Meanwhile, the outbreak response efforts in Mekembo were not going well. Power struggles, politics, and infighting among the team members, both expatriate and Gabonese, were deteriorating morale and reducing the team's effectiveness. Furthermore, the outbreak team and their public health prevention messages were generally not being welcomed by the local population. A history of suspicion of white foreigners dating back to colonial times, intertribal frictions, and distrust of the government in Libreville (who had met the outbreak with measures such as cancelling scheduled elections, presumably intended to prevent virus transmission facilitated by the gathering of large groups of people, and imposing a quarantine on the implicated provinces) were among the factors that led to significant resistance by the community. The cancelling of elections seemed proof that political forces were at work. Rumors circulated that Ebola virus was intentionally planted in the nonhuman primates as a diabolical plan to introduce it into and wipe out the local population through hunting. Furthermore, the fact that the malady seemed to concentrate only in certain families was taken as evidence that witchcraft might be at the heart of it, rather than viruses which "should affect everybody equally." To date, virtually all of the patients who had gone into the isolation ward, run in part by the Gabonese military, had died, again arousing suspicion, fueled still more by rumors, that patients were simply being left in their beds to die.

Persons thought to have Ebola increasingly refused to be admitted to the isolation ward. Families refused to cooperate with the outreach teams. Contacts could not be traced. At one point, villagers felled trees along major routes to prevent the outreach team vehicles from reaching the villages. A key meeting of the response team was held in late January. With control efforts ground to a halt and increasing risk of violence, it was decided to suspend operations.[18] Experts in communications and social mobilization were brought in to try to diffuse the tense situation with the community. Operations eventually resumed, but the control of the outbreak definitely suffered a setback. We learned a hard lesson about the dangers of underestimating the importance of building trust and a solid relationship with the local community before delving into outbreak response measures.

THE END OF THE OUTBREAK AND HUNT FOR THE EBOLA VIRUS RESERVOIR

After the convention in filovirus outbreaks of declaring them over when a period of two times the longest incubation period (i.e., 2×21 days = 42 days) has past, the outbreak in Gabon was declared over in May 2002, with a total of 65 cases and 53 deaths (case fatality of 82%). Another 59 cases and 44 deaths occurred across the border in the adjacent Cuvette Ouest region of the Congo.[5] The international team was involved in field activities for nearly 5 months in the two countries and included over 70 representatives from 17 institutions. The first human case, retrospectively identified, was a hunter reported on October 25, 2001, 47 days before the outbreak was officially declared on December 11.[1,5] Four distinct primary foci were identified together with an isolated case noted in Franceville in the southeast of Gabon, 580 km away from the epicenter, who subsequently traveled by airplane to Libreville (Figure 18-2). No secondary transmission occurred in Libreville. In addition to the human toll, Ebola was likely responsible for a great number of animal deaths, especially great apes and duikers (small- to medium-size antelopes) in the surrounding forest[5,9,19–21] with animal deaths reported as far back as

August 2001. Samples taken from their carcasses confirmed a concomitant animal epizootic (i.e., an epidemic in animals).[22]

Because the reservoir for the filoviruses is unknown, environmental investigations, usually entailing the trapping of a wide range of animals for future laboratory analysis, is often a component of the outbreak response (Figure 18-3). These usually occur toward the end of the outbreak, even after it has concluded, because of the obvious priority of first combating the spread of disease in humans. Field collections in Gabon in the wake of the outbreak resulted in the identification of Ebola virus sequences by PCR and antibodies to Ebola in fruit bats.[23] Because a virus itself was not isolated (PCR identifies a portion of the virus' nucleic acid, but does not always indicate the presence of viable virus capable of replicating), these findings should be considered suggestive, but not definitive, of fruit bats being the reservoir for Ebola. Notably, Ebola's cousin, Marburg virus, has recently been isolated from bats trapped in Uganda.[24]

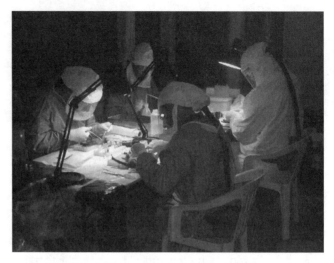

FIGURE 18-3 An ecological investigation team harvests tissues from bats in the Democratic Republic of the Congo in 1999 to test for the presence of Marburg virus. Courtesy of Pierre Rollin.

SOME LESSONS LEARNED

The outbreak in Gabon was one point on the continuum of piecing together the natural history of Ebola virus transmission, both from the natural reservoir to humans and subsequent person-to-person transmission. Major lessons that this outbreak taught us include a greater appreciation of the risk and role of nonhuman primates in the transmission of Ebola to humans. That nonhuman primates could be infected with Ebola and that humans could catch it from them were already known, but these had been isolated incidences. The experience in Gabon and Congo in 2001–2002 helped us understand the much broader scope of human–animal interactions in the context of Ebola, and the danger it poses to both.

> *The outbreak in Gabon was one point on the continuum of piecing together the natural history of Ebola virus transmission, both from the natural reservoir to humans and subsequent person-to-person transmission.*

Harder lessons were also learned, with issues that remain to be solved. The years of cultural clashes, tension of the populations under pressure, and lack of clinical management options came to a violent head in Gabon. Violence has been seen in subsequent filovirus outbreaks, at times again threatening to derail control efforts. Although these events have engendered a greater appreciation of the need to specifically address issues of communication and cross-cultural understanding, progress must still be made in this regard, perhaps with a renewed focus on the well-being of the individual patient, as opposed to viewing the patient as mainly a source of infection to be isolated for reasons of outbreak control.[25] Although there have been significant research advances on the treatment and vaccine prevention of the filoviruses, no products are yet licensed for use in humans, which continues to pose a major obstacle to the management of outbreaks.[17]

As for me, I still have vivid and surreal memories of spending New Year's Eve 2001 transferring patients to the newly opened isolation ward in Makokou, gowned, gloved, and masked and riding in the back of a pick-up truck that served as a make-shift ambulance. I suspect that villagers in Makokou who witnessed this strange and probably terrifying spectacle also recall the occasion. I also remember, much later that night, Dr. Abessolo Mengue, a good man doing his best with a difficult situation who also tried to make us feel at home, inviting the outbreak team over to his house for drinks. I could not tell you where I was at the stroke of midnight—might have been still hanging on to a beer at his house or maybe already given into exhaustion and sleep.

I eventually did make it back to Switzerland and London, a couple months late for the Christmas celebration or to help my fiancée move. I stuck around the

CDC for another year or two after the outbreak in Gabon, continuing to participate in response to outbreaks of hemorrhagic fevers and other virulent viruses, including hantavirus in Bolivia in 2002 and SARS in Vietnam in 2003, as well as work in the laboratory in Atlanta. Although I learned an immense amount from these experiences, I began to feel frustrated by their short-term nature, the feeling that I and the other members of these large international teams, while effective in what we were doing, were inevitably only offering a quick fix for a chronic problem. Without taking more concerted steps to improve the every day capacity on the ground in Africa to respond to outbreaks of all etiologies, we would still be doing the same thing decades from now.

I decided that academia gave me more freedom to pursue some of the goals that I felt important in the field of hemorrhagic fevers, as well to work in aspects of my career that were important to me but largely lacking in my government job, including teaching and interacting with students, more clinical medicine and patient care, expanding the domain of my research to other pathogens, and being able to address more broadly related issues of development, health, and human rights. In 2003, I moved back to New Orleans to rejoin the faculty at the Tulane School of Public Health and Tropical Medicine. At Tulane, one of my major activities is to direct, in contract with the WHO, the Mano River Union Lassa Fever Network (http://www.sph.tulane.edu/ManoRiverLassa), a project to build laboratory and public health infrastructure for the research and control of Lassa fever, a viral hemorrhagic fever prominent in West Africa.[26] I remain interested in the filoviruses, especially directing my attention to how patient care can be improved[25] and how capacity can be built to conduct clinical research in the field on Ebola and Marburg and to translate the laboratory research advances on these viruses through to improved treatment and control in sub-Saharan Africa.[17]

DEDICATION

This chapter is dedicated to my wife, Dr. Frederique Jacquerioz, who admirably weathers the unenviable position of being married to someone interested in field work in the viral hemorrhagic fevers.

ACKNOWLEDGMENTS

The author thanks Katie McCarthy and Catherine Pruszynski for careful review of the manuscript.

REFERENCES

1. Bausch D, Rollin P. Responding to epidemics of Ebola hemorrhagic fever: progress and lessons learned from recent outbreaks in Uganda, Gabon, and Congo. *Emerg Infect* 2004; 6:35–57.
2. Bausch DG, Towner JS, Dowell SF, et al. Assessment of the risk of Ebola virus transmission from bodily fluids and fomites. *J Infect Dis* 2007;196(Suppl 2):S142–S147.
3. Dowell SF, Mukunu R, Ksiazek TG, Khan AS, Rollin PE, Peters CJ. Transmission of Ebola hemorrhagic fever: a study of risk factors in family members, Kikwit, Democratic Republic of the Congo, 1995. Commission de Lutte contre les Epidemies a Kikwit. *J Infect Dis* 1999;179(Suppl 1):S87–S91.
4. Bausch D. Of sickness unknown: death, and health, in Africa. *United Nations Chronicle* 2001;38:5–13.
5. Nkoghe D, Formenty P, Leroy EM, et al. Multiple Ebola virus haemorrhagic fever outbreaks in Gabon, from October 2001 to April 2002. *Bull Soc Pathol Exot* 2005;98: 224–229.
6. Khan AS, Tshioko FK, Heymann DL, et al. The reemergence of Ebola hemorrhagic fever, Democratic Republic of the Congo, 1995: Commission de Lutte contre les Epidemies a Kikwit. *J Infect Dis* 1999;179(Suppl 1):S76–S86.
7. CDC and WHO. *Infection Control for Viral Haemorrhagic Fevers in the African Health Care Setting.* Atlanta: Centers for Disease Control and Prevention, 1998.
8. Bausch DG. Ebola and Marburg Viruses. In *PIER: The Physicians' Information and Education Resource.* Philadelphia: American College of Physicians, 2008 (http://pier.acponline.org/physicians/diseases/d891/d891.html).
9. Walsh PD, Abernethy KA, Bermejo M, et al. Catastrophic ape decline in western equatorial Africa. *Nature* 2003;422: 611–614.
10. Georges AJ, Leroy EM, Renaut AA, et al. Ebola hemorrhagic fever outbreaks in Gabon, 1994–1997: epidemiologic and health control issues. *J Infect Dis* 1999;179(Suppl 1):S65–S75.
11. Formenty P, Hatz C, Le Guenno B, Stoll A, Rogenmoser P, Widmer A. Human infection due to Ebola virus, subtype Cote d'Ivoire: clinical and biologic presentation. *J Infect Dis* 1999;179(Suppl 1):S48–S53.
12. Monath TP. Ecology of Marburg and Ebola viruses: speculations and directions for future research. *J Infect Dis* 1999;179(Suppl 1):S127–S38.
13. Johnson ED, Gonzalez JP, Georges A. Filovirus activity among selected ethnic groups inhabiting the tropical forest of equatorial Africa. *Trans R Soc Trop Med Hyg* 1993;87: 536–538.
14. Leroy EM, Baize S, Debre P, Lansoud-Soukate J, Mavoungou E. Early immune responses accompanying human asymptomatic Ebola infections. *Clin Exp Immunol* 2001; 124:453–460.
15. Leroy EM, Baize S, Volchkov VE, et al. Human asymptomatic Ebola infection and strong inflammatory response. *Lancet* 2000;355:2210–2215.
16. Baize S, Leroy EM, Georges-Courbot MC, et al. Defective humoral responses and extensive intravascular apoptosis

are associated with fatal outcome in Ebola virus-infected patients. *Nat Med* 1999;5:423–426.
17. Bausch D, Sprecher AG, Jeffs B, Boumandouki P. Treatment of Marburg and Ebola hemorrhagic fevers: a strategy for testing new drugs and vaccines under outbreak conditions. *Antiviral Res* 2008;78:150–161.
18. Larkin M. Ebola outbreak in the news. *Lancet Infect Dis* 2002;3:255.
19. Lahm SA, Kombila M, Swanepoel R, Barnes RF. Morbidity and mortality of wild animals in relation to outbreaks of Ebola haemorrhagic fever in Gabon, 1994–2003. *Trans R Soc Trop Med Hyg* 2007;101:64–78.
20. Rouquet P, Froment JM, Bermejo M, et al. Wild animal mortality monitoring and human Ebola outbreaks, Gabon and Republic of Congo, 2001–2003. *Emerg Infect Dis* 2005; 11:283–290.
21. Leroy EM, Rouquet P, Formenty P, et al. Multiple Ebola virus transmission events and rapid decline of central African wildlife. *Science* 2004;303:387–390.
22. Leroy EM, Souquiere S, Rouquet P, Drevet D. Re-emergence of Ebola haemorrhagic fever in Gabon. *Lancet* 2002;359:712.
23. Leroy EM, Kumulungui B, Pourrut X, et al. Fruit bats as reservoirs of Ebola virus. *Nature* 2005;438:575–576.
24. Towner JS, Amman BR, Sealy TR, et al. Isolation of genetically diverse Marburg viruses from Egyptian fruit bats. *PLOSPathos*, 2009; Jul 5(7): e1000536.
25. Bausch D, Feldmann H, Geisbert T, et al. Outbreaks of filovirus hemorrhagic fever: time to refocus on the patient. *J Infect Dis* 2007;196(Suppl 2):S136–S41.
26. Khan S, Goba A, Chu M, et al. New opportunities for field research on the pathogenesis and treatment of Lassa fever. *Antiviral Res* 2008;78:103–115.

LEARNING QUESTIONS

1. What are the primary control measures used for outbreaks of diseases like Ebola for which there is no effective vaccine or antimicrobial? Is there historical precedent that these measures are effective?
2. The author explains that the community was not comfortable with the idea of patients suspected of Ebola being placed in an isolation ward. What are some of the considerations that field epidemiologists must keep in mind when creating an isolation ward in a setting such as the one where this Ebola outbreak occurred? When answering this question, keep in mind the importance of being sensitive to the concerns and fears that may be present in the community and among healthcare or political leaders.

CHAPTER 19

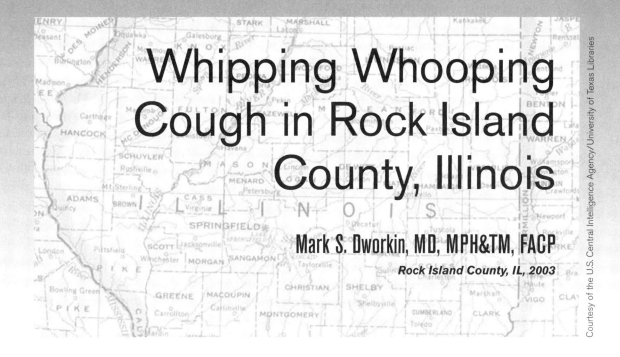

Whipping Whooping Cough in Rock Island County, Illinois

Mark S. Dworkin, MD, MPH&TM, FACP

Rock Island County, IL, 2003

INTRODUCTION

In 2003, I was the state epidemiologist for the Illinois Department of Public Health (IDPH). One of the many interesting and challenging parts of my job was leading the state health department's rapid response team (RRT). This team was created as a response to several highly publicized infectious disease outbreaks that had occurred in the late 1990s. When Illinois was dealing with those events, I was in Atlanta working at the Centers for Disease Control and Prevention (CDC) as a medical epidemiologist in the Division of HIV/AIDS Prevention in the Surveillance Branch. Working at the CDC was my first job after the long but interesting training of medical school, internal medicine residency, infectious diseases fellowship, and the CDC's Epidemic Intelligence Service (EIS) (where I was stationed in Seattle at the Washington State Department of Health).

Among the Illinois outbreaks that preceded my arrival was a large outbreak of gastroenteritis from *Escherichia coli* O157:H7 among attendees of a big outdoor rural event in which a lot of meat was cooked and served in a cow pasture. Consumption of inadequately cooked ground beef that had been contaminated with cow feces was a well-recognized mode of transmission of this foodborne disease, partly because of the highly publicized Jack in the Box hamburger outbreak in the early 1990s. In the case of the Illinois rural outbreak, the mystery of what precisely caused the outbreak was summarized by one epidemiologist as "hamburger patty or cow patty?" because it was not perfectly clear whether the burgers or the unwashed hands that were holding them were contaminated. Another newsworthy Illinois outbreak involved participants in a triathlon who swam in Lake Springfield and then became ill with leptospirosis.[1] There is something humbling about the ability of one of the tiniest life forms (the bacteria) to bring the strongest athletes down with complaints of feeling weak. There was also a Chicago area outbreak of streptococcal disease that included cases of necrotizing fasciitis (the bacterial disease inaccurately named by the media as the "flesh-eating virus"). I was told that this latter outbreak received a lot of newspaper and television coverage. These and other publicized outbreaks served to increase recognition of the importance of infectious diseases and the state health department's need to respond. Legislation was passed that provided funding to IDPH to create an RRT to help fight these emerging threats to public health and to assist local health departments during these events.

The initial RRT was hired before my arrival. The intention was that a physician hired as the state epidemiologist would be the team leader. The RRT was created as a multidisciplinary group of public health personnel. In addition to being led by a medical epidemiologist, it included a regional communicable disease representative, a veterinarian knowledgeable in animal slaughter and meat processing, a sanitarian with environmental health and restaurant and food establishment inspection expertise, a microbiologist with a PhD and experience working with pathogens that may be used in bioterrorism, an infection control nurse, and someone experienced in data systems and data analysis. With the exception of myself and an infection control nurse, the individuals that were hired were not trained in epidemiology; therefore, an important part of the meetings that I led every 1 to 2 months included epidemiology training and review of published outbreak investigations. What this team may have lacked in epidemiology training, it made up for with terrific enthusiasm to do what needed to be done and an eagerness to learn and apply that learning. Later, the team gained CDC EIS officers and public health fellows that I recruited to train at IDPH. The team also benefited from its collaboration with enthusiastic members of various sections within the health department who volunteered on outbreaks on an as-needed basis and the program staff who had experience managing outbreaks before there was the RRT. Many of these health department volunteers had experience working on outbreak investigations before the RRT was created, although their job duties did not allow them to focus on such work. The RRT helped to augment the work of experienced program staff members who were spread thin. Most program staff could not spare the time to get out into the field as often as would benefit the local health departments of the state, and thus, the RRT helped to fill this gap.

By September 2003, the team had already gained experience working on many outbreak investigations. Our first experience with pertussis (whooping cough) occurred in 2001 when Coles County in rural eastern central Illinois requested assistance with a rise in pertussis. We provided onsite assistance with the outbreak and observed that a large proportion of the cases that were reported were in adults. Because many people, including in the health care profession, had written pertussis off as a childhood disease that was largely controlled in the United States, the finding of many adult cases attracted my attention. I will not soon forget one man who came to the health department after he learned of the local rise in pertussis. A photograph was taken of him because of the impressive sequelae of the chronic cough that he was manifesting. When he walked into the health department, I was told the first impression was that he had been in an automobile accident because both of his eyes looked purplish red as if he had been struck on the back of the head; however, he met the case definition for pertussis, and had no other condition that would explain his facial change. The man had bilateral subconjunctival hemorrhages (Figure 19-1). This ocular finding is not specific to pertussis but is one of its possible complications. Other diseases that cause spasmodic coughing for prolonged periods of time are also capable of doing this.

Pertussis is caused by infection with the bacterium *Bordetella pertussis* and is notorious for causing prolonged coughing fits that can occur on and off for weeks or months, vomiting after one or more of these fits, and an inspiratory gasping sound that is known as the whoop. If someone has been previously exposed to pertussis either from a history of having whooping cough or being immunized, they might have a milder illness less likely to be recognized as pertussis but no less deadly to a susceptible infant. Infants are the most likely to be hospitalized or killed by this disease; therefore, control of an outbreak could interfere with transmission to infants and thus prevent hospitalization and death.

In 2002, an outbreak of pertussis occurred in an oil refinery in another downstate rural location, Crawford County. Our CDC EIS officer (Greg Huhn) and others published that outbreak in MMWR,[2] and it served as another nail in the coffin of the myth that pertussis is just a disease of childhood. No children were working at an oil

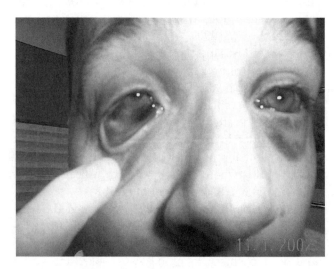

FIGURE 19-1 Man with subconjunctival hemorrhage secondary to paroxysms of coughing.

refinery! My experience with an outbreak among office workers when I was an EIS Officer in Washington State during 1994 to 1996,[3] the Coles County outbreak, and this additional work place outbreak, and reviewing the published literature on pertussis in adults had convinced me that pertussis was not just a disease of childhood. It was a disease of all ages despite widespread immunization with pertussis vaccine for decades. The incidence of pertussis had been gradually rising for 2 decades (Figure 19-2).[4] In 2003, pertussis was the only disease with a rising incidence among the diseases for which there was a recommendation for universal childhood immunization.

In late September 2003, I was called by the administrator of the Rock Island County Health Department, Wendy Trute. Rock Island County is in western Illinois on the Mississippi river and had a population of approximately 148,000 at this time. This region is mostly rural but also is known for its "Quad Cities" (Rock Island and Moline in Illinois, Bettendorf and Davenport in Iowa). The IDPH regional immunization and central office staff were aware of a rise in the number of cases reported from there through their recent communication with the Rock Island County Health Department. As for verifying that there was indeed an outbreak, a review of surveillance data revealed that only 15 cases of pertussis had cumulatively been reported in Rock Island County in the past 8 years; however, between July 1 and September 26 (just a 3-month period), 11 cases had been reported to the health department. It was definitely a situation worthy of additional investigation.

My partner in crime for this outbreak was a seasoned member of the immunization section of IDPH, Chuck Jennings. When he was not in his office, he rode around the state in a well-worn Ford van with a personalized license plate that said "CNTAGN 1." At first, I struggled to figure out how to read it until Chuck pronounced it for me, "Contagion 1." He was soft spoken and balding but with a pony tail. Idealistic, passionate about his work, and schooled in the 60s, Chuck began working with immunization preventable disease in the 70s during the "swine flu" vaccine campaign. Only someone who had spent their career excited about the field of immunizations could reveal with great pleasure that he knew where the long since retired jet injectors from the swine flu campaign were stashed.

Chuck recognized the power that our response team could bring to an outbreak. He was eager to apply the enthusiastic personnel resources to fighting the good fight of beating back a disease such as pertussis, and he was a perfect match for the RRT. He knew his way around the state and the subject matter. Despite his experience with pertussis investigation, he very much welcomed having a partner with a different background but equal enthusiasm and at times complementary knowledge about the pathogen and its manifestations. How we related to each other was a critical feature of the outbreak investigation's ability to succeed.

As the state epidemiologist and a physician, I was an unusual member of a field work team. Many local health department investigations are handled without a physician. Although I knew of several physicians that

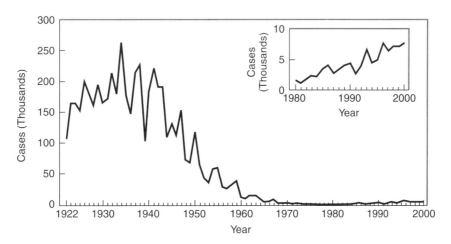

FIGURE 19-2 Number of reported pertussis cases by year—United States 1922–2000. Adapted from Zanardi L, Pascual FB, Bisgard K, Murphy T, Wharton M, Maurice E. Pertussis—United States, 1997–2000. *Morb Mortal Wkly Rep* 2002;51:73–6.

were warmly regarded years after their assistance, more than once I had been told by local and state health department and hospital staff in Illinois and other states about medical epidemiologists who came in to assist and were condescending, competitive, or left behind a feeling that they were out of touch in some way. I suspect that these ill-remembered medical epidemiologists may have meant well but were ignorant about how they were perceived and the missteps they were taking. The relatively academic culture of medical institutions where physicians are schooled and trained is unlike what one often finds in many state and local health departments and in many community hospitals.

As an example, I recall when I was an EIS officer, a microbiologist in Spokane, Washington told me of his experience with a CDC investigation some years earlier. He had been working with others at his hospital on an investigation of an outbreak of *Pseudomonas cepacia*. The CDC was called to discuss it, and although a breach of good practices related to a medical device was already identified, a CDC investigator requested sending out an EIS officer, as it would be a good training experience. The officer arrived along with his supervisor and additional epidemiologic work was performed without problems.

The point of the story as it was related to me, however, was that another more senior epidemiologist at the CDC had hoped that the Spokane microbiologist would authorize the CDC team to take the investigation data, and then they could publish it themselves. The CDC field supervisor had shared this unsavory plan with the microbiologist, as she had no interest in helping make this happen and was uncomfortable with her requested role. Having not been a part of this investigation or personally knowing the senior epidemiologist, I can not say what was his true intention. In this case, however, it does not matter what his true intention is, because the perception of what he was doing was that he was going to publish someone else's data without giving them credit for it. In a phone call that apparently had become an oft-told tale, the senior epidemiologist back at the CDC was on the phone with the field supervisor in Spokane (and the microbiologist was listening in on another line as invited to by the field supervisor so the microbiologist could hear for himself if the issue of taking over control of the outbreak data came up). When the senior epidemiologist asked whether the field supervisor had gotten a release for them to have the data, the field supervisor said that he should ask him himself because he was on the line. This led to an uncomfortable pause and a kind of "gotcha" moment. This story underscores the importance of good communication and the ability for perception (or misperception) to undermine current and future public health work. Needless to say, the microbiologist was hesitant about inviting staff coming from the CDC to assist in an investigation in the future and perhaps others that he may have told the story to retained the same concern.

It is important for anyone, medical or nonmedical, who becomes a guest in a community where they will provide assistance, to be clear and focused on the mission of their work but to maintain an attitude that it is a team effort and not just an opportunity to publish a scientific article as a lead author. Even if one is in the lead of the team, one is also a member of the team. With that thought in mind, Chuck Jennings and the local health department administrator were co-team leaders in this pertussis outbreak investigation. I made it clear very early on that I was not swooping in to take control. I was there to assist them with their efforts. In this and other outbreak investigations at local health departments, this approach was consistently successful.

The conversation with the health department administrator centered primarily on my gathering the facts as known at that time, determining whether onsite assistance was desired (which it was), and outlining what might be done upon arrival of the RRT. The primary work would be (1) to enhance surveillance in order to better determine the extent of the outbreak through case ascertainment and descriptive epidemiology and (2) to control the outbreak through the established public health actions that accompany the identification of a case including antibiotic prophylaxis of close contacts of cases. For my first visit to Rock Island County, to save time, I arranged to fly rather than drive. I was met at the small airport by Chuck Jennings who had a smile on his face like a kid in a candy shop. He really loved the work.

Chuck drove me to the Rock Island County Health Department in his well worn van, and on arriving, we held a meeting of the participating RRT members supplemented by regional immunization section staff, recently hired IDPH bioterrorism preparedness staff (including Judy Conway, an excellent nurse, and Pat Welch, an experienced former environmental health worker from another Illinois county), and local health department staff. This was a crucial meeting because it established what work we would do, allowed for staff to question and then better understand the rationale for the work, and set the tone for organization in the days to come. A "to-do" list was essential, as it laid out what was in front of us and allowed us to see where we were at in the investigation at any given time. A list of everyone relevant to the investigation was also created with contact information including telephone numbers (cell and land lines), pager numbers, and e-mail and text-pager addresses. This was copied and distributed to all of us at the end of the meeting without delay because soon many of us would be going in different directions, including my returning to Chicago where communication would typically be with the staff by phone. Such basic organizational tools as a list of names and how to reach each other should not be overlooked within the design of a successful outbreak investigation. There was a palpable feeling of relief and excitement by the staff that we had a clear direction to what we each needed to do and where it fell into the big picture.

SURVEILLANCE

Case ascertainment was at the top of our "to-do" list. Passive reporting had allowed for recognition of the pertussis outbreak. Active case finding would benefit our attempt to describe the epidemiology of the outbreak and to control it. The RRT including our communicable disease staff member, Dorian Robinson, and our veterinarian, Karnail Mudahar, helped the local health department to respond to the rise in case reports that followed by performing telephone case investigations on the suspect cases.

Surveillance is information for action.

Surveillance is information for action. I had emphasized this to the RRT so many times by this point that one day, as we were assembling the team to meet with the Rock Island County staff, Judy walked into the room and stood at attention while saluting, "Judy Conway reporting for duty. Surveillance is information for action!" That action includes respiratory precautions to prevent droplet spread from cases, treatment of cases, and prophylactic treatment of close contacts of the cases. These are the primary methods used to interrupt transmission. It is also important to ensure that the antibiotic used is appropriate for treatment of *B. pertussis* because not just any antibiotic that might get prescribed for a cough illness will reliably kill this organism.

The first way to increase reporting was to enhance the passive reporting system by increasing awareness and encouraging reporting of suspect and confirmed cases. The main reporters of pertussis were physicians and laboratories; therefore, a memorandum was drafted and sent to the local laboratories and to the hospitals for distribution to the physicians. Memorandums were also sent to local day care centers (including one for directors and a separate one for parents), schools, urgent care centers, and chiropractors. There was also communication with neighboring county health departments, including across the river in Iowa (Scott County), to make them aware of the situation and to encourage sharing of information when appropriate. A rise in pertussis was occurring in this part of Iowa which was not a surprise because in this Quad City area some people lived in one state but worked, recreated, or received medical care in the other. After the administrator of the Rock Island County Health Department and the Scott County Health Department spoke, it was agreed that they meet monthly in the future.

In addition to paper communication, I paid a personal visit to several health care facilities to underscore the importance of reporting cases and to provide an opportunity for answering questions that physicians or laboratory personnel might have. I gave a brief lecture on pertussis (including our initial outbreak data) in a doctor's dining room at the Trinity Regional Health System's east campus; met privately with the head of the emergency department, the laboratory director, and then later the adult and pediatric infectious disease physicians at Illini hospital; visited another emergency department at Trinity West; and also visited a community health practice. I made sure that for every visit, I traveled with a health department staff member. I wanted to be certain that the state health department was not given sole credit for the outbreak investigation work. Such a misperception could have undermined the credibility of the local health department. I would come and go, but they would remain in the community. It was therefore very important to boost their credibility and not appear like a "white knight" that came in to save the day. The health department and I both recognized that having a physician knowledgeable in the clinical and epidemiologic side of the pertussis outbreak going out and personally speaking to other health care staff (especially other physicians) was a rare opportunity to bolster the health department surveillance and investigation efforts. Many health departments outside the largest urban areas of a state lack such a resource, although they may have a community physician who they call on from time to time to assist with medical-related public health decisions. I have had local health department staff confide in me that doctors in their community may dismiss the local health department recommendations because they are coming from a nonphysician.

Another activity was to make the IDPH Division of Laboratories aware of the situation in an effort to increase the speed of communication between the laboratory and the county health department. One of our team members was tasked with being in phone contact with the laboratory regularly. At first, it was daily communication. It was possible to learn of unreported suspect cases by reviewing the state laboratory's list of pertussis tests and comparing the names with the county's list of cases under investigation. When testing was being performed on Rock Island County residents that had not been reported to the Rock Island County Health Department, an investigation was launched to gather information and verify that those persons met the case definition. We used the case definition that was recommended by the Council of State and Territorial Epidemiologists (Exhibit 19-1).

The concepts of sensitivity and specificity come to life within the pertussis case definition because this definition provides for a very sensitive and nonspecific alternative for use during an outbreak. This alternative case definition requires that the case only have cough illness for at least 2 weeks and be reported by a health care provider. It is a great way to catch a lot of cases. The question at this point was whether this case definition is intended for a community outbreak. With a population of approximately 148,000 people, the application of this very sensitive definition could lead to a substantial and even dramatic rise in case reporting with the potential to include large numbers of persons who have other cough illnesses; therefore, a case definition such as this is most useful in a community setting when used for identifying possible cases in order to investigate further whether they satisfy the probable or confirmed case definition and for selective use in outbreaks in special settings such as among a well-defined population rather than the entire county.

We also performed active case finding by sending some of our team members to review the medical records of the emergency department at Trinity West. We picked a limited time period of records to review based on two factors. The first was personnel. Judy Conway and Pat Welch who were primarily assigned to this task were available to realistically perform it for approximately 3 or 4 days at the most. The second factor was the likelihood that we could perform useful actions after identifying cases retrospectively. Perhaps we could have examined records going several months back in time, and in theory, we might have identified additional persons who met our case definition and populated an epidemic curve of the outbreak; however, for every medical record that we screened where their symptoms lasted at least 7 days and were consistent with the possibility of pertussis (such as cough illness but without an obvious explanation), we contacted the patient to interview them with questions to determine whether they met the pertussis case definition. If we had gone back 3 or perhaps 4 months, not only would we have created a huge mound of records to review and had a problem with recall, we would also have identified cases that were no longer contagious and whose close contacts were also unlikely to be contagious because of how long ago their infections had started; therefore, we reviewed emergency

---

EXHIBIT 19-1 Council of State and Territorial Epidemiologists' 1997 Case Definition for Pertussis

Clinical Case Definition

A cough illness lasting at least 2 weeks with one of the following: paroxysms of coughing, inspiratory "whoop," or posttussive vomiting, without other apparent cause (as reported by a health professional)

Laboratory Criteria for Diagnosis

Isolation of *Bordetella pertussis* from clinical specimen

Positive polymerase chain reaction (PCR) for *B. pertussis*

Case Classification

Probable: meets the clinical case definition, is not laboratory confirmed, and is not epidemiologically linked to a laboratory confirmed case

Confirmed: a case that is culture positive and in which an acute cough illness of any duration is present; or a case that meets the clinical case definition and is confirmed by positive PCR; or a case that meets the clinical case definition and is epidemiologically linked directly to a case confirmed by either culture or PCR

Comment

The clinical case definition above is appropriate for endemic or sporadic cases. In outbreak settings, a case may be defined as a cough illness lasting at least 2 weeks (as reported by a health professional). Because direct fluorescent antibody testing of nasopharyngeal secretions has been demonstrated in some studies to have low sensitivity and variable specificity, such testing should not be relied on as a criterion for laboratory confirmation. Serologic testing for pertussis is available in some areas but is not standardized and, therefore, should not be relied on as a criterion for laboratory confirmation.

Both probable and confirmed cases should be reported nationally.

department records of patients presenting with cough illness during the previous 2 months starting with the most recent cases.

A spreadsheet of possible cases was generated from this review and health department staff performed the follow-up telephone calls after they cross-referenced with the spreadsheet with cases already reported (to avoid duplication of effort). A similar medical record review was also performed at a local urgent care clinic. Seven suspect cases were identified among the emergency department records reviewed (although the denominator is not available to determine what fraction that was of all reviewed records); however, among 250 urgent care records reviewed, five were suspect cases (2%). Given that our goal was to control a disease that could be passed from person to person to person to infant (whom it could hospitalize or kill) and because we had adequate personnel resources at the beginning of the outbreak investigation, we believed that this was an acceptable, although low, yield for this record review.

To help us determine the scope and the impact of the outbreak, we also surveyed local pharmacies. We had an interest in exploring syndromic methods of surveillance to gain experience with these issues. There were no electronic methods in place that obtained data representative of the region so Pat Welch gathered the information directly from pharmacies. She contacted nine large pharmacies to identify what was their experience with sales of over the counter cough medicine and antibiotics that would likely be used to treat pertussis (specifically, erythromycin, clarithromycin, and azithromycin). This identified a modest increase in over-the-counter sales and the antibiotics, but nothing dramatic. We were satisfied to have gone through this exercise to demonstrate what we were capable of doing, but we did not find it very useful as the outbreak was already established; however, if we had identified a marked increase in the sales of these pharmaceuticals, we would have hypothesized that the outbreak might be impacting the community to a greater degree than we currently had recognized, and we would have questioned the sensitivity of our surveillance system efforts. Additional investigation would then have been performed.

The county's outbreak data was maintained using an Epi Info database that RRT member Roland Lucht helped to set up and maintain. Chuck made sure that the data were reported to the Immunization Section at IDPH. As we examined the data regularly throughout our surveillance efforts, there were several factors we had to consider that could influence the case count. The first was heightened awareness. Our efforts led to an increased likelihood that physicians would think of pertussis when a compatible case presented to them. Of course this was an intended result that we hoped would increase reporting so that we could ensure control measures were undertaken for each case; therefore, a rising case count early on would not indicate an outbreak that we were failing to control but more likely an outbreak that we were more accurately capturing through surveillance. There was media coverage as well, and thus, the community was learning about pertussis from their local newspaper and other media outlets. As a result, persons with a cough illness might bring up the possibility that they had pertussis to their health care provider and even could request testing. Given that pertussis was recognized to be circulating among the U.S. population before the outbreak, we had to consider that some of the rise in cases was actually an uncovering of the endemic disease secondary to heightened recognition and increased testing practices. We did not have a way to quantify this issue because we did not have data that defined the true background rate of pertussis in this community. We only had historic passive pertussis surveillance data that are known to underrepresent markedly the true incidence of disease.

Another important factor that impacted on our data was diagnostic testing. Culture of *B. pertussis* is considered the gold standard, but the organism can easily die, which may lead to false negatives. The organism requires a special transport medium that is not as widely available as a rapid test for strep throat or a transport medium used to swab an ordinary wound for culture. Thus, a special effort was made to supply and resupply the local laboratories with plenty of this transport medium and to educate the local physicians that it was needed for accurate diagnosis. A nasopharyngeal swab is performed to collect the specimen; however, not all physicians are aware of this, and therefore, a throat swab can be incorrectly submitted. In addition, the choice of swab used to obtain a nasopharyngeal specimen could also impact on the yield of culture and the more sensitive molecular-based PCR. Dacron and calcium alginate swabs are preferred for culture because cotton swabs can inhibit the growth of *B. pertussis*. Calcium alginate swabs inhibit PCR. When culture and PCR are planned, Dacron

> *Thus, there were many factors competing to undermine our confirmation of cases, including trying to get physicians, including many unfamiliar with pertussis, to perform the nasopharyngeal swab using the right kind of swab and sending it with the special transport medium.*

and rayon swabs are the best choice.[5] Thus, there were many factors competing to undermine our confirmation of cases, including trying to get physicians, including many unfamiliar with pertussis, to perform the nasopharyngeal swab using the right kind of swab and sending it with the special transport medium.

The timing of the nasopharyngeal swab is also important. The yield is highest in the first 2 weeks after the onset of illness.[6] It may not be worthwhile testing several weeks into the cough illness, although that is when pertussis is most likely to be considered in sporadically occurring cases. Age also impacts on yield. Adults and immunized persons mount an immune response that suppresses the number of organisms more quickly after onset of illness so that diagnostic yield is less with increasing age. What this meant to our outbreak was that we were likely to have a lot of negative specimens because we were observing a large proportion of cases in adolescents and adults and who had been coughing for weeks before being recognized as cases.

Laboratory confirmation is a subclassification of the case definition but is not required for case reporting if the patient met the clinical case definition; however, reporting is affected by the factors that can increase the likelihood of a negative laboratory result in a true case because physicians commonly view negative test results for a pathogen as a rule-out procedure for that diagnosis. Therefore, a patient could meet the clinical case definition and their physician could think of pertussis and even decide that it was worth the extra effort to submit a specimen for culture or PCR; however, if the swab chosen was not the optimal swab for the test being ordered or they swabbed the throat, if the transport medium was not correct, if the patient was several weeks out since onset of illness or was an adolescent or adult, if the specimen was mishandled in transport, or if laboratory difficulties with the specimen were to occur, a negative result would later be received by the health care provider, and no report would follow. As if these were not enough issues with laboratory diagnosis, serology is also another point for confusion. A reliable and Food and Drug Administration (FDA) approved serologic test for pertussis was not available for use during this outbreak investigation; however, serologic tests (not FDA approved) were available to health care providers and were being obtained. As a result, serologic test results could not guide definitive conclusions about whether a person had been infected with pertussis, but lack of awareness of this could have caused some physicians to use them as a definitive answer. For this reason, it is important during pertussis outbreaks to stress to health care providers that reporting should not be dependent on the laboratory results. If their patient meets the clinical case definition (or the outbreak case definition in the setting of an outbreak), then the case should be reported. It should also be recognized that there are situations where local or state health departments may decide to limit reporting of cases to only those meeting the confirmed case classification because of the department's inability to handle the volume of probable cases that would result.

THE CONTROVERSY OF DEFINING A CLOSE CONTACT

In the midst of all the surveillance activities, we were made aware of an adult football coach who was positive by PCR for *B. pertussis*. An investigation was begun, and it was learned that the coach had extensive face-to-face contact with others (which, of course, was not unexpected). Interviewing of approximately 110 students and other contacts of the coach at the high school one evening identified 26 persons with an active cough illness. The team physician elected to give chemoprophylaxis to the entire team. Practices continued, and they planned to postpone their next game by 3 days; however, the competing team, apparently driven by fear, would not play their perceived to be contagious competitor, and a forfeit was arranged. The rationale for providing prophylaxis to the team was explained by the Rock Island County Health Department administrator in a local newspaper article entitled "Whipping whooping cough": "...If you think about a football team, being in a locker room together, on a bus together, three or four hours everyday together in practice, the coach being positive, there's a lot of reasons why the players would be more susceptible." The finding of this cluster of potential cases within the community illustrates another example of the value of heightened surveillance within an outbreak. It allows for recognition of situations in which additional investigation may be needed such as this football coach or a health care provider or hospital employee who might have routine close contact with patients.

In this and other pertussis outbreaks I have been involved in, how to define a close contact has been controversial. Often there has been a general rule applied but judgment has been allowed on a case-by-case basis. I have seen it defined as prolonged face-to-face contact versus being within 3 feet some period of

> *In this and other pertussis outbreaks I have been involved in, how to define a close contact has been controversial.*

time, such as at least 10 minutes versus much longer. The questions will come up: "What about the child who sits directly behind the case in the classroom? Does that child need prophylaxis?" "What about the other children in the classroom for whom we don't know exactly how much contact they might have had with the child during the day?" "How do we handle the situation where a student does not stay in one room most of the day (such as the high school student) but sits in multiple classrooms of different students throughout the day, leading to a huge number of potential close contacts?" "How about those who ride on the bus with the child?" The more questions asked and answered liberally to try to interrupt transmission completely, the more prophylaxis might be dispensed to the point where it seems excessive. As a result, some health departments have changed their recommendation for close contacts to be only those at highest risk for morbidity or mortality or contributing to the morbidity and mortality of others (such as reserving it for pregnant women and others who are likely to expose infants).[7]

THE IMPORTANCE OF AGE

By October, a preliminary look at the epidemiology demonstrated some interesting findings that illustrated the importance of this disease in the adolescent and adult population. Recalling that the case definition included two classic features of the disease that were typically thought to occur mainly in children and the unimmunized (posttussive vomiting and whooping), we examined the data collected from the cases by age group to understand better the distribution of these symptoms in adolescents and adults. The hypothesis was that these symptoms would be uncommon but present; therefore, I was surprised to observe that posttussive vomiting occurred as frequently as 20% to 60% in those older than 21 years of age. Even more surprising was that whooping occurred in 33% to 88% of those older than 21 years of age (Figure 19-3).

When we later examined nearly all of the cases, it was clear that the majority (70%) were in adolescents and adults (Figure 19-4). This was yet another example of the important role of the older population as a reservoir of pertussis for infants who were most vulnerable to its more severe complications. Our active case finding had identified many persons in the community that met the case definition who otherwise would have gone unrecognized.

Given that these cases were occurring in persons basically with a history of pertussis immunization as children or old enough to have likely had pertussis in the prevaccine era, the lesson learned here was that the vaccine does not provide lifelong immunity. This was not new information, but given that many vaccines do appear to provide long lasting immunity (such as measles vaccine), it can be overlooked that pertussis vaccine-induced immunity begins to decline relatively soon after completion of the pertussis immunization series of vaccines. The duration of immunity after vaccination ranges from approximately 4 to 12 years and for infection-acquired immunity ranges from 7 to 20 years[8]; therefore, a vaccinated child can be fully susceptible as

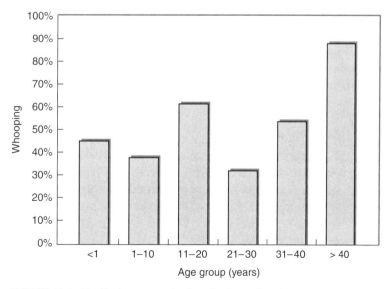

FIGURE 19-3 Preliminary analysis of whooping by age among the first 66 cases reported, Rock Island County, Illinois, 2003.

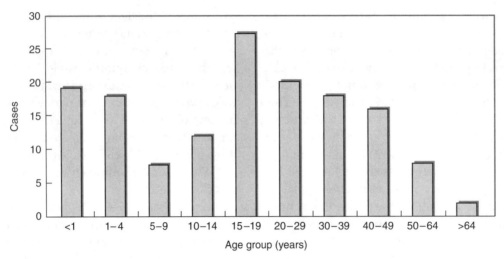

FIGURE 19-4 Distribution by age of 148 cases of pertussis, Rock Island County, Illinois, 2003.

early as 9 or 10 or during their adolescent years. What was nicely illustrated here was that adults with surprising frequency could get the more classic symptoms such as whooping rather than only very mild illness, as had been the common anecdote when I interacted with a variety of physicians in various settings over the years. Certainly, adults can and do get mild illness, but I had not before seen documented such a relatively high frequency of these more severe symptoms. I recall one of the investigation staff commenting that an adult patient was having a coughing fit and whooping during their telephone interview with them.

COMMUNICATION

Finally, a variety of communications issues had to be dealt with during this outbreak investigation. Communication targets included the media (and through them to the public), other public health jurisdictions, and others who can be viewed as stakeholders of the investigation and pertussis surveillance system, including health care providers, laboratories, and the local college, schools, and day care facilities. In addition, internal communications were vital, including among the investigation staff and with personnel off site within the state health department, including program staff and those higher up the chain of command.

> *Communication with the media should be handled with forethought and ideally is performed by someone with experience.*

Communication with the media should be handled with forethought and ideally is performed by someone with experience. Although health departments in jurisdictions with large populations may have a public information officer whose role can be critical during outbreaks, emergencies, and day-to-day communication with the media, most health departments do not have this luxury and the Rock Island County Health Department fell into this category of serving a moderate sized population; however, we were able to consult with IDPH on these issues and also found that once we had our overriding communications objectives decided on, the anxiety of communicating with the media decreased.

A concern with communicating with the media about an outbreak is primarily that, although you can control what you write in a press release or speak in an interview, what the journalist does with the information after that is completely out of your control. As a result, they could choose to write an article about how the health department is incompetent, or they can make heroes out of the staff, or something in between. In one outbreak investigation, the local newspaper referred to our investigation team as a "crack team" of experts who "descended" on the local jail where the outbreak was occurring. They made us sound like a bunch of superheroes. I have been fortunate not to have the other extreme, but I have seen news that put health departments in an unfavorable light.

The media can play a vital role within the response to the outbreak. They can help disseminate prevention information and calm fears about the emerging problem. You do not usually see public health prevention as front-page news, but if it is going to occur, an outbreak is a likely time for it. Therefore, we made how to prevent disease transmission and advocacy for disease reporting among our major communications objectives in interviews with local newspapers and other journalists who contacted the health department. We were pleased to see information about the disease symptoms, who was susceptible, and how to prevent it on the front page of the Quad City Times (Exhibit 19-2). Wendy, the local health department administrator, had not been on the job very long when this outbreak occurred, but she and her staff did a great job with handling it, as well as with communicating with the media. I made myself available for some interviews, especially when it would lend credibility to the dissemination of medical information; however, as mentioned earlier, it was important to have the local health department speak for themselves to the media with assistance from the state as needed rather than giving the unhelpful impression that the state deserved all the credit for the control of the outbreak.

Another of the important messages to impart through the media was that the case count was expected to rise. Communicating this properly was of great importance because as we performed case ascertainment successfully, the number of cases reported would rise sharply. If not forewarned that this was a planned outcome, the media could issue news reports that the outbreak was worsening despite health department efforts. The last thing we wanted to see was a headline such as "Cases of Whooping Cough Soar Despite Health Department's Attempts at Control." This would undermine credibility and be inaccurate; therefore, we made it clear during early interviews that our efforts would likely lead to a rise in case counts and that this was our intended result.

As mentioned earlier, the Rock Island County Health Department maintained regular contact with their colleagues across the river in Iowa. They also shared information with other health departments in their region of Illinois. Within Illinois, these activities were facilitated by a regional IDPH employee who also shared information with the central office at IDPH. This kind of communication with other jurisdictions was especially important to minimize the chance of inconsistent information being released. The media could go to other jurisdictions and to the state health department for information on this outbreak because it was not exclusively involving Rock Island County. With so many potential voices, it would be easy for inconsistent messages to be released.

Appropriate prescription of antibiotics for prophylaxis of all close contacts was another important communications issue. Prophylaxis has been a routine part of pertussis control for many years (although recently its efficacy as a control measure has been called into question). In outbreaks of limited size, it may be feasible to treat all close contacts with an antibiotic that is effective at killing *B. pertussis*. Some health care providers enthusiastically attempted to comply with this recommendation, and we even heard from one physician that there was a shortage of erythromycin at one or more of the local pharmacies; however, in conflict with this kind of recommendation was the recent public and health care provider targeted campaign by authoritative organizations such as the American College of Physicians and the CDC aimed at minimizing inappropriate prescription of antibiotics.[9,10] This campaign was an effort to respond to the rising rates of antibiotic resistance among bacterial pathogens. As a result, there was a lot of pushback on the recommendation to treat asymptomatic children and adults with the drug of choice at that time (erythromycin). It did not help that the drug needed to be given for 14 days and was known to cause an upset stomach; therefore, our communication needed to stress the rationale for the recommendation and to explain that prophylaxis was indicated for close contacts regardless of age and even if they had a history of pertussis immunization.

Although I am now less convinced that every single "close contact" of a pertussis case needs to receive prophylaxis as part of the control of a pertussis outbreak, during this outbreak I spent a great deal of time talking to individuals and groups of physicians explaining the rationale for this policy. It was intended to aggressively interfere with the spread of pertussis; however, as a policy, it was difficult to enforce and ensuring that close contacts took the antibiotic for the full 14 days was not even a part of the activities of the outbreak response. Although there is biologic plausibility to a policy like this and I assumed it must have been derived from some carefully performed population studies of pertussis, I have not seen such studies and am not certain there are any. I now endorse the more prioritized policy of focusing on those most likely to spread the disease to infants and those who are more likely to have severe disease,[11] as well as a case-by-case judgment call for other situations.

Communications with the local laboratories was another important activity. They were highly impacted by the outbreak. Testing for pertussis increased substantially as we advocated for increased awareness of the disease as a means of increasing case ascertainment and the media further increased awareness among health care providers and the public. Testing was occurring in persons who had the classic clinical presentation, persons

EXHIBIT 19-2 Newspaper Article in the Quad City Times, Including Information on Transmission and Prevention of Pertussis as Front-Page News

Friday, September 26, 2003

WHOOPING COUGH STRIKES Q-C

LOCAL AUTHORITIES CONFIRM 22 CASES OF DEADLY DISEASE

By Cherie Black
QUAD-CITY TIMES

An outbreak of a disease many thought was no longer a threat has invaded the Quad-City area.

Pertussis, more commonly known as whooping cough, has appeared in a cluster of cases throughout Rock Island and Scott counties in recent months, prompting local health departments to begin investigating the extent of the outbreak and educating physicians and residents of the possible dangers.

Since July 1, there have been 11 confirmed cases among Rock Island County residents between the ages of two months and 37 years old with more than a dozen other cases being investigated. This compares with just 15 cases reported between 1995 and 2002.

In Scott County, 11 cases have been diagnosed since Aug. 1, including one confirmed Thursday. Nine of the cases came from the same day care facility. Last year, 25 cases were diagnosed; there were six in 2000 and 2001.

"Even though pertussis is an old disease, it is considered to be making a comeback," said Chuck Jennings, a member of the Illinois Department of Health Rapid Response Team, which has teamed with the Rock Island County Health Department to investigate the outbreak. "We now see that adults serve as a reservoir for this bacteria. Ten to 12 years ago, we didn't think adults could get this."

Whooping cough is a highly contagious bacterial infection that causes coughing and gagging with little or no fever. An infected person has cold-like symptoms and prolonged cough episodes that may end in vomiting or cause a "whoop" sound when the person tries to breathe in. Once diagnosed by a nasal swab or a DNA-type test, whooping cough can be treated with a 14-day dose of antibiotics. Household contacts who may have also been exposed are also asked to be tested. Although it is a disease most people have been vaccinated against, it is more dangerous in infants 12 months and younger and can be fatal.

"Because it's a vaccine-preventable disease, we don't expect to see it as much as we have in our population," said Roma Taylor, a clinical services counselor with the Scott County Health Department. "But the effectiveness of the vaccine tends to wane in teenagers and adults."

Because of this, health officials are encouraging residents and especially physicians [to be aware] of the symptoms to avoid the spread of the disease.

"We're into allergy season and also going into flu season, and we want physicians to be thinking of whooping cough as a possibility and not just think patients just have allergies or bronchitis," Taylor said.

Rock Island County Health Department administrator Wendy Trute and state epidemiologists have been visiting hospitals, schools, day care facilities and health care clinics to make sure staff is aware of symptoms.

"I think a lot of them were surprised this wasn't even on their radar," Trute said. "This spreads from person to person to person and is highly contagious. We want to try and stop the spread and break that chain of development."

BY THE NUMBERS

Pertussis is a highly contagious bacterial infection that causes coughing and gagging with little or no fever. An infected person has cough episodes that may end in vomiting or cause a "whoop" sound when the person tries to breathe in.

THE SYMPTOMS: Symptoms appear between 6 to 21 days after exposure to the bacteria. The disease starts with cold symptoms like a runny nose and a cough. Sometime in the first two weeks, episodes of severe cough develop that can last one to two months. The infected person may look and feel fairly healthy between these episodes. During bouts of coughing the lips and nails may turn blue for lack of air. Vomiting may occur after severe coughing spells. During the severe coughing stage, seizures or even death can occur, particularly in an infant.

WHO GETS IT: Anyone who is exposed can get pertussis. Unimmunized or inadequately immunized people are at higher risk for severe disease. Many cases occur in adults because protection from the vaccine lasts only 5 to 10 years.

TREATMENTS: The vaccination against pertussis is included in the DTP and DTaP vaccines. Before age 7, children should receive 5 doses of the DTP or DTaP vaccine. These usually are given at 2, 4, 6, and 15–18 months of age and 4–6 years of age. Persons with pertussis should avoid contact with others until no longer contagious. If you live with someone who has pertussis or are exposed in any way, antibiotics are necessary.

Reprinted with permission of the Quad City Times.

who had some overlapping clinical presentation but were not highly likely to be true cases, and even some who were asymptomatic (apparently the worried well); therefore, there was an influx of inappropriate testing going on and the local laboratories (as well as the more distant reference laboratories) observed a large increase in their workload including acquiring the appropriate test kits with the transport media, processing the samples, notification of laboratory test results, sending samples to the state laboratory, and reporting results to the county health department. It was clear in one of my meetings with a local hospital laboratory manager that they were upset about the situation, and it was my impression from them that they felt as if I and the health department had been overreacting leading to their having to deal with the consequences. This was understandable given that their staff had not previously dealt with a pertussis outbreak like this one, that they had not been forewarned of what to expect nor explained the rationale for the activities, and that they were witnessing a large number of negative results (as so many of the specimens submitted were from low likelihood clinical scenarios combined with the relatively low yield for pertussis culture and PCR in the setting of advanced illness and older age). They were processing lots of samples from patients who did not have pertussis and from patients who probably had it but it was too late into their illness to identify it. All in all, it was an unsatisfying experience for the laboratory. Our state laboratory was also unenthused with the situation; therefore, communication with the laboratory was important throughout the outbreak. The investigation team needed to be aware of the laboratories' concerns and to respond to them by encouraging appropriate testing by the affected health care community (which we did).

FINAL THOUGHTS

It should be emphasized that during the first 2 weeks of our assistance with this outbreak, it felt like there was nonstop activity. Serving as the lead consultant to the health department, there were numerous questions and issues that needed to be settled. One moment someone interviewing a possible case needed clarification, and then there might be an interview with the media, then a visit to a hospital, then review of some data, again more questions. At one point, to lighten things up a bit, I asked that some of the health department personnel and RRT members hold one of our daily update meetings at a local old famous ice cream parlor in Moline. One of the things I enjoyed about being state epidemiologist was visiting the many small towns and finding pearls of history or local culture. I drove thousands of miles of Illinois highway during my approximately 5.5 years in this job and loved the big skies, migrating birds, and the variety of small towns and their characteristics. A few months before this outbreak I had received a magazine in the mail that mentioned that in Moline, Illinois was an ice cream parlor in business for 100 years named Lagomarcinos. I had clipped the little story of this place and saved it. When I realized I was working nearby, I decided it would be a great place for our meeting. We sat in a cramped mahogany booth with a Tiffany-style lamp overhead. From the unique floor to the metal ceiling, it was a great place to go over data and enjoy each other's company. The hot fudge sundaes were fantastic, and who knows, maybe the "sugar rush" enhanced our epidemiologic minds.

The number of cases with onset of illness had declined by early November. The state health department needed to have its staff members resume their routine duties. The local health department that experienced

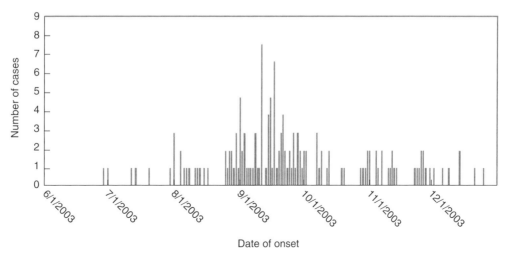

FIGURE 19-5 Epidemic curve of 151 pertussis cases by date of onset, Rock Island County, Illinois, 2003.

three retirements around this time needed to stop performing active surveillance work. The outbreak response was then largely completed in November with ongoing passive surveillance demonstrating relatively low level continued community transmission in December (Figure 19-5).

This outbreak investigation illustrates some of the many issues that are relevant to the response to a community outbreak of a respiratory illness. Unlike some outbreaks where the expected final outcome is an eradication of the disease in the impacted population, for a community-wide outbreak where endemic low level disease is the norm, a more modest outcome is acceptable. Pertussis continues to be a problem nationwide; however, I am optimistic that since the approval of licensure by the FDA in 2005 of two booster vaccines (one initially licensed for use in adolescents and the other for adolescents and adults) the burden of pertussis in the United States will fall to hopefully historically low levels in the coming decades, and pertussis outbreaks will be less frequent.

REFERENCES

1. Morgan J, Bornstein SL, Karpati AM, et al. Outbreak of leptospirosis among triathlon participants and community residents in Springfield, Illinois, 1998. *Clin Infect Dis* 2002; 34:1593–1599.
2. Skaggs P, Jennings C, Hunt K, et al. Pertussis outbreak among adults at an oil refinery—Illinois, August–October 2002. *Morb Mortal Wkly Rep* 2003;52:1–4.
3. Dworkin MS, Spitters C, Kobayashi JM. Pertussis in adults. *Ann Intern Med* 1998;128:1047.
4. Zanardi L, Pascual FB, Bisgard K, Murphy T, Wharton M, Maurice E. Pertussis—United States, 1997–2000. *Morb Mortal Wkly Rep* 2002;51:73–76.
5. Cloud JL, Hymas W, Caroll KC. Impact of nasopharyngeal swab types on detection of Bordetella pertussis by PCR and culture. *J Clin Microbiol* 2002;40:3838–3840.
6. Sotir MJ, Cappozzo DL, Warshauer, et al. Evaluation of polymerase chain reaction and culture for diagnosis of pertussis in the control of a county-wide outbreak focused among adolescents and adults. *Clin Infect Dis* 2007;44: 1216–1219.
7. Pertussis prophylaxis passé? CD Summary. Retrieved September 18, 2008, from www.oregon.gov/dhs/ph/cdsummary/ 2005/ohd5409.pdf.
8. Wendelboe AM, Van Rie A, Salmaso S, Englund JA. Duration of immunity against pertussis after natural infection or vaccination. *Pediatr Infect Dis J* 2005;24:S58–S61.
9. Centers for Disease Control and Prevention. Get smart. Know when antibiotics work. Available June 4, 2008, from http://www.cdc.gov/drugresistance/community/faqs.htm.
10. Maguire P. Your patients are sick but do they need antibiotics? *ACP-ASIM Observer* November 2001. Retrieved June 4, 2008, from http://www.acponline.org/clinical_information/ journals_publications/acp_internist/nov01/antibiotics.htm.
11. Pertussis. Oregon Public Health Division. Oregon Department of Human Services. 2007:1–10 (see page 5). Retrieved June 4, 2008, from http://www.oregon.gov/DHS/ph/acd/ reporting/guideln/pertussis.pdf.

LEARNING QUESTIONS

1. Case ascertainment was a priority in this outbreak in part because there were important public health actions that would follow as a result of the notification of a case of pertussis. What were these actions and what was the rationale for performing them?
2. The investigation team did not have access to any electronic syndromic surveillance system that could aid them with suspect case ascertainment. What did they do in order to attempt to enhance recognition of suspect cases syndromically? Was this activity fruitful?
3. What was the controversy over how to define a close contact of a pertussis case?

CHAPTER 20

Emergency Yellow Fever Mass Vaccination in Post-Civil War Liberia

Gregory Huhn, MD, MPH&TM
Liberia, 2004

INTRODUCTION

The Call

The last few months of employment at the Epidemic Intelligence Service (EIS) are usually set aside as wrap-up time for the officer. Their supervisors usually divert new assignments to others as we double check analysis of surveillance projects, write and edit manuscripts (if not already plunged in the dreadful purgatory of the Centers for Disease Control and Prevention [CDC] clearance process), and perhaps most importantly, cobble together enough annual leave to catch a sunset or two while sipping caipirinhas on a Brazilian white sand beach. Nevertheless, as commissioned officers with our own public health service march,* we know that any expectation of a reserved sabbatical at the end of our tour of duty is a sucker's bet. We can get "the call" at any time. On March 8, 2004, with less than 4 months remaining in my EIS fellowship, I did not get the call. I made a call, and suddenly I was cashing in my chips on a new outbreak.

I was stationed with the state branch at the Illinois Department of Public Health, revising a manuscript describing the first human outbreak of West Nile virus in Illinois in 2002 when I needed clarification of a new term that the CDC had developed, "neuroinvasive disease," for surveillance purposes in categorizing West Nile virus meningitis or encephalitis cases. I called the guy who I knew would give me a straight answer, Dr. Tony Marfin, deputy director of the Division of Vector-Borne Infectious Diseases in Ft. Collins, Colorado. Both Tony and I have San Diego roots, so, not only did I trust his acumen in all things arboviral, but I also enjoyed just catching up with him. "So what's new, Tony?" "We just got a report this week from a UNICEF representative that there may be a yellow fever outbreak in Liberia." Yellow fever, how fascinating. Liberia, how sublime. A country under United Nations security protectorship with a transitional government 5 months removed from the end of a macabre 14-year civil war, this small nation of 3 million people was awakening from the devastating rule of warlord president Charles Taylor that witnessed 250,000 killed, millions uprooted

---

*"In the silent war against disease no truce is ever seen; we serve on the land and sea for humanity." Available at: http://coa.spsp.net/phsmusic.html.

as refugees or internally displaced persons (IDPs), and nearly all institutions ruinous. Most physicians are asked at some point when or why they first wanted to become doctors. For me, the answer was Liberia.

In 1990, 25 years old and seeking some sort of muse beyond the borders of my job as a research assistant at the Research Institute at Scripps Clinic, I volunteered as a clinical lab technician with a Spanish order of Brothers who operated St. Joseph's Catholic Hospital in the capital of Monrovia. By my fifth month, we were the only hospital functioning in the city, as the genesis of the civil war rapidly spilled into Monrovia. Two factions of rebel forces led by Charles Taylor and Prince Johnson battled the government soldiers of President Samuel K. Doe. By this time, Medicins Sans Frontieres (MSF) had established a field surgical unit within our compound, and I had redirected my job description to start a blood bank for which I exchanged 5 cups of rice, valuable currency in this time of desperation and starvation, plus iron and folate tablets, for a unit of blood from community donors. By mid-August, my nascent apprenticeship in Liberia was vanquished when our hospital was bombed behind two battle lines by government soldiers. We were forced to evacuate within a matter of hours. Mortars blasts had damaged much of our transportation vehicles; however, we quickly repaired a cadre of cars and rolled out in the Charles Taylor rebel-controlled streets. After a 2-day journey through the bush, the last I saw of Liberia was the shores of a rebel training ground lined with young fighters lying prone on the sand, with their AK-47s aimed toward the helicopters of the unarmed U.S. Marines who had been hastily deployed to pick us up and fly us off into safe waters.[1–3]

From this experience, I decided to enter medical school and study tropical medicine. I did not elaborate all of this to Tony; I simply told him that I had worked previously in Liberia and was familiar with the people and political situation. To investigate this yellow fever outbreak would be an opportunity of a peaceful homecoming, I thought. Tony said, "You know, it might be useful to have an EIS officer who knows the lay of the land over there." UNICEF was initiating an emergency yellow fever immunization program and requested assistance from the CDC. A year beforehand, the UNICEF representative in Liberia had been supervising UNICEF's aid program in Afghanistan. An EIS team had established a surveillance system for unexploded ordinance throughout the country after the U.S. military involvement. Pleased with the performance of the EIS, the representative felt confident that the CDC could provide expertise in controlling this yellow fever outbreak. Before acting on the invitation, however, we still needed to invoke the first rule of outbreak investigations—verify that there is an outbreak.

THE OUTBREAK

On January 1, 2004, a 26-year-old male living in an IDP camp in Totota, Salala District, Bong Country, Liberia (Figure 20-1), one of roughly 531,600 Liberians[4], or one-sixth of the nation's estimated population living in such camps throughout the country, returned from his work as a day laborer in a nearby rural farm complaining of fevers, chills, headache, and muscle aches. Over the next week, he had transient fever and chills with a persistent headache and abdominal pain. He continued to work in the fields. By day 8 of his illness, he was unable to work, as the fevers, chills, and headache continued, the abdominal pain worsened, and he developed nausea and back pain over the next 3 days. From days 11 to 13, he noted an onset of epistaxis (bleeding from the nose), emesis, and weakness, with ongoing constitutional symptoms. On day 14, he was seen by Dr. Hansel Otero of MSF at the camp clinic. Vital signs recorded a temperature of 39°C, hypotension with a blood pressure of 90/50 mm Hg, a heart rate of 80 beats per minute, and noticeable jaundice. The patient was confused and was vomiting blood. The patient was admitted to the field hospital on site, which consisted of a large tent with rows of beds separated by white cloth curtains. Blood was drawn for laboratory testing. Intravenous fluids were administered, and the patient was treated empirically for malaria. By the next day, the patient developed progressive confusion with seizures, had profuse bloody vomiting, and his fevers were unrelenting. He died within 24 hours of admission.

Dr. Otero was a relatively recent graduate of the Universidad Central de Venezuela medical school, class of 2002. After graduation, he worked for 1 year in a small town on the Caribbean coast in Venezuela, and then he joined forces with MSF France. His first assignment was delivering basic health care to the IDPs of Bong County in the interior of Liberia. On the job for approximately 6 weeks, he suspected that the young rural farm laborer he encountered with fevers, jaundice, and apparent hemorrhage might be suffering from a disease that he had never seen before but that he had read about in his medical texts. Nearly everyone in West Africa presenting with fever and headache is treated for malaria. Dr. Otero made this perfunctory step in his treatment plan; however, he knew that his diagnostic plan demanded a more critical

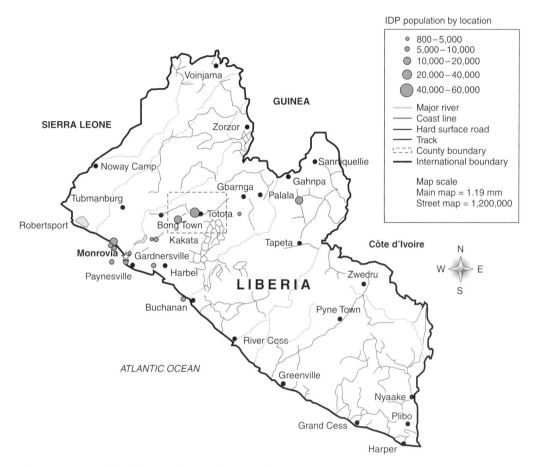

FIGURE 20-1 Salala District, Bong County, Liberia. From Humanitarian Information Centre of Liberia. Available at http://www.humanitarianinfo.org/liberia/mapcentre/catalogue/index.asp. Accessed November 4, 2008.

exercise. Dr. William Osler once said, "The value of experience is not in seeing much, but in seeing wisely." As an astute clinician (and most all outbreaks, before they are realized as outbreaks, start with the "astute clinician" type, ranging from medical professionals to even concerned parents), processing the constellation of signs, symptoms, and setting—the nosebleed, the bloody vomit, the fever and jaundice—this he insisted appeared to go beyond the commonplace malaria that he was already accustomed to seeing in a healthy young man. In medicine, "zebras" are the rare diagnoses. Clinicians are cautioned not to seek them out without due cause. So, Dr. Otero went zebra chasing, as he began to piece together these tropical hoof beats while perhaps hearing echoes of Dr. Osler's edict. He ordered a blood test that he knew would take several weeks to finalize a result and probably would not save his patient's life.

In 2003, during the scare of SARS, the New York Times published "The Epidemic Scorecard" (Figure 20-2). Ensconced in the bottom right-hand corner among 10 other deadly diseases sat yellow fever, with 30,000 deaths and 200,000 new cases per year worldwide. Although viral diseases such as Ebola and Marburg may grab more headlines, yellow fever is the "original" viral hemorrhagic fever, untreatable in its clinical course and responsible for over 1,000 times the number of infections and death than these more recent emerging diseases. Yellow fever has been described for centuries, dating back to the 17th century Mayans, who inscribed a manuscript detailing an epidemic of *xekik*, the black vomit. The virus likely evolved from other mosquito-borne viruses approximately 3,000 years ago, probably from Africa from which it was transported to the New World through the slave trade. Despite an effective vaccine, first introduced in the 1930s as derived from the 17D strain from a patient from Ghana, with over 400 million immunized hence worldwide, yellow fever continues to inflict endemic and epidemic disease in sub-Saharan Africa and South America, where vaccination programs are lacking. This is the case in countries such as Liberia. Within the yellow fever belt in Africa (latitude 15° north to 10° south), these developing countries

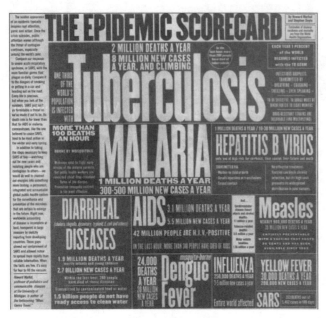

FIGURE 20-2 "The Epidemic Scorecard." *New York Times*, Op-Ed Section, April 30, 2008.

have been targeted by the World Health Organization (WHO) Expanded Program on Immunization (EPI) for decades to support sustainable efforts against a wide range of vaccine-preventable diseases, including yellow fever. Analytic models since the 1990s have advocated for inclusion of yellow fever vaccination in EPI in endemic areas.[5] In Liberia, however, 14 years of civil war through 2003 devastated much of the country's health care infrastructure and severely disrupted public health disease surveillance and immunization programs. Since 1999, Liberia has had a surveillance system sanctioned by the Liberia Ministry of Health (MOH) for eight diseases: acute flaccid paralysis, neonatal tetanus, meningitis, bloody diarrhea, cholera, Lassa fever, measles, and yellow fever. Weekly reports from county health centers filter into Monrovia, comprising an early warning system to monitor incidence patterns of these diseases. Because of ongoing civil conflict, the system had never been fully operational. Laboratory support for the system was minimal, with yellow fever diagnostic capacity first initiated in 2001 through grants from the WHO and the Global Alliance for Vaccine Initiatives. Crippled by lack of reagents, however, testing had never been performed in the country. A resurgence of vaccine-preventable diseases would not be surprising and in reality likely expected.

> *A resurgence of vaccine-preventable diseases would not be surprising and in reality likely expected.*

During the last couple of weeks in January, initial reports of suspected yellow fever in Dr. Otero's patient began to filter back to MOH and aid agencies such as UNICEF and the WHO in Monrovia, prompting the MOH to alert all IDP camp medical personnel, government-run clinics, and nongovernmental organization (NGO) health care systems throughout the country to report all suspected cases with appropriate serum testing to the MOH. By February 13, 2004, the WHO declared an outbreak of yellow fever in Liberia following laboratory confirmation of four cases, three fatal, all with onset of illness between January 1 to 9, 2004, in Bong County and Nimba County, near the Côte d'Ivoire border. The first case as cared for by Dr. Otero had a blood specimen shipped to the nearest diagnostic laboratory for yellow fever at the Institut Pasteur de Côte d'Ivoire in the capital Abidjan. The preliminary serology was negative for IgM anti-yellow fever antibody. A positive anti-yellow fever IgM enzyme-linked immunosorbent assay result in late acute or early convalescent phase, which peaks by the end of the second week of illness and was the time point for which Dr. Otero's patient had his blood drawn for testing, provides a presumptive diagnosis. Demonstration of a rising antibody response from two blood samples collected several weeks apart from each other beginning after onset of illness is confirmatory. This was not an option for Dr. Otero's patient. IgM antibody testing for yellow fever requires exquisite laboratory technique, and the sensitivity of IgM enzyme-linked immunosorbent assay serology is approximately 70%; thus, Dr. Otero's patient's blood was then sent to the Institut Pasteur in Dakar, Senegal for more advanced polymerase chain reaction (PCR) testing. In early February, the PCR test for yellow fever was positive, and by the second week in February, all four cases were likewise confirmed. The WHO considers even one case of confirmed yellow fever worthy of outbreak investigation because of the concern for human-to-human transmission, particularly in urban areas. Two of the four cases occurred in men aged 19 years and Dr. Otero's 26 year old patient living in densely populated IDP camps in Bong County. The WHO announcement of a yellow fever outbreak set in motion an international response to control the epidemic quickly to prevent potential rapid spread to surrounding areas and urban settings.

In the early stages of the outbreak, it was uncertain just where the mosquito-borne sources for yellow fever truly lied. In West Africa, the virus is transmitted in three cycles—a sylvatic or "jungle" cycle, in which transmission occurs between forest-dwelling mosquitoes and nonhuman primates; an intermediate cycle, in which transmission occurs between mosquitoes and both nonhuman primates and humans in moist savanna areas referred to as "emergent zones"; and an urban cycle where it causes large epidemics (Figure 20-3). Urban cycle epidemics develop from anthroponotic, also known as human-to-human, transmission in which humans serve as the sole host reservoir of the peridomestic *Aedes aegypti* mosquito vector. Urban epidemics occur when persons who do not have the tell-tale sign of jaundice but do have virus circulating in their blood (and are not yet severely ill) travel from emergent zones of transmission in jungles and savannas to cities where they infect local *A. aegypti* mosquitoes. This species of mosquito is abundant in urban areas and in areas where humans store water. It was well known that thousands of men in the IDP camps would travel routinely to Monrovia in search of work. Low background prevalence of neutralizing antibody to yellow fever virus in the population because of lack of previous vaccination or naturally acquired infection and poor disease surveillance systems are also contributing factors to epidemics in West Africa. Human-to-human transmission to an urban area such as Monrovia could be ominous. The last urban yellow fever outbreak to hit West Africa occurred in neighboring Abidjan, Cote d'Ivoire just 3 years before in 2001, claiming 14 lives and requiring an emergency immunization campaign to vaccinate 2.6 million people over a 4-week period. Dr. Muireann Brennan, a veteran CDC epidemiologist dispatched to Liberia in late 2003 to supervise EIS officers during a mass immunization campaign of children against measles after the fall and exodus of the Charles Taylor regime, recognized the urgency of this threat. In a February 9 e-mail to Dr. Barry Miller, a director of the arbovirus diseases branch of the CDC in Ft. Collins, CO, Dr. Brennan wrote,

> "Greetings from Liberia. I have a vector question that I hope you can help with. We have suspected yellow fever in Monrovia. We are concerned about 200,000 IDPs living in camps in very crowded conditions with poor sanitation. We also have the population of greater Monrovia. Less crowded but still poor sanitation. We are wondering what would be the most effective vector control measures. We have eight trained sprayers and spraying equipment. What is the best use of these people? How many gallons of 'stuff' do we need and what is the best chemical? Should we save spraying for the IDP camps, near drains and water outlets? Do you have a number I could call you at? My number is *** 47 525 *** thanks, Muireann."

Dr. Miller replied one hour later,

> "Dear Dr. Brennan. I assume you are worried about *Aedes aegypti*. The only effective means of controlling this mosquito is to cover water storage containers and to dump all containers on property that hold water. Spraying is a last ditch effort and it only helps if every residence is sprayed inside. Outdoor spraying is not very effective. Although covering containers that hold water seems simple, getting the population to implement it is not. Mass vaccination with 17D is your best bet in my opinion."

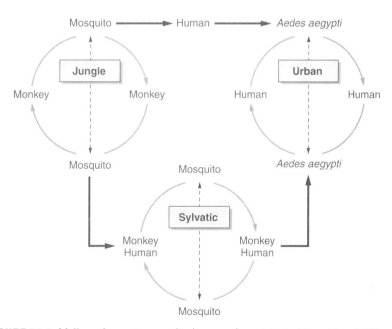

FIGURE 20-3 Yellow fever transmission cycles. Adapted from Monath TP. *Lancet Inf Dis* 2001;1:11–20.

This dialogue is instructive to our understanding of outbreak investigation. Dr. Brennan, in the final throes of the measles mass vaccination campaign, has been watching another soon-to-be-confirmed outbreak unfold and believes identifying, controlling, and eliminating the source of the outbreak should be a top priority. In most classic settings, controlling the source of the epidemic is generally a critical component in outbreak investigations. Dr. Miller, a wisened entomologist, counters though that the source, the ubiquitous *A. aegypti* mosquito, is an entrenched menacing force that will not back down even if a gazillion gallons of "stuff" were carpet-bombed on every field, house, spare tire, and tin can in the area. He essentially tells Dr. Brennan that if you want to best protect the people, do what you do best and start mass immunization with yellow fever 17D vaccine.

CONTROL THE OUTBREAK— YELLOW FEVER MASS VACCINATION

After the worldwide announcement of a yellow fever outbreak on February 13, UNICEF, the WHO, and MSF convened with the Liberian MOH on February 18 to draft an emergency vaccination proposal to immunize the approximately 722,000 Liberians aged 6 months or older at risk for yellow fever in Bong and Nimba counties. The WHO and UNICEF would fund and supervise the effort, whereas MOH, MSF, county public health departments, and other NGOs would implement the campaigns. The plan was split into two phases. Phase I was termed outbreak intervention and divided into two steps. Step 1 encompassed mass vaccination in Salala District IDP camps and their host communities in Bong County, and step 2 outlined mass vaccination for two districts from which two of the confirmed and fatal cases originated in Nimba County. Phase II was designated outbreak prevention to later canvass remaining areas within Bong and Nimba counties for mass immunization not covered during phase I. Though there were many obstacles, two issues predominated before the vaccination campaign launched into action. Where was Liberia going to get the money, and did the country have enough vaccine for such an undertaking? The country was nearly completely dependent on outside aid for most aspects of civil services, including health care, and the Liberia MOH only had 80,000 doses of yellow fever vaccine in stock. As the number of suspect cases climbed to nine (symptoms compatible with yellow fever, but not yet laboratory confirmed), UNICEF and the WHO released a joint statement on February 25 through the WHO Disease Outbreak News network on ProMED mail (a global electronic reporting system for outbreaks of emerging infectious diseases and toxins, http://www.promedmail.org/pls/otn/f?p=2400:1000). They appealed for $1.3 million to cover costs for vaccine and injection materials, operational logistics, and the strengthening of epidemiological surveillance and public awareness.[6] The situation was described as "urgent" with a potential for "exploding to larger populations in displaced persons camps and urban areas" and "even more favourable (conditions) for the disease with the onset of the rainy season in April." The governments of Ireland and Norway pledged financial commitments and the WHO set aside 400,000 doses, approximately one tenth of its entire worldwide supply, for the campaign. The next day, MSF France received 72,000 vaccine and syringe doses with official Liberia Yellow Fever vaccination verification cards from the WHO. UNICEF provided 2 refrigerators, 4 deep freezers, 15 cold ice-pack containers, 32 cool boxes, 991 ice packs, and syringe safety disposal boxes for the initial phase of the campaign at MSF IDP camp clinic facilities and surrounding villages to implement the first phase of the campaign in Bong County, the epicenter of the outbreak. Essential elements to emergency mass vaccination quickly took form.

Operations and Organization

Nine vaccination teams each with six members and one supervisor, comprising public health officials from MSF France, the district hospital, Save the Children, and the Bong County Health Department, were formed and trained in appropriate techniques in yellow fever immunization. Vaccination centers within the four IDP camps where two of the confirmed cases originated, Totota and Maimu I, II, and III, were set up with a registration table, vaccine administration area, and an exit station where vaccine verification cards were documented and distributed. There were two vaccinators per team, with a goal of 300 immunizations delivered per vaccinator. Each member of the team was paid 5 U.S. dollars per day.

Cold Chain System

The yellow fever vaccine is manufactured from live-attenuated virus and unstable at room temperature; maintaining a functional cold chain for vaccine storage between 2°C and 8°C is vital to ensuring potency of the vaccine. Cold chain systems are a series of storage and transport links through a network of refrigerators, freezers, and cold boxes that keep vaccines at a safe temperature throughout their journey (Figure 20-4).

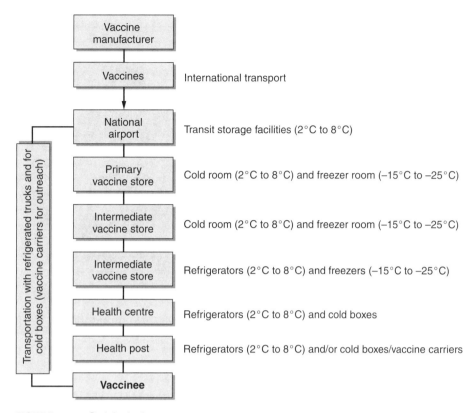

FIGURE 20-4 Cold chain system.

A generator was secured to provide electricity from 5 a.m. to 11p.m. to maintain temperatures in the refrigerators between 0°C and 8°C and < 0°C for the freezers. Supervisors delivered ice packs from the freezers to the field vaccination teams at 2-hour intervals to maintain the cold chain. Each cold box was affixed with a 3M MonitorMark card that served as an in-field alarm system in case the cold box reached temperatures beyond the range recommended for usable vaccine. A cold chain coordinator recorded the temperature of each cold box daily each morning and evening (Figure 20-5).

Social Mobilization

> *Social moblilization is a process that is used to increase awareness of a program and stimulate community participation.*

Social moblilization is a process that is used to increase awareness of a program and stimulate community participation. Social mobilization brings a marketing atmosphere to generate community interest in mass vaccination campaigns. This enterprise began one week before the immunization kick-off date and continuing throughout the campaign. Messengers with megaphones delivered announcements throughout the camps, villages, and even by shelter-to-shelter visits describing the symptoms of yellow fever, modes of spread of the disease, methods to eliminate household mosquito breeding sites, and the need for vaccination. The vaccines were advertised as free of charge. These messages were translated in English and five different local languages (Kpelle, Mende, Loma, Vai, and Southern Kisi). In the town of Totota, a local radio station transmitted details of the disease and campaign. The social mobilization efforts were reinforced midway through the campaign with testimonials by church elders, heads of schools, and other leaders of local institutions. Signs were posted as guideposts to the vaccination sites (Figure 20-6).

Adverse Events Following Immunization

The day before the campaign launch date, vaccination team supervisors were briefed on recognition and reporting of adverse events following immunization (AEFI) by MSF campaign managers. AEFI surveillance is important to preserve the integrity of the campaign and cultivate public confidence overall in immunization programs. Monitoring events related temporally to immunization enable campaign managers to reduce

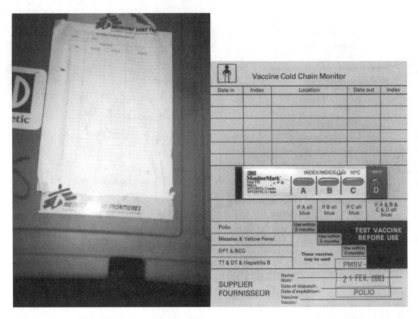

FIGURE 20-5 Cold chain cold boxes and temperature monitoring card.

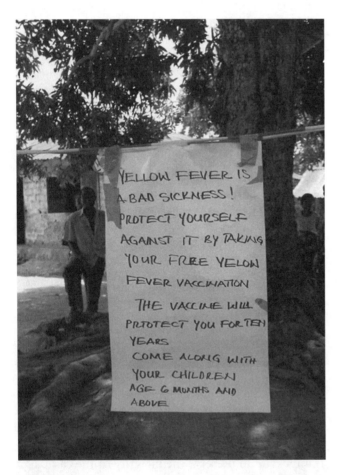

FIGURE 20-6 Social mobilization. Yellow Fever mass vaccination campaign, Liberia, February–March 2004.

risks even further as AEFI are investigated in search of idiopathic reactions versus potential program-related discrepancies in storage and handling of the vaccine, or inconsistencies in vaccine administration technique. Supervisors were instructed to be vigilant for all injection site abscesses, severe reactions such as anaphylaxis, toxic shock, sepsis, encephalitis, febrile jaundice illnesses, and deaths potentially related to immunization within 4 weeks of vaccine receipt. Although rare, viscerotropic and neurotropic reactions, or a fulminant yellow fever infection from the reactivated live attenuated 17D vaccine strain, have resulted in death following yellow fever immunization, primarily in immunocompromised or elderly persons receiving vaccine.[7–16] Given the urgency of the campaign and because screening every vaccine recipient for HIV was not feasible, AEFI surveillance was important to ensure safety and public acceptance of the campaign.

The campaign lasted 10 days, from February 26 to March 6. An extension of the campaign occurred from March 16 to March 20 in two additional Bong County IDP camps, Salala and Tumutu, as well as the town of Salala. Outreach vaccination teams also immunized persons living in outlying villages in Bong County. Two vaccinees developed mild self-limited facial rashes after immunization, and there were no serious AEFI reported. Among the estimated 87,000 population living in the IDP camps, only 47,763 (56.8%) were vaccinated. The vaccination coverage fell far short of the 80% goal, which is believed to be a threshold level for immunoprotection within a community to limit person-to-person transmission of yellow fever.

What happened? The MSF coordinators had several theories. Insecurity in the area with unconfirmed rumblings of rebel activity contributed to lower campaign turnout. Some outlying communities could not be accessed. The rainy season perhaps had restricted movement of some people, and some IDPs and villagers may have been absent from the area as itinerant farmers. The overriding suspicion, however, was that the original target population estimate was too high. Julie Gerberding, director of the CDC, once said in a lecture of the principles of epidemiology, "Anyone can count numbers for the numerator, but the real skill of what makes an epidemiologist a scientist is determining the correct denominator." If the denominator is wrong, then the most well-designed plans, as apparently engineered during this first phase of the emergency yellow fever vaccination campaign, can appear fruitless in the end. Meanwhile, in the middle of the vaccination campaign, before all the final tallies were in, another missive was posted from the WHO Disease Outbreak News network on ProMED Mail on March 11: "A total of 39 suspected cases including 8 deaths are reported to WHO from 5 counties."[17] The outbreak was not yet over and appeared to be claiming more victims.

THE CDC RESPONSE

On February 25, the day before the first phase of the mass vaccination campaign, Angela Kearney, the UNICEF representative to Liberia e-mailed Tony Marfin at the CDC requesting "urgent technical assistance from CDC and specifically the Division of Vector Borne Diseases in controlling a yellow fever outbreak in Liberia, in particular, support in planning and implementing a mass vaccination campaign." Ms. Kearney had already conferred with the WHO and the Liberia MOH, agreeing to a 6-week time period for CDC involvement "as soon as possible."

Tony replied that day after reading the WHO/UNICEF joint proposal that Ms. Kearney had attached to her e-mail:

> I think that you have done a very good job to cover all the aspects of the mass campaign and certainly have addressed the more pressing needs in terms of operational research issues such as AEFI. I see that MOH, WHO, and UNICEF have covered the majority of the work tasks and that the plan enlists the assistance of multiple groups, such as MSF, Africare, and the International Red Cross. With all of this expert assistance already in place, I am a little confused as to what you see as the function of CDC personnel that may participate. I suspect that we are not being asked to partake as another independent partner (too many partners can be as big a problem as too few). It seems that you may be asking us to participate as a UNICEF resource that is being contributed to this effort and that we would be working more directly with UNICEF. That would be a fine paradigm, but I just want to more fully understand if that is correct and what you see as the scope of work. If you would, please clarify for me to whom a senior yellow fever subject matter expert would be reporting. Please pardon my caution. We are always ready to pitch in; it is just when there are so many organizations that we must be sure that we actually have a function when we arrive. One thing that Dr. Brennan may not have mentioned to you was that most of the people in our division work on the surveillance, epidemiology, laboratory, and ecology aspects of yellow fever—more research aspects of the disease and vector control than operational aspects of running a mass yellow fever vaccination campaign. Still, we have some people (including me) that have also overseen the operation of such campaigns and set up surveillance for adverse events. Because we do not have anyone that has regularly performed the logistical activities, our division may be able to provide the senior staff subject matter expert and possibly an experienced EIS officer as team leaders. Then we would work closely with other CDC groups to find people that are much more experienced in the logistical aspects of these campaigns. I will work to get you an answer as quickly as possible.

As a seasoned CDC epidemiologist, Tony exhibits a prescient assessment of UNICEF's request for CDC assistance. One of the CDC's unspoken ground rules for accepting invitations from outside organizations to help investigate outbreaks is that unless otherwise explicitly stated, the locals are in charge. Local officials are central stakeholders in outbreak settings, and the CDC is exquisitely mindful of avoiding any perceptions of commandeering an investigation and undermining the authority of on-the-ground forces and institutions. In seeking clarification of the CDC's proposed role, Tony wanted to ensure that he lined up the right people for the right reason. EIS officers, with burgeoning epidemiologic skills and energy, are usually the right answer. Indeed, Ms. Kearney wanted to bolster UNICEF's support system with EIS officers, a blueprint that had worked so effectively for her in Afghanistan 1 year prior and most recently with measles mass vaccination in Liberia. Tony identified two EIS officer veterinarians from the CDC arboviral branch in Ft. Collins, Colorado, Drs. Susan Montgomery and Jennifer Brown, for the assignment. Both had worked tirelessly in the United States on surveillance for West Nile virus that was sweeping the country during 2002 to 2003 and were ready for an international field experience. Sue was in my EIS class, and I knew her well from shared experiences with West Nile virus. I had not yet worked with Jen. Both were scheduled to arrive in the capital Monrovia on Monday, March 15. As the senior EIS officer, Sue would assist in the interpretation of the yellow fever surveillance data, review appropriateness of the response, coordinate activities among Liberia MOH, UNICEF, the WHO, and any other partners, and assess laboratory capacity for in-country diagnosis of acute yellow fever—all in 8 days. Conversely, Jen had a 33-day itinerary to more intensely participate in yellow fever disease surveillance activities and enhance AEFI surveillance, as well as assist in any possible vaccine coverage surveys. Once travel documents and security clearance were obtained for Sue and Jen, Tony replied to Ms. Kearney on Friday, March 12, "We have had some difficulty identifying someone with campaign experience who could help in performance of the vaccination campaign for 4–6 weeks, but we will keep working on this part this weekend." Tony had told me to keep my bags packed later that week after our serendipitous phone conversation on May 8. The "shoe-leather epidemiology" that the EIS prides itself often allows officers to assert themselves in unfamiliar situations. Tony assured me, "I know you can handle it. You know the place." Apparently I was the guy with mass vaccination campaign experience. I had never seen, let alone helped organize, a mass vaccination campaign as far as I was aware.

The duo from Ft. Collins had 3 weeks to prepare for the deployment. I had 1 week, tentatively scheduled to depart March 15. The day after my initial phone conversation with Tony, I drove up to the Great Lakes Naval Training Base, about 30 miles north of Chicago, which was considered the commissioned corps' local health center. Along with malaria prophylaxis, I received three catchup vaccines, quadrivalent meningococcal, typhoid, and of course, yellow fever. I needed emergency visas and country clearance from the respective embassies of Côte d'Ivoire and Liberia (there were limited commercial flights into Liberia and local air carriers usually routed through Côte d'Ivoire or Ghana), government travel orders from the United States (granted only after country clearances were obtained), and a seat on a flight. For a tour of duty slated for 30 days, I packed rather light—some clothes, cash (no traveler's checks, Liberia was a cash economy, with the U.S. dollar as the hard currency), bug spray and a mosquito net, 90 energy bars (three a day, just in case), my laptop with the season 1 DVD collection of "Curb Your Enthusiasm," and my old St. Joseph's Catholic Hospital ID card for those unforeseen instances when I might need a little "street cred" (Figure 20-7). By the morning of March 15, I had no Liberian country clearance and therefore no travel orders. A cable from Monrovia was sent to the CDC at 11:54 a.m. for my country clearance. At 12:20 p.m., my travel orders were secured. On a freezing day in Chicago at 2:00 p.m., I was out the door and on a 5:45 p.m. flight to Paris and then on to Abidjan for an overnight stay until touching down in Monrovia 2 days behind Sue and Jen on March 17. As I looked down from my window seat on the plane flying over the tropical savanna into Liberia, I felt a sense of hopefulness.

UNICEF had arranged rooms at the Mamba Point Hotel, in the heart of the diplomatic district in Monrovia. Bungalow style, it was nice and clean, with air conditioning, satellite television, and a full-service restaurant. The spread probably ranked between 2 to 3 stars by U.S. standards. It was touted as one of the premier hotels in Liberia. At $120 U.S. a night, it was outlandishly expensive. Despite the breezy beaches across the street, this stretch of real estate, or really anywhere else in Liberia, could not be considered a tourist destination. Most guests were foreign aid workers, journalists, or diplomats, with governments or NGOs footing the bill. A good proportion of the room rate was in fact for shadow security, imperative in this still volatile country. Romeo, an engaging Liberian in his 30s, was

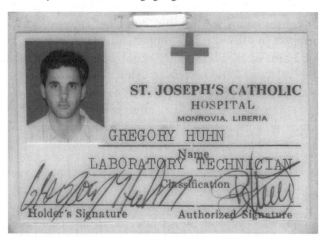

FIGURE 20-7 St. Joseph's Catholic Hospital identification card, 1990.

the desk manager and chief broker agent for the folk art street hawkers outside the lobby. His easy smile and animated graciousness brought back my recollections of an otherwise friendly people who were pulled and mangled by tribal-based conflicts, ultimately manipulated into brutality by ruthless and greedy warlords.

I checked in, took a quick shower, and headed to the UNICEF compound down the street to start digging into our roles in the yellow fever outbreak. I first met with Dr. Bjorn Forssen, the UNICEF emergency medical officer from Sweden, and Ms. Carmen Michielin, the UNICEF staff security officer from South Africa, for a security briefing. An international peacekeeper force, with the characteristic blue helmets, patrolled most all major cities in Liberia, including Monrovia, as authorized by the United Nations Mission in Liberia (UNMIL). UNMIL was established by the U.N. Security Council resolution 1509 in late September 2003 to support the ceasefire agreement and peace process; protect United Nations staff, facilities, and civilians; support humanitarian and human rights activities; as well as assist in national security reform, including national police training and formation of a new, restructured military.[18] In Monrovia, the national police force had disintegrated, replaced by an international civilian police contingent called CIVPOL.[19] There were reports of kidnappings and even cannibalism of both Liberians and expatriates, so, Carmen encouraged us to always use a UNICEF security escort when walking or traveling at night in Monrovia. Eleven thousand peacekeepers were in place by the time we arrived, but 15,000 were needed to secure the borders. There were still active rebel incursions from the Côte d'Ivoire border in Nimba County in the eastern part of the country, where the other two confirmed yellow fever cases were detected. To implement the next step of the mass vaccination campaign, targeting the population of Nimba County, we would need an UNMIL military escort while in the field. The Bangladeshi UNMIL unit stationed in the Nimba County capital of Sanniquellie was alerted of our intention to start the campaign imminently. Radio call-ins every hour to UNICEF offices in Monrovia would be required to provide updated security situation reports (known as SitReps) during our field operations. I left the meeting with a UNICEF symbol embossed certificate stating, "Gregory Huhn has successfully completed Basic Security in the Field—Staff Safety, Health, and Welfare" and quickly realized why we received an extra few hundred bucks in commissioned corps hazardous incentive pay for "hostile fire/imminent danger" during our assignment here in Liberia.

During the first couple of days before I arrived, Sue and Jen had been reviewing the line list of suspected yellow fever cases reported since January. A suspect case was defined as acute onset of fever followed by jaundice within 2 weeks of onset of first symptoms. Several were already IgM antibody negative for yellow fever, yet were still counted as suspect cases. The chief WHO surveillance medical officer, Dr. Mekonnen Admassu from Ethiopia, maintained that these may have been true yellow fever infections with IgM antibodies that had waned. The IgM antibodies usually persist for 30 to 60 days after acute illness and then decline over several months.[20] The case definition for confirmed cases used by WHO in Liberia also included an "epidemiologically linked" category. To EIS officers disciplined in precision in tracking West Nile virus cases, this extension of the case definition appeared unsound in the arboviral world and prone to over inflation of the true case rate. Tony was in daily e-mail communication with our team for the first week and put this practice into context:

> This is exactly what many countries do. They use a syndromic case definition for surveillance to add cases, but do not use serology or PCR results to remove cases. This is the way you end up with a lot of P. *falciparum* malaria on the list. Epi-linked is exactly as you state.... There is a geographic and temporal relationship between a person who meets the surveillance case definition and a person with a serologically confirmed case of yellow fever.... This is the part that is often left out. What happens is you have someone with fever and jaundice and they get added to the case list. Then the sister or some other family relative gets ill (not always fever and jaundice) a week later and they get added to the list because of the relationship to a case that was never confirmed. It is not wrong to continue to emphasize the importance of lab confirmation. If there were many hundreds of cases and the first 25–50 cases were serologically confirmed as the "real deal," then no one would have a problem doing syndromic surveillance beyond that point. But, what happened in Cote d'Ivoire and it sounds like it may be happening here is there are 'some' cases and only some of those are serologically or PCR confirmed. Then syndromic surveillance with a highly sensitive and unspecified specificity starts to run the program...even though many of them turn out to be negative on serology.

By the time I arrived to meet Sue and Jen at the UNICEF offices, the two of them had pressed the WHO and UNICEF surveillance leadership, which also included Dr. Nuhu Maksa from Nigeria, UNICEF Project Officer for Nutrition and Health, on tightening up to a more specific case definition, to delete at least the IgM-negative cases. Our overtures we could sense hovered among this multinational team with mild skepticism (change can sometimes move as slow as a goat roast in this equatorial land). We were nonetheless ready to then concentrate our efforts on the second step of immunization campaign targeting high-risk populations in Nimba County. Two days into my time in Liberia, Jen and I had finished a new case investigation form emphasizing duration and onset of symptoms and dates for yellow fever acute and convalescent serology submission for public health officials in Nimba County. I had the opportunity to pilot this form as I was called to investigate a case of a 2-year-old boy from Monrovia hospitalized at an MSF clinic down the road from the UNICEF office. Five days after onset of symptoms, primarily dyspnea, the boy developed fevers and then 7 days later jaundice and hematemesis. He died 1 day later. Yellow fever serology was submitted to MOH on the day of death. I spoke with his parents just after he died. The boy did not spend any recent time outside Monrovia. The working diagnosis was pneumonia. We learned later that the yellow fever serology was negative.

Within the first couple of days in Liberia, I bought a cell phone. Minutes could be bought freely from calling cards on sale at many outposts throughout the city without a contract. Although much of the country was physically in decay, Liberia was as wireless as any developed nation. Advances in communications technology, from our Internet hookups at our UNICEF office to our slick cell phones, were quite a revelation for me when looking back to my past experience in the country 14 years prior. We were without any communications except for a fuzzy ham radio for my last 6 weeks during the battles around our hospital in 1990. Now I was able to call my wife daily from most anywhere (except the deepest parts of the bush), preferably from across the street of the Mamba Point Hotel, on the beach next to a lobster shack. With our reliable Ethernet connection, I also downloaded and printed a chapter from a WHO website on how to organize a mass vaccination campaign. Acquiring on-the-fly expert-level knowledge by sometimes unconventional means becomes almost instinctual for EIS officers in the field. I read it on the 6-hour jeep ride out to Nimba County to commence our roles as supervisors in phase I, step 2 of the campaign.

As Sue wrapped up her reports on yellow fever surveillance and a summary of diagnostic laboratory capacity she had researched in Monrovia (there essentially was none, so Dr. Juliet Bryant, an arboviral biochemist from Ft. Collins, was summoned later in April to revive the yellow fever lab), Jen and I set out for Sanniquellie on Sunday, March 20 after receiving UNICEF security travel clearance. We went shopping the day before at a Monrovia market as if we were provisioning for a Yosemite hiking trip. We bought a camping stove, canned and dried foods, peanut butter, cheese sticks, crackers, bottled water, and toilet paper. I also brought along a good bulk of my energy bars. We stayed at a hostel across the street from the Bangladeshi UNMIL compound. The place was fairly sparse, outfitted with a few single bedrooms with plug-in fans, clean sheets, and a shared hallway bathroom. Electricity ran during the day, but not at night. A patio out front served as our commissary where we sparked up our stove for bean or soup dinners. Our hostel hosts provided a cooler of cold beers, which actually creates a relaxing tonic as you snooze away under the mosquito net in the humid hot nighttime air. The buzz also probably took the edge off those vivid dreams that usually accompanied my weekly dose of mefloquine malaria prophylaxis.

On Monday, March 22, we met up with the Bangladeshi UNMIL team and traveled out with our WHO and UNICEF colleagues to supervise the mass vaccination activities just underway as coordinated by MSF Holland and Swiss, Liberia MOH, and the Nimba County public health department. As compared with the recent mass immunization in Bong County, there were no IDP camps in Nimba County. Rather, vaccination sites were decentralized throughout towns and villages in the two high-risk districts of Zoegeh and Gbehleygeh. The Zoegeh district was demarcated into two zones based on security factor; a western zone comprised an estimated population of 35,000, and an eastern zone was bordering Côte d'Ivoire with an estimated 15,000 target population. The eastern zone was essentially off-limits to foreign NGOs and international aid groups such as UNICEF and the WHO because of ongoing cross-border armed skirmishes; therefore, the MOH conducted the immunization campaign in this area. The target population for the Gbelaygeh district was 75,000 for a planned 10-day campaign. The WHO provided vaccines, and the same mass vaccination organization structure employed in Bong County was instituted in the Nimba County campaign; however, the nature of village life provided obstacles not encountered in the Bong County IDP camps. Terrain was rugged and there were no paved roads village to village (Figure 20-8). The largest towns along the perimeter of the district

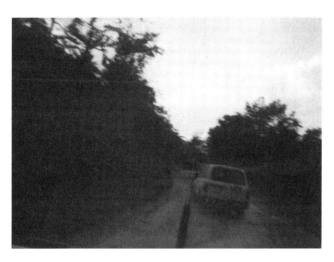

FIGURE 20-8 UNMIL Bangladeshi unit escort in Zoeheh District, Nimba County, Liberia.

zones were selected as vaccination sites to create accessibility to the villages' populations. Still, many villagers had to walk 2 hours to get to a vaccination center, particularly taxing on older people. Satellite vaccination sites were then created by mobile vaccination teams to reach out to some of these outlying villages (Figure 20-9).

There were disagreements over money transfers between UNICEF and the WHO to the MSF, MOH, and local public health department teams that did the actual implementation of the mass vaccination in the western Zoegeh district. Rumors stirred that some county public health vaccinator teams "boycotted" the campaign over these financial disputes, resulting in poor social mobilization and low campaign turnout rates in some areas.

Inconsistencies in vaccine delivery systems were uncovered. Standard multidose vials for WHO 17D yellow fever vaccines are reconstituted with 10 cc of diluent and administered as 0.5-cc subcutaneous injections. Vaccinators in the Gbelaygeh district campaign disclosed to supervisors 3 days into the campaign that the diluent vials contained 12 cc of solution, allowing 24 injections per vial. After consultation, we recommended that vaccinators first draw up 2 cc from the diluent vial, waste it, and then proceed with resuspension with 10 cc for proper dilution concentration. Vaccinators in the Zoegeh western district were already

> *Inconsistencies in vaccine delivery systems were uncovered.*

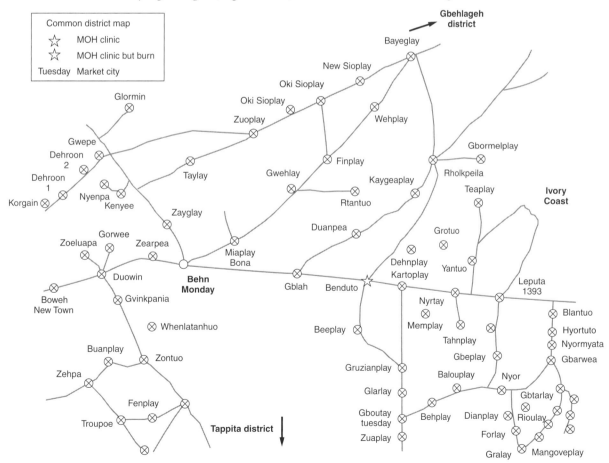

FIGURE 20-9 Map of towns and villages, Zoegeh District, Nimba County, Liberia.

6 days into the campaign, and 49% of target population had been immunized by this time, when this correction was applied in that campaign as well. Minimal potency requirements established by WHO for standard yellow fever vaccine exceed the 90% immunizing dose by fivefold; therefore, it was unlikely that the excess dilution affected vaccine immunogenicity.[21]

The cold chain system in Gbehlaygeh campaign was particularly imperiled. "Running on the limits of what was acceptable," according to Steven de Bock, chief logistician for MSF Holland. Approximately one third of the large cold boxes supplied by the public health department for vaccine storage in the field vaccination sites were defective and could not close and lock properly. Six different sizes of ice packs, rather than a uniformly sized ice pack, made loading of the cold boxes awkward, leading to "unnecessary delays, confusion, and inefficient use of the cold chain equipment," by De Bock's account. Perhaps most distressing was the mystery surrounding the whereabouts of essential heavy equipment. UNICEF apparently promised MSF Holland a freezer and generator to be stationed in the district capital town of Karnplay, population 11,000, as the central ice pack and vaccine storage center. They never showed up. (We were later informed that the equipment had been destroyed in heavy fighting in the rebel stronghold town of Ganta in 2003). MSF Holland improvised, renting two freezers and a generator at a local bar, but they were in need of renovation. De Bock rehabbed the equipment, but the generator broke down after the first day of the campaign. The head MSF office in Monrovia quickly sent a new generator up to Karnplay the next day; however, the largest refrigerator on site gave out by the third day of the campaign. De Bock simply stated, "There was no room for error." As supervisors, we observed watery ice packs shuttled from Sanniquellie every 2 hours by car to Karnplay and then onto to vaccination sites in villages by car or bicycle. There were no temperature-monitoring cards on the cold boxes, and only a few thermometers were spotted to accurately record cold box temperatures. Even our jeep limped into one of the villages with a flat tire, burning fumes on a near empty tank of gas. Pulling up to a lean-to gas station, a jack and a patch, along with petrol poured from recycled beer bottles that were sitting on a rickety table, got us back on our way (Figure 20-10). Through improvisation and grit, the logisticians displayed the resiliency and resourcefulness vital to public health emergency operations.

In regards to AEFI, surveillance was erratic, and some public health department vaccination teams believed that an emphasis on AEFI reporting actually un-

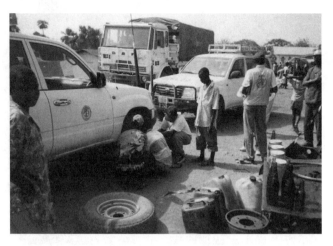

FIGURE 20-10 Gas station in Gbehlaygeh District, Nimba County, Liberia.

dermined their credibility as protectors of public health and deterred villagers from participating in the immunization campaign. We attempted to reinforce the importance of AEFI surveillance with tutorials on proper case form completion during our daily supervisory visits to vaccination centers. Ultimately, there were no AEFIs reported nor any other suspect yellow fever cases identified during the western district Zoegeh and Gbehlaygeh campaigns. We were not in communication with the MOH campaign in the eastern district of Zoegeh. We felt that no news was probably good news. If there happened to be an unfortunate breach in safety, we thought we would have heard about it.

Despite setbacks, there was success. Vaccinations started promptly at 6:30 a.m. at most sites. With four vaccinators per site, people sped through waiting lines and could make it back off into the farms for their usual daily routine (Figure 20-11). Among the target population of 75,000, 66,469 (87%) people were immunized.

By March 25 in the western Zoegeh district, 23,680 among the 35,000 target population (67.5%) had been immunized. There had been efforts to mobilize the population to get vaccinated (social mobilization). We were uncertain how adequate those efforts had been. Jen and I developed a rapid coverage survey to determine whether lapses in social mobilization efforts may have given rise to disproportionate vaccination rates among various communities. A survey such as the one we performed here is useful to better understand the initial tally data collected at the vaccination site registration tables because it is important to ensure that resources have adequately been dedicated to all at-risk populations. We selected three villages within a 45-minute to 2-hour walking distance from one of the five main vaccination sites as a convenience sample (Figure 20-9). Holding true to our principle that the locals always need to be en-

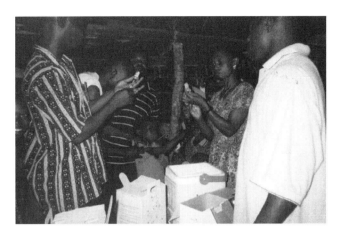 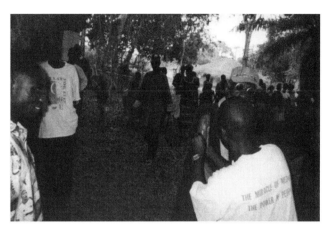

FIGURE 20-11 Young boy and elderly man immunized with 17D Yellow Fever Vaccine in Gbehlaygeh District, Nimba County, Liberia, in March 2004.

gaged and sign off on our activities, we met with village elders in roundtable sessions to explain our intentions and reinforce the importance of controlling yellow fever in their communities. We visited 10 houses in each village. We asked the head of the household how many people lived in the house 6 months of age or more, if they heard about the yellow fever vaccination campaign, whether they did get vaccinated, and if not vaccinated, what were the reasons. Two villages ranked 86.8% and 99.2% vaccination coverage, respectively. A mobile vaccination had been deployed to each of these communities for at least one day. A third village, Gweley, showed a dismal vaccination rate, 2.4%, primarily because of lack of awareness of the campaign, inaccessibility to a vaccination center, and the expectation that vaccination teams would come to their community as had previously occurred during polio eradication campaigns year ago (Table 20-1). Our suspicions were confirmed. Based on

TABLE 20-1 Yellow Fever Convenience Coverage Survey, Zoegeh District, Western Zone, Nimba County, Liberia

	GWELEY VILLAGE				
Number	Number of Family Members Older than 6 Months	Is the Family Aware About the Ongoing Yellow Fever Campaign?	Number of Family Members Vaccinated with Card	Number of Family Members Unvaccinated	Core Reason for Nonvaccination
1	15	Y	0	15	Access
2	7	Y	1	6	Waiting for vaccinators
3	8	Y	1	7	Access
4	20	N	0	20	Do not know about it
5	8	N	0	8	Access
6	10	N	0	10	Access
7	15	N	1	14	Access
8	29	N	0	29	Access
9	5	N	0	5	Access
10	7	N	0	7	Access
Total	124	3	3	121	Access
Percentage	100	30.00	2.42	97.58	Access

(continues)

TABLE 20-1 Continued

ZAYGLAY VILLAGE

Number	Number of Family Members Older than 6 Months	Is the Family Aware About the Ongoing Yellow Fever Campaign?	Number of Family Members Vaccinated with Card	Number of Family Members Unvaccinated	Core Reason for Nonvaccination
1	12	Y	12	0	N/A
2	8	Y	7	1	Was absent
3	9	Y	9	0	N/A
4	10	Y	10	0	N/A
5	15	Y	15	0	N/A
6	8	Y	8	0	N/A
7	10	Y	10	0	N/A
8	20	Y	20	0	N/A
9	20	Y	20	0	N/A
10	12	Y	12	0	N/A
Total	124	10	123	1	N/A
Percentage	100	100.00	99.19	0.81	N/A

GBLAH VILLAGE

Number	Number of Family Members Older than 6 Months	Is the Family Aware About the Ongoing Yellow Fever Campaign?	Number of Family Members Vaccinated with Card	Number of Family Members Unvaccinated	Core Reason for Nonvaccination
1	14	Y	14	0	N/A
2	7	Y	6	1	Was absent
3	7	Y	7	0	N/A
4	6	Y	6	0	N/A
5	6	Y	6	0	Was absent
6	12	Y	10	2	N/A
7	10	Y	6	4	Were absent
8	15	Y	15	0	Access
9	25	Y	25	0	Access
10	27	Y	17	10	Were absent
Total	129	10	112	17	Were absent
Percentage	100.00	100.00	86.82	13.18	

these results, MSF Swiss agreed to provide vaccine and cold chain supplies to the MOH to extend the campaign during March 27 to 29 for these uncovered communities, resulting in 32,318 persons (92.3%) overall receiving immunization. For me, a truly astonishing figure emerged from our study—the absolute value of our coveted denominator. As epidemiologists, we treasure the denominator, but sometimes lose sight of the intimate witness that it may bear. Through our treks into rather sparse and withered two to three room homes, the median household size was about 12 people. Households numbering 20 or more residents were not uncommon. Village life, the poverty, and the family commitments that solidify a community in times of strife, peace, and disease can be breathtaking.

REASSESSMENT–BACK TO BONG COUNTY

After 8 days supervising the campaign in Nimba County, Jen and I returned to our UNICEF base in Monrovia to update ourselves on case surveillance and review options for a catchup campaign in Bong County, where coverage rates fell far below threshold goals. Sue had flown back to the United States during our sojourn in Sanniquellie, and as she regrouped with the CDC powers in Ft. Collins, an understanding of where our Liberia work fit into a bigger picture, with global political implications, began to emerge.

Liberia was still smoldering with guns and disillusionment. Young uneducated fighters had spent most of their formative years simmering in a cesspool of violence, without the moral playbook that formal schooling can often provide. Quickly after Charles Taylor's exile in late 2003, the United Nations Development Programme established a multidisciplinary international mandate, DDRR (Disarmament, Demobilization, Reintegration, Rehabilitation), to disarm the approximately 80,000 combatants throughout the country to reeducate and reintroduce these factions into society. Launched in December 2003, DDRR's credibility had been challenged by the time we showed up in mid March with a high number of ex-fighters registered, exceeding preparatory estimates, although with a sub par number of weapons confiscated.[22] With few weapons confiscated, the term "disarmament" became a worrisome misnomer within the international donor community.

Sue was now preparing to testify with Muireann Brennan and Tony in Washington, DC to a USAID Office of Foreign Disaster Assistance (OFDA) panel on the success of yellow fever control in Liberia and need for long-term support of vaccine-preventable disease programs. OFDA had also been keeping close tabs on DDRR and was concerned that DDRR had thus far failed. UNICEF, United Nations Development Programme's subsidiary, was largely responsible for executing many of DDRR's objectives. Thus, funding of our work depended on perception from those far away. There was concern that DDRR was not getting its job done. Therefore, reassurance was needed that we were getting our job done. Sue wrote in a March 29 e-mail to us, "My impression was that OFDA was reluctant to fund UNICEF since they seemed to be dropping the ball on that program so why would the vaccine program be a success?" As UNICEF received extensive funding from USAID for their overall activities in Liberia, offering a compelling narrative from U.S. commissioned corps officers on the scene could prove persuasive. Yet could we really call our efforts a success with the wimpy Bong County numerators dangling like stale cassava in a dry harvest line? Recall that among the estimated 87,000 population living in the IDP camps of Bong County, only 47,763 (56.8%) were vaccinated and that the vaccination coverage goal was at least 80%.

Dr. William Perea, from the communicable diseases emergency operations division of the WHO, had just arrived in Monrovia from Geneva, Switzerland to provide further expertise on control of the epidemic. The question now was if there was still an outbreak? This was an issue because by March 30 the WHO reported 46 suspect cases from eight counties; however, 31 cases were IgM negative, and the initial four confirmed cases from the first 2 weeks in January were the only confirmed cases. The outbreak may have been over; therefore, a shift toward absorbing yellow fever immunization resources into routine EPI throughout the country began to germinate among the WHO and UNICEF leadership. Jen compiled a summary presentation of the mass vaccination campaigns, and I was designated to create a strategic plan with a budget for yellow fever immunization EPI integration. I had some bystander experience at the Illinois Department of Public Health in pandemic influenza planning, which accelerated during 2003 with the SARS experience, although now potentially millions of dollars in funding appeared riding on my rudimentary bookkeeping aptitude. Yet, being epidemiologists, we were still hung up on the less than satisfying numbers calculated out of the Bong County campaign. We needed some rational consensus before we could sensibly close the book on Bong County and declare victory.

Toward the end of the perceived finish line in outbreak investigations, fatigue often sets in among the pertinent players. You just want to move on to the next outbreak, those unfinished manuscripts lingering on your desk, or that cold caipirinha your wife poured up that's tantalizingly within reach back home. Dr. Perea reenergized our focus to examine the attributes of the campaigns and take one of the last steps in an outbreak investigation, the outcome assessment. He encouraged formulating a strategy to formally survey vaccination coverage in Bong County. On April 1, Jen and I met for the first time with Dr. Otero, who too was troubled with the low calculated vaccination rate. He spent 3 days after the campaign going shelter-to-shelter looking for yellow vaccination cards and found most occupants had one. The IDP camps were built in 2002 and administered by the Liberian government through the Liberia Refugee Repatriation and Resettlement Commission. Food was supplied by the World Food Programme (WFP). The last government census in Liberia occurred in 1984.[23,24] MSF France wanted to perform a census of the Bong County IDP camps, but was not granted permission by the Liberia Refugee Repatriation and Resettlement Commission or the WFP. A WFP formula of five persons per shelter was used to estimate the camp population. But how was this formula derived?

As a denominator detective, I finally learned of its rather imprecise origins about 6 weeks after we left Liberia in an e-mail reply to my inquiry with the WFP. "There seems to be a general agreement that the average family size in Liberia is 5 to 6," and "on average, the shelters in Liberia IDP camps are 4 × 5 meters, well below recommended area per person," according to Alfred Nabeta, a representative for the WFP director in Liberia (Figure 20-12). Mr. Nabeta added this:

> In the camp environment, there are some cases of families that are compelled to occupy more than one shelter because they cannot fit in one single shelter. In addition to the prevalence of large nuclear families, perhaps the other thing that tends to have a bearing on the family sizes in reality is the very strong bond between the nuclear family and the extended family.

Long ago I realized that if you want the real dirt on a new town, ask a cab driver what's really going down in the place. Jefferson Cooper, our trusted driver from UNICEF, took an interest in what we were doing in these IDP camps. When we told him we wanted to survey people in their shelters, he said, "If you want to really know how many IDPs actually occupy a shelter, ask them how many people sleep there overnight. Otherwise, if you ask them how many people just live there, they're used to getting that question from the WFP and will always give a higher number because more people means more food rations." In developing countries, a reliable driver can be more

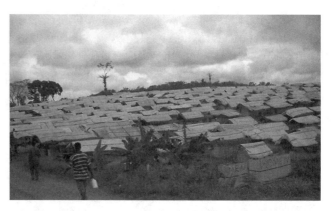

FIGURE 20-12 Physical design and spatial location of shelters in IDP camps, Salala District, Bong County, Liberia.

> *If you want to really know how many IDPs actually occupy a shelter, ask them how many people sleep there overnight.*

valuable to your well-being than potable water, vaccines, or the "tourista" antibiotics you pack along. Road accidents kill more expatriates than exotic diseases. Thus, Mr. Cooper was doing double duty for us as both our eyes on the road and epidemiologic mole. I felt like deputizing him as an honorary EIS officer for his inscrutable insight.

Jen and I devised a two-prong attack to determine vaccination coverage in IDP camps and outlying host communities. For the IDP camps, I designed a two-stage cluster sampling survey with the assistance of local maps and registration logs of habitable shelters in each of the six camps.[25] Each camp was partitioned into alphabetical blocks, and each shelter within each block was given a sequential integer number. Each of the 17,384 total shelters in these six camps had a unique identification that included the camp name, a block letter, and a shelter number. Sample size was calculated based on 5% allowable margin of error. The design effect was equal to one because one person per shelter cluster was to be randomly selected for the survey. We chose the conjectured vaccination coverage rate to be 80%, the threshold that is believed to eliminate the likelihood of human-to-human transmission.[26,27] Sample size was calculated by a standard random cluster formula[28]:

$$(t^2)(\text{design effect})(\text{coverage rate})(1 - \text{coverage rate})/(\text{margin of error})^2 =$$
$$248 \text{ persons } [t = 1.96 \text{ for } 95\% \text{ level of confidence}]$$

As a contingency for missing persons in selected shelter households, an additional 5% (12 persons) were added for a total sample size of 260.

The sum total of all shelters ($n = 17{,}384$) served as the overall denominator for the population. At the first stage, we constructed a single sampling frame (x) among all six camps by using an alphabetical and numerical hierarchy of shelter addresses to create a linear list of all shelters. Thus, the first cluster on the list was shelter A1 from Totota camp and the 17,384th and final cluster was shelter D361 from Tumutu camp (Figure 20-13). We divided the total number of shelters by the sample size ($17{,}384/260 = 67$) to determine an interval-sampling instrument (r) to select shelter clusters systematically. A two-digit number x, between 01 and r, from a random number table was chosen as the first sampling point on the frame, with subsequent points provided by $x + r$, $x + 2r$, $x + 3r$, etc., until $x + 259r$. Wherever a point fell on the cumulative shelter population list, that shelter was assigned as a cluster. The number of clusters chosen per camp was proportional to camp size.

The second stage sampling was performed on site. Persons aged 6 months or more living in the shelter were assigned a number based on their height, from the shortest person in the shelter to the tallest. We invoked the newly minted "Jefferson Cooper" definition of a person considered to be a household member if he or she routinely slept overnight in the shelter during the vaccination campaign. Household members present during the survey supplied height estimates for absent persons who lived in the shelter. One person per shelter cluster was randomly chosen for the survey using a random number table. No replacement of shelters or persons in shelters occurred during the survey.

Approval for the survey was granted by local authorities in the Liberia Refugee Repatriation and Resettlement Commission. A standardized questionnaire in English eliciting demographic information, household size, awareness of the yellow fever vaccination campaign, yellow fever vaccination status, and reports of AEFI was distributed to 12 teams of interviewers. In addition, a signed and dated yellow fever vaccination card was requested from each person who was interviewed. Each team consisted of three to four interviewers proficient in English and at least five of the other local languages spoken by a substantial majority of IDPs in the camps. We formed one team from each camp among local MSF and county public health department workers and trained them in the use of the questionnaire by role playing on April 4. Our UNICEF and WHO colleagues joined us as supervisors on the teams. On my team, I had two local MSF workers who were also IDPs in one of the Maimu camps. Both were college educated, yet their career paths had been derailed by the civil war. They told me that the IDPs were issued tarpaulins, and then each had to build their own shelters to reside in the camps (Figure 20-14).

During April 5 to 7, teams conducted face-to-face interviews with randomly selected survey participants. Questionnaires were translated as needed. If an absent adult was selected, the survey team queried present household members to schedule a return appointment based on the availability of the selected adult. If after 3 consecutive days the selected adult remained unavailable, a present household member was surveyed as a proxy regarding the adult's information. If a young child was selected, a present adult household member was surveyed as a proxy about the young child's information. Oral, informed consent was obtained from all respondents before interviews. To minimize response bias of

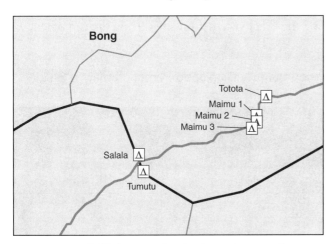

FIGURE 20-13 IDP (internally displaced person) camps, Salala District, Bong County, Liberia.

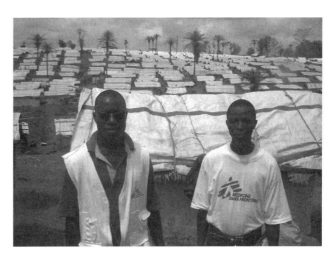

FIGURE 20-14 Medecins Sans Frontieres survey team, Maimu IDP camp, Salala District, Bong County, Liberia.

overreporting household size, respondents were clearly informed that the survey was not linked to a registration or food-distribution process.

Of the 260 shelters we visited, one of the 260 shelters did not exist. Among the 259 existing shelters, 22 were either unoccupied for 3 successive days during the survey (15 shelters) or were incomplete shelters that were not yet inhabited (seven shelters). Data were analyzed for 237 survey respondents (one person per shelter). There were no missing data from IDPs surveyed and no AEFI reported.

We drove in and out from Monrovia daily for about a 2.5-hour trip each way, and thus, I was able to enter data from our survey forms and analyze it in real time using Epi Info.[29] The median number of household members living in a shelter was four (range, 1–8). We estimated that 69,536 persons lived in these six camps, or 20% less than the WFP-based estimate of 87,000 used before the campaign. This disparity in the denominator was the greatest factor in the low vaccination rates initially tabulated through the onsite administrative tally data sheets. The median age of respondents was 20 years (Table 20-2); of the 237 respondents, one half ($n = 119$) were aged 15 to 44 years. Females outnumbered males by an almost 2:1 ratio (Table 20-3).

Of the 237 respondents, 230 (97.6%) were informed of the vaccination campaign; 215 (91.9%) had been vaccinated during the campaign by their self-report, and 196 (83.5%) possessed a signed and dated vaccination card from the recent campaign. Self-reported vaccination rates were highest in the 5- to 14-year age group (94.8%) and lowest in the 15- to 44-year age group (89.7%) (Table 20-4). Gender distribution was similar among vaccinated versus unvaccinated respondents ($P = 0.63$), and no difference existed in the median age among respondents reporting vaccination (aged 20 years) during the campaign compared with unvaccinated respondents (aged 21 years) ($P = 0.86$).

Among 22 unvaccinated respondents, 8 (38%) did not participate in the campaign because of prior yellow fever vaccination within the past 10 years; 5 (24%) stated that they were unaware of the campaign, and 5 (24%) stated that vaccination was "inconvenient." Two respondents were absent from the IDP camps during the campaign, and one respondent had no access to the vaccination site. One respondent provided no explanation. Including respondents reporting prior yellow fever vaccination within the past 10 years with the persons with self-reported recent vaccination, 223 respondents (94.8%) were immunized against yellow fever.

Our study had at least four limitations that may have affected data interpretation. First, some interviews were conducted by proxy; however, proxy interviewees were members of the same shelter and usually very familiar with the demographic and vaccination status of the selected person. Second, proof of vaccination was not obtained from 19 persons (9%) who claimed to have been immunized during the campaign, which may have introduced recall bias. This occurred most commonly when an absent person was selected and their vaccination card was unavailable either because the card was locked with their personal belongings inside the shelter or the absent person had taken the card with them outside the camp for documentation if traveling on main roads, registering for school, or seeking medical treatment. Also, because no other vaccination programs occurred within the IDP camps during the yellow fever immunization campaign, bias by inadvertently attributing yellow fever immunization to another vaccine was likely diminished. For these reasons, self-report or proxy report of vaccination was considered an adequate indicator of immunization status. Third, although we verified the dates and county of vaccination in 2004 for nearly all (> 90%) survey participants because data were not available on the validated vaccination cards specifying the exact vaccination site during the campaign, we

TABLE 20-2 Age and Yellow Fever Vaccination Status Among Internally Displaced Persons Living in Salala District, Bong County, Liberia, 2004

Population (Number)	Age (Years)*		
	Median	Range	Interquartile Range (25th and 75th percentile)
Total sample (237)	20	1–87	10, 36
Vaccinated (215)	20	1–87	10, 37
Unvaccinated (22)	21	1–62	16, 31

* No significant difference between vaccinated and unvaccinated; $p = 0.86$.

TABLE 20-3 Yellow Fever Vaccination Coverage Estimates Using Administrative and Survey Methods Among Internally Displaced Persons Living in Bong County, Liberia, 2004

Characteristic	Number Total	Vaccinated in 2004	Coverage (%)	95% CI
Administrative				
Total	87,000	47,676*	54.8	NA†
Age group (%)				
6 months to 4 years	13,920 (16.0%)	9,422	67.7	NA
5–14 years	25,230 (29.0%)	12,238	48.5	NA
15–44 years	34,800 (40.0%)	18,427	53.0	NA
> 44 years	13,050 (15.0%)	7,589	58.2	NA
Gender				
Female	NA	NA	NA	NA
Male	NA	NA	NA	NA
Survey				
Total	237	215	91.9	88.4–95.5
Age group (%)				
6 months to 4 years	28 (11.8%)	26	96.2	90.9–101.6
5–14 years	54 (22.8%)	51	94.8	89.0–100.7
15–44 years	119 (50.2%)	105	89.7	84.1–95.2
> 44 years	36 (15.2%)	33	91.5	81.2–101.9
Gender‡				
Female	151 (63.7%)	138	92.7	88.6–96.9
Male	86 (36.3%)	77	90.2	84.2–96.8

*An additional 1,719 IDPs reported YF vaccination within the past 10 years and did not participate in the 2004 campaign. Ages of previously vaccinated IDPs were not collected. The total number of IDPs considered appropriately immunized using the administrative method was 49,395 (56.8%).
†NA = not applicable.
‡No significant difference between vaccinated females and males; relative risk = 1.0 (95% confidence interval 0.94–1.1, $P = 0.63$).

could not quantify estimates of IDPs vaccinated outside the camps in 2004. Finally, the reason for the low proportion of males surveyed remains unclear. More men may have moved from IDP camps in search of employment near the capitol city Monrovia since the civil war ceasefire. Of the estimated 200,000 Liberians killed during the civil war, most were male combatants,[30] which may have changed the distribution of gender in the country overall.

As lords of the denominator, we were confident now that the mass vaccination campaign in IDP camps in Bong County did in fact meet its target goal. In addition, we were able to determine that there was near-universal knowledge and broad acceptance of the campaign among IDPs, which highlights the high degree of yellow fever disease awareness in this population generated through effective social mobilization. We were able to avoid a costly and unnecessary mass immunization

TABLE 20-4 Survey Results of Yellow Fever Vaccination Coverage Survey for 237 Internally Displaced Persons, Bong County, Liberia, 2004

Characteristic	Positive Response	Percentage	95% Confidence Interval
Knowledge of campaign	230	97.6	95.5–99.6
Vaccinated, 2004	215	91.9	88.4–95.4
Possessed 2004 vaccination card	196	83.5	78.6–88.5
Vaccinated, 1994–2003	8	2.9	0.9–5.0
Appropriately vaccinated*	223	94.8	92.0–97.7

* Vaccinated either in 2004 or within past 10 years.

mop-up campaign in the IDP camps through our rapid assessment coverage study. We then looked to the surrounding villages to fill in the missing pieces of the Bong County coverage data.

LOT QUALITY ASSURANCE SAMPLING

In the host communities surrounding the IDP camps, where 24,866 persons were vaccinated during the Bong County campaign, we did not have the luxury of a documented address system as we had had in the camps. We therefore could not perform a similar survey format as conducted in the IDP camps. Because of population upheavals from the civil war, even rough estimates of village populations collected as recently as 2002 were considered inaccurate by local officials. For these host communities, Jen opted for a lot quality assurance sampling (LQAS) survey to assess communities.[31] This technique was originally developed by Westinghouse in the manufacturing industry in the 1950s for quality control purposes. To determine whether a batch, or lot, of light bulbs met desired specifications, a sample of light bulbs from each lot was inspected for defects. If the number of defective items in each sample exceeded a decision value, then the entire lot was rejected. The sample size and decision value are based on user-defined risks of type I and type II errors. The WHO adopted this method in the 1990s to assess vaccination coverage rates. When delivered in the context of an immunization coverage survey, the "lot" is a community and a "defective item" is an unimmunized person. The LQAS method has been used to identify communities with inadequate coverage without the need for precise population denominator verification. It can also estimate the overall immunization coverage in a group of communities by taking a weighted average of the estimated coverage in each community.

The sample size and decision value were calculated using WHO guidelines. The desired level of accuracy for the survey results was ± 8% and the desired level of confidence for the survey results was 95%. Given these levels of accuracy and confidence, the required sample size according to WHO guidelines was 150 households. MSF France and the Bong County public health department supplied us with maps with labeled villages of the surrounding area. All communities were eligible for the survey, but major population centers had a higher probability of being identified. Ten communities were systematically selected and the size of each relative to the others was used to determine the weight of its contribution to the overall target population (Table 20-5). The minimum lot sample size was therefore 15 households per community. The low threshold level, at which immunization coverage was judged "unacceptable," was set at 50%. The high threshold level, at which immunization coverage was judged "acceptable" was set at 80%, as this was the goal set by campaign coordinators. Given these thresholds, the decision value, the number of unimmunized persons necessary to call coverage "unacceptable" in a specific community was 4.

The same survey teams used in the IDP camps study ventured into the communities on April 7 and 8. Teams first visited the village chief to request permission to conduct the survey, ask for an estimate of the population of the community, and seek guidance on what time was best to start the intervention. The teams walked to the center of each community or at focal points such as schools, places of worship, or health facilities. The teams then determined a vector direction at random by spinning a

> *To determine whether a batch, or lot, of light bulbs met desired specifications, a sample of light bulbs from each lot was inspected for defects.*

TABLE 20-5 Estimated Weighted Populations, Host Communities LQAS Study, Salala District, Bong Country, Liberia

Community	Estimated Population	Weight
Central Totota	5,000	0.23
New Totota	3,000	0.13
Maimu	4,000	0.18
Salala	4,000	0.18
Frelela	3,000	0.13
A-99	1,000	0.04
Tumutu	1,000	0.04
Wreputa	1,000	0.04
Tokpaipolu	500	0.02
Velengai	250	0.01
Total	22,750	1.00

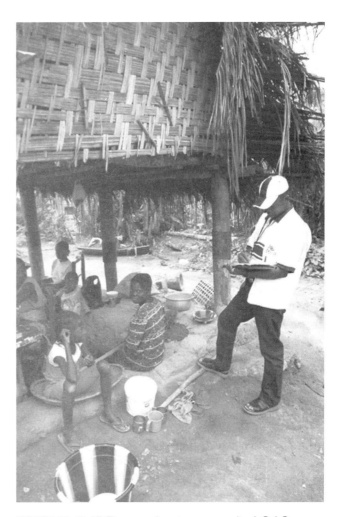

FIGURE 20-15 IDP camp host community LQAS Survey, Salala District, Bong County, Liberia.

pencil on the ground and proceeding outward to the first house in the selected direction.

At noon on April 7, we all suddenly stopped and fell silent for one minute. It was the International Day of Reflection on the Genocide in Rwanda, marking the 10th anniversary of beginning of the massacre. U.N. Secretary General Kofi Annan called on people of the world "everywhere, no matter what their station in life, whether in crowded cities or remote rural areas" to observe this somber memorial.[32] To be in Liberia at this moment doing what I was doing struck me with solemn pause that just perhaps as a global community we have grown in solidarity to offer empathy and protection to the world's vulnerable and suffering whether by conflict or disease.

One person from each household in the vector line was asked for the names of all of the residents in the house aged 6 months or more, including anyone not present at the time of the survey. Each name was assigned a number. One number was then selected using a random number table. The person whose number was selected was the person for whom the survey was administered (Figure 20-15). The standardized questionnaire used in the IDP camps study was the same survey tool used for the LQAS study. If the person selected was too young to answer the survey, then the questions were directed to his or her parent. If the person was not present, then a proxy interview was conducted with another member of the household. When the interview was completed, the protocol was repeated at the next house, following in the same vector that was pinpointed by the spin of the pencil.

One person was surveyed in each of a total of 158 households across the 10 communities. The median household size was 10 people (range, 1–32). Eighty seven (55%) of the residents randomly selected were female. Fifteen (9%) were 6 months to 4 years old. Thirty three (21%) were aged 5 to 14 years. Seventy nine (50%) were aged 15 to 44 years, and 31 (20%) were 45 years or older. There were no AEFI reported. An estimated 95% of the population of the 10 communities was aware of the 2004 immunization campaign. If self-report of immunization was used as an indicator of campaign coverage, then an estimated 89% of the population was immunized in the campaign. If proof of immunization by yellow card was used as an indicator of campaign coverage, then an estimated 71% of the population was immunized. The self-report figure we believed was a fairly accurate portrayal of the true vaccination rate for the same reasons also illustrated in the IDP camps study. Immunization coverage in the overall target population was estimated by calculation of a weighted average of the proportion of people reporting that they were immunized in each sample. When weighted according to the rough figures provided by town chiefs and public health department personnel of community densities, the overall immunization coverage was 89% (95% confidence interval, 0.84–0.94), similar to the IDP camps survey and again indicating that the target levels of immunization were achieved.

There were differences, however, in vaccination coverage in discrete villages. Using the binary decision value established at four, 4 of the 10 communities were "rejected" as not achieved adequate vaccination coverage (Table 20-6). Two of these communities, Frelala and A-99, were located on the main road between camps but somewhat distant from major immunization sites. The two other communities, Tokpaipolu and Velengai, were less populated and very remotely isolated within the district. Because of their distant locations, social mobilization was challenging, limiting the duration of the campaign in these areas. These neighboring communities also hosted weekly market days attracting many IDPs. Numerous IDPs were reportedly vaccinated at community sites on market days and not in the camps. This would have resulted in extra doses being administered in the villages, but not necessarily to town residents, further deflating the actual coverage rates in some host communities.

TABLE 20-6 Level of "Acceptable" Vaccination Rates in Host Communities, LQAS Study, Salala District, Bong Country, Liberia

Community	Number Not Immunized	Sample Size	80% Coverage
Central Totota	1	16	Yes
New Totota	0	15	Yes
Maimu	1	17	Yes
Salala	1	15	Yes
Frelela	5	16	No
A-99	7	17	No
Tumutu	1	17	Yes
Wreputa	1	15	Yes
Tokpaipolu	5	15	No
Velengai	4	15	No

One of the disadvantages of the LQAS sampling method is that there is no measure of magnitude in unacceptability of individual lots. Although this survey design did provide information on deficiencies in some communities, the overall vaccination rate revealed in the study enabled us to finally conclude that the Bong County mass vaccination campaign successfully met target goals.

Concerns with the quality of administrative data used to estimate vaccine coverage have prompted several retrospective surveys after National Immunization Days in other settings[33–40]; however, to our knowledge, this was the first reported survey to evaluate yellow fever vaccination coverage in IDP or refugee camps. Worldwide, nearly 35 million refugees (9.7 million) and IDPs (25 million) existed by 2004; more than 7 million of these persons have been warehoused in camps and settlements for at least 10 years.[41–43] Our studies underscored the importance of accurately estimating the population at risk for yellow fever to assist programmatic decisions regarding future vaccination strategies.

FINAL RECOMMENDATIONS

Jen and I returned to our Monrovia office on April 9. With information on phase I activities now fully complete, I finalized a revision of the WHO and UNICEF Response to Yellow Fever Outbreak Control in Liberia, along with a new draft budget. An overall total of 199,729 persons were immunized against yellow fever in Bong and Nimba counties during February 26 to March 31. We reviewed the document with Dr. Forssen, Dr. Maksha, and Ms. Kearney of UNICEF, who were in agreement with its content. We presented our findings to a group meeting among WHO, UNICEF, and MSF, in particular to answer this question: Now should we move on to phase II of the original plan targeting an additional 320,000 persons in Bong and Nimba counties? The group agreed that "catch-up" immunization campaigns are important to boost background immunity in endemic areas where yellow fever immunization is not yet routinely administered as part of EPI; however, the group also agreed with our conclusions that the implementation of phase II should be deferred in favor of investing resources in reinforcing yellow fever immunization integration in EPI in Liberia. The demographic distribution and stagnant number of confirmed cases—no other cases had been confirmed since early January—suggested that the outbreak was over. Mass immunization campaigns would require the reallocation of already limited health care resources and might preclude control of other causes of morbidity and mortality. We identified yellow fever outbreak preparedness as a priority by bolstering the fledgling MOH surveillance system and strongly recommended that provisions for outbreak preparedness be supported to ensure in-country readiness and capacity to respond to future outbreaks immediately. With lessons learned and laid forth from implementation of phase I, this response capacity included a capital and technical network to vaccinate rapidly and efficiently a population of 200,000 persons. Funding requirements within our draft budget to maintain outbreak preparedness were $396,000 and were requested by UNICEF from donor agencies throughout the international community.

BRINGING IT ALL HOME

I had the opportunity to twice visit St. Joseph's Catholic Hospital on the other side of town from the diplomatic district in Monrovia. As I first approached the entrance, the compound looked about the same as I recalled before mortar shells had torn holes in the building and ripped off one of the roofs. They had been firmly repaired, and the adjacent coconut grove, stripped bare for firewood after all the coconuts had been consumed by a starving population during the war, had grown back. I recognized one of the hospital's drivers named Lhame standing out front. He looked at me as if I was a ghost (well, my hair had grayed a little bit over the past 14 years). I flashed my old ID card. He smiled, gave me one of those rhythmic African handshakes, and then took my card and ran into the back administrative offices. Brother Justino Izquierdo, the long-standing chief operating officer, came barreling through the hallway and threw out a big bear hug. We spent the next couple of hours reminiscing of those hospital workers who died during the war, the survivors, and the dedication of the staff throughout the war (after they came back about a month after our evacuation, they never left again). It was the homecoming I had wished for, filled with fondness, regret, and hope. My next and last visit was on the request of Angela Kearney to consult on a French expatriate employee of UNICEF hospitalized with malaria. I assured her that St. Joseph's Catholic Hospital was still regarded as the best medical center in the country.[44] Her care was excellent, and she was recovering.

I am now an assistant professor in the division of infectious diseases at the John H. Stroger Jr. Hospital of Cook County and Rush University Medical Center in Chicago. The last I searched proMED mail as of August 2008 with the words "yellow fever" and "Liberia" I found no other accounts, neither cases nor outbreaks, announced since the 2004 epidemic. A long list of outbreaks in neighboring West African countries in the interim 4 years popped up, so perhaps our presence in 2004 and recommendations for enhanced surveillance and EPI uptake have paid off. I present this investigation as an example not only of an international public health response to an isolated outbreak of yellow fever in a small tropical country, but as a paradigm to the obstacles both practical and political that need to be addressed if a viable vaccination strategy for HIV were ever to take hold in Africa. I am often reminded of our mission as epidemiologists to protect populations at risk of injury or diseases, whether ancient afflictions such as yellow fever or new threats such as HIV, when I look at a watercolor portrait hanging on my otherwise nondescript office wall in Chicago. As I stepped out of the Mamba Point Hotel on April 11, 2004, to throw my bags into Jefferson Cooper's jeep for a lift to the airport, Romeo was behind the front desk and made sure that I met an artist friend of his named Mitchell before I vanished. I handed over 8 U.S. dollars and rolled up one of his paintings. A traditional Liberian couple is dancing, smiling, celebrating (Figure 20-16).

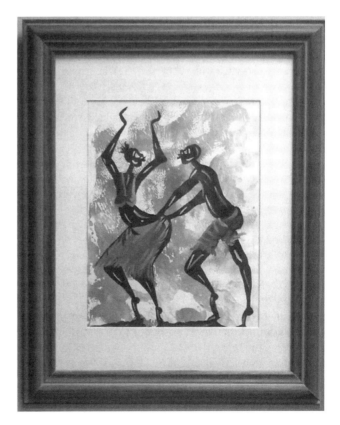

FIGURE 20-16 Painting of traditional Liberian couple dancing.

REFERENCES

1. Evacuees from Liberian capital city describe battles, bodies in streets. *The Washington Post*, August 15, 1990, A18.
2. Liberians' brutality stuns U.S. volunteer. *The Chicago Tribune*, August 15, 1990, 3.
3. San Diego lab tech helped in Liberian evacuation. *Los Angeles Times*, August 21, 1990.
4. United Nations. Office for the Coordination of Humanitarian Affairs. December 18, 2003. Retrieved August 19, 2008, from http://www.humanitarianinfo.org/liberia/.
5. Bryce JW, Cutts FT, Saba S. Mass immunization campaigns and quality of services. *Lancet* 1990;335:739–740.
6. ProMED mail. Retrieved August 19, 2008, from http://www.promedmail.com/pls/otn/f?p=2400:1202:3246059765909252::NO::F2400_P1202_CHECK_DISPLAY,F2400_P1202_PUB_MAIL_ID:X,24586.
7. Robertson S. Yellow fever: the immunological basis for immunization. Document WHO/EPI/GEN/93.181993.
8. Merlo C, Steffen R, Landis T, Tsai T, Karabatsos N. Possible association of encephalitis and 17D yellow fever vaccination in a 29-year-old traveler. *Vaccine* 1993;11:691.
9. Kengsakul K, Sathirapongsasuti K, Punyagupta S. Fatal myeloencephalitis following yellow fever vaccination in a case with HIV infection. *J Med Assoc Thai* 2002;85:131–134.
10. Centers for Disease Control and Prevention (CDC). Adverse events associated with 17D-derived yellow fever vaccination—United States, 2001–2002. *Morb Mort Weekly Rep* 2002:51;989–992.
11. Chan RC, Penney DJ, Little D, Carter IW, Roberts JA, Rawlinson WD. Hepatitis and death following vaccination with 17D-204 yellow fever vaccine. *Lancet* 2001;358:121–122.
12. Vasconcelos PF, Luna EJ, Galler R, et al. Serious adverse events associated with yellow fever 17DD vaccine in Brazil: a report of two cases. *Lancet* 2001;358:91–97.
13. Martin M, Tsai TF, Cropp B, Chang GJ, Holmes DA, Tseng T, et al. Fever and multisystem organ failure associated with 17D-204 yellow fever vaccination: a report of four cases. *Lancet* 2001;358:98–104.
14. Adhiyaman V, Oke A, Cefai C. Effects of yellow fever vaccination. *Lancet* 2001;358:1907–1908.
15. Troillet N, Laurencet F. Effects of yellow fever vaccination. *Lancet* 2001;358:1908–1916.
16. Werfel U, Popp W. Effects of yellow fever vaccination. *Lancet* 2001;358:1909.
17. ProMED mail. Retrieved August 19, 2008, from http://www.promedmail.com/pls/otn/f?p=2400:1202:3246059765909252::NO::F2400_P1202_CHECK_DISPLAY,F2400_P1202_PUB_MAIL_ID:X,24687.
18. United Nations Mission in Liberia. Retrieved August 19, 2008, from http://www.un.org/depts/dpko/missions/unmil/index.html.
19. International Civilian Police. Retrieved August 19, 2008, from http://www.civpol.org/portal/html/index.php.
20. Monath TP. Yellow fever: An update. *Lancet Infect Dis* 2001;1:11–20.
21. *Prevention and Control of Yellow Fever in Africa*. World Health Organization, Geneva, 1986.
22. Liberia Disarmament Demobilisation and Reintegration Programme (DDRR) Activity Report, United Nations Development Programme Administered Trust Fund—December 2003 to August 2004. Retrieved August 19, 2008, from http://www.lr.undp.org/DEX/DDRR%20Trust%20Fund%20%20Report.pdf.
23. Ministry of Planning and Economic Affairs. *1984 Population and Housing Census of Liberia: Summary Results in Graphic Presentation, PC-1*. Monrovia, Liberia, 1986.
24. Population Reference Bureau, Washington D.C. Retrieved August 19, 2008, from http://www.prb.org/Articles/2008/liberia.aspx.
25. Huhn GD, Brown J, Perea W, et al. Vaccination coverage survey versus administrative in the assessment of a mass yellow fever immunization in internally displaced person camps—Liberia, 2004. *Vaccine* 2006;24:730–737.
26. Brés P. Benefit versus risk factors in immunization against yellow fever. *Dev Biol Stand* 1979;43;297–304.
27. Monath TP, Nasidi N. Should yellow fever vaccine be included in the Expanded Program of Immunization in Africa? A cost-effectiveness analysis for Nigeria. *Am J Trop Med Hyg* 1993;48:274–299.
28. Lemeshow S, Robinson D. Surveys to measure programme coverage and impact: a review of the methodology used by the Expanded Programme on Immunization. *World Health Stat Q* 1985;38:65–75.
29. Dean AG, Dean JA, Coulombier D, et al. Epiinfo Version 6: A Word Processing, Database, and Statistics Program for Public Health on IBM-Compatible Microcomputers. Atlanta, GA: Centers for Disease Control, 1996.
30. United Nations, United States, World Bank. International reconstruction conference on Liberia. June 2–3, 2003. Retrieved June 6, 2005, from http://www.un.org/News/Press/docs/2004?ARF827.p2.doc.htm.
31. Brown J, Huhn G, Perea W, et al. Yellow fever immunization coverage in host communities for internally displaced persons—Liberia, 2004. 53rd Annual Meeting of the American Society of Tropical Medicine and Hygiene (abstract 989), Miami Beach, Florida, USA, November7–12, 2004.
32. United Nations General Assembly resolution A/RES/58/234. International Day of Reflection on 1994 Genocide in Rwanda. Retrieved August 25, 2008, from http://www.un.org/events/rwanda/.
33. Reichler MR, Aslanian R, Lodhi ZH, et al. Evaluation of oral poliovirus vaccine delivery during the 1994 National Immunization Days in Pakistan. *J Infect Dis* 1997;175(Suppl 1):S205–S209.
34. Reichler MR, Darwidh A, Stroh G, et al. Cluster survey evaluation of coverage and risk factors for failure to be immunized during the 1995 National Immunization Days in Egypt. *Int J Epidemiol* 1998;27:1083–1089.
35. Rojas JC, Prieto FE. National immunization day evaluation in Columbia, 2001: an ecological approach. *Rev Salud Publica* 2004;6:44–62.

36. Bhattacharjee J, Gupta RS, Jain DC, Devadethan, Datta KK. Evaluation of pulse polio and routine immunization coverage: Alwar District, Rajasthan. *Indian J Pediatr* 1997;64:65–72.
37. Guyer B, Atangana S. A programme of multiple-antigen childhood immunization in Yaounde, Cameroon: first year evaluation 1975–76. *Bull World Health Organ* 1977;55:633–642.
38. Borgdorff MW, Walker GJ. Estimating vaccination coverage: routine information or sample survey? *J Trop Med Hyg* 1988;9135–9142.
39. Tawfik Y, Hoque S, Siddiqi M. Using lot quality assurance sampling to improve immunization coverage in Bangladesh. *Bull World Health Organ* 2001;79:501–505.
40. Cutts FT, Othepa O, Vernon AA, et al. Measles control in Kinshasa, Zaire improved with high coverage and use of medium titre Edmonston Zagreb vaccine at age 6 months. *Int J Epidemiol* 1994;23:624–631.
41. United Nations High Commissioner for Refugees. Refugees by numbers, 2004. Geneva, Switzerland. October 14, 2004. Retrieved June 6, 2005, from http://www.unhcr.ch.
42. United States Committee for Refugees. World refugee survey 2004. Washington, DC. May 24, 2004. Retrieved June 6, 2005, from http://www.uscr.org.
43. Global IDP Project. Internal displacement: Global overview of trends and developments in 2004. March 2005. Retrieved June 6, 2005, from http://www.idpproject.org/publications/2005/Global_overview_2004.final.high.pdf.
44. From Liberian war, tales of brutality. *New York Times*, July 9, 1990.

LEARNING QUESTIONS

1. What is social mobilization and how was it applied in this yellow fever mass vaccination campaign?
2. The author and his colleagues performed a study to determine vaccination coverage in IDP camps and outlying host communities. What were the limitations of this study?
3. What is lot quality assurance sampling and how was it applied in the public health setting?

CHAPTER 21

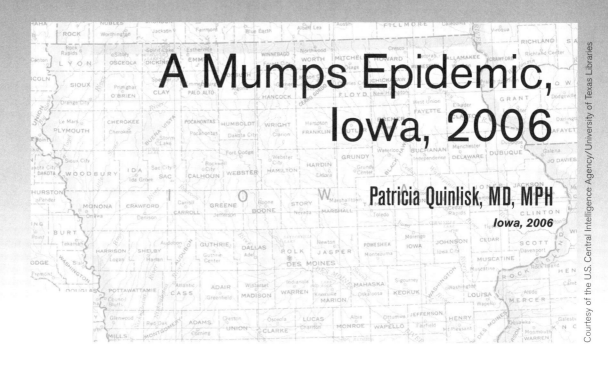

A Mumps Epidemic, Iowa, 2006

Patricia Quinlisk, MD, MPH
Iowa, 2006

INTRODUCTION

Outbreaks often begin with obvious circumstances. For example, you get a call on Friday afternoon reporting that almost everyone who ate at the church supper Wednesday night now has diarrhea, but sometimes these outbreaks, as Carl Sandburg once said about fog, "come on little cat feet," and not until some time has passed do you realize that you are at the beginning of a very large epidemic. This one was like that.

A BRIEF HISTORY OF MUMPS

Hippocrates described mumps in the 5th century BCE, and its correlation with orchitis (testicular inflammation) was noted in the 1700s. Before the vaccine era, mumps was endemic in the United States, with spring and early summer seasonality. The mumps virus is spread by airborne transmission, respiratory droplets, and direct contact with saliva from an infected person. It was one of the most common causes of deafness in the prevaccine era and was associated with sterility in men. Since 1967, after the introduction of a live mumps vaccine, there has been more than a 99% decline in the annual incidence of mumps with seasonal variation no longer occurring. Before this epidemic, the most recent large U.S. outbreak had occurred in Kansas in 1988–1989 in school children, with 269 cases.[1] Because of outbreaks of vaccine-preventable diseases that occurred in the late 1980s (primarily of measles), in about 1990, the national recommendation changed from one dose of measles containing vaccine to two doses, most of which was given as the MMR (measles, mumps, and rubella) vaccine (Figure 21-1). States changed their child care and school entry laws to reflect this.

During the 15 years after the two-dose vaccine recommendations, no large outbreaks of mumps were reported in the United States, and by 2005, only 906 cases of mumps were reported nationally; however, in less vaccinated populations in other parts of the world, outbreaks had continued. The United Kingdom experienced a very large epidemic of mumps between 2004

> *The mumps virus is spread by airborne transmission, respiratory droplets, and direct contact with saliva from an infected person.*

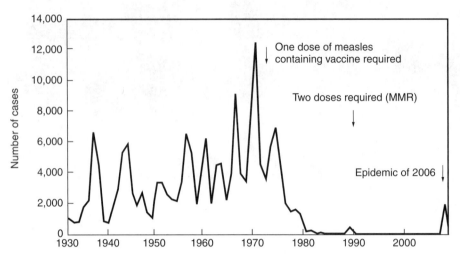

FIGURE 21-1 Number of cases of mumps, Iowa, 1930–2007.

and 2007 with over 56,000 cases, primarily occurring in poorly vaccinated young adults (see http://www.cdc.gov/mmwr/preview/mmwrhtml/mm5507a1.htm). This outbreak was caused by a serotype G mumps virus. An introduction into the United States of mumps from this outbreak had occurred in the summer of 2005 at a camp in New York, resulting in a contained outbreak of 31 cases (see http://www.cdc.gov/mmwr/preview/mmwrhtml/mm5507a2.htm).

Before this epidemic, Iowa's children were highly vaccinated, with over 97% of children starting school in 2004 having received two doses of MMR vaccine; however, because the mandatory second dose of vaccine for school entry didn't start until 1991 in Iowa, many of those in college, particularly juniors and seniors, had only received one dose.

THE IOWA EPIDEMIC

In the early winter of 2005, a cluster of possible mumps cases in eastern Iowa were reported to the health department. Earlier cases may have occurred, but it is difficult for health care workers or public health personnel to identify cases of diseases that only rarely occur and are not expected because of widespread vaccination. Also, health care workers lose experience in diagnosing these diseases as they become so rare. Testing was done for mumps on two people in this cluster, and they had positive mumps IgM tests (but because of the low positive predictive value of tests when disease prevalence is low, these could have been false-positive tests). It was not unusual for a few cases of mumps to be reported. Since the beginning of the 1990s, Iowa had about five cases of mumps reported to the state health department each year, with most of the recent cases having been imported. Thus, at this point, the normal public health follow-up investigation by the local health department was performed, but not much else.

By January of 2006, seven more cases of mumps-like illness had been reported to the public health surveillance system, which were more cases than expected, meeting the definition of a possible outbreak. Because we wanted to confirm that the symptoms of these cases were actually caused by the mumps virus (see Exhibit 21-1), we arranged for clinical specimens (both blood and cheek swabs) to be taken from these patients and sent to Iowa's public health laboratory, the University Hygienic Laboratory (UHL). Mumps viruses were isolated from the cheek swab samples of two patients, and several of the other patients in this cluster had mumps IgM antibodies in their blood. The isolated mumps viruses were sent down to the Centers for Disease Control (CDC) for further identification; the viruses were found to be serotype G (similar to the virus causing the U.K. outbreak). All of these patients were considered to be confirmed cases of mumps using the case definition at the time (see Exhibit 21-2). At this point, we knew we were having an unusual number of mumps cases, so several public health actions were taken:

1. Free laboratory testing began being offered to any Iowan with symptoms consistent with mumps to decrease economic barriers to diagnosis and to assure the identification and reporting of all cases.
2. Messages were sent out to Iowa's health care providers warning them that mumps was spreading in the state and to laboratorians on the process for

having laboratory specimens tested (see http://www.idph.state.ia.us/adper/common/pdf/epi_updates/epi_update_060906.pdf for Iowa's weekly EPI update, a newsletter on health events in Iowa).
3. A review of all public health department mumps information material was updated, which included a new case report form (revised to ensure information pertinent to this outbreak was collected).
4. Follow-up investigation of each case was performed.

By late February, with over 20 reported cases via our standard passive disease surveillance system, we were seeing the beginnings of the largest outbreak of mumps to occur in the United States in decades, although we were still unaware of that at the time. Because many of Iowa's early cases occurred in college age students (Figure 21-2) and transmission was occurring on several college campuses, we responded by starting active surveillance in five Iowa counties (including those with the three largest universities and the three colleges where transmission was already confirmed) (Exhibit 21-3). To do this, we coordinated with the local health departments to contact local hospitals and clinics, student health services, and similar health care facilities, and asked that anyone with possible mumps be immediately reported. Education of health care workers and college authorities was expanded across the state. On all college campuses, we recommended[1] education of all students on the symptoms of mumps, the

---

EXHIBIT 21-1 Laboratory Issues

The University Hygienic Laboratory (UHL), Iowa's public health laboratory, provided almost all of the laboratory support during this epidemic. Unlike what might be seen in a clinical trial, the laboratory methods chosen to confirm mumps cases evolved with the outbreak.

The first IgM-positive laboratory tests were thought to be possible false positives because the laboratory reagent used to perform the IgM serology test was not Food and Drug Administration approved (validation had been done with a minimal number of samples). At the UHL, as the outbreak swelled, the large volume of serologic testing for IgM (testing for acute disease) resulted in the decision not to accept specimens for IgG testing (testing for immunity). Thus, when hospitals and clinics began testing their staff for immunity, these specimens had to be sent to reference laboratories. Although all of the mumps tests performed at UHL were done free of charge, those sent to reference labs were not.

Viral cultures were desirable, but the virus is known to be difficult to grow. The cell cultures using primary rhesus monkey kidney (PRMK) cells were used. Because PRMK cells in tubes were in short supply, UHL converted to using PRMK shell vials on April 4. When the outbreak escalated, the demand for any PRMK cells became too great for the suppliers to provide enough; therefore, UHL switched to vero cells (after performing the necessary validation to confirm that vero cells would support the growth of the mumps virus). Vero cells are also of monkey kidney origin.

In the beginning of the outbreak, the patients were asked to provide both urine and buccal swab specimens, but weeks later, after analysis of the data, it was determined very few positives were being detected from the urine cultures; thus, from then on, only buccal swabs were requested.

At the start of the outbreak, the laboratory questioned whether developing a test using the newer technology of a polymerase chain reaction (PCR) assay for mumps virus should be developed. As the outbreak continued to escalate, it became obvious that the culture method needed to be abandoned because of the amount of labor and time involved; thus, a PCR method was developed. After validation of the test (in collaboration with the CDC), proving that this method was as sensitive as a culture, it became the method of choice. The method was then posted on the Association of Public Health Laboratory's website to make it available to other states.

EXHIBIT 21-2 Case Definitions

1999 National clinical case definition: An illness with acute onset of unilateral or bilateral tender, self-limited swelling of the parotid or other salivary gland, lasting longer than or equal to 2 days, and without other apparent cause. *Laboratory criteria for diagnosis:* (1) isolation of mumps virus from clinical specimen or (2) a significant rise between acute- and convalescent-phase titers in serum mumps IgM antibody level by any standard serologic assay, or (3) a positive serologic test for mumps immunoglobulin (IgM) antibody. A "case" could be a person with positive laboratory test(s) but no clinical symptoms.

As a consequence of this epidemic, it changed to the following:

Iowa's outbreak case definition in 2006: Because of variation of the symptoms patients with mumps were presenting with and because of limited supplies of mumps laboratory reagent, we modified the 1999 clinical case definition to include only those with symptoms consistent with mumps, which could include no salivary gland involvement but other glandular involvement such as testicular inflammation (orchitis), and the patient had to have a laboratory test positive or be epi-linked to a confirmed case.

2007 National clinical case definition: An illness with acute onset of unilateral or bilateral tender, self-limited swelling of the parotid and/or other salivary gland(s), lasting at least 2 days, and without other apparent cause. *Clinically compatible illness:* Infection with mumps virus may present as aseptic meningitis, encephalitis, hearing loss, orchitis, oophoritis, parotitis or other salivary gland swelling, mastitis or pancreatitis. *Laboratory criteria:* (1) isolation of mumps virus from clinical specimen or (2) detection of mumps nucleic acid (e.g., standard or real time RT-PCR assays), or (3) detection of mumps IgM antibody, or (4) demonstration of specific mumps antibody response in absence of recent vaccination, either a fourfold rise in IgG titer as measured by quantitative assays or a seroconversion from negative to positive using a standard serologic assay of paired acute and convalescent serum specimens. A "case" must have clinically compatible symptoms. This was changed because of experience with the 2006 epidemic.

For more information on case definitions, see http://www.cste.org/Positionstatement.asp.

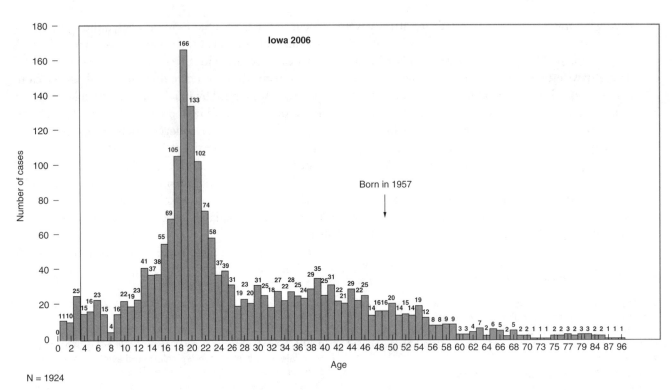

FIGURE 21-2 Age distribution of mumps cases, Iowa 2006.

importance of isolation for ill persons, and how to seek medical care if symptoms are suspected. We also recommended that all students be assessed for vaccine status and vaccines be given to any student or staff without two documented doses.

With control measures in place, we hoped to interrupt transmission of the virus; however, on college campuses, student's adherence to the isolation recommendations was sporadic and difficult for the student health center staff to enforce. (We had symptomatic students admitting to attending beer parties where they "shared saliva" via glasses of beer and other behaviors: there were three beer parties where the spread of mumps virus was confirmed.) Mumps continued to spread on college campuses and into communities around these campuses. Because the spread was occurring and research on mumps had not been feasible for decades because of low numbers, the epidemiologists at the CDC asked whether they could come into Iowa to do a special study on these college campuses looking at transmission of the virus and immunity. We agreed, and by early March, three CDC investigators had arrived, met with IDPH staff, and were conducting their study on a couple of the affected eastern Iowa college campuses.

> With control measures in place, we hoped to interrupt transmission of the virus; however, on college campuses, student's adherence to the isolation recommendations was sporadic and difficult for the student health center staff to enforce.

Quarantine for the public was not used for several reasons, unlike during a measles outbreak in Iowa 2 years earlier. Those reasons included: (1) 20% to 30% of cases are asymptomatic, (2) mumps virus can be spread up to 3 days prior to symptoms, (3) some mumps cases are so mildly ill that they do not seek medical attention, thus they are not reported to public health, and (4) mumps is generally a mild illness. Isolation and work quarantine (i.e., restrictions on patient contact during the incubation period), however, were used for health care workers because of the risk of spread to vulnerable patients. We did recommend at this time that all health care workers in Iowa be assessed for immunity and offered vaccination (two doses of MMR were recommended for anyone without documented immunity; this was defined as laboratory evidence of antibodies, documented receipt of two doses of MMR or physician diagnosed mumps).

In February, we knew that everyone in the state needed to be aware of the situation, and thus, getting information out was of critical importance. When looking at a response to an outbreak, epidemic, or any other biologic emergency, the most challenging aspect is almost

EXHIBIT 21-3 Outbreak Data Management

At the beginning of the epidemic, we quickly realized that the mumps investigation form used for routine reports of mumps disease would not be sufficient. We had to quickly assess what questions in a form would answer the many questions surrounding this outbreak.

- Was this due to improper handling of the vaccine causing inactivation? Were there one or a few medical clinics that could be pin-pointed as the source?
- How many doses did our mumps cases receive and when, where, and from whom?
- Were these cases related to travel?
- What mild symptoms and complications were patients experiencing that we did not capture with the old form?
- Were the cases occurring in college students? If so, what types of colleges (e.g., private, public)? What exposures on college campuses would lead to mumps disease?
- What laboratory tests were being done to confirm disease?
- What occupations did our cases have?

Because we initiated active surveillance, we were able to have those sites complete a supplemental form. From that, we determined improper handling of the vaccine was not an issue, neither was timing or dosage of the vaccine. We then modified our standard mumps investigation form to include expanded demographics, specific and numerous manifestations of clinical symptoms, several options for laboratory testing, and extensive vaccine and travel history.

Creating the form was the easy part. Entering every form into a database with epidemiology staff already stretched beyond capacity was the next challenge. Approximately 1 month into the epidemic we started prioritizing daily disease reports. Those with the potential to cause outbreaks were processed with mumps (e.g., *Salmonella, Shigella*), and those that were not spread person to person (e.g., Lyme disease) were held until everything else was processed. We hired and trained temporary data entry staff. Everyone took turns entering follow-up forms.

On a typical day, we might process 20 reports of all reportable communicable diseases covered by the Iowa Administrative Code. During the mumps epidemic, we handled up to 20 cases of only mumps in addition to the normal number of reports for other diseases. After the outbreak was over, we determined that the number of mumps cases in Iowa nearly doubled the disease reports processed by the Iowa Department of Public Health for 1 year.

EXHIBIT 21-4 Communications in Iowa

The communication pathways used in this situation included the following:

Face to face: Conferences were held at IDPH each morning to review what had happened the day before and to determine the actions to be taken that day. This was attended by IDPH staff, visiting CDC consultants, and UHL staff (public health laboratorians).

Telephone: Conference calls were held weekly with the local health department officials and as needed with Iowa's Infectious Disease Advisory Committee. Also, regular conference calls were done with the CDC, and as the outbreak spread, to involved states, and then to all states.

E-mail: Electronic methods were used to send documents and other information to public health and health care workers, particularly the "Epi Update," a weekly IDPH newsletter. Colleges used their student e-mail systems for getting information to their students on symptoms of mumps, and where vaccine clinics were held.

HAN: The Health Alert Network, a statewide alerting system, was used to both alert public health and health care workers around the state about new events and as a secure, password-protected website for accessing confidential information.

IDPH website: Biweekly updates on numbers of cases, the process for submission of clinical specimens, worksheets for patient assessment, forms for reporting of cases, mumps information sheets in various languages, and other information were placed on the website. This information was used by Iowa's health care workers and newspaper reporters and, as the outbreak spread beyond Iowa, by public health officials in other states as a template for addressing their communication needs. We also posted a running list of the most frequently asked questions and their answers (access this website at http://www.idph.state.ia.us/adper/mumps.asp).

Media: Newspapers, radio, television, and nontraditional media (websites) were used to get information out to the public. Seven official press conferences/news releases occurred during this time with the last one on August 21. IDPH's public information officer worked full time for weeks on this issue alone because the need to get information out and to respond to media inquiries was so critical.

CDC: The *Morbidity and Mortality Weekly Report* (MMWR) published several articles on this situation, the first as it started in Iowa (see http://www.cdc.gov/mmwr/preview/mmwrhtml/mm5513a3.htm), the second as it spread (see http://www.cdc.gov/mmwr/preview/mmwrhtml/mm5520a4.htm), and a third update as the epidemic wound down (see http://www.cdc.gov/mmwr/preview/mmwrhtml/mm5542a3.htm). On this site is also found the Advisory Committee on Immunization Practice's recommendations for use of vaccine to control mumps (see http://www.cdc.gov/mmwr/preview/mmwrhtml/00053391.htm).

---

always communication. Getting the right information to the right audience at the right time can be difficult. Thus, it was at this point that the communications aspects of this outbreak really began (Exhibit 21-4).

During outbreaks like this, you have exportation of the disease that must be followed up on to contain spread. Early in the outbreak, several business travelers from eastern Iowa went to Washington, DC to visit politicians on "the hill." A couple days later, it was determined that one of them was infectious during those visits. IDPH contacted the offices of both of the Senators and Representatives that were visited and the Washington, DC Health Department. The Washington,

> *During outbreaks like this, you have exportation of the disease that must be followed up on to contain spread.*

DC Health Department worked with the Medical Director of Congress and quickly offered vaccine to all the potentially exposed nonimmune persons. No mumps cases were identified as a result of this incident.

In other examples, there was fear of the spread of mumps when a bus load of eastern Iowa college students traveled down to Missouri for an athletic competition. They were not allowed off the bus and were sent back to Iowa by local college officials immediately, even though no one on the bus had mumps. When a wrestling tournament occurred between Nebraska and Iowa, mumps was spread not among the athletes, but among spectators and parents in the bleachers, beginning an outbreak in Nebraska among non-college-aged adults.

In March, the number of cases began skyrocketing; by the end of the month, over 300 additional cases had been reported, mostly in eastern Iowa, and another 14 possible cases were being investigated in the bordering states of Illinois, Minnesota, and Nebraska (Figures 21-3 and 21-4).[2] This compares with an annual average of 265 cases reported in the entire United States between 2001 and 2005. By March 15, eastern Iowa papers were printing: "Mumps making comeback." By April 5, the outbreak was on the front page of Iowa's largest newspaper, the *Des Moines Register*, above the fold. (Of course, the *Des Moines Register* headline "Mumps cases have doctors confounded" would not have been my choice, but at least the word was getting out to the public.) Other *Des Moines Register* articles included "Health Officials: Mumps vaccine still effective" (April 7, 2006) and "Young adults targeted in Mumps fight" (April 21, 2006). We even made page 3 in *USA Today* on April 3 and page 13 in the *New York Times* on April 1.

More control measures were instituted in March. They included targeting health care workers with immunity assessments (either checking for documented doses of MMR, or serologic testing for immunity—primarily used with the older members of this population because they grew up in a time when mumps was quite common in the community and no vaccines were available). We also changed the recommendations for isolation of case-patients to be reduced from 9 days after onset to 5 days. This was done because of the difficulty of ensuring isolation of college students for 9 days and because the science was showing almost all of the transmission was occurring early in the illness; thus, we felt we would get better compliance with the 5 days, and this could help us slow the transmission of the virus. Our web page on mumps was expanded, and given its own specific site, HAN (health alert network); messages were used as a means to keep public health officials and medical personnel across the state up to date on the epidemic. Questions about vaccine efficacy were common (Exhibit 21-5).

We also began regular conference calls with each of our partner groups: local health departments, infection-control professionals in hospitals, and bordering state health departments/the CDC (which very quickly were

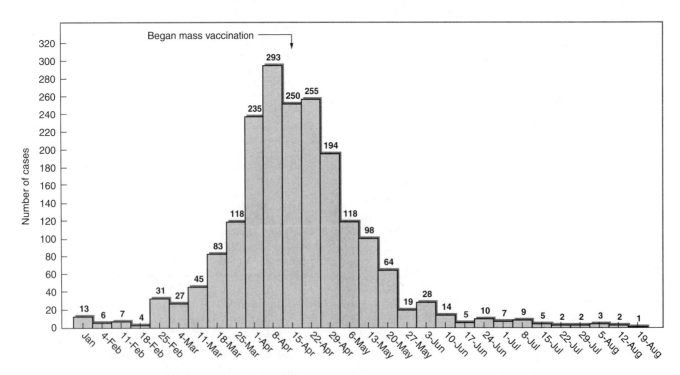

FIGURE 21-3 Number of cases of mumps, by date of onset—Iowa, January 1–August 22, 2006.

■ The Iowa Epidemic   251

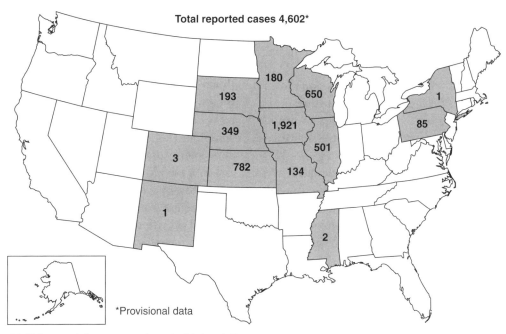

FIGURE 21-4 Mumps outbreak, United States 2006.

EXHIBIT 21-5   Vaccine Efficacy

As the public became more aware of the outbreak and the fact that many of those with mumps had been vaccinated, questions arose about whether or not the vaccine was effective at preventing disease. Because we did not want people to falsely use this situation as a reason to not vaccinate their children, we provided information and examples of why this was occurring. (This was created early in the outbreak when vaccine efficacy was still thought to be around 95% after two doses of MMR.)

Examples Explaining Mumps Vaccine Effectiveness

Or Why Are So Many Mumps Cases Occurring in Vaccinated People?

There have been many questions about why people, who have been vaccinated, are getting mumps. As you read through the examples that follow, keep these key points in mind.
- The mumps vaccine (part of the MMR vaccine) is about 95% effective.
- This means out of every 100 people vaccinated, 95 will be protected; however, the vaccine will not "take" in 5 people, and these people will remain susceptible to the disease.
- By comparison, the measles vaccine (also part of the MMR vaccine) is about 98% effective and the annual influenza vaccine is about 70% to 85% effective.

Example 1

In a community of 100 people, 100% have been vaccinated. Everyone is exposed to mumps. What happens?
- Ninety-five people (95%) in the community are protected by the vaccine and do not get mumps.
- Five people (5%) in the community become ill with mumps because the vaccine did not "take."
- Of the 5 people who get mumps, all (100%) have been vaccinated.

Example 2

In a community of 100, 98% have been vaccinated (a similar rate to what is being seen today in Iowa's K-12 schools and some colleges). Thus, 98 people are vaccinated, and 2 people are not. Everyone is exposed to mumps. What happens?
- Ninety-three people (95% of the 98 who are vaccinated) in the community are protected by the vaccine and do not get mumps.
- Five people (5% of the 98 who are vaccinated) become ill with mumps because the vaccine did not "take."
- Two people who have never been vaccinated get ill because they have no immunity to the disease.
- Of the 7 (5 vaccinated + 2 unvaccinated) people who get mumps, 71% (5 of 7) were vaccinated (similar to what is happening now in Iowa)

Thus, a large percentage of the people with mumps have been vaccinated. This is expected in a highly vaccinated population when dealing with a vaccine that is 95% effective and a contagious disease like mumps. This does not mean that the vaccine is not working; in fact the mumps vaccine is working as expected (http://www.idph.state.ia.us/adper/common/pdf/mumps/explaining_effectiveness.pdf).

expanded to all affected states, then to all states). All of these groups were encouraged to copy any of the information/forms/fact sheets that we had produced, to use it however they might need. When you are busy with follow-up investigations and outbreaks, you don't need to reinvent the wheel. Because many similar questions were coming into our hotline system, we began keeping a list of the common questions and how we answered them on our website—a "running Q&A."

By April, the outbreak had reached epidemic levels, and over 50 cases were being reported each working day (Exhibit 21-6). The epidemic was no longer contained in any localized area but had spread across Iowa (Figure 21-5) and to several neighboring states. When situations such as this occur, the importance of good relationships cannot be emphasized enough. Relationships, not only with your public health partners like the local health departments, other state health departments and the CDC, but with other state agencies like emergency management, the governor's office, the legislature, and the media are critical. If you have good relationships, the issues are resolved quickly, and you are able to focus your time and efforts on stopping the epidemic. If your relationships are poor, you may find your time being spent on side issues, stalling your efforts. These relationships are best forged prior to any emergency and are based in understanding each others assets/abilities and roles and responsibilities.

At this point, we began using the incident command system (Figure 21-6). I will be honest—a decade ago, when I began to realize that the incident command system was going to be used during outbreaks and epidemics, I was not thrilled. I was concerned that this system would get in the way of the science and epidemiologic response; however, after several large outbreaks, including this one, I am a believer. This system was first put into place to deal with forest fires and allows those knowledgeable in emergency response, administration, and intra-agency coordination to deal with those issues, allowing the epidemiologists/scientists to focus on the epidemic and medical aspects of the situation. The result is a better handled situation and more effective epidemiologists. One of the first things completed under this system was the establishment of a phone bank to deal with all of the calls coming into the health department. Most of the calls were from health care providers; very few were from the public. Thus Iowa's phone bank was used only to deal with the medical issues (because we could answer the situation specific questions best), and the public was sent to the CDC's answering system where their more general questions could be answered (although the public probably didn't realize this was happening), freeing up our people to deal more directly with the response issues.

Since the beginning of the epidemic, a targeted vaccination strategy had been used; vaccinating college students and health care workers, for example; however, as the disease expanded across the state and showed no signs of slowing, various options were considered. Because there had been no outbreaks of mumps for almost 20 years, I had no experience with outbreaks of mumps and wanted the advice of someone with experience at the state level. It took some effort to find epidemiologists experienced with mumps control efforts. I am still grateful to the three state epidemiologists who gave up a Saturday afternoon to have a conference call with me. In the end, with the advice of these epidemiologists and the CDC and lots of discussion at the state level, mass vaccination of the whole state was considered (Exhibit 21-7). This is obviously a very difficult strategy; there were issues of vaccine supply, payment of vaccine purchased, distribution of the vaccine to each county, determination of the amount needed by each county, getting the word out about the program, and efforts to have clinics in the midst of the highest risk groups (such as on college campuses). A special committee meeting of legislators with the Director of the Iowa Department of Public Health was needed to release the emergency funds required to buy the vaccine. (For the best uptake of vaccine, it had to be offered free of charge; thus, public funding for the vaccine had to obtained.) This whole process took about 10 days from the decision to do a statewide mass vaccination program, purchase the vaccine, have it shipped to Iowa, distribute it to the local health departments, and have vaccination clinics. In the end, a total of 37,500 doses of

---

EXHIBIT 21-6   What Is an Epidemic

Epidemic definition [from the Greek *epi* (upon), *d_mos* (people)]: the occurrence in a community or region of cases of an illness...clearly in excess of normal expectancy. The community or region and the period in which the cases occur are specified precisely. The number of cases indicating the presence of an epidemic varies according to the agent, size, and type of population exposed; previous experience or lack of exposure to the disease; and the time and place of occurrence. Epidemicity is thus relative to usual frequency of the disease in the same area, among the specified population and the same season of the year.

Outbreak definition: An epidemic limited to localized increase of a disease, for example, in a village, town, or closed institution.

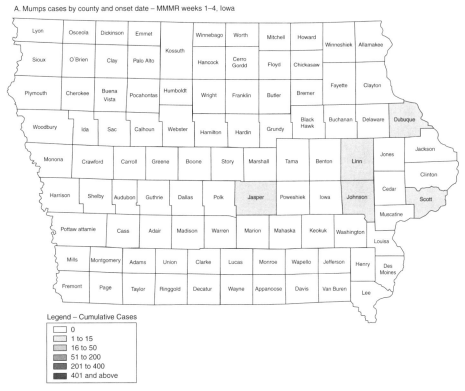

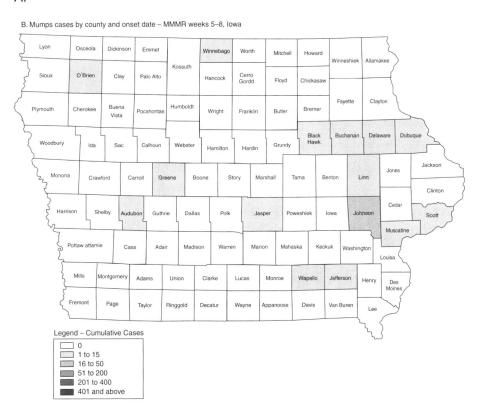

FIGURE 21-5 A. Mumps cases by county and onset date—MMMR weeks 1–4, Iowa. B. Mumps cases by county and onset date—MMMR weeks 5–8, Iowa.

(continues)

CHAPTER 21 ■ A Mumps Epidemic, Iowa, 2006

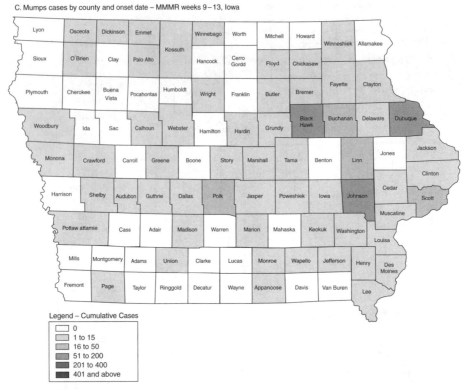

C.

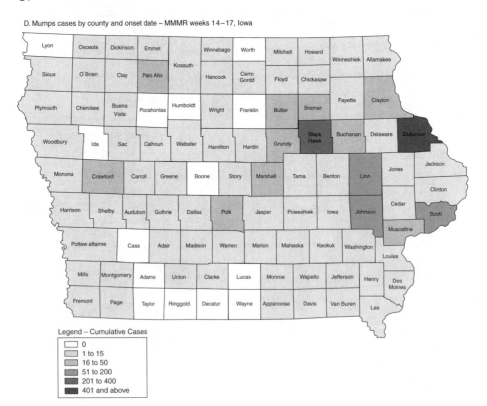

D.

FIGURE 21-5 C. Mumps cases by county and onset date—MMMR weeks 9–13, Iowa. D. Mumps cases by county and onset date—MMMR weeks 14–17, Iowa.

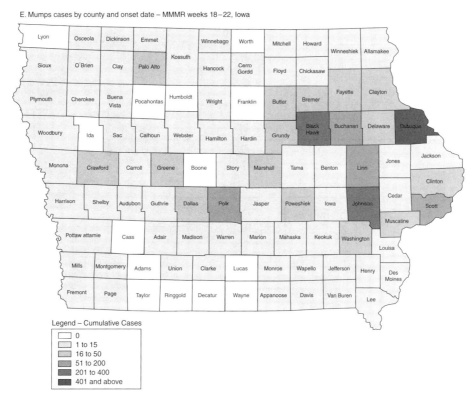

E.

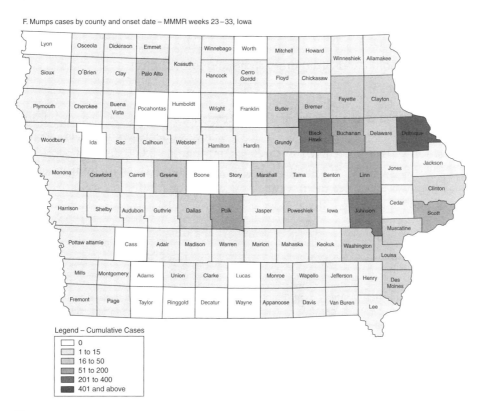

F.

FIGURE 21-5 E. Mumps cases by county and onset date—MMMR weeks 18–22, Iowa. F. Mumps cases by county and onset date—MMMR weeks 23–33, Iowa.

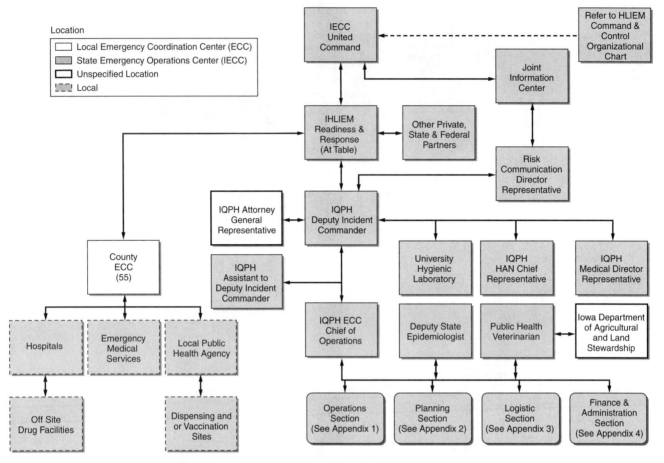

FIGURE 21-6 IDPH Incident Command Structure–Command and Control.

MMR vaccine were purchased and made available. This was no small task.

The mass vaccination program occurred in three stages: the first stage was vaccination of young adults ages 18 to 22 years, which was expanded the next week to ages 18 to 25 years, and 2 weeks later, the ages were expanded to 18 to 46 years. We found it difficult to get college students to go and get vaccinated, and in the end only about 10,000 doses of vaccine were used in Iowa's 99 counties. (The remaining vaccine did not go to waste as large quantities of vaccine were sent to the East Coast

---

EXHIBIT 21-7 Policy Issues

Whenever complicated situations such as this occur, there will always be issues that require far-reaching decisions, or "policy decisions." These decisions have to be made carefully because they not only impact the present situation, but also will effect future situations. When these types of decisions needed to be made, usually one person proposed it, and it was discussed over a period of time with the appropriate people, such as the director, our public health lawyer, and other department directors that might be affected by this policy. Invariably, it was modified, and then the director would "sign off" on it. When the first MMWR article was published on April 7, and the word "epidemic" was used in the title, there were concerns expressed about the political ramifications of using the word "epidemic" rather than "outbreak." Thus, I had to explain the scientific difference between epidemic and outbreak and why we used the word epidemic.

One example of these policies involved mass gatherings. The First National Special Olympics were to be held in central Iowa on a college campus in the summer of 2006, and our public health department was asked for their advice. After discussion, our policy was that persons traveling to Iowa for events like this were advised not to change their plans but instead to ensure that they were fully vaccinated against mumps prior to arrival. This policy was then placed on our website (see http://www.idph.state.ia.us/adper/common/pdf/mumps/mass_gathering_041806.pdf).

a couple months later in response to an outbreak of measles.)

Between the mass vaccination program, college spring semesters ending, and the natural decrease of mumps in late spring, the epidemic began to slow down in late April and early May. By late May, we were saying that the epidemic was waning, and on June 2, it was publicly announced that the epidemic was contained.

Over the summer, we continued to encourage vaccination and recommended that all students planning on attending college that fall ensure that they had two doses of MMR. There was concern that mumps would re-emerge during the next school year, causing new outbreaks. Fortunately, Iowa had no further outbreaks of mumps, but unfortunately, several college campuses in other states were not as lucky.

We never did figure out how mumps got started in Iowa, although we looked hard for the index case. Our best guess is that it was brought in from the United Kingdom, probably by a college student(s). This outbreak tested Iowa's public health system and cost us over 1 million dollars. The many lessons learned will be put to use in our next public health emergency. Today, Iowans are better vaccinated, public health is better prepared, and the medical community is more aware that these vaccine-preventable diseases can come back; in addition, the role of public health is better understood. It is unlikely that this large a mumps outbreak will ever happen again in Iowa.

This mumps epidemic also served as a "natural experiment," and consequently, research into mumps occurred with many issues being better understood (Exhibit 21-8).

This was the largest epidemic that I had ever been involved with. Fortunately, mumps is typically a mild disease and one for which we have a relatively effective vaccine. Only one death occurred in Iowa (in someone with other more serious medical problems), and very few people needed hospitalization. There were reports of temporary deafness, but it appears that most, if not all, have regained their hearing. Had this been a disease such as measles or SARS, the outcome could have been devastating.

In the end, we learned a lot about how to respond to biologic emergencies and used this experience to improve our response system. I believe that should Iowa be faced with a similar biologic emergency situation in the future, we will be better prepared because of this mumps epidemic and have a more effective response.

REFERENCES

1. Hersh BS, Fine PE, Kent WK, et al. Mumps outbreak in a highly vaccinated population. *J Pediatr* 1991;119:187–193.
2. Dayan G, Quinlisk P, Parker AA, et al. Recent resurgence of mumps in the United States. *N Engl J Med* 2008;358:

EXHIBIT 21-8 Mumps Research

Several studies were performed during this mumps epidemic and some of these have been published:

1. A study of transmissibility of the mumps virus among college students found that two dose vaccine efficacy was only 76% to 80% among college students (most vaccinated >10 years prior).[3]
2. A study of transmission of mumps among airplane passengers found that mumps does not spread to any significant degree on planes. Thus, today when passengers infectious with mumps are found to have traveled on an airline, the other passengers are NOT notified. (see http://www.cdc.gov/mmwr/preview/mmwrhtml/mm5514a6.htm)
3. An economic impact study was done, which determined that this epidemic cost over 1 million dollars to Iowa's public health system alone.
4. A small health care worker study found that although over 80% of health care workers who thought that they were immune to mumps were immune, approximately 20% were not.
5. A study was done on viral shedding by the UHL and the University of Iowa, which found that patients continued to shed the virus for up to 9 days, but that the most significant shedding occurred during the 5 days after onset of symptoms.[4]
6. Laboratory-based studies:
    a. The method for the new PCR test was developed by UHL during this epidemic.[5]
    b. A model was developed to predict the duration of viral shedding (http://www.idsociety.org/WorkArea/showcontent.aspx?id=8412).
    c. An analysis of the geospacial relationship of the spread of mumps was performed (see http://www.cdc.gov/eid/content/14/3/ICEID2008.pdf).
7. National recommendations of use of vaccine were changed by the Advisory Committee on Immunization Practices, particularly for all health care workers to be vaccinated with one to two doses of MMR (unless proved immune) (http://www.cdc.gov/mmwr/preview/mmwrhtml/mm5522a4.htm).

1580–1589. Available from http://content.nejm.org/cgi/content/short/358/15/1580.
3. Marin M, Quinlisk P, Shimabukaro T, et al. Mumps vaccination coverage and vaccine effectiveness in a large outbreak among college students—Iowa, 2006. *Vaccine* 2008;26:3601–3607.
4. Polgreen PM, Bohnett LC, Cavanaugh JE, et al. The duration of virus shedding after the onset of symptoms. *Clin Infect Dis* 2008;46:1447–1449.
5. Boddicker JD, Rota PA, Kreman T, et al. Real-time reverse transcription-PCR assay for detection of mumps virus RNA in clinical specimens. *J Clin Microbiol* 2007;45:2902–2908.

Note: MMWR weeks roughly correspond to months of the year, such that weeks 1 to 4 refers to January, 5 to 8 refers to February, and so on.

LEARNING QUESTIONS

1. Although mumps was a reportable disease in Iowa in 2006, the rise in mumps cases necessitated the collection of supplemental information beyond that collected on the routine mumps case report form. What information did they need to collect on this supplemental surveillance form?
2. What methods of communication were used to disseminate the information about this epidemic of mumps and who is the audience for each of these methods?
3. A large proportion of the mumps cases in Iowa were among vaccinated persons. Why wasn't it concluded that the vaccine was not working?

PART III

Outbreak Investigations of Intoxications and Other Noninfectious Causes

CHAPTER 22

Something Borrowed, Something Blue: A Wedding to Remember

Cortland Lohff, MD, MPH; Tom Boo, MD; and Patricia Quinlisk, MD, MPH

Iowa, 2003

AN UNLIKELY SOURCE REPORTS AN OUTBREAK

Cortland Lohff: In March of 2003, I was the deputy state epidemiologist at the Iowa Department of Public Health (IDPH), located in Des Moines. Prior to joining the IDPH, I completed a residency in General Preventive Medicine and Public Health, training that would provide me with the academic and practical experiences that would be useful for a career in public health.

At the IDPH, I worked with a team that included other physicians, nurses, veterinarians, epidemiologists, and administrative staff to conduct statewide disease surveillance and to respond to possible public health threats. We worked closely with the 99 county and 2 city health departments to receive reports on diseases and outbreaks, investigate the reports, and use the information learned to inform prevention and control strategies. The day-to-day work tended to focus on communicable diseases, but at times we confronted diseases and outbreaks with non-infectious or unknown causes. Some of these proved to be quite extraordinary.

It was a Saturday afternoon in March of 2003 when the IDPH first received a report of one such extraordinary outbreak. I happened to be in my office when the IDPH public information officer telephoned. He had just been called by a reporter from a local television station, who wanted to know why numerous ambulances were flooding the emergency departments at the three hospitals in Des Moines. Not knowing the reason, he called me and I began calling the emergency departments.

My calls verified what the reporter had said. All three emergency departments were indeed being flooded by ambulances, as well as by individuals transporting themselves, their friends, or their family members. I also learned where the people were coming from. They were not being brought from a "usual" mass-casualty event, such as a massive car pile-up or natural disaster. Instead, they were being brought from a wedding at a local church. I was also informed that some of the patients were cyanotic, or blue, and were having trouble breathing.

At this point, I knew that a fairly dramatic outbreak of unknown cause had occurred among people attending a wedding. Most interesting was that some of these ill people had turned blue, which is not at all common. I did not know at that time what caused this outbreak, nor did I know whether it was confined to the wedding or

> *At this point, I knew that a fairly dramatic outbreak of unknown cause had occurred among people attending a wedding. Most interesting was that some of these ill people had turned blue, which is not at all common.*

whether a broader public health threat might exist. Whatever the cause or the extent of the outbreak, it was clear that an immediate investigation was needed.

I first called one of our nurses, one of our epidemiologists, and one of our physicians, and asked that they each go to one of the three hospital emergency departments to gather more information. I also called a sanitarian and a public health nurse from the county health department to inform them of the situation and to ask that they meet me at the church to assist in the investigation. I will discuss the findings at the church later, but first I want to bring in one of the co-authors—Tom Boo—who will discuss his findings at one of the local emergency departments.

AN INVESTIGATION BEGINS AND CONTROL MEASURES ARE IMMEDIATELY INSTITUTED

Tom Boo: Cortland called me late that Saturday afternoon and informed me of the situation. I was especially struck by the reports that some of the ill were cyanotic, or blue. When I got to one of the emergency departments, it was busy, full of sick and anxious people. By that time, the treating physicians had determined that the cyanosis seen in some of the patients was due to methemoglobinemia, which had been laboratory-confirmed in numerous patients. Physicians also noted blood from some of the patients to be chocolate-colored, a classic finding for this condition, and the sicker patients had presented with symptoms that were consistent with this diagnosis, including headaches, dizziness, and shortness of breath. Some of the patients, especially those more seriously ill, were being treated with intravenous methylene blue, which acts as an antidote, and were responding favorably.

I had never encountered methemoglobinemia during my training as a family physician or during the 6 years I practiced before becoming an Epidemic Intelligence Service (EIS) officer with the Centers for Disease Control and Prevention. As an EIS officer, I was assigned to the IDPH for a 2-year on-the-job training program in applied epidemiology. It was in this capacity that I arrived at one of the local emergency departments.

In addition to speaking with the emergency department physicians, I spoke with some of the patients and other wedding guests. I asked them to describe what had happened, what they thought might have caused themselves or others to become ill, and what symptoms they experienced, if any. I stayed in close contact with Cortland, reporting my initial findings, as did our colleagues at the two other hospitals, who were speaking with other patients and wedding guests.

We learned some of the details of the wedding. The wedding ceremony took place earlier that afternoon and was attended by approximately 500 people. Following the ceremony, guests came down to the basement, where the reception was held, with food and beverages available from a self-serve buffet. At this point, patients and other guests began to recount the sequence of events that led them to the hospital. At the reception, "wedding punch" was served. Some who had recalled drinking the punch reported to us that it "tasted funny." Others recalled that they heard that one of the first persons to get sick was the photographer, who had been one of the first to arrive at the reception and one of the first to drink the punch.

Accounts such as these are common during outbreak investigations. In some cases, when many people implicate a specific source (such as a food or beverage), they may turn out to be correct. The fact that many people believed the punch "tasted funny" was a big clue for us. However, we could not rely on these anecdotal reports alone as the basis for our response. We recognized that people's impressions about what made them sick can often be mistaken, but if the punch was not the source, then what was? Even if it was the source, could other patients who were not affiliated with the wedding have consumed this punch? Or, could other beverages and even food served at the reception been involved as well? And what was the full extent of the outbreak? How many people got ill, and what were their symptoms and outcomes? How much of the punch and other beverages and foods served at the wedding did they consume? These questions and more prompted us to proceed with an investigation.

Our first step was to continue to interview those patients and other guests at the hospitals, and to do so in a more systematic way. One of our colleagues obtained the menu identifying the food and beverages served at the reception and quickly put together a questionnaire. In addition to asking about the food and beverages consumed, if any, this questionnaire also asked about basic demographic information (name, age, address, phone number) as well as any symptoms experienced and when they started. After this questionnaire was developed, she faxed it to me and our other colleague, and we proceeded to formally interview the patients and other wedding guests who were still at the hospitals.

> *Methemoglobinemia can be an adverse effect of numerous drugs, both therapeutic and recreational, but outbreaks are not typically seen with these.*

In addition to speaking with the physicians, patients, and other guests, I also spoke with the state poison control center. They were already aware of the outbreak, having been consulted earlier by the emergency department physicians to help identify the illness and to discuss the appropriate treatment. Together, we identified a number of compounds that can cause methemoglobinemia, with nitrates and nitrites being the most common causes of the occasional outbreaks that occur. Methemoglobinemia can be an adverse effect of numerous drugs, both therapeutic and recreational, but outbreaks are not typically seen with these. For example, methemoglobinemia is a well-recognized side effect of local anesthetics at high doses, especially in children, leading to recent calls to abandon the use of benzocaine, a fairly common topical agent.[1] Other prescription drugs commonly implicated are dapsone and primaquine. Some recreational drugs, such as inhaled nitrates, or poppers, can cause methemoglobinemia.[2]

We also determined that, depending on the compound, methemoglobinemia can be caused by ingestion, inhalation, or cutaneous exposure. From what we knew, it appeared that whatever the compound (and the source of the methemoglobinemia), people were exposed to it at the wedding and ingestion appeared to be the most likely route of exposure.

Cortland Lohff: I arrived at the church early that evening and met the sanitarian and the nurse from the county health department. The scene was relatively calm, which I learned was in stark contrast to what it had been like a few hours earlier. By the time of my arrival, all the guests were gone. Remaining at the church were a handful of public safety officials—police officers, firefighters, and emergency medical personnel—and some kitchen staff.

The public safety officials recounted what happened earlier that afternoon. Shortly after the wedding reception began, the first call came to them from the 911 dispatcher, requesting an ambulance at the church to respond to one ill individual. This first ambulance arrived within 5 minutes, by which time two more people were ill and two more ambulances were called. No sooner had this request been made than more people became ill, with some collapsing and having trouble breathing. Within 10 minutes of the first call, ambulances were being requested from neighboring jurisdictions. Soon, a mass casualty incident was declared and a unified command was established to coordinate the response. Officials were designated to direct triage and ambulance staging operations; traffic in the vicinity of the church was diverted to enable response personnel to move to and from the scene. In total, the response involved more than 60 public safety officials from eight agencies. In addition to those who drove themselves (or were driven by others), 18 persons were transported by ambulances to area hospitals.

While addressing the needs of those who were ill, public safety officials sought the cause of the mass casualty event. Given some of the signs and symptoms, including breathing difficulties and collapse, officials initially suspected carbon monoxide poisoning. This was ruled out after tests of the indoor air and a few patients were negative. Public safety officials had to also consider that this mass casualty event might have been due to some criminal action—that someone or some group was intent on deliberately causing harm to the bride or groom, the wedding participants, or the guests. Though not likely, the scene had to be treated as a crime scene and the investigation (including our public health investigation) had to follow established procedures so that any evidence gathered would be admissible in court.

Following the discussions with the public safety officials, I joined the sanitarian and nurse in performing the public health investigation. By this time, we had heard from our colleagues at the emergency departments that methemoglobinemia was the probable diagnosis, that this illness was likely due to the ingestion of one of the many types of compounds known to cause this condition, and that some guests suspected the punch served at the reception. Knowing this, we interviewed the kitchen staff to learn the details of how the food and beverages (including the strange-tasting punch) were prepared and served. We learned that some of the food and beverages, like the punch, were prepared elsewhere and brought to the church, whereas others were prepared on-site. We then collected samples of everything served, being careful to establish a legal "chain of custody," documenting the personnel and methods that collected, transported, and tested the samples. Such documentation would be crucial if any litigation were to arise. After collecting these samples, all the remaining food and beverages were thrown away (much to the chagrin of the kitchen staff, who had labored long hours in their preparations) to prevent any additional illness from occurring.

Suspecting the punch, the sanitarian and I investigated the preparation and serving of the punch at the church and began to trace its origins. Our immediate actions were to determine whether others, apart from those who attended the wedding, might have purchased it. If so, we could alert them to the possibility that the punch might be contaminated, which might help them avoid meeting the same fate as some of the wedding guests.

Members of the bride's family informed us that they purchased the punch ready-made from a local vendor—a couple who made and sold it out of their home. We were also informed that this particular type of punch was well known locally, popular for events as well as for individual consumption. This, of course, was worrisome to us because it suggested that others, possibly many others, could be at risk if the punch was indeed contaminated.

We immediately called the couple that made this punch. They informed us they had already talked to the mother of the bride, who had called earlier in the day about her concerns with the punch. Hearing this concern, one of them had tasted the punch from the same lot as the punch sold for the wedding and was able to confirm that the punch did not taste "right."

We first asked for the names and contact information of anyone who purchased punch from the same lot that was served at the wedding. They identified three purchasers and we immediately attempted to contact them. We were able to reach two of the three, and were gratified to find out that they had not yet consumed any of the punch. We advised them not to drink any of it, of course, but asked them to hold on to the punch for now, in case it was needed for testing. Unfortunately, despite repeated attempts and the assistance of the local police, we were not able to reach the third person who had bought punch—a young woman who had bought 2 gallons of it for a baby shower. (Two days later we found out that the punch was served at a baby shower attended by 15 people. Of these people, 8 developed symptoms consistent with those experienced by the ill wedding guests, but none sought medical attention. They told us that because the punch tasted funny, they did not consume much of it.)

We all worked rather late into the night. By the time we quit for the day, we had an initial understanding of the nature of the outbreak, its extent and severity, and some leads as to the cause. We had also instituted some interim control measures. We had learned that an outbreak of methemoglobinemia had occurred among people attending a wedding, and that dozens had been seen in three local emergency departments, with 16 admitted to the hospital. (Thankfully, there were no deaths, although we understood that the condition of one of the older patients was guarded that evening.) We suspected that one or more of the foods or beverages at the reception had been contaminated by a compound that could cause methemoglobinemia, and we had collected samples of all the foods and beverages for laboratory testing. Through interviews of patients and other guests, we had evidence supporting a hypothesis that the punch was the source of the outbreak. We needed more information to test this hypothesis, but, based on the information available, we had taken steps to prevent others from consuming the suspect punch.

Before we discuss the next steps in the investigation, it is worthwhile to review the pathophysiology of methemoglobinemia.

METHEMOGLOBINEMIA

Tom Boo: Oxygen from the lungs is carried by red blood cells to cells of the body. Oxygen attaches to the hemoglobin molecules within the red blood cell; the iron atom at the center of each hemoglobin molecule is the key to this binding. Hemoglobin can only bind and carry oxygen if the iron is in the reduced or ferrous (Fe^{++}) state. If the iron atom is in the opposite state (i.e., oxidized to Fe^{+++}), this nonfunctional hemoglobin molecule is called methemoglobin. The oxidation of hemoglobin is a reversible reaction and occurs normally at low levels as red blood cells are exposed to oxidant chemicals from dietary or other sources. Red blood cells contain antioxidant compounds that reverse the formation of methemoglobin, thus maintaining the hemoglobin in its functional state. If red blood cells are exposed to higher

> *If red blood cells are exposed to higher amounts of oxidizing chemicals, more than they can compensate for, a larger than normal proportion of the hemoglobin in the bloodstream will be converted to methemoglobin.*

amounts of oxidizing chemicals, more than they can compensate for, a larger than normal proportion of the hemoglobin in the bloodstream will be converted to methemoglobin. Methemoglobinemia is usually defined as the condition in which greater than 1–2% of the hemoglobin in the body has been oxidized and cannot carry oxygen.

The effects of methemoglobinemia depend upon the proportion of the body's hemoglobin that is in the oxidized state, the rate at which the oxidation has occurred (a slow, chronic oxidization process may be much better tolerated than a sudden one), and of course, the age and general condition of the affected person. Table 22-1 shows some of the signs and symptoms associated with methemoglobinemia, with more severe symptoms associated with greater levels of methemoglobinemia. Methemoglobinemia is potentially fatal, but death is uncommon in otherwise healthy people, in part because the condition is readily treatable.

Milder levels of methemoglobinemia are reversible without treatment. Generally, after the exposure to the causative agent is removed, the body's normal compensatory mechanisms will suffice. In more serious cases, methylene blue can be administered intravenously, rapidly returning the oxidized hemoglobin to its normal reduced state. Within minutes of administration to a distressed cyanotic patient, the recipient begins to turn pink and breathe normally.

TABLE 22-1 Signs and Symptoms of Methemoglobinemia

Cyanosis (pale-blue discoloration of the skin)
Headache
Shortness of breath
Lightheadedness
Weakness
Confusion
Heart palpitations
Chest pains
Altered mental status
Seizures
Coma
Death

THE EPIDEMIOLOGIC INVESTIGATION CONTINUES

Tom Boo: Sunday morning, we sat down to discuss the investigation and plan our next steps. We needed to determine as quickly as possible whether there was an ongoing public health threat to more people, and if so, prevent others from becoming ill. We also needed to determine what caused this outbreak and use this information to prevent such outbreaks in the future.

We determined that the investigation would need to have three components: epidemiologic, laboratory, and environment. The epidemiologic component would allow us to describe the outbreak—how many people got ill, when they got ill, and their symptoms and clinical course—as well as identify what caused them to become ill. The laboratory component would allow us to identify the compound that caused methemoglobinemia, the foods and beverages that were contaminated with this compound, and the amount of contamination. The environmental component would allow us to determine how this compound was introduced into the foods and beverages.

We wanted to interview more of the wedding attendees than just those who were at the hospital the night before. We discussed how we might select a sample of attendees, but in the end decided that it would be feasible to try to interview all of the people who attended the wedding. We reviewed and made refinements to the questionnaire that we had used the night before. This revised questionnaire asked basic demographic information (age and sex), body weight (a possible predictor of illness because low-weight individuals might be at greater risk for illness than high-weight individuals if they both consumed the same amount of contaminant); illness information (presence or absence of illness, presence or absence of certain signs and symptoms suggestive of methemoglobinemia, and whether a person was treated or hospitalized); and exposure information (whether a person consumed specific foods or beverages served at the reception and if so, how much).

While working on the questionnaire, we obtained the wedding invitation list from the bride's family and the guest book from the church in order to contact all of the wedding guests. Even with this information, it was challenging because many people on the invitation list had not attended the wedding, the signatures in the guest book were frequently hard to read and correlate with the invitation list, and neither source provided phone numbers. While we began looking up phone numbers and calling people, we also sent letters to everyone on the invitation list (we had their addresses from the invitation list), asking them to call us if they had not already been contacted. I also went back to the three hospitals to collect clinical information from the medical records using a standard form we developed to extract patient data.

This effort to gather as much data as possible took several weeks. However, as data began to accumulate, we got a clearer understanding of the range of symptoms reported and used these data to establish case definitions. Case definitions are used by investigators to categorize interviewees as cases (i.e., cases had the illness being investigated and others did not). They also are used to classify interviewees according to the investigator's level of confidence that they are cases (the reason behind the commonly used nomenclature confirmed, probable, and suspect cases). Case definitions are developed based on the understanding of the signs and symptoms of the disease and the timing of the onset of illness. They can also include references to the results of clinical laboratory tests, if such tests are available. We compiled a list of the symptoms reported by at least three wedding attendees; those who reported one or more of the symptoms within 8 hours of the reception were classified as "suspect cases" and those with one or more of the symptoms within 8 hours of the reception *and* methemoglobin levels greater than 1% were classified as "confirmed cases" (see Table 22-2). Following completion of the interviews and the medical record review, data were entered into *Epi Info 2002* and were analyzed using *Epi Info 2002* and *SAS 4.0*.

After several weeks of trying to make contact with all of the wedding attendees, we ultimately succeeded in interviewing 258 persons, representing about half of the estimated number of people in attendance. Among those who were interviewed, 41 met the confirmed case definition and 89 met the suspect case definition, for a total of 130 cases. Sixty-three people had sought emergency department care and 20, including 14 people younger than 15 years of age, were hospitalized. Thirty-five people were treated with methylene blue. Fortunately, there were no deaths.

> *Case definitions are developed based on the understanding of the signs and symptoms of the disease and the timing of the onset of illness. They can also include references to the results of clinical laboratory tests, if such tests are available.*

TABLE 22-2 Case Definition Used in an Iowa Outbreak of Methemoglobinemia

Criteria
Clinical criteria: Collapse, cyanosis, headache, dizziness, palpitations, shortness of breath, nausea, vomiting, weakness, fatigue, chest discomfort, or chills within 8 hours of the wedding reception.
Laboratory criteria: Methemoglobin level >1%
Case definitions
Suspect case: Attendee with one or more clinical criteria.
Confirmed case: Suspect case meeting laboratory criteria.

Those who met the case definitions experienced a variety of symptoms, which are listed in Table 22-3 with data on the frequency of these symptoms.

An epidemic curve (epi curve), showing confirmed cases in light gray and suspect cases in dark gray, is presented in Figure 22-1. The reception began at about 1415 hours (2:15pm), as indicated by the arrow. Almost immediately, some people developed symptoms. Thirty people reported onset of symptoms within 15 minutes,

TABLE 22-3 Frequency of Symptoms Reported Among 130 Cases

Symptom	Number	Percentage
Headache	77	59
Dizziness	77	59
Nausea	49	38
Vomiting	28	22
Palpitations	28	22
Weakness	28	22
Fatigue	22	17
Shortness of breath	20	15
Cyanosis	12	9
Collapse	9	7
Chest discomfort	5	4
Chills/sweats	4	3

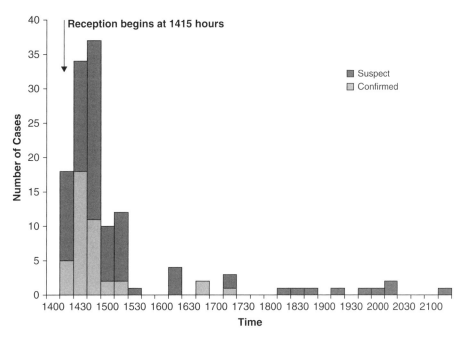

FIGURE 22-1 Epidemic curve of time from reception to onset of symptoms.

most within one hour, and all confirmed cases within 3 hours.

These data allowed us to determine any associations between illness and consuming specific foods or beverages. Consuming the punch was statistically associated with illness (relative risk 18.2 (95% C.I. 5.9–55.4)), meaning that a person who consumed punch had an 18-fold greater risk of developing illness compared to someone who did not. Among the 180 persons who reported drinking any amount of punch, 70% of them became ill; thus the attack rate was 70%.

We also wanted to see if there was a dose–response relationship (i.e., was the risk of illness higher with higher amounts of exposure to the punch). If so, this would strengthen the statistical association between punch consumption and illness. In the questionnaire, we asked each person who had consumed one or more of the menu items to try to quantify how much they ate or drank, and from this we calculated an estimated dose in cc/kg of body weight. Although the estimates of quantity were subjective, the results did show a clear dose–response effect, with the attack rate increasing as the dose of punch consumed increased (chi-square for trend, suspect cases – 5.7; p-value 0.02; confirmed cases – 28.1; p-value <0.01).

THE ENVIRONMENTAL INVESTIGATION CONTINUES AND A TRACEBACK OCCURS

Cortland Lohff: On the Monday following the outbreak, we made our first visit to the couple's house where the punch was made. In describing how they made the punch, they told us it had three ingredients: a flavoring agent, sugar, and citric acid. The flavoring agent, which the couple referred to as their "secret ingredient," had been purchased a few years before and was stored in the basement of their home. When they wanted to prepare some powdered punch mix, they provided some of the secret ingredient to a local food processing facility. The food processing facility, supplying the sugar and citric acid, would mix the three ingredients according the couple's recipe, and package the powdered mix in 18-ounce foil packages. These were packed into boxes, shipped to the couple's home, and stored in the garage.

Upon receiving orders from consumers, the couple would take one 18-ounce package of the powdered punch mix, mix it with water and ice in a one gallon container, freeze the liquid, and sell the frozen punch with instructions to thaw it overnight and serve it in a slushy consistency (Figure 22-2). These preparations were done is a separate room off of the garage.

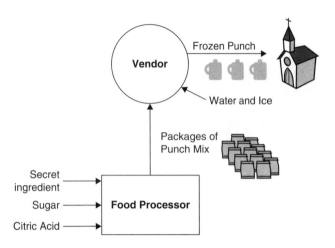

FIGURE 22-2 A generalized pathway from punch creation to consumption.

We visited the couple's house several times over the following days, accompanied by an inspector from the Department of Inspections and Appeals (the state agency responsible for the licensing and inspection of restaurants, other food vendors, and food processors). We gathered the details about how the implicated lot of punch was made, learning that this lot included a total of 1,420 pounds of powdered punch mix in cases containing the 18-ounce foil packages. We also inspected the site where the powdered punch was mixed with water and ice, and took samples of everything for laboratory testing: packages of the powdered punch mix, the secret ingredient, water, and ice.

The couple was very cooperative throughout the investigation, providing full access to their premises and records. Our inspection of the couple's home revealed no findings that suggested the contamination occurred there. Knowing this, our attention then shifted to the food processing facility.

Tom Boo: Within days following the outbreak, investigators from the Department of Inspections and Appeals and the federal Food and Drug Administration inspected the food processing facility. During their inspection, they interviewed the owner and some of the supervisors, reviewed pertinent records, and inspected the facility. The owner and the supervisors explained how the powdered punch mix was prepared, and inspections were done in the parts of the facility where the different steps in the preparation of the mix had occurred: the warehouse where the ingredients were stored, the mixing room, and the packaging room. They learned that the facility's practice was to bring the ingredients from the warehouse to the mixing room, where the ingredients were weighed. Then, these measured ingredients were held for 5 days before they were mixed; the secret ingredient and the citric acid were held in separate labeled plastic bags atop the sugar, which was in a large wheeled-tub. They scrutinized the records of the production of the implicated lot of the punch mix. These records showed that the punch order had been mixed in two separate batches because of its size, though each was assigned the same lot number.

During the first inspection, samples of the citric acid were collected for laboratory testing. However, because the turnover of the sugar stock was high, none remained from the time when the implicated lot of punch mix was made.

THE LABORATORY INVESTIGATION BEGINS

Tom Boo: The specimens of foods and beverages collected at the church were sent for analysis to the University of Iowa Hygienic Laboratory (UHL), which is the state's public health laboratory. In the days that followed, we sent additional specimens—the samples collected from the home of the couple who made and sold the liquid punch, samples of punch that had been recalled from other buyers, and samples of the citric acid collected from the food processing facility. In total, more than 70 specimens were tested.

In the beginning of this investigation we did not know the compound that caused methemoglobinemia, so the UHL tested for a number of compounds known to cause this condition using a variety of tests—light microscopy, rapid test strips, ion chromatography, liquid chromatography mass spectrometry, inductively-coupled plasma (ICP) atomic emission mass spectroscopy, and ICP mass spectrometry. Quantitative testing was subsequently performed using ion chromatography and automated colorimetry.

The results of all these tests revealed high levels of sodium nitrite (500–800 mg/kg) in samples of the punch served at the wedding and in samples of the punch from the same lot that had been sold to another consumer. Similarly, testing showed high levels (3200–6000 mg/kg) of sodium nitrite in the unopened 18-ounce packages of powdered punch mix obtained from the couple's home. No sodium nitrite was found in other foods from the wedding or in the water, ice, or secret ingredient obtained from the couple's home.

THE ENVIRONMENTAL INVESTIGATION CONTINUES

Tom Boo: As soon as the UHL informed us that sodium nitrite was the contaminant, I went to the food processing facility with the state and federal inspectors to determine how this contamination might have occurred. The inspector from the Department of Inspections and Appeals was familiar with the food processor and knew that they used sodium nitrite in some of their cured meat products. During our record review, we looked to see whether any foods containing sodium nitrite had been processed during the period the implicated lot of punch was prepared. None had been. The last order containing sodium nitrite had been processed 5 days before they started the punch mix.

THE LABORATORY INVESTIGATION CONCLUDES AND A HYPOTHESIS DEVELOPS REGARDING THE REASON FOR THE CONTAMINATION

Tom Boo: In addition to finding sodium nitrite, the UHL determined that there was no citric acid in any of the samples where sodium nitrite was found—there was no citric acid in the punch served at the wedding or sold to another consumer, nor was there any citric acid in the unopened 18-ounce packages of the powdered punch mix. Based on these results, we considered the possibility that sodium nitrite may have been added instead of citric acid to prepare the powdered punch mix. Both were white powders and one could have been substituted for the other, either intentionally or unintentionally. To know if this substitution did in fact occur, I sought further assistance from the UHL to determine if the amount of sodium nitrite that had been added was equivalent to the amount of citric acid that should have been added. I asked the chemists to help me calculate backward from the concentration of sodium nitrite in the punch mix to the amount of citric acid that should have been added at the time of mixing. The calculation demonstrated that the measured concentrations of sodium nitrite were consistent with someone having added the right amount of the wrong substance. To me, this suggested a mistake, rather than an intentional act, but it was impossible to know. With this information, we then turned our attention back to the food processing facility.

THE INVESTIGATION CONCLUDES

Tom Boo: Having determined that the punch mix contained sodium nitrite instead of citric acid, we inspected the food processing facility again. In the warehouse, we looked to see how the sugar, citric acid, and sodium nitrite were stored. Although the sodium nitrite and citric acid looked pretty similar—both were white crystalline substance—the containers were quite different and located on opposite sides of the same shelf, accessed from different aisles. It was not clear how someone might have inadvertently substituted one for the other. We asked whether there were any disgruntled employees who could have intentionally put sodium nitrite into the punch mix, but the management assured us there were not. They hypothesized a language barrier might have played a role in this substitution because some of the key staff were less than fluent in English.

We never determined how sodium nitrite was substituted for citric acid in the punch mix. We learned nothing that made us suspect this was done maliciously and we assumed, at the time, that the substitution had been accidental.

> *In retrospect, inviting law enforcement officials to be part of the inspection at the food processing facility might have been helpful because their inquiries may have helped to uncover some additional details that were unknown to us.*

However, in retrospect, inviting law enforcement officials to be part of the inspection at the food processing facility might have been helpful because their inquiries may have helped to uncover some additional details that were unknown to us.

DISCUSSION

Patricia Quinlisk: Like Tom, I was an EIS officer (many years earlier) and completed my training at a state health department prior to eventually taking my present position as state epidemiologist and medical director for IDPH. However, despite my years of experience, I too had never responded to an outbreak of methemoglobinemia. I had encountered cases of "blue baby syndrome." This is a form of methemoglobinemia that occasionally occurs in infants after they are fed baby formula made with well water contaminated with nitrites, a byproduct of agricultural fertilizers.

These concentrations of nitrites can sometimes cause symptoms in infants, even though older children and adults will not get ill.

Outbreaks of methemoglobinemia due to contamination of foods with nitrates or nitrites have been known to occur as a result of mistaking one white powder with another (Figure 22-3). In fact, one of the most famous descriptions of an outbreak investigation found in the literature is told by the medical journalist Berton Roueché in his book *Eleven Blue Men*.[3] This book recounts the story of a 1944 outbreak in which 11 homeless men in New York City turned blue after eating oatmeal served at a run-down café. They had developed methemoglobinemia and turned blue (cyanotic), hence the title of the book. An investigation revealed that the oatmeal had been made in a 6-gallon batch using oats, water, and a handful of salt. The salt was taken from a gallon container labeled "salt," which happened to be sitting right next to a similar gallon container with a different type of white crystalline substance—sodium nitrate (saltpeter)—that was used by the café in corning beef and pastrami. The person preparing the oatmeal grabbed a handful of sodium nitrate, mistaking this for the regular salt, when preparing the oatmeal. Additionally, some of the saltshakers placed on the tables had been filled with sodium nitrate, explaining why those who had additionally sprinkled what they believed to be common table salt on their oatmeal were more likely to become ill. One of the 11 men died.

An outbreak of methemoglobinemia affecting members of a single household in New York City in 2002 was similar in origin, but involved concerns of terrorism.[4] After preparing a meal using a white crystalline substance found in a bag labeled in English and Arabic as "refined iodized table salt," five adults became acutely ill, experiencing dizziness, lightheadedness, and cyanosis. Upon presentation to a local emergency department, all were markedly cyanotic and blood drawn for testing was noted to be dark-colored. All were treated with methylene blue and within minutes their cyanosis resolved. Public health and law enforcement officials investigated because sodium nitrate can be used as an antidote by persons handling sodium cyanide and, suspiciously, a shipment of sodium cyanide had recently disappeared. The investigation determined that a previous tenant had left behind some sodium nitrite (that he used to preserve meat) in a bag labeled "refined iodized table salt."

Tom Boo: Nitrates and nitrites are also used in plumbing because they retard corrosion, and some significant outbreaks have occurred when drinking water became contaminated. Outbreaks have been reported at a school and an office in which drinking water from a municipal source was contaminated by boiler additives due to defective backflow valves.[5] At the school, 29 students were found to have methemoglobinemia, some with quite high levels. Industrial exposures have also caused outbreaks of methemoglobinemia. Linz and colleagues reported the investigation of methemoglobinemia in five workers at a rubber plant that was attributed to handling an adhesive containing dinitrobenzene.[6]

CONCLUSIONS

Patricia Quinlisk: As illustrated in this report, outbreaks do not occur in isolation. Outbreaks can, and

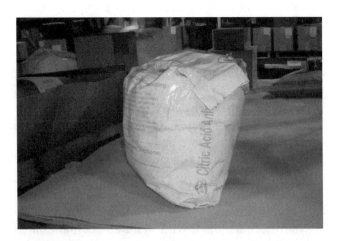 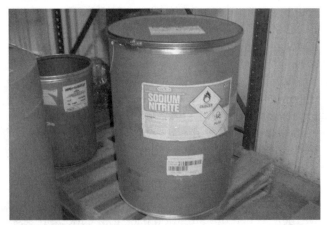

FIGURE 22-3 Photos taken of citric acid in a bag, and sodium nitrite in a barrel. These two white powder substances are quite similar in appearance.

often do, have widespread implications—sometimes on a community, as reported here, and other times on the whole nation (e.g., an outbreak of *E. coli* caused by contaminated spinach). In this investigation, all of those attending the wedding were impacted (regardless of whether or not they became ill), three emergency departments were inundated with patients (with a very unusual disease), public safety officials had to respond, and the news media was involved. A good epidemiologist is aware of all the partners involved and understands their respective roles.

I admit that of all the outbreaks I have been involved with in my career, this is the one that I felt the most sympathy for the affected persons. It is hard to imagine a worse ending to your wedding than having 11 ambulances arriving at the church, the fire department setting up incident command, and half of your family and friends seeking medical care. I hope that they at least had an uneventful honeymoon!

Cortland Lohff: Good communication between public health officials and healthcare providers is critical. Although public health officials would like to hear about outbreaks from healthcare providers as soon as healthcare providers recognize one, unfortunately, this is not always the case. Epidemiologists and other public health officials need to do a better job of keeping healthcare providers informed of their obligations to report outbreaks and teaching them how to report. Healthcare providers need to do a better job of meeting these obligations. Healthcare providers are legally required in all states to not only report certain diseases, but also to immediately report outbreaks and other public health emergencies (this is especially true for diseases or outbreaks secondary to an act of terrorism).

In this case, I am very grateful to the news reporter. Although her call put us in an awkward position (her question could not be answered because we did not know anything about the outbreak), she did "tip us off" and we were able to respond.

Tom Boo: Outbreak investigations are challenging and exhilarating experiences. They force the epidemiologist to put into practice their knowledge and skills, often under very stressful conditions. At the same time, they can be frustrating experiences. Despite all the effort one may put into an investigation, there are times when epidemiologists are not able to understand everything. In this investigation, despite conducting a very comprehensive investigation that included epidemiologic, laboratory, and environmental components, in the end, we never did determine the reason why the sodium nitrite was substituted for the citric acid. Not knowing, we were unable to offer specific recommendations to the food processing facility to prevent this from ever happening again.

LEARNING QUESTIONS

1. Outbreak investigations commonly have three components. List each of these components and discuss how they contribute to the investigation.
2. Case definitions are useful for outbreak investigations. Describe what a case definition is and how they are used in these investigations.
3. How could you edit the investigators' case definition to make it more specific (and therefore less sensitive)?
4. The investigators were concerned that the punch might have been contaminated intentionally. What did they do to try to determine if there was intentional versus unintentional contamination? What did they find? How comfortable are you with their conclusions?
5. During outbreak investigations, those affected may report what they believe to be the cause of the outbreak. Under what circumstances can such reports be useful to the investigator? Despite these reports, why must the investigator continue to conduct the full investigation?

REFERENCES

1. Ash-Bernal R, Wise R, Wright SM. Acquired methemoglobinemia: a retrospective series of 138 cases at 2 teaching hospitals. *Medicine (Baltimore)*. 2004;83(5):265–273.
2. Romanelli F, Smith KM, Thornton AC, Pomeroy C. Poppers: epidemiology and clinical management of inhaled nitrite abuse. *Pharmacotherapy*. 2004;24(1):69–78.
3. Roueche B. *Eleven Blue Men and Other Narratives of Medical Detection*. New York, NY: Berkley Publishing Group, 1965.
4. Methemoglobinemia following unintentional ingestion of sodium nitrite—New York, 2002. *MMWR Morb Mortal Wkly Rep*. 2002;51(29):639–642.
5. Methemoglobinemia attributable to nitrite contamination of potable water through boiler fluid additives—New Jersey, 1992 and 1996. *MMWR Morb Mortal Wkly Rep*. 1997;46(09):202–204.
6. Greenham RK, Fallon LF Jr. Methemoglobinemia: an industrial outbreak among rubber molding workers. *J Occup Environ Med*. 2006;48:523–528.

CHAPTER 23

Toxic School Lunch: Chemical Poisoning of Elementary School Children in Joliet, Illinois

Alpesh Patel, MBBS, MPH, CERC, CPHA and
Mark S. Dworkin, MD, MPH&TM, FACP

Illinois, 2002

INTRODUCTION

Alpesh Patel: The events of September 11, 2001 (9/11), the ensuing anthrax scare, and fears of smallpox and other bioterrorism attacks shook the U.S. public health system. During 2002, more than $1 billion flowed from the federal government to the states and from there to some of the more than 3,000 local public health jurisdictions. This money was aimed at strengthening and preparing public health systems to cope with the emerging threat of bioterrorism. In November 2002, I began working at my first real job as an epidemiologist with one of the local health departments in northern Illinois. Before this job, the only experience I had was working in the HIV/AIDS section of the Illinois Department of Public Health and assisting with the department's rapid response team (RRT) in limited capacity. As a trained medical doctor in India, I had been taught about diseases and biological agents of terrorism. I graduated from the Baroda Medical College, Maharaja Sayajirao University of Baroda, Gujarat, India in 1997 and came to the United States in October 1998 as a graduate student with the hope of acquiring higher education in medicine and public health and begin a career as an epidemiologist. I was very excited to have a real job at the Will County Health Department as their lead epidemiologist where I could apply my knowledge and the little experience that I had recently acquired while assisting the RRT at my previous job.

Mark S. Dworkin: In November 2002, I was the Illinois Department of Public Health's state epidemiologist. In this position, I was the team leader for the RRT, which provided onsite assistance to local health departments that requested help with outbreak investigations. I also led related field epidemiology training at a regional level throughout the state.

I met Alpesh when we both were working for the state health department in their downtown Chicago office. At first, I thought Alpesh was a program staff level epidemiologist working in the HIV section. While that was true, by talking to him and going out to lunch a few times I learned that Alpesh was much more than that and he was employed far below his level of capability.

Sometimes, we would go to a nearby Indian restaurant that had old Bollywood movies distractingly blasting from a TV. It was what most would describe as a "hole in the wall" and the place literally looked like it was falling apart, which just gave it that much more of a mystique and attracted me to return many times. Over naan and curry dishes, we talked of infectious diseases, health department politics, and a little about his life in India. I learned that he had a medical degree and a Master's degree in public health. What a potential resource. I enthusiastically offered him the opportunity to assist with the RRT and to work with me on some data analysis of laboratory results related to salmonellosis and a particularly concerning antibiotic-resistant strain of *Salmonella typhimurium* referred to as DT104. I hoped that he would get promoted. Before that could happen, he was offered a job with the Will County Health Department.

Alpesh Patel: It was my first week at the new job; I was introduced to various staff that I would be working with directly and indirectly on a daily basis. Some of them had never heard of a professional title called "Epidemiologist." They thought I held some special knowledge and expertise dealing with biological agents that were so much in demand after 9/11. I was not even a part of the health department's communicable disease program because my new position had not existed before. I was placed in the Information Technology department because they thought that I had a lot to do with data. They were right, to a certain extent, in their assumption that I had a lot to do with data, but they were not sure about what department I should be placed in. I explained that I would be working with the communicable disease staff, area hospitals, and healthcare providers on a daily basis to acquire disease information to perform my duties. Just as they were learning about me in the first week, I learned a lot about local health departments and their capabilities. Most surveillance done at the local level is relatively passive. It was often a paper process that required full clinical confirmation of a fairly narrow set of specific diseases. In many large communities, such as nearby Cook County (where Chicago is located), a syndromic surveillance model was being implemented. This costly, but potentially useful, active surveillance system employed ongoing communication. Access to the funding for such a system was limited and acquiring this real-time capability would be time consuming and labor intensive with uncertainty about the future funding and efficacy of the system in real life. I decided to strengthen the existing systems by opening the communication channels among our local surveillance stakeholders so that information could be reported immediately and followed up on in a reasonable amount of time.

The nation barely had time to catch its breath after the 9/11 attacks and the intentional anthrax outbreak where spores were sent to various politicians and reporters through the U.S. mail. It was not unusual to receive a call from a concerned citizen about a suspicious package or letter with one of the hallmarks of concern, including white powder, excessive postage, handwritten or poorly typed addresses, incorrect title, title without a name, misspelled common words, oily stains, odors, discoloration or lopsided appearance of the envelope, missing return address, excessive weight, protruding wires or aluminum foil, or excessive security measures such as string, masking tape, and so on. Even letters marked "personal" or "confidential" and letters that had a city or state in the postmark that didn't match the return address were suspect.

Mark S. Dworkin: It had been an incredibly busy 12 months. The attack on the twin towers in New York City and the anthrax investigations led to an unprecedented amount of bioterrorism preparedness and response work at the national, state, and local level. Everything from anthrax and plague to chemical poisoning and smallpox vaccination was being considered or, in the case of smallpox vaccination, dealt with. (These were all diseases that we normally had little to nothing to do with before this new age of bioterrorism.) I was lucky to be assigned an Epidemic Intelligence Service (EIS) officer from the Centers for Disease Control and Prevention (CDC), who arrived in August just as Illinois experienced its first summer and fall of human West Nile virus fever, meningitis, and encephalitis. Illinois had more than 800 cases reported that year in just a 3-month time frame and it became a huge part of our workload on top of everything else we had been dealing with. The RRT was part of the health department's massive planning for a high-level weapons of mass destruction exercise called TOPOFF II (top officials, second exercise) that would, in one way or another, involve the Department of Homeland Security, the governor's office, and high- and low-level officials at the state and local level in Illinois. It was scheduled for May 2003. All things urgent and emergent were very much on our minds at this time.

THE NOTIFICATION

Alpesh Patel: It had been just 2 weeks since I started this job. On November 25, 2002, the Will County Health Department was notified of illness among several dozen school children, many within 1 hour of eating lunch prepared by the Laraway Elementary School kitchen (grades 3–8) in Joliet, IL. This school's kitchen had also prepared lunch for nearby Oak Valley Elementary School (grades K–2). The illnesses were characterized primarily by stomachache, nausea, and headache. Onset of illness was very fast and many students were reported to have vomited in the bathrooms and hallways of the school. Understandably, this created some panic because things had progressed quickly and dramatically. Eighteen ambulances took 42 children and two adults to five local hospital emergency departments. Due to the recent anthrax attack and potential bioterrorism threat, the school and area hospitals notified the health department immediately about this unusual explosion of illness. They shared with us that this illness started immediately after the school lunch was served. We knew that the nature of the illness would catch the attention of the local and national media due to the ongoing threat of terrorism.

It was like I was having an out-of-body experience: I had just started working as an epidemiologist and barely started establishing contacts with internal and external partners, when an outbreak of unusual illness landed in my lap. I knew that I would be asked to lead the investigation, but it had a public health magnitude of importance that I had never encountered in my training and brief public health career. I feared I could lose my position if the investigation of this outbreak did not identify the cause of the illness, but at the same time it was a great opportunity for me to utilize my epidemiologic skills and knowledge and prove my ability. My experience working with the Illinois RRT came in handy. The Communicable Disease section and Division of Food, Drugs, and Dairies at the Illinois Department of Public Health were immediately notified about the incident. I was afraid that I would not have enough individuals available to conduct interviews, enter data, answer phone calls, collect specimens, and test specimens as quickly as the situation warranted. It was not an ideal way to start a new job, but it was very important that I fulfill the expectation of the health department and perform my job. I made up my mind before the end of the day to ask my superior to allow me to seek assistance from the RRT.

Mark S. Dworkin: When I received the telephone call from Alpesh that there was an outbreak with such a sudden onset and that it was in a vulnerable population (young school children), I was both eager to provide assistance and uncertain what to expect. I was reassured that at the time he called me, he knew that many of the children were already recovering and no one required life support. But, the image of ambulances rushing children from the school to emergency departments at the local hospitals gave the outbreak a sense of immediacy and urgency that was above and beyond most of the outbreaks I had experienced. I also wanted to dismiss the possibility that this could be intentional poisoning because I did not want such a major incident to have occurred, but I knew that it would have to be considered.

This outbreak did not need a step to verify that it was indeed an outbreak. Baseline absenteeism rates were irrelevant when ambulances show up to carry away dozens of ill students. Confirming the diagnosis would come later because at this time we had only a gastrointestinal syndrome, but nothing definitive. In preparing for the field work, I quickly performed a PubMed search on the Internet about school lunch and outbreaks just in case it would be helpful. It was uninformative, but it reassured me to go through the motions just in case it might be helpful.

FIELD INVESTIGATION–THE DAY OF THE INCIDENT (NOVEMBER 25, 2002)

Alpesh Patel: It was just another regular autumn day at the school. The Laraway Elementary School has a large kitchen and prepares lunches for themselves and Oak Valley Elementary School in the same district. The school receives their supplies for lunch under the National School Lunch Program (NSLP) through the Illinois State Board of Education. It is a voluntary program available to all public schools, private schools, and residential child care institutions that agree to operate a nonprofit program offering lunches meeting federal requirements to all children in attendance. The lunch arrives in packed boxes and is stored in school refrigerated or frozen storage at the recommended temperature until prepared and served. The kitchen staff knows the routine and prepares the lunches according to the recommended oven temperatures; the result is a hot lunch. We were told that within a few minutes after the lunch was served, a few students and teachers started smelling an unusual odor coming from the lunch, but the cafeteria staff decided to continue serving the lunch and asked students to eat. It was unfortunate that the early warning signal was ignored under the assumption that kids make excuses about a bad smell or taste, or suddenly and conveniently have a stomachache when the food served is not their choice or to their liking. It was very obvious from the complaint that something was wrong with the food, but it was believed that the food in the school comes from a highly regulated lunch program run by state and federal authorities.

Mark S. Dworkin: In an interview with one of the children held at the Will County Health Department the day after this event, Alpesh and I asked a boy if he had smelled anything unusual. He said that it smelled like they had cleaned the cafeteria because of the odor of window cleaner. He said his chicken smelled unusual and he told one of the lunch monitors. The reply was to just put more barbecue sauce on it and to go ahead and eat it. He complied.

Alpesh Patel: Within one hour after eating the lunch, 42 students and 2 adults started complaining of a combination of one or more symptoms, including mouth burning, dizziness, headache, nausea, and vomiting. A total of 335 students and teachers at the schools were served lunch prepared at the Laraway Elementary School kitchen to students at both schools in two lunch periods (11:00 a.m. to 11:30 a.m. and 12:00 p.m. to 12:30 p.m.). A total of 122 lunches were served to students at Laraway Elementary School in the second lunch period. The illness was mainly reported from students and teachers who ate lunch in the second period. The other school had only one lunch period that coincided with Laraway's first lunch period. Laraway Elementary School immediately called 911, the emergency response service, so that the students who were sick would get immediate medical attention. Forty-two students and two teachers were taken to five area hospital emergency departments via ambulance for further evaluation. Most were treated and released; none was admitted for any life-threatening injury caused by the illness. School was cancelled for the rest of the day because of the magnitude of the unexplained sickness. The news about an unusual illness making dozens sick after eating lunch at the school was spreading rapidly in the community and to local and national news media. The school parking lot was filled with local media vans and camera crews waiting for any possible information regarding the incident.

An outbreak of foodborne illness is not uncommon in school settings, but the magnitude and nature of this one was unusual at the time when local communities feared a possible bioterrorism attack. Local residents were concerned about the incident and the safety of their children and families. The health department was flooded with calls from the community and media about the incident. Local communities were worried and scared because of the nature of the outbreak when the threat of bioterrorism was high. It was very obvious to me that I would be asked to initiate the investigation immediately. It was very important that I coordinate the investigation with local partners (our Division of Environmental Health and the Communicable Disease program) and state partners (the Illinois Department of Public Health and the Illinois State Board of Education) so that information could be gathered and shared in a timely manner. We hypothesized that food was a source of the outbreak and the school administration suspended serving lunch prepared from the supply they received under the NSLP.

Mark S. Dworkin: The initial hypothesis that the source of the outbreak was the school lunch that the students had just eaten seemed reasonable. However, it was important to entertain alternative hypotheses to ensure we did not overlook another plausible source of these illnesses. Outbreaks caused by infectious diseases can have onset of illness from hours to days after consumption of the meal. Could the students who became ill have eaten a shared meal in the morning, perhaps at a Head Start program? Or could they have possibly eaten a contaminated lunch the day before with a 24-hour incubation period? Technically, these possibilities were not completely excludable. However, the apparent clustering of so many ill persons in such a narrow time period (within an hour of the school lunch) was uncharacteristic of an infectious disease, with the exception of one that makes a preformed toxin, such as from *Staphylococcus aureus* (30 minutes to 8 hours) or *Bacillus cereus* (30 minutes to 6 hours). However, the illness observed with those organisms would more likely have a spectrum of cases where some might have onset in an hour or two after eating the meal and others might have onset a few hours later. The same reasoning can be applied to the hypothesis that a shared lunch the previous day was the source. If it were an organism with a mean incubation period of 24 hours that had caused the outbreak, its natural history would have been to have many cases with onset during the lunch hour, but also many cases with onset in the hours preceding lunch and in the hours following lunch. We would be able to validate that this distribution of onset of illness had not occurred as we gathered data from interviews of the lunch attendees. Also, a peculiar odor had been reported during this lunch and that was uncharacteristic of reports of outbreaks of infectious diseases.

Alpesh Patel: The health department's environmental health sanitarian was sent out to perform a thorough inspection of the school kitchen and cafeteria so that any potential food items remaining could be embargoed and secured for testing and tracking of its origin. An inspection of Laraway's kitchen was performed late afternoon on November 25 and previous inspection reports were reviewed. Sanitarians from our health department identified the brand and source of all the foods prepared for the implicated school lunch, including their pathway from packaging to supplier and storage facilities before delivery to the school. So far, no smoking gun was detected and all paper trails suggested that the food supply came from an approved facility and was inspected by an appropriate regulatory agency before being shipped. The state health department's Division of Food, Drugs, and Dairies (including RRT member Karnail Mudahar) determined that the food from the same lots had been delivered to other schools in Illinois and those schools were surveyed for information on quantity received, date received, date served, any product remaining, and illness reported if product was served. Their food was also embargoed with the plan to either save it for testing or destroy it. It was strange in the sense that the same food lots were distributed to other schools in the state, but illness was reported from only one school district. It raised some questions and concerns about possible contamination locally at the school, which kept alive initial concerns about intentional poisoning. Local law enforcement was informed of the outbreak.

By late afternoon, we had valuable pieces of information from the environmental health inspection, emergency department visits, and calls received from concerned parents. To restore confidence and faith in the public school system, it was necessary that we investigate and identify the cause of illness in a short period of time so that parents and local leaders could go back to their routines.

FIELD INVESTIGATION—DAY 1 (NOVEMBER 26, 2002)

Alpesh Patel: Upon request, three members of the Illinois RRT, with EIS officer Greg Huhn, arrived at our health department the morning after the event. By now, the story was already out in local and national media. We knew that the nature of the illness could raise questions and concerns among the general public if a possible cause of illness was not determined in a matter of days, if not hours. During the first hour after the RRT arrived, we reviewed the information from the environmental health inspections of the school kitchen and information collected through calls and emergency department visits. We collected enough information to plan steps that we would follow in terms of environmental, laboratory, epidemiologic, and field investigations. We had valuable information available, such as symptoms, onset of illness, illness duration, and outcome of illness to narrow down our suspicion and formulate a hypothesis to initiate an investigation with a questionnaire distributed to this school cohort.

Through brainstorming based on the available data, we recognized this was not likely to be an illness caused by a bacterial pathogen; it was possibly a commonly used chemical, cleaning agent, or heavy metal contamination. Outbreaks of foodborne illness caused by chemical agents are uncommon and rarely reported in school settings.

Mark S. Dworkin: In assembling the team, I knew that our EIS officer was spread thin with other duties, but I wanted him to at least have a chance to be on the ground for a day with this unusual outbreak, so I invited him out just to help for that brief time. In addition, Dorian Robinson, a Communicable Disease section regional staff person who covered all the local health department jurisdictions within Cook County, and I were the main members of the RRT to go on site. I was offering a public health infectious disease elective for Rush Medical College at the time and had a student who was with me for just 2 weeks. He really got lucky that an outbreak occurred during his short time and he assisted with the investigation.

The administrator for the Will County Health Department led a meeting in his office with our RRT, Alpesh, and other relevant staff. Early in the meeting, Alpesh showed me that the sanitarian had returned with some of the uneaten lunch. Of particular interest was a baggy with uncooked chicken tenders. The administrator, Alpesh, and the sanitarian all seemed pretty confident we were dealing with a chemical agent because of the smell of the chicken. They seemed biased to me and I hesitated to trust their hunch because it had been ingrained in me to assume nothing. Alpesh held up the baggy with a smile and said, "Do you want to smell it?" My initial reaction was to decline, but he encouraged me again with a knowing smile. "C'mon. It has a strong smell of ammonia." I thought this was too good to be true and with everyone in the room watching me, I took the baggy and opened it. Right away, a whiff of ammonia hit me, leaving no doubt that I was now among the converted. This was some sort of chemical. Alpesh volunteered as he smelled it again, "It smelled stronger yesterday."

Alpesh Patel: None of us were experts in chemical foodborne intoxication. We decided to search and review professional publications and literature on foodborne outbreaks caused by chemical agents. Some of the known chemical agents involved in chemical foodborne illness are beneficial and essential in the diet as nutrients; others serve to preserve food or improve food quality, while others are beneficial in food production or used to ensure a clean and sanitary food handling environment.

Chemicals are present all around us. We use them for refrigeration, cleaning, disinfecting, and preserving. They are commonly found in our kitchens and often within close proximity of our food, despite their warnings of toxicity with the potential to result in chemical poisoning. Contamination can occur anywhere from farm to fork. That includes where it was manufactured and stored as well as during transport. It may also be contaminated in a market or in the home, school, restaurant, or other kitchen. The symptoms, severity of symptoms, illness onset, and duration of illness are different among the agents.[1]

The information collected through calls and emergency department visits was really helpful to compare with the literature and further narrow down our suspicion to a potential cause of the outbreak. We were also interested in looking at foodborne illness caused by chemical agents or heavy metal in school settings.

After an extensive search, we were able to find only one foodborne outbreak caused by chemical agents in school settings reported in the United States.[2] That outbreak involved milk contaminated by liquid ammonia that was served to Wisconsin schoolchildren in their lunches; 20 children became ill within 60 minutes of drinking the milk. Ammonia levels greater than 50 ppm can cause immediate irritation of the nose and throat; acute exposure to highly concentrated aerosols can cause cardiovascular problems, including tachycardia, bradycardia, hypertension, cardiac arrhythmia, or in severe cases, cardiac arrest. Burning of the lips, oral cavity, and pharynx can result from exposure to anhydrous ammonia.[3]

Through an online search of medical literature and other publications, you can find some information about almost anything! Unfortunately, your search is fruitless if it doesn't provide you with what you need to do to solve your problem. "What are we going to do?" you may puzzle to yourself. "How are we going to figure out what is making these people sick?" The combination of our new knowledge of ammonia and the results of the environmental investigation from the previous day provided valuable information to consider when we initiated the epidemiologic and laboratory investigation.

Epidemiologic Investigation

Mark S. Dworkin: We knew we needed to interview the students and teachers who had eaten lunch. Determining the descriptive epidemiology is a basic objective in outbreak investigations. With reportable diseases (such as salmonellosis or measles), there are standardized case report forms that guide what information to collect for each case. In our situation, we had neither the diagnosis of a reportable infectious disease nor the belief that we were encountering one. Therefore, we needed to create a data collection instrument that would allow us to describe the distribution of disease. However, we also wanted to try to determine what caused it or at least to provide some evidence for any potential hypothesis about the cause. I was concerned that if we waited to ask those kinds of questions until after we had laboratory confirmation of a chemical, it might be too late to get good cooperation from the school or the children. Sometimes, follow-up studies are undermined by apathy from those involved in the outbreak because they have fully recovered from the illness. This leads to lower participation rates. Because studies like these are limited by the sample size that nature provides rather that the optimal sample size, it can be quite problematic when individuals tell you not to bother them anymore. In addition, cases may be willing to participate early in an outbreak investigation, but may seek legal counsel as time goes on in order to pursue a lawsuit. It has been my experience that often such individuals are advised not to provide any more information to the health department. Therefore, the information we gleaned from our Internet search, the environmental investigation up to this point, and a desire to try to determine all we needed to know quickly were kept in mind as the questions were quickly drafted.

> *A case was defined as a student or teacher who ate food prepared in the Laraway kitchen on November 25, 2002 and developed a headache or symptoms of gastrointestinal tract irritation, including the mouth, throat, or stomach, within 180 minutes of eating lunch.*

Alpesh Patel: A questionnaire was developed using all available information. We decided to administer it to each student in attendance at the two schools on the day of the outbreak. A case definition was developed. A case was defined as a student or teacher who ate food prepared in the Laraway kitchen on November 25, 2002 and developed a headache or symptoms of gastrointestinal tract irritation, including the mouth, throat, or stomach, within 180 minutes of eating lunch. A time period of 180 minutes was chosen because almost no medical literature was available to guide the time period to choose and to provide the most sensitive case definition as possible. It was very important that we interview the students as quickly as possible because we were concerned about difficulty with recall. Interviewing minors about illness is a very tough job because they may forget or change their stories. We wanted to interview more than 300 students at two locations before the end of the school day, which typically ends at 3:00 p.m. We needed patient and skilled personnel. While a final questionnaire was being prepared, an effort was already launched by the health department administration to draw additional staff from other programs. Within a reasonable time, we were able to add 10–12 nurses to the investigating team. With the additional help from school administration and teachers, we were able to interview all of the students before the end of the day.

Mark S. Dworkin: We had good cooperation from the schools. This allowed quick access to interview the students and their faculty about food consumption. Recall bias can be a significant problem in foodborne outbreak investigation, especially when the consumption of the implicated food was days or weeks earlier. Sometimes, asking children about food preferences helps to implicate certain foods when their precise knowledge of what they ate is expected to be poor (such as very young children in a daycare or kindergarten outbreak). In this case, because of the very short time from food consumption to onset of illness, we were able to begin interviewing while recall would still be fairly good. We had a clear hypothesis that the chicken tenders were responsible because they had a chemical smell and the other foods served did not. In addition, the school menu was limited, unlike what is encountered at many restaurants where there may be a dozen or even a hundred different items that can be ordered. Basically, if the student did not eat the entrée (chicken tenders) and the few sides served at the school that day, then they brought their own lunch from home. This advantage of a limited menu was also a potential disadvantage. If most of the students ate the chicken tenders entrée, and there was only one entrée, we might have trouble demonstrating an association with consuming it unless it had an overwhelming attack rate because there could be many persons who ate the chicken tenders but did not get sick. To increase the likelihood we could implicate the chicken tenders if they were truly responsible, we made sure to include a question that asked if they ate "chicken tenders that smelled funny." We also asked how many chicken tenders they ate because we hypothesized that there could be a dose response effect to consuming more chicken (i.e., more ammonia).

Alpesh Patel: While the team out in the field was collecting valuable epidemiologic data, the rest of the members of the RRT at the health department started exploring options to get the environmental and food samples collected from the previous day tested either at the state health department's laboratory in Chicago or at reference laboratories elsewhere. We had no familiarity with how to get food tested for chemical contamination.

Laboratory Investigation

Alpesh Patel: Frozen chicken tenders, as well as samples of those that had been heated but not served, were submitted to the Illinois Department of Public Health laboratory in Chicago for testing. Even though we suspected chemical and heavy metal agents, we decided to request additional testing for staphylococcal toxin and *Bacillus cereus* as potential causative agents because they tend to cause illness of a similar nature. Three tenders were submitted to a reference laboratory in Portland, Oregon for ammonia testing. Testing was performed for staphylococcal toxin by TECRA immunoassay (TECRA International Pty. Ltd., New South Wales, Australia) and for ammonia by spectrophotometry after extraction of meat tissue was submitted to the U.S. Department of Agriculture's Food Safety and Inspection Service (FSIS) laboratory in Athens, Georgia.

With a coordinated effort and support from the health department, school, and the RRT, the field investigation was completed. We used Epi-Info 6.04 software for data entry to calculate frequencies, relative risks, P values, and 95% confidence intervals (CI). The communicable disease staff started data entry immediately. To speed up the data entry process, I took home some completed questionnaires to work from home.

FIELD INVESTIGATION-DAYS 2 AND 3 (NOVEMBER 27-28, 2002)

Epidemiologic Investigation

Alpesh Patel: We were running some preliminary numbers while the data entry was continuing. By the end of the day, we had a significant amount of data entered and available for preliminary analysis to test our hypothesis. On day three, we were able to put together the details of our investigation and successfully identify the cause of the illness.

Among 312 students (median age 10 years), ranging in age from 6 to 14 years, and 18 teachers interviewed at the schools, 157 persons (151 students and 6 teachers) became ill on November 25, 2002 after eating the school lunch. One hundred ten persons satisfied the case definition. Time was the major reason that ill persons did not meet our case definition (Figure 23-1). The time of onset of illness after eating was missing for 36 ill persons and many of the others did not satisfy the case definition because time of onset was beyond our requirement of 180 minutes after eating.

For Laraway, the attack rate was 41% overall—15% for the first lunch period (11:00 a.m. to 11:30 a.m.) and 56% for the second lunch period (12:00 p.m. to 12:30 p.m.). Fifty-seven percent of all cases among the students and 50% of all cases among the teachers ate during the second lunch period at Laraway. The attack rate for Oak Valley was 11%. The lunch included only one main dish (chicken tenders), which was eaten by 99% of cases and 91% of persons who were not ill. The attack rate for those who ate the chicken tenders was 51% (relative risk 7.1, 95% CI 1.0 to 48.3, $P < 0.05$).

The attack rate for those who ate chicken tenders that smelled unusual was 63% (relative risk 9.2, 95% CI 1.4 to 62.6, $P < 0.05$). Ninety-one percent of students that had the school lunch reported their chicken tenders smelled unusual and 55% of students complained of an unusual taste. Descriptions of the odor were highly variable, but many reported a window-cleaning agent odor. The attack rate increased with increasing number of chicken tenders eaten (zero tenders, 1 of 5 [20%]; one tender, 15 of 51 [29%]; two tenders, 36 of 91 [40%]; three tenders, 33 of 80 [41%]; more than three tenders, 23 of 51 [45%]).

For a foodborne illness, time of onset of symptoms after lunch was very short, compatible with a chemical agent (Figure 23-1); some of the cases had onset of illness within only 10 minutes! Symptoms among cases included stomachache (82%), headache (61%), nausea (41%), and vomiting (23%). The interview form did not specifically ask about dizziness, diarrhea, or mouth burning, but 14, 5, and 4% reported these symptoms, respectively. No one was hospitalized despite all emergency department evaluations. Duration of illness was not precisely measured, but many cases reported feeling well within hours of onset.

Review of medical records of 44 students seen in four of the emergency departments identified no fevers,

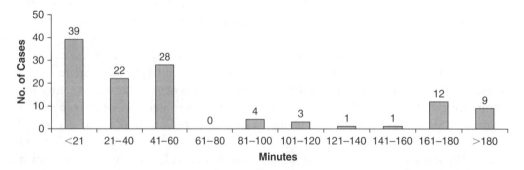

FIGURE 23-1 Histogram of time of onset of illness from ammonia poisoning after eating school lunch among 119 ill students and teachers (110 who met the case definition and 9 additional ill persons). Reprinted with permission from the Journal of Food Protection. Copyright held by the International Association for Food Protection, Des Moines, Iowa, USA.

median pulse rate of 84 (range of 62 to 136), median systolic blood pressure of 116 mm Hg (range of 92 to 165 mm Hg), and median respiratory rate of 20 breaths per min (range of 16 to 32). The medical history of seven (15%) of the students indicated asthma. One student had an asthma exacerbation, but it was not determined whether it was caused by the lunch. However, this student's symptoms included mouth burning, nausea, stomachache, dizziness, and headache. No intravenous fluids were administered.

Environmental and Food Investigation

Alpesh Patel: The school kitchen was inspected on November 25 and no critical violations were identified. A review of recent routine inspections also revealed no critical violations. The meal included chicken tenders, barbecue sauce, green beans, dinner rolls, apricots, milk, and other beverages. The chicken tenders had arrived in a box containing six 5 lb. clear plastic bags of product on October 15, 2002; the boxes were discarded, and the product stored in the school kitchen freezer until served on November 25. No food preparation logs were available; however, kitchen staff recalled that the chicken had reached an acceptable temperature of 168°F during preparation. It is generally recommended that poultry should be cooked to at least 165°F (74°C) for at least 15 seconds. Each of the 335 lunches prepared that day included a serving of three chicken tenders; additional tenders could be purchased. Remarkably, kitchen staff did not report detecting an unusual odor during preparation.

Mark S. Dworkin: The finding that the kitchen staff did not smell the chemical odor despite so many children complaining about it was hard to believe. However, it did not surprise me. My experience with outbreak investigations involving food handlers in restaurants had left me suspicious of the accuracy of the responses to questions that could implicate them as partly or completely responsible for illnesses. While I would hope that responses to a government health official's questions would be honest in this setting, I could understand why a frightened food handler, possibly with few skills, would be unwilling to say that yes indeed they had smelled the odor but served it to the children anyway. They probably feared public humiliation in the press and on television, loss of their job without much chance of getting hired someplace else in any hurry, and a fine or imprisonment. We assumed that they smelled it and saw nothing to gain at this point in pursuing the matter further.

Alpesh Patel: An investigation of the source of the chicken revealed that, after production by a large commercial poultry company, the chicken was sold to the Illinois State Board of Education and stored in a warehouse facility in St. Louis, Missouri. While at this facility, the chicken was exposed to a liquid ammonia spill in November 2001. Three hundred sixty-one cases of the product were considered unsafe for distribution; these cases were stored for approximately 10 months (apparently as part of a reconditioning process) before being distributed to 49 schools throughout Illinois, including Laraway Elementary School. A survey of the schools that had received product from the same lot was completed for 35 schools. Twelve had served chicken tenders from this lot and 11 still had unserved product in their freezers. This product was embargoed and transported back to the distributor before it was destroyed. At least four schools had noticed an ammonia smell from the chicken and one had served the product on October 2, 2002; none noted any unusual illnesses.

Mark S. Dworkin: The state health department's Division of Food, Drugs, and Dairies was instrumental in this traceback activity that helped to establish how contaminated chicken could have entered the school because we had no evidence ammonia had contaminated the product at the school itself. We learned through them that the Illinois State Board of Education has a warehouse facility in Illinois where large quantities of food are stored until they are scheduled to be shipped to the schools. When needed, there is an overflow warehouse near St. Louis, Missouri for additional storage. It was in this overflow warehouse that these chicken tenders originated and were exposed to the leaked ammonia that was used as a refrigerant. Such a leak would have likely been a major event at the warehouse, given the potent odor of ammonia. Apparently, the ammonia had sprayed onto the boxes, because we later learned that rather than discard the chicken, the boxes were repackaged. I read in a publication by the Agency for Toxic Substances and Disease Registry (ATSDR) that plastic films, such as cryovac, are considered less permeable to ammonia than paper products, but more permeable than metal or aluminum foil.[2] Therefore, ammonia must have penetrated the box and then passed through the plastic bag in which the tenders were packaged. I also learned that you can store food contaminated with ammonia for months and the ammonia should leach back out.[4] Maybe that is true in an experimental situation with food at room temperature. However, this chicken was stored in the overflow warehouse freezer for a year after the leak and repackaged before being shipped out to the schools. A fumigation process was performed, but in retrospect it seems the best practice would have been to discard all potentially contaminated food. Clearly, it was still a public health threat.

As for the repackaging of the chicken (thus concealing that anything had happened to it), this action was illegal. The warehouse manager responsible for this was later sentenced to a year and a day in prison. Two Illinois State Board of Education employees were also somehow caught up in this bad error of judgment about the chicken and ended up in court too (Figure 23-2). This outbreak led to a lot of media coverage from initial recognition to the trials of the warehouse manager and Board of Education employees (Exhibit 23-1).

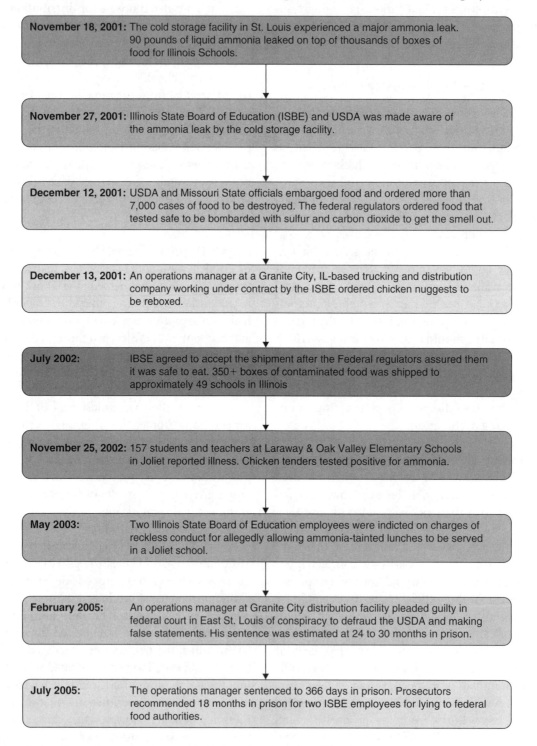

FIGURE 23-2 A timeline of events: Ammonia Poisoning in Joliet, Illinois.

EXHIBIT 23-1 Selected local newspaper headline coverage of the ammonia poisoning outbreak

"Sickness strikes students: Food poisoning? Dozens rushed to hospital from Laraway school" November 26, 2002, *The Herald News*.

"Ammonia found in meat at school—42 students been sickened at Laraway facility" December 5, 2002, *The Herald News*.

"Ammonia-contaminated food was served to Illinois students after fumigation" December 12, 2002, *Chicago Tribune*.

"Officials knew of contaminated chicken—meat fumigated, sent to schools" December 12, 2002, *The Herald News*.

"Tainted meat subject of grand jury—students got ill: school, health officials answer questions" December 19, 2002, *The Herald News*.

"Two school officials charged in tainted chicken case—Food contaminated with ammonia sickened Joliet kids" May 1, 2003, *Chicago Sun-Times*.

"USDA named in tainted chicken lawsuit—Seattle firm hits failure to release documents" May 8, 2003, *The Herald News*.

"Warehouse manager admits sending school bad chicken" February 25, 2005, *St. Louis Post-Dispatch*.

"Penalty for food danger—Downstate man gets prison for lying to federal authorities" July 31, 2005, The Associated Press and *The Herald News*.

Laboratory Investigation

Alpesh Patel: Ammonia was detected in three uncooked chicken tenders (from Laraway Elementary School) and two heated unserved chicken tenders (from Oak Valley Elementary School) at 552 parts per million (ppm), 1,605 ppm, 2,468 ppm, 880 ppm, and 1,076 ppm, respectively. Additional testing performed by the FSIS laboratory detected ammonia at similar levels and also documented levels as high as 256 ppm and 138 ppm in unserved frozen chicken tenders obtained from two other schools that had not reported illnesses.

CONCLUSIONS

Alpesh Patel: This was the first report of an outbreak of ammonia poisoning associated with a solid food. The only other outbreak previously identified was caused by a beverage (milk) contaminated with ammonia among 20 Wisconsin schoolchildren.[5] A chemical agent was the etiologic agent for only seven percent of foodborne outbreaks in U.S. schools with a known cause.[6] The total number of students reported ill from a non-heavy metal chemical source from 1973 through 1997 was only 98 (eight outbreaks)—fewer than the total number ill in our investigation.

Ammonia is a common industrial chemical used for refrigeration, fertilizer manufacturing, and production of dye, synthetic fiber, plastic, nitric acid, and explosives production.[5,7] It is a colorless gas with a sharp odor. However, in water, it changes to ammonium ions, which do not have an odor.[2] Therefore, when ammonia penetrates a frozen food, it may be absorbed by water glaze or ice on the food and lose its odor.[1,4] Ammonia can cause death from airway obstruction with exposure to 5,000 to 10,000 ppm.[7] Levels greater than 50 ppm cause immediate irritation of the nose and throat; acute exposure to highly concentrated aerosols may cause cardiovascular problems, including tachycardia, bradycardia, hypertension, and cardiac arrhythmia, or in severe cases cardiac arrest. Burning of the lips, oral cavity, and pharynx may result from exposure to anhydrous ammonia.[7]

Mark S. Dworkin: In food, ammonia present at greater than 15 ppm is considered abnormal, so even the lowest level identified in the chicken (138 ppm) was concerning and the highest level (2468 ppm) was alarming.[5] Most of the levels identified in the tested chicken were much higher than the levels reported in the Wisconsin outbreak caused by contaminated milk. Also, in this investigation, the attack rate was as high as 56% among students eating during the second lunch period compared to only 3.9% in the Wisconsin outbreak. This difference could be related to several factors: differences in concentration of ammonia in the contaminated product; quantity of contaminated product consumed; dilution of product in a beverage compared to possibly uneven contamination in a solid food; and, perhaps, acidity, alkalinity, or other properties of the food or beverage contaminated or ingested with the contaminated product. Among the analyses we performed, we explored the effect of milk consumption on likelihood of being a case. Milk is a beverage with pH 6.6 and buffering properties.[8] We found that consumption of milk was associated with a protective effect, but the results were of only borderline statistical significance and the frequency of symptoms among cases was not affected by milk consumption.

This outbreak is illustrative of differences between chemical and biological (bacterial, viral, parasitic) food-borne outbreaks. Chemical outbreaks, such as this one, do not rely on immune system activation, organism reproduction, or toxin production time to cause symptoms. Therefore, they have the shortest incubation periods, typically measured in minutes.

One possible limitation of our investigation was the choice of 180 minutes in our case definition, rather than

60 minutes. Recall bias, perhaps related to children feeling ill as part of a second wave of hysteria, could have been responsible for cases with onset greater than 60 minutes. However, little is known about the time from ingestion to onset of illness for ammonia poisoning to determine whether our case definition was more sensitive than needed.

While even bacterial pathogens with preformed toxins, such as *Staphylococcus aureus* and *Bacillus cereus*, have incubation periods as short as 30 minutes to 8 hours and 1 to 6 hours, respectively,[9] for most of the cases in our investigation and in the Wisconsin outbreak caused by contaminated milk, the time from eating until symptoms was within 60 minutes.[5] Other chemical foodborne outbreaks have reported median times of 45 minutes (aldicarb)[10] and 40 minutes (methomyl).[11]

Alpesh Patel: The aldicarb outbreak occurred in July 1998 in Louisiana. Fourteen out of 20 employees who attended a company lunch that included homemade pork roast, boiled rice, cabbage salad, biscuits, and soft drinks became ill. The illness consisted of gastrointestinal (abdominal cramps—93%, nausea—93%, diarrhea—86%) and neurologic (dizziness—93%, sweating—86%, muscle fasciculations—86%, eye twitching—57%, and blurred vision—43%) symptoms with onset shortly after eating the lunch contaminated with aldicarb (organic phosphates and carbamates). Improperly stored and labeled aldicarb had been used mistakenly in food preparation. The duration of illness was 1–8 hours (median of 4 hours) and the duration of onset ranged from 40 minutes to 3 hours (median of 45 minutes). Two persons were hospitalized because of a heart rate abnormality. It seems that someone used a can labeled "black pepper" to prepare cabbage salad. This can had been found 6 weeks before the lunch in a deceased relative's truck; apparently, the diseased relative had used this mislabeled can of aldicarb on bait to prevent destruction of his crawfish nets, ponds, and leaves by wild dogs and raccoons. The contents of the black pepper container were tested and found positive for organophosphorous and carbamate pesticides.[10]

In the other report, an outbreak of gastrointestinal illness associated with the consumption of food seasoned with methomyl-contaminated salt occurred in 1998–1999 in Fresno County, California. This outbreak involved a Thai restaurant and led to 107 patrons developing nausea (95%), vomiting (51%), dizziness (72%), abdominal cramps (58%), headache (52%), chills (48%), and diarrhea (46%) within 2 hours of eating. Several persons were treated at emergency departments, although no one was hospitalized. Ill persons recovered in less than 1 day. The median duration of onset was only 40 minutes (range, 5–120 minutes) and the median duration of symptoms was 6 hours (range, 1–168 hours). The restaurant had added salt, glutamate, and sugar to almost all of its dishes. The more salt consumed, the stronger became the association with being a case.

In our outbreak of ammonia poisoning, unlike many foodborne and waterborne outbreaks, there was no significant morbidity (or mortality) beyond the immediate symptoms that occurred during the initial hours after ingestion. Although one asthma attack did occur during this outbreak in a child with a history of asthma, it could have occurred that day regardless of the ammonia exposure. Alternatively, it may have been precipitated by the ingestion of ammonia or possibly by the inhalation of fumes in the cafeteria.

Mark S. Dworkin: One of the mysteries of the outbreak was how the ammonia contaminated such a large number of chicken tenders in the warehouse, but no one smelled it until it was being cooked and served. We knew that quite a lot of chicken had been contaminated because when we tested chicken from the schools both in Joliet and in other parts of the state, positive samples were identified. In other words, we did not have to work very hard to prove that other packages of the chicken were contaminated. The biologically plausible explanation for the lack of detection of ammonia's notorious odor is caused by a property of ammonia that I only learned of during our research into ammonia as a result of the outbreak. The ammonia likely sprayed from the pipes or vessel it was stored in as a refrigerant onto the boxes. Then, it soaked through the boxes and also evaporated, becoming a gas. The gas and/or the liquid penetrated through the cardboard and then the plastic bag. After it came into contact with the water and ice glaze on the surface of the chicken tenders, it was absorbed. In this frozen ice crystal state, it was odorless. So, during transport, no one would be concerned and, in the warehouse, they could have been lulled into the false assumption that the ammonia had leached out. Heating the chicken brought the odor back out so the lunch room smelled like window cleaner; however, heating did not reduce the ammonia concentration to safe levels.

Alpesh Patel: This investigation has implications for chemical bioterrorism preparedness. Although the model for public health reporting of notifiable disease, including unusual cases or clusters of illness, is from healthcare providers (such as emergency departments or hospitals) to local health departments (and subsequently to the state health department), in this outbreak the school notified the local health department and the latter then informed the local emergency departments to help prepare them for the arrival of students with an unidentified illness. Public health bioterrorism preparedness communication plans should include two-way notification (between emergency departments and health departments) because it could save lives by allowing emergency department personnel potentially valuable minutes to prepare for relatively large numbers of patients and possibly to quickly review textbook, Internet, or other educational material that might allow a more rapid diagnosis of unfamiliar conditions and potential delivery of an antidote if one is available.

LESSONS LEARNED

Mark S. Dworkin: Several lessons can be learned from this experience with foodborne ammonia poisoning:

1. This outbreak is a reminder of the vulnerability of the U.S. food supply; even food contaminated with a chemical known to have an unpleasant and recognizable odor may pass from storage to the table and be eaten, given the right circumstances.

2. Foodborne outbreaks caused by a chemical agent are uncommon. However, prompt recognition could be lifesaving. It was fortunate that this outbreak did not lead to any deaths or even hospitalizations. However, increased awareness of the characteristics of chemical poisoning may save lives or prevent morbidity if they involve agents for which there is an antidote and if early recognition leads to avoidance of exposure by others.

3. Ammonia should be considered among the causes of chemical food poisoning when an outbreak of gastrointestinal illness has a very short incubation period. Ammonia contamination of food is periodically reported through the U.S. Consumer Product Safety Commission (http://www.cpsc.gov/cpscpub/prerel/prerel.html), the U.S. Food and Drug Administration (http://www.fda.gov/safety/recalls/default.htm), and Food Safety.gov (http://www.foodsafety.gov).[12–14] Since 2000, such recalls have included contaminated sparkling soda, burritos, diet cola, and ice cream. Ammonia contamination of water has also been reported in livestock, which caused six deaths in these animals at an Illinois county fair.[15]

4. Intact packaging can contain contaminated food or beverage. Plastic packaging may be porous to some contaminants. When a food or beverage does not taste or smell right, this should be taken seriously and not dismissed.

5. When a large number of a cohort under investigation has been exposed to the hypothesized source of the outbreak, consider examining the data for a dose response effect to establish or validate the association with the exposure.

LEARNING QUESTIONS

1. In what ways are chemical poisoning outbreaks similar to and different from infectious disease outbreaks?
2. What aspects of this poisoning event overlap with important issues of bioterrorism preparedness?
3. What foodborne infectious diseases have a very short incubation period and, therefore, should be considered when encountering an outbreak with a short time from ingestion of the implicated food until the onset of illness? How are the manifestations of those diseases similar to and different from ammonia poisoning?

ACKNOWLEDGMENTS

The authors gratefully acknowledge assistance with this investigation from Gregory Huhn, Kuo-Jen Kuo, Glen Yoshimura, Marlena Bordson, James Zelko, Seth Baker, Connie Austin, Suresh Dua, David Goldman, and staff of the USDA laboratory in Athens, Georgia.

REFERENCES

1. Tybor PT, Hurst WC, Reynolds AE, Schuler GA. *Preventing Chemical Foodborne Illness*. Georgia: The University of Georgia College of Agriculture & Environmental Sciences, Cooperative Extension Service. http://pubs.caes.uga.edu/caespubs/pubcd/b1042-w.html. Accessed September 10, 2009.
2. US Department of Health and Human Services. *Toxicological Profile for Ammonia*. Draft for Public Comment. Atlanta, GA: Agency for Toxic Substances and Disease Registry; 2002:1–10, 19–107.
3. Agency for Toxic Substances and Disease Registry. ToxFAQs for Ammonia, CAS#7664-41-7. Centers for Disease Control and Prevention Web site. http://www.atsdr.cdc.gov/tfacts126.html. Accessed September 10, 2009.

4. Massachusetts Department of Public Health Food Protection Program. Guidelines for evaluating food products for salvage and reconditioning. http://www.state.ma.us/dph/fpp/web-fp-01.pdf. Published April 30, 1998. Accessed September 10, 2009. No. FP-01.
5. Centers for Disease Control and Prevention. Epidemiologic notes and reports, ammonia contamination in a milk processing plant—Wisconsin. *MMWR Morb Mortal Wkly Rep.* 1986;35(17):274–275.
6. Daniels NA, MacKinnon L, Rowe SM, Bean NH, Griffin PM, Mead PS. Foodborne disease outbreaks in United States schools. *Pediatr Infect Dis J.* 2002;21(7):623–628.
7. Koren H. *Illustrated Dictionary of Environmental Health and Occupational Safety*. Boca Raton, FL: CRC Lewis Publishers; 1996:22.
8. O'Mahony F. *Rural Dairy Technology*. Addis Ababa, Ethiopia: International Livestock Centre for Africa; 1998: Milk chemistry—an introduction. http://www.ilri.org/InfoServ/Webpub/Fulldocs/ILCA_Manual4/Milkchemistry.htm. Accessed September 10, 2009.
9. Chin J, ed. *Control of Communicable Diseases Manual*. 17th ed. Washington, DC: American Public Health Association; 2000:202–208.
10. Centers for Disease Control and Prevention. Aldicarb as a cause of food poisoning—Louisiana, 1998. *MMWR Morb Mortal Wkly Rep.* 1999;48(13):269–271.
11. Bucholz U, Mermin J, Rios R, et al. An outbreak of foodborne illness associated with methomyl-contaminated salt. *JAMA*. 2002;288(5):604–610.
12. US Consumer Product Safety Commission. Recalls and product safety news. US Consumer Product Safety Commission Web site. http://www.cpsc.gov/cpscpub/prerel/prerel.html. Accessed September 10, 2009.
13. US Food and Drug Administration. Recalls, market withdrawals, & safety alerts. US Food and Drug Administration Web site. http://www.fda.gov/safety/recalls/default.htm. Accessed September 10, 2009.
14. FoodSafety.gov. http://www.foodsafety.gov. Accessed September 10, 2009.
15. Campagnolo ER, Kasten S, Banerjee M. Accidental ammonia exposure to county fair show livestock due to contaminated drinking water. *Vet Hum Toxicol.* 2002;44(5):282–285.

CHAPTER 24

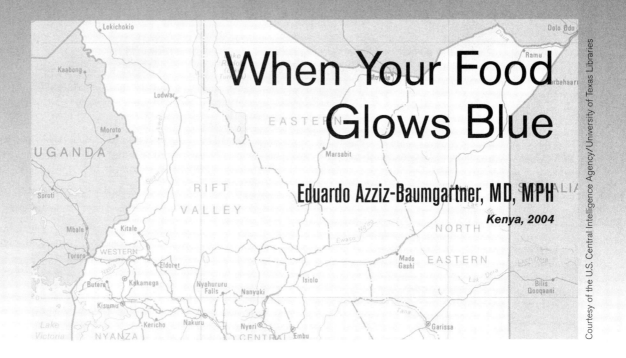

When Your Food Glows Blue

Eduardo Azziz-Baumgartner, MD, MPH

Kenya, 2004

THE CALL

It must be an unwritten universal law that any outbreak of magnitude must be reported to health authorities Friday afternoon, usually after 3:00 p.m. The 74th CDC EPI-AID in 2004 was no exception. As I was sitting in my office sifting through paperwork, my supervisor leaned in through the door, said, "Call in Carol's office," and disappeared. For a few seconds, I stared at the empty doorway and then at the large clock on the wall. It was 3:47 p.m., and a call in the branch chief's office could not be good news.

In Dr. Carol Rubin's office, a small group of some of the best environmental epidemiologists and toxicologists at the Centers for Disease Control and Prevention (CDC) sat around a small circular table that held a speaker phone. Their heads leaned toward the phone. Some were scowling in concentration while others took notes. A tired male voice sounded through the speakerphone, "[The] hospitalized patients with acute jaundice were tested for yellow fever; Rift Valley fever; dengue; acute hepatitis A, B, and C; West Nile virus; and Chikungunya and Bunyamwera virus...but all samples were negative." I found an empty chair and wondered who was calling and why we were talking about viruses. After all, we worked at the Health Studies Program of the National Center for Environmental Health.

As it turns out, a colleague of our branch chief called from Foodborne Diseases to pass on a request for assistance from the CDC-Kenya to investigate a suspected acute jaundice outbreak. Alerted by hospital authorities in eastern Kenya of an unusual number of cases of acute jaundice, the local Ministry of Health and CDC field teams tested the serum of seven patients for a variety of viruses endemic to Kenya that can cause acute hepatitis. All results were negative and local health authorities were now inclined to believe that the timing of the outbreak might be suggestive of an intoxication with aflatoxins—potent colorless, odorless toxins formed by the Aspergillus fungus (Exhibit 24-1). As the only Epidemic Intelligence Service (EIS) officer in the room, I listened and took notes. I had never heard of Chikungunya, Bunyamwera virus, or aflatoxins.

As Carol hung up the phone, she turned to the team leaders and formulated the questions. All investigations worth their salt are designed to answer a set of

> **EXHIBIT 24-1** Selected facts about aflatoxins and aflatoxicosis
>
> **Aflatoxins**
>
> Aflatoxins have the following characteristics:[2]
> - They are a family of toxic compounds produced by mold.
> - They may cause liver cancer.
> - An estimated 4.5 billion persons are chronically exposed in developing countries.
> - They affect immunity and nutrition.
> - They are produced as metabolites by *Aspergillus flavus* and *Aspergillus parasiticus*.
> - Favorable conditions include warm temperature (24(to 35(C) and moisture.
> - Common foods implicated are peanuts, maize, and beans.
>
> **Aflatoxicosis**
>
> Aflatoxicosis has the following characteristics:[1]
> - It may be caused by either acute intoxication with liver damage or chronic exposure.
> - Approximately 25 percent of acute poisonings result in death.
> - It is more likely to occur when food is scarce and people are living in poverty.

specific questions. The questions for this investigation were, in order of importance:

1. Was this a real outbreak (i.e. were there really more jaundice cases than usual in eastern Kenya)?
2. If there was an outbreak of acute jaundice, was it caused by aflatoxicosis (i.e. mass intoxication with aflatoxins)?
3. If there was a mass intoxication with aflatoxins, what was the source of the aflatoxins?

A priori, one hypothesis was that people were eating food contaminated with aflatoxins. For example, maize is a staple of the diet in eastern Kenya and maize contaminated with *Aspergillus* fungus that produces aflatoxins may not be visibly moldy or taste different from uncontaminated maize. Cooking the maize does not destroy aflatoxins. People who eat contaminated maize rapidly absorb aflatoxins in the gut, where they are transported through the circulation to the liver. In the liver, a fraction of the aflatoxins bind to proteins and DNA, destroying their natural function and creating aflatoxin adducts. Adducts are complexes that form when a chemical binds to a biological molecule. We were fortunate that a team of chemists at the CDC had recently developed a blood test to quantify the presence of aflatoxins in serum that could be used to test if participants had been exposed to aflatoxins during the past 20–60 days. This would be the first investigation where aflatoxins were recovered from case-patients' food and aflatoxin adducts were recovered from case-patients' serum, thus making a very compelling argument that we were dealing with an outbreak of aflatoxicosis. I took notes in my standard government-issue green notebook.

Formal requests for assistance to the CDC, where an EIS officer and CDC staff are dispatched to provide technical epidemiologic assistance or "EPI-AIDS," vary in scope according to the severity of the public health emergency and the eagerness with which partners seek assistance. This particular EPI-AID proceeded with the pace of a national emergency. One day, I was planning my weekend in the fiendishly dull suburbs of Atlanta and the next, I was counting socks for a trip of undetermined duration to Africa. Less than 36 hours later, my supervisor, a PhD analytical chemist who was a mycotoxins expert, and I were lugging enormous black plastic suitcases. These were filled with needles, syringes, assorted test tubes, cryovials, packing material, commercial aflatoxin test kits, centrifuges, UV lights, and personal protective equipment to augment the CDC-Kenya's supplies. A nondescript government van was packed with the equipment by well-wishing colleagues and we were off.

GETTING ORIENTED

My supervisor and I finally arrived at the Hartsfield-Jackson Atlanta International Airport, lugged in the suitcases, paid an extra baggage fee, and sighed with relief. From Terminal E, I called my wife at home and then pulled out a large stack of journal articles on aflatoxicosis onto the black vinyl seats of Gate 6. Flights are ideal for catching up on technical reading material. I couldn't believe we were on our way to Kenya. Reality seemed an ocean away. After wandering aimlessly through Amsterdam's Schiphol Airport, we boarded the flight to Nairobi. The flight was cramped, but we could see the blue and white of the Mediterranean and later the tan undulation of the Sahara below. By the time we touched down, it was dark. The airport in Nairobi was crowded with passengers; we followed our fellow passengers through nondescript corridors and shuttered shops to passport control. Only one of us was asked to pay for an entry visa. We collected our massive load and, after exchanging money for Kenyan shillings, we pushed our carts past the sliding glass doors to the crowd waiting outside. A tall gentleman in a white shirt stood holding a sheet of paper with our names printed on it in large black letters. Minutes later, we were hurtling through the dark Nairobi streets.

The next morning, I woke disoriented and wandered over to the breakfast buffet. The dining room was breezy and we could see the bougainvilleas and the pale blue skies through the open windows. Businessmen and women dressed in colorful garb were clustered among the tables, chatting quietly. The buffet tables were laden with papayas, pineapples, and a variety of unidentifiable dishes. We briefly debated whether to risk gastroenteritis (e.g. traveler's diarrhea). Later, we loitered by the hotel and thumbed through the *Kenya* Lonely Planet guide before a white van arrived to take us to the CDC-Kenya.

We drove into the CDC Nairobi compound, a series of low-slung buildings that sit on a hill facing the sea of tin roofs and crooked alleys of the Kibera slums. The inside of the offices is clean, spare, and unassuming. Five office staff greeted us politely. We needed an appointment with the very busy country director. For an EIS officer, who is in essence a fellow training in field epidemiology, the demands on a country director's time are unfathomable. It would take me years to understand all the information needed for Dr. Kevin DeCock to manage millions of dollars and dozens of public health initiatives in this east African country of approximately 38 million people. Regardless, he made time for us and we met later that afternoon in a large office decorated with old black-and-white photographs of aristocratic-looking people (his relatives), gigantic maps, and stacks of books and journals. We sat around another round table with a laminated wood top—a twin replica of the one in Atlanta.

Kevin DeCock has a career that might excite anyone interested in global health. He trained in infectious diseases and held a faculty appointment at the London School of Hygiene & Tropical Medicine. He has worked in Africa and served as the CDC's Division of HIV/AIDS director. In Kenya, his responsibilities included overseeing the Global AIDS Program (GAP) and the International Emerging Infections Program, as well as collaborating on polio eradication. (He now serves as the director of the Department of HIV/AIDS for the WHO.)

DeCock reiterated the situation to date. Thirty some case–patients had been identified and a dozen were reported to have died. The epi-graph, compliments of Karen Gieseker, can be found under the Samples and Additional Resources tab at http://www.jblearning.com/catalog/9780763778910/. My supervisor suggested the first course of action should be to confirm the preliminary results of the government of Kenya's National Public Health Laboratory that suggested that dry pulses (i.e., leguminous crops) and maize samples obtained from decedents were contaminated with aflatoxins.

The next morning, I struggled to remain alert. It was 3:00 a.m. in Atlanta and my body had not adjusted to the local time. We briefly met with the laboratory director. He spoke to my supervisor with the familiarity of a kindred spirit recognizing another laboratorian. We then walked across the campus to the laboratory buildings. I was completely unprepared for what I saw. The laboratory buildings seemed derelict. I recognized the black bench tops, but not much of the ancient laboratory equipment or the glassware marred and scratched by decades of use. Past the threshold of the door, I immediately noticed a peculiar odor reminiscent of guano. "Bats?" I wondered. Searching to identify the source of the smell, I looked around the room and then finally at the ceiling. Pale sunlight streamed into the room where portions of the roof had caved in. I suppressed a glance at my supervisor and followed the director as if a laboratory with holes in the roof was the most natural thing in the world.

> *I looked around the room and then finally at the ceiling. Pale sunlight streamed into the room where portions of the roof had caved in. I suppressed a glance at my supervisor and followed the director as if a laboratory with holes in the roof was the most natural thing in the world.*

In the afternoon, we met with more of the laboratory staff, identified the remains of pulses and maize samples obtained from decedents, and discussed methods to identify aflatoxins in food. The staff seemed thoroughly knowledgeable, but my supervisor suggested more robust methods to confirm the presence of aflatoxins (provided they have access to modern testing equipment). By 2:30 p.m., three of us were in the supply closet of the government laboratory, crouching around a battered paper bag. The bag, which had recently been brought from the house of a case–patient in Mtito Andei, smelled of dusty maize. I held the bag open while my supervisor held a portable UV light over the battered looking kernels inside. Our Kenyan colleague closed the closet door. Illuminated only by the violet light of the lamp, we peered inside. Speckles of blue light reflected from the kernels of maize indirectly suggested the presence of fungus toxins aflatoxins.

I was thrilled by our preliminary findings, but these were insufficient to implicate, let alone quantify the aflatoxin levels in the maize. We arranged to have grain samples tested for aflatoxins at the CDC laboratory in Nairobi. We called Atlanta. It was arranged that the U.S.

Food and Drug Administration would send a team from the Center for Food Safety and Applied Nutrition to bring commercial test kits and train Kenyan laboratory staff to quantify the amount of aflatoxins in food consumed by people with acute jaundice. Next, we explored the situation in the affected community. We arranged to travel with our local counterparts from the Ministries of Health and Agriculture to eastern Kenya. It was time to meet those affected, refine our differential diagnoses, and generate hypotheses as to why people may have become intoxicated with aflatoxins. As we loaded our equipment into another white van early next morning, I fretted that I had never seen a case of acute aflatoxicosis.

GENERATING HYPOTHESES

Rural Kenya is very beautiful. After traveling hours down a rutted road, we escaped the sooty Nairobi sprawl and made our way onto the undulating plains. "Masai lands," Mary Onsongo, our Kenyan counterpart, told us as she pointed out the car window. Outside, ochre fields spread out into the distance, the shadow of clouds adding texture to the plains. We bounced up and down with our equipment, our voices nearly drowned by the sound of the tires and the frenetic squeaks and bumps of the suspension. Soon, we drove past a herd of gazelles. From afar, they moved with surreal grace. Hours later, I saw the flat top of Mount Kilimanjaro, just visible under the waning moon. We were driving past the "bread basket" of Kenya. But, by then, I had lost feeling in my legs and the jetlag had returned to mar the afternoon. I was infinitely grateful when the car stopped at Hunter's Lodge.

Hunter's Lodge sat on a large plot of land with an artificial pond, expansive lawns, and groomed trees that hosted a troop of Rhesus monkeys. We stood at the dark registration desk, waiting for an old gentleman arduously processing our reservations in dog-eared triplicates. As I waited for my room key, I looked for a place to sit. Behind me were a dusty side table and a strange-looking stool. The stool looked like a round wrinkled drum with crescents around the edge. I wondered if it could hold my weight. As I got near, I registered what I was seeing. It was the severed and stuffed leg of an elephant, cursed, no doubt, by angry pachyderm gods.

The next morning, we wolfed down stale toast and scrambled eggs and drove to the local hospital. We pulled into a dusty driveway that ended in a cluster of one-story buildings. Our Ministry of Health colleague impressed upon us the importance of following protocol. We were instructed to meet with hospital authorities, introduce each other, share business cards, indicate why we were there, and ask permission to enter the wards. After what seemed like an eternity of appraising each other in the cramped office of the administrators, we followed the head matron to the male ward. It was a long barrack-like building across from the female ward. As we got closer, the smell of perspiration, clotted blood, urine, and feces became stronger. The head matron and I stood at the threshold of the open ward. Cots that held one or two emaciated patients lined both sides of the building. The breeze wafted through the open windows and doors. There was little movement inside.

We were led to the bedside of a young man, either sleeping or comatose, on one of the metal cots. The physician greeted the patient who nodded silently in reply. Then, the physician placed a hand on the patient's forehead and lifted his eyelid. The patient's sclera was neon yellow. I asked permission to palpate his liver and spleen. The liver was 4 inches below the costal margin (so very enlarged) and seemed tender. I turned to wash my hands in the sink in the middle of the ward. There was soap, but no connection to water pipes. As we walked away from the bed, the physician told us that the hospital had few options for even the most basic supportive care, and he did not know if the patient would live or die. We visited one patient after another with equally flagrant jaundice and ended our tour at the pediatric ward. A small toddler was lying listlessly in a crib. The nurse told us that most of his family had died and that they did not know if he was going to survive. If he did survive, she did not know who would take care of him. Overwhelmed, we asked if they had stored any of the case–patients' sera and then escaped to the emotional safety of the clinical laboratory.

The next morning, we again headed for the field. We drove for more than an hour past commercial flower nurseries, charcoal mounds, and finally open fields. The few other vehicles on the road barreled past us at improbable speeds. I checked my seatbelt. After a while, we finally pulled off the road and into a dirt lane by a general store. There, we got out and followed the local health officer onto a foot path that wound through the plains. We trudged on the soft dust and sand, enjoying the sunshine, and the buzzing of the insects. Near a plot of tall maize, we found a small hut cobbled together from corrugated tin, old plywood boards, and woven sticks. In front of the shack stood a young woman wearing a traditional dress and holding a 6-month old baby in a soiled T-shirt.

The local health officer spoke to her quietly in Kikamba, the Bantu language of these Akamba people. Her replies were muted, her face expressionless. Her other child was still in the hospital and she did not know if he was going to survive. We asked about the maize in the field. The agriculture officer translated that she used to sun dry her maize on mats outside her home before storing it in a well-ventilated granary woven out of sticks. This year, however, the rains came early and she had to store the wet maize as she scrambled to prepare the fields for planting.

We asked, "Where did she store her maize?" She replied that it was stored inside her house, of course, where she could keep it safe from hungry neighbors who might pilfer it at night. Here was an uncomfortably real example of food insecurity. With an almost imperceptible nod, she allowed us to see her maize stores. I stooped to enter the hut. As the door opened, warm sodden air wafted over me. Inside, it was dark with an odor like a barnyard. Under wooden cots were gurney sacks with maize, maize flour, and dry pulses. My supervisor pulled out her UV light and the maize kernels fluoresced with blue light.

> *We asked, "Where did she store her maize?" She replied that it was stored inside her house, of course, where she could keep it safe from hungry neighbors who might pilfer it at night. Here was an uncomfortably real example of food insecurity.*

THE CASE-CONTROL STUDY

The next morning, we returned to the CDC-Kenya office to meet the rest of the local team that had been working on the outbreak. A conference call was held with Atlanta to talk over our preliminary findings. After much discussion, we settled on the following strategy: use commercial test kits to confirm the presence of aflatoxins in food eaten by cases, obtain serum from case–patients to test for aflatoxin adducts as evidence of exposure to contaminated food, and explore risk factors for exposure to aflatoxins through a case–control study (Exhibit 24-2).

We were fortunate to have two PhD epidemiologists from the CDC-Kenya, who had started working on a study protocol and had done much groundwork. The first was Dr. Lindblade working on malaria and other endemic diseases at the Kisumu field station. The second was an Epidemic Intelligence Service (EIS) classmate, Dr. Gieseker, who was helping the CDC-Kenya teach its Field Epidemiology and Laboratory Training fellows in 2004. The protocol and its accompanying instruments were finalized in a flurry of activity and the package was sent for expedited ethical review. We settled on a case definition that was restricted to acute jaundice of unknown origin leading to hospitalization during the peak of the epidemic in the areas most affected by the outbreak. The cases could not have a history of cirrhosis or obstructive liver disease. There would be 40 patients and 80 controls.

Within days, we were able to mobilize to the field. We deployed to the field in half a dozen vehicles with teams of Field Epidemiology and Laboratory Training Program (FELTP) fellows to canvas the study communities. The FELTP is a training program, like the EIS program, that is intended to help countries develop their public health system and infrastructure. The fellows have signed on for a 2-year full-time training and service commitment, including classroom instruction, fieldwork, and often supervision from CDC staff (especially

TABLE 24-1 Risk factors [n (%)] for jaundice among case patients (n = 28) and controls (n = 43) who ate maize kernels grown on their own farms, Kenya, 2004.

Characteristic	Case patients	Controls	OR (95% CI)
Initial dryness of stored maize			
Wet	15 (53.6)	11 (25.6)	3.5 (1.2–10.3)
Dry	13 (46.4)	32 (74.4)	1.0
Storage location			
House	22 (81.5)	23 (53.5)	12.0 (1.5–95.7)
Granary	5 (18.5)	20 (46.5)	1.0
Preservatives added to storage			
Ash	6 (15.4)	13 (17.6)	1.6 (0.4–5.6)
Insecticide	9 (23.1)	21 (28.1)	0.6 (0.2–1.8)

*Reproduced with permission from *Environmental Health Perspectives*[1]

> **EXHIBIT 24-2** Plan for additional studies during an investigation of aflatoxicosis in Kenya
>
> The plan consisted of the following steps:
> - Confirm that aflatoxin was present in the food eaten by case–patients.
>   - Use commercial test kits to test food.
> - Provide evidence that exposure to contaminated food caused disease.
>   - Test case–patient serum for aflatoxin adducts.
> - Explore risk factors associated with exposure to the aflatoxin.
>   - Perform a case–control study.

during the first years when the FELTP program has begun).

We unloaded boxes of equipment and supplies at the previously empty parking lot of the Hunter's Lodge. The boxes containing stacks of questionnaires weighed as much as the centrifuges and I thought how easy it would be to enter participants' responses directly into laptops. Then, a dose of reality hit as someone shook his head and said, "and when the batteries run dry…" The team scurried about in a frenzy of activity, crowding the hallways and preparing for tomorrow's data collection. Breakfast the next day was boisterous and we lined the benches of the dining room. We reviewed the study questionnaires one final time to ensure all were asking the questions in the same way.

Most case–patients affected were Akamba, an ethnic group of subsistence farmers who live in some of the most arid lands in Kenya. When the rains do not come, Akamba lands do not yield. This year, there was a shortage of 156,000 metric tons of maize. Outside the hospital we were told that around here, people pick through moldy maize or starve. I drove to the hospital with Dr. Patrick Nguku, a pleasant and insightful Akamba FELTP fellow. Again, we met hospital administrators, followed protocol, and then were allowed to enter the wards. As we walked from building to building, Nguku gave me a brief tutorial on the microeconomics of health care in rural Kenya, which dispels my misconceptions about why there are 2 or 3 patients per cot, sinks without piped water, and scant medicines for patients. Nguku spoke with a young man in Kikamba. He held the patient's hand, his voice gentle, quiet, and sad.

After each interview, we obtained venous blood to test for aflatoxin adducts. As a medical student, I had a summer job as a phlebotomist. In Kenya, I was out of practice. Three times, I inserted the tip of a 23-gauge butterfly needle into the arm of a stoic case–patient but, each time, only drops spurted into the test tube. Fortunately, Nguku obtained blood from even the most dehydrated person. I collected the test tubes, labeled them, and placed them in the cool box. Because the aflatoxin adduct assay developed by the CDC's Drs. McCoy, Schleicher, and Pfeiffer was new, we needed to preserve the samples' integrity because we did not know how hemolysis, for example, might affect the test results. I carried the cool box gingerly and periodically checked the ice packs. They felt soft and cool. While the samples needed to be kept at ~4°C, the only freezer available for miles did not seem to freeze the icepacks each night.

When the sun had set and we only had civil twilight, we drove on to Mutomo. The hotel we were taken to was in a compound surrounded by pink sun-bleached walls and a giant sheet metal gate. Inside was a series of low-slung buildings. We went to the little reception desk and, for the first time, saw metal bars on the windows. I watched the FELTPs pay the equivalent of US $4 for their room. I was given a key to the "London Suite." The innkeeper gesticulated with her hand that it was around the corner. I nodded and walked around the building, past a small courtyard and a series of large cement cisterns, until I found the doors to the rooms. It was very dark, but eventually I found my suite conveniently located next to the "New York" suite, where my supervisor was staying. I opened the padlock that led to my room and let the heavy wooden door swing open.

Now, I have stayed in many places throughout my tenure at the CDC, but never in a suite quite like this one. In front of me was a cot with remarkably stained sheets. A dusty blue mosquito net hung over the bed, its weave full of small tears. I stepped inside and wondered why it smelled powerfully of urine and feces. I followed the smell to a doorway on the left of the cot. In the adjacent room, there was a sink whose piping was not connected to anything. A plastic water pitcher sat on top. In the center of the room, I found two strips of what appeared to be giant boot prints and in the middle, a 6-inch hole (Figure 24-1). I leaned forward to peer into the impenetrable darkness of the hole and was repulsed by the strong stench. It was my first encounter with the squat toilet.

We washed up and ate as a team while we debriefed. The FELTP fellows ordered chicken and mutton that was brought in large bowls bathed in a vegetable broth. To my horror, the food smelled faintly of urea. I watched Nguku tuck in with relish while I wrung my hands. We had spent all day with people who were just like us but who had little to eat. While I felt very guilty at the thought of rejecting food, I couldn't bring myself searching for words. Her expression belied the vast experience gap between me, an EIS officer based in Atlanta, and her, a seasoned PhD epidemiologist living in the field. I regretted my question and sat on a box of questionnaires.

As we went through the schedule and matched case and control questionnaires with food and blood samples, the importance of the task soon became obvious. Some case–patients did not have a blood sample, others were missing randomly selected controls, and some food samples were inappropriately wrapped. Until the team became familiar with the routines of study collection, these nightly quality control meetings would become essential. We wrote down feedback for the team and planned tomorrow's logistics.

Finding case–patients' homes in rural Kenya was a logistic feat (Figure 24-2). One may travel 3 hours down a dirt road, clouds of dust billowing behind you, before getting anywhere close to the village. Occasionally, you may pass a troop of baboons walking next to the road. Once or twice, your vehicle may puncture a tire on the giant acacia thorns. Then, the road will inevitably narrow to a dirt track. Then, the driver will stop the vehicle and turn to look at you—your cue that it's time to walk (Figure 24-3). You then pile out of the car and collect the equipment, sling the cool box over your shoulder with bags full of phlebotomy equipment and stacks of

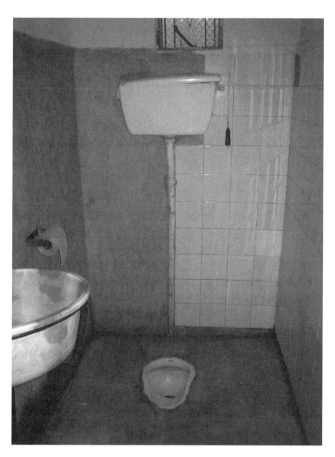

FIGURE 24-1 Field epidemiology is not always glamorous. Boldly going where I had never gone before, at my hotel.

to eat the chicken. Gastroenteritis in the field is a real curse and I was already out of Ciprofloxacin from a previous bout in Nairobi. I settled for sukumawiki (i.e., steamed kale) and chapattis for the rest of the trip, but held off the third vegetarian option, ugali (i.e., maize mash). It would be poor form to unwittingly become a case–patient during the outbreak investigation.

> *I settled for sukumawiki (i.e., steamed kale) and chapattis for the rest of the trip, but held off the third vegetarian option, ugali (i.e., maize mash). It would be poor form to unwittingly become a case–patient during the outbreak investigation.*

Later that night, I met with Dr. Kim Lindblade, the driving force behind the case–control study. She sat on a cot surrounded by stacks of questionnaires, checking each of them against a line-list and the blood samples in the cool boxes. It seemed late and I asked her if we could sort through these in the morning. She looked at me quizzically,

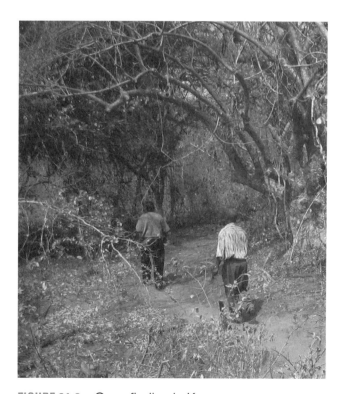

FIGURE 24-2 Case finding in Kenya.

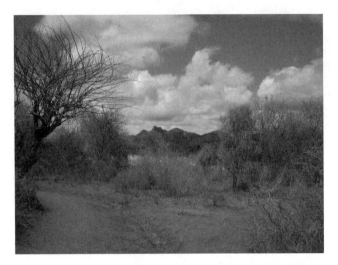

FIGURE 24-3 Where the road ends, you must walk.

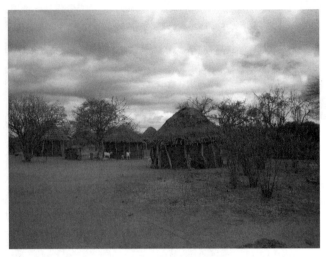

FIGURE 24-4 Typical huts observed during an investigation of aflatoxicosis in Kenya.

questionnaires gritty with dust, and head out. You may then walk into footpaths of soft rust-colored sand, past hills full of brambles, bottle trees, dry river beds, empty water wells, and parched fields.

Children may peer at you shyly from behind a granary as you enter a cluster of huts (Figure 24-4). Someone will quickly bring out rickety chairs, benches, or wooden stumps and arrange them in a circle in the dusty space between the huts. Everyone sits in a circle while the local health officer and a village elder who has come with your team introduces you to the family. Consent forms are reviewed by someone who speaks the local language (such as the FELTP fellow). Sometimes, families grieving for the ill or the dead immediately consent and the FELTP fellow launches into the questionnaires. At other times, your hosts may be suspicious or angry. The health officer and the village elder will then try to convince them that it is important to learn what is causing people to get *muku* (i.e., jaundice) to prevent others from getting sick. In the end very few refuse.

As I sat on a tree stump and watched the team administer the questionnaire in Kikamba, I tried to justify to myself why it was important to trouble these people who were grieving and had already gone through so much. Much of their maize and pulse stores looked spoiled, their fields parched, and their maize wilted and stunted in the sun. During the walk here, the Kenyan government agricultural officer, who had joined us during the field visit, explained how maize, imported from the Americas, was ill-suited for eastern Kenya. Maize requires a lot of water to grow. Plants raised during drought are stressed and more susceptible to invasion by insects and *Aspergillus* fungus. Drying maize well is critical, but because of the insufficient and untimely rains, there was a maize shortage of 156,000 metric tons of maize throughout Kenya (Figure 24-5). People were reluctant to leave their maize to dry in a granary because of the risk of having it taken by another hungry family.

Later, we walked over to a young woman digging in the field with a sharpened stick. Our footsteps crunched on the octagons of dried mud that covered the field. "No," she replied, there was no irrigation system there. "No," she said, the well went dry several years ago. She daily walked her donkey 4 hours to bring water for her family (Figure 24-6). She pointed at the faded yellow plastic water drums stacked against the wall of one of the huts; they were old oil containers. We asked for a sample of her maize and gave her a 1 kilogram bag of commercial maize flour in exchange. As we left, the agricultural

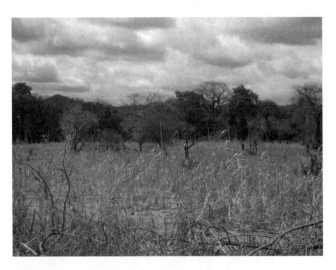

FIGURE 24-5 Dry maize fields in rural Kenya.

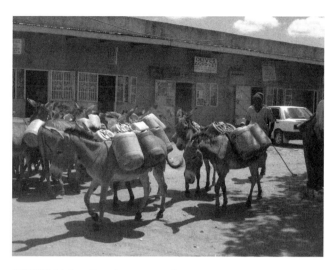

FIGURE 24-6 Donkeys used to transport water containers in rural Kenya.

officer turned to her to discuss burning her maize stores. Disheartened, I reminded myself that although by now we strongly suspected maize was the culprit of the identified 125 acute jaundice deaths, we had yet to prove our case.

After we left her house, we went in search of another control family for the study. For each case–patient family we interviewed, we also needed to select two random controls from their village. Controls were to come from the same village because we expected that these individuals would share similar soil, microclimate, and farming practices. To accomplish this, we use one of the empty soda bottles from the back of the truck. Near a case family home, we crouched on the road and spun the glass bottle. We looked to see where the bottle was pointing, shouldered our gear, and then set off in search of controls. We skipped the first two houses we passed because we did not want to be too close to the case household. If we obtained information from neighbors who were too close to case households, we risked obtaining controls who likely shared too many behaviors with cases compared to other randomly selected controls, thus decreasing our ability to identify potential risk factors for aflatoxicosis. Instead, we walked farther. Sometimes, we got lucky and found houses relatively close. Other times, the third house in the general direction indicated by the bottle was out of sight and we resigned ourselves to a long walk. At the household, we identified all residents who had slept in the house the night before and then we used a random number sheet to select one household member to interview. Infants that were solely breastfeeding were excluded because they would not have consumed maize. This process was repeated during the next weeks.

During our second week in the field, we were scheduled to find the family of a case–patient who had survived his acute episode of jaundice. We walked down a dirt road as Dr. Sopiato Likimani, today's CDC-Kenya counterpart, explained how villages in this region make decisions through consensus during a baraza or gathering. During the daily calls with Nairobi, we heard that the CDC lab had identified elevated aflatoxin B1 levels in maize grown by subsistence farmers. Some of the maize samples from case–households had aflatoxin-B_1 levels as high as 4000 ppb, orders of magnitude higher than the safety limit imposed in the United States of 20 ppb (Figure 24-7). Dr. Likimani suggested we should request village elders to call a baraza to discuss potential prevention measures. Listening to the cadence of our footsteps on the gravel road, we mulled over her recommendation. Soon, we passed a large tree with a rounded canopy and small waxy leaves. The locals had become so familiar with the periodic outbreaks of acute jaundice that they identified a local remedy for it and used the tree's leaves to make a drink like tea.

As we rounded the top of the hill and entered a cluster of houses, I noticed something was off. The compound looked unusually still; there were no children

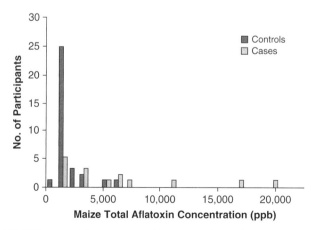

FIGURE 24-7 Frequency of total maize aflatoxin concentrations for participants. Reproduced with permission from *Environmental Health Perspectives*[1]

playing among the houses; there was no smoke from the fire pit. The place looked deserted. Near the houses were mounds of recently turned dirt. We wound around the back of the compound, taking in the stillness. I listened for voices, but could hear only the wind as it rustled the leaves on the trees. Peering into the darkness of one of the huts, the healthcare worker waved and greeted someone. The healthcare worker gently coaxed an elderly man into the bright sunlight. The man shuffled toward us, stooped and seemingly disoriented. Dr. Likimani and the elderly man spoke for a long time. Although I could not hear them well, I sensed the sadness in their voices. Then he pointed an emaciated arm towards the mounds next to the huts. He and a hospitalized grandchild were the last to survive the jaundice. The others were buried where the man was pointing.

Invariably, these outbreaks occur among the impoverished and marginalized. Food insecurity, poor infrastructure, and limited resources predispose them to outbreaks of disease. When locals prepare the little maize available, it is impossible to tell contaminated maize from safe maize. There is a terrible divide between our lives and theirs. Typically, the epidemiologist operates within a different world, a world of comparative wealth and technical resources. One could just as easily have been born to these circumstances. Between meetings, while walking or driving from site to site, and at the end of the day, I have to remind myself that I get to go home after the study is over. This helps me to not become despondent and to stay focused on the task at hand.

When we returned from the villages, the team gathered for dinner at Hunter's Lodge, my hotel, or wherever we were collecting data. Dinner conversation would often be lively and boisterous. We would talk about food habits, cultural norms, and the mundane (e.g., who got a flat tire that day). I suspect it was to suppress what we had witnessed during the day. If there were Rhesus monkeys on the roof of the hotel, someone might bring out handfuls of bread to toss to them. At dusk, I would search for troops of baboons (Figure 24-8) walking single-file down the road. Of course, attempting to feed a baboon would just be tempting fate. As the days passed, however, the monotony of our data collection routine and the long days were a sufficient distraction.

After 3 weeks of data collection, the teams were tired and less talkative. Finally, it was our last day in the field. I had skipped breakfast and, cursing my poor judgment, was looking forward to lunch. As the only medical person in that day's field team, I knelt in front of a young woman of about 16 years of age who was offering her left arm for a blood sample. She sat on a tree stump with

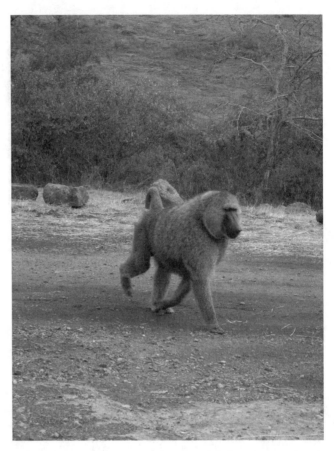

FIGURE 24-8 One of many baboons of rural Kenya.

the elbow of her outstretched arm supported by her right hand. I inserted the cannula of the 23-gauge butterfly needle into her cubital vein and then inserted the test tube into the other end of the tubing. I relaxed when I saw blood dribbling into the vacuum of the red top tube. During the past days, it was difficult to predict who would be an easy stick, given everyone's general dehydration. Distracted, I waited for the tube to fill while the young woman sat immobile. As soon as the tubes filled, I pulled out the needle from her arm and placed gauze in her decubital fossa. As I turned away from her and palmed the rest of the tubes, I felt a sharp pain. The needle was jabbed upright on my outstretched index finger.

I, like many other medical officers, have had many needle sticks, but that was in the United States and not in Kenya where the prevalence of HIV is substantial. I blanched and gently pulled out the needle. Then, I walked away and, without saying a word, started sucking the wound. Disorganized thoughts clamored in my head. What was the probability of getting HIV from one needle stick? What were the chances of getting Hepatitis B or C? I wandered toward the car to find the satellite radio. I gripped the black rubbery casing and pointed the antenna at the sky. I dialed the only number I could remember under the circumstances, the CDC operator. It was after-hours, but after several attempts, she was able to contact the physician on call for the occupational health clinic. She was reassuring, but advised me to start antivirals immediately. Then, we could wait and see. I did not want to become a cautionary tale. I should have eaten breakfast and brought some water. No matter now. I was infinitely relieved when the blood sample tested negative for HIV and viral hepatitis several days later.

We spent the next several days at the CDC-Kenya offices further cleaning the data and preparing to scan questionnaires. The blood samples needed to be aliquoted into cryovials, one aliqout to remain in Kenya and two for shipment to the United States. I borrowed an ill-fitting laboratory coat from one of my Kenyan colleagues and sat on a stool on the black bench with a rack of test tubes on my right, a bag of single disposable pipettes in front of me, and boxes of empty 4-milliliter test tubes on my left. I uncorked the test tube tops into the garbage can by my leg, pipetted the serum, taking care not to disturb the precipitated red blood cells, and emptied the content of the pipettes with satisfaction into the cryovials. Each cryovial required labeling with a marker. A duplicate entry was entered into the laboratory sample line–list. It was slow, but cathartic work.

Outside, in a grassy spot between the laboratory and the main CDC building, a colleague from the FDA, Dr. Henry Njapau, and his local counterpart were taking turns lunging a 4-foot long wooden pestle into a giant mortar to grind the maize samples. From the window of the lab, I could see one of them as he raised the pestle above his head and swiftly brought it down. Both laboratorians looked tired and hot in their green lab coats, the noon sun beaming down on them with characteristic apathy. Beside them were three abandoned grinders that they had burned through in their attempts to get the maize to the proper grain size. The commercial aflatoxin kits required finely ground maize so the toxins could be efficiently eluted from the sample, but dry maize was tough stuff. The dry maize kernels had already destroyed our coffee grinders, large manual and motorized commercial grinders, and now "we" had resigned ourselves to go at it Neolithic style. I watched Dr. Njapau, a serious scientist, pounding on the maize.

By the end of field work, the days and nights ran together in the constant minutia of wrapping food samples, entering sample questionnaires, and preparing preliminary "exit reports." Fortunately, the CDC had sent Drs. Lauren Lewis and George Luber, who have a wealth of field epidemiology experience, to initiate the next phase of the investigation, a sampling of aflatoxin in commercial maize. When I finally arrived home, exhausted and rumpled after 27 hours on various flights, I could not adequately explain to my family what I had seen or done. Showing trip photos to coworkers and family only reminded them that they had to pick up the slack during my absence. To many, the trip seemed to be little more than medical adventurism and did not outweigh its perceived risks. It was best to quietly return to the routine and the improbably long list of unanswered emails.

The day the laboratory results arrived had all the qualities of a major holiday. For the epidemiologist, the laboratory is where magic happens—where all those little vials are processed and a spreadsheet is returned to you with the long anticipated results. Will your cases indeed have higher aflatoxin levels than the controls? Will you have to scramble to test the samples for something else you had not considered? The branch chief called us over to the office as soon as the spreadsheets arrived from the laboratory. Upon hearing the news, I ran back to my office around the corner and opened her forwarded emails. The spreadsheets were coded so that the laboratory folks were blind to who was a case and who was a control; in this way they are not tempted to interpret marginal results in favor of cases or controls. I matched our participant identification numbers with those on the spreadsheets and identified which results belonged to cases and which belonged to the controls. Then, I sorted the spreadsheets and calculated some arithmetic averages. It is a quick and dirty method of exploring the data, but within minutes I could clearly see that mean aflatoxin-B_1 adduct levels in case samples were much higher than that of controls (Figure 24-9). Relieved, I ran back to Carol's office to report my finding. At the threshold of Carol's office stood the statistician, nodding her head and smiling. The data, like that of many biomarkers of environmental exposure, were skewed data and were better compared as geometric means after accounting for clustering. For the moment, however, we were all satisfied with the findings.

The secret value of the EIS officer is his or her focus on a single task. While the real clinicians, epidemiologists, statisticians, and laboratorians have multiple duties, the EIS officer can remain focused on the analyses, interpretation, and dissemination of his or her project. Few EIS officers can do these tasks well without a lot of help, but with the invaluable help of the statistician, toxicologists, epidemiologist, and mathematicians, our

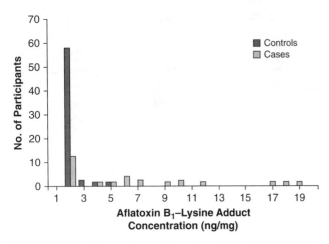

FIGURE 24-9 Frequency of serum aflatoxin B1-lysine albumin adduct concentrations for participants.
Reproduced with permission from *Environmental Health Perspectives*[1]

team confirmed that aflatoxin levels were higher in maize samples obtained from case households and that aflatoxin-B_1 adduct levels were higher in case–patient's serum. Having confirmed the outbreak findings, the team then set out to identify the risk factors by exploring the data in the case–control questionnaire. A detailed analysis, accounting for clustering, determined that storing wet maize and doing so in unventilated dwellings (as opposed to dry maize in well-ventilated granaries) were important risk factors for exposure to aflatoxins. That day, the findings of the investigation were relayed to the CDC-Kenya so that prevention measures could take place. The findings provided the government of Kenya with the necessary evidence to mobilize a logistically challenging and expensive maize replacement campaign. Within months, the findings were also presented at the Epidemic Intelligence Service conference in Atlanta and attracted much attention from public health colleagues because of the magnitude of the outbreak (314 cases, 127 dead) and its novel methods. In fact, this outbreak resulted in the largest number of fatalities ever documented in an aflatoxicosis outbreak. Thanks to the methods developed by the laboratory colleagues, this is the first time that aflatoxin-B_1 adduct levels were recovered from humans during an acute aflatoxicosis outbreak. The inevitable question then became how do we prevent such outbreaks from occurring again?

> *The findings provided the government of Kenya with the necessary evidence to mobilize a logistically challenging and expensive maize replacement campaign.*

During that spring, the Health Studies Branch applied for funding from the CDC Foundation and other groups to disseminate the findings of the study at the WHO offices in Geneva at a conference and formulate a strategy for the prevention of future outbreaks. The work of organizing the meeting was then transferred to the energetic and well-organized Heather Strosnider at the Office of the Director. In the meantime, epidemiologists like Dr. Lauren Lewis and toxicologist Dr. Manish Patel planned a series of sophisticated studies to further explore issues of aflatoxin contamination in commercial food supplies, its effects on children, its association with endemic viral hepatitis, and its potential role in the high hepatocellular carcinoma incidence in the region. I spent the next several weeks completing applications for funding and writing study protocols. Before I knew it, our team was in Europe trying to decipher how to get tokens from the automatic ticket machine at the Geneva airport for a train ride into WHO headquarters.

Walking around one of the countless auditoriums of the WHO offices with the ninth cup of coffee of the morning, it seemed strange that we would be meeting here, in Geneva, when the root of the aflatoxin problem was one of food insecurity in Kenya. Our colleagues from agriculture reminded us that aflatoxin contamination was preventable through proper crop selection, irrigation, pest control, and post-harvest processing of grains and pulses. They had explored the issue of aflatoxin contamination for decades and suggested several agricultural solutions to the issues of food security and aflatoxin contamination. I wondered how much we could do from Geneva, even with our outlined research agenda, tentative liaison with policy makers in Kenya, and good intentions. I wondered how many commercial grain driers and wells the monies from the conference could pay for. The morning of my presentation, I sat on the steps of the hotel entrance wondering about the role of public health in improving the lives of marginalized communities that live in degraded environments. The situation of aflatoxicosis in Kenya seemed like a case study from Jared Diamond's *Collapse*, a book that discusses factors that have historically contributed to the collapse of past societies and that presents the buildup of toxins in the environment as a new factor to consider.

During the talk, I found that there were colleagues from many countries who had been wrestling with the same issues. They talked of contamination in Benin, about pilot interventions, and of what remains to be done. Developing effective prevention efforts is challenging work. First, the communities affected have next to nothing. Health promotion is perceived as a luxury and only acute illness motivates individuals to seek medical care that they know may be ineffective and bankrupt the household. Second, even if there are obvious solutions, behavior change is hard. It requires great expertise and resources to establish new habits in a population. Nevertheless, it is obvious from listening to the discussion in the packed auditorium that colleagues have been thinking creatively about cost effective, culturally appropriate ways to tackle the issue. It took me years to understand that for our branch, this outbreak was an overture into addressing the issue of aflatoxin contamination. From this overture, it is the patient work of people like Dr. Lauren Lewis and others that truly furthers our understanding of how to prevent aflatoxin exposure in Sub-Saharan Africa.[3] With each field investigation, hopefully we get closer to controlling this public health threat.

LEARNING QUESTIONS

1. The author mentions that several viral infectious diseases were tested for early in this investigation. They included yellow fever, Rift Valley fever, dengue, acute hepatitis A, B, and C, West Nile virus, Chikungunya and Bunyamwera virus. How are the diseases caused by these viruses similar to and different from aflatoxicosis?
2. What are the environment and human factors that promote risk for aflatoxicosis? Do these factors promote the risk for any other infectious diseases of public health importance?
3. When asking to interview and bleed persons who had a family member recently die, the author questions why they need to disturb these grieving villagers. How would you justify "disturbing" them, given that it is too late to save their deceased loved one?
4. Laboratory staff were blinded to the status of the persons who had donated blood for testing. In other words, they did not know if the donor was a case–patient or a control. What was the rationale for blinding the laboratory staff to case status?
5. Why did this study plan to report geometric means rather than just reporting the mean aflatoxin-B_1 adduct levels?
6. The author was concerned that friends and family perceived his field investigation as "medical adventurism." Summarize in just a few sentences the investigation and its importance.
7. Needle sticks are a hazard to healthcare workers and field investigation staff involved in drawing blood. Using the Internet or scientific journals, try to identify the prevalence of HIV in Kenya. What is the source of data for that prevalence? What should be considered when trying to estimate the risk of transmission of HIV, hepatitis B, and hepatitis C to the author from a needle stick in Kenya when the blood came from a person of unknown serostatus for these viral infections?

ACKNOWLEDGMENTS

Kimberly Lindblade, Karen Gieseker, Helen Schurz Rogers, Stephanie Kieszak, Henry Njapau, Rosemary Schleicher, Leslie F. McCoy, Ambrose Misore, Kevin DeCock, Carol Rubin, Laurence Slutsker, Lorraine Backer, the Aflatoxin Investigative Group including J. Nyamongo, C. Njuguna, E. Muchiri, J. Njau, S. Maingi, J. Njoroge, J. Mutiso, J. Onteri, A. Langat, I.K. Kilei, G. Ogana, B. Muture, J. Nyikal (Kenya Ministry of Health); P. Tukei, C. Onyango, W. Ochieng (Kenya Medical Research Institute); I. Mugoya, P. Nguku, T. Galgalo, S. Kibet, A. Manya, A. Dahiye, J. Mwihia, S. Likimani, C. Tetteh (Kenya Field Epidemiology and Laboratory Training Program/Kenya Ministry of Health); J. Onsongo, A. Ngindu (World Health Organization, Kenya Country Office); P. Amornkul, D. Rosen, D. Feiken, T. Thomas (CDC-Kenya); P. Mensah, N. Eseko, A. Nejjar (World Health Organization, Regional Office for Africa); M. Onsongo, F. Kessel (Foreign Agricultural Service, U.S. Department of Agriculture); D. L. Park (Center for Food Safety and Applied Nutrition, Food and Drug Administration); C. Nzioka (Office of Global Health, CDC); L. Lewis, G. Luber, C.D. Powers, C. Pfeiffer (National Center for Environmental Health, CDC); W. Chege, A. Bowen (Epidemiology Program Office, CDC) and our hosts in Kenya.

The views and opinions expressed by the author do not necessarily represent the official views of the CDC. The use of trade names is for identification only and does not imply endorsement by the Centers for Disease Control and Prevention, the Agency for Toxic Substances and Disease Registry, the Public Health Service, or the U.S. Department of Health and Human Services.

REFERENCES

1. Williams JH, Phillips TD, Jolly PE, Stiles JK, Jolly CM, Aggrawal D. Human aflatoxicosis in developing countries; a review of toxicology, exposure, potential health consequences, and interventions. *Am J Clin Nutr*. 2004;80(5): 1106–1122.
2. Azziz-Baumgartner E, Lindblade K, Gieseker K, et al. Case–control study of an acute aflatoxicosis outbreak, Kenya, 2004. *Environ Health Perspect*. 2005;113(12):1779–1783.
3. Lewis L, Onsongo M, Njapau H, et al. Aflatoxin contamination of commercial maize products during an outbreak of acute aflatoxicosis in eastern and central Kenya. *Environ Health Perspect*. 2005;113(12): 1763–1767.

CHAPTER 25

What Do People Eat When They Have No Food? A Tragic Story of Poverty, Monsoon Floods, and Weeds

Emily S. Gurley, MPH
Bangladesh, 2007

AT THE ICDDR,B

I have many fond memories of living in Bangladesh. I lived there from 1986 to 1988 when my father served as the physician at the U.S. Embassy in Dhaka. As a child of about 12 years of age leaving the United States for the first time, I was immediately struck by the heat, strong smells, and strong tastes of Bangladesh. I found the extreme poverty troubling, but learned that beauty is ever-present in the cooling monsoon rains, kind people, and never-ending green countryside. This early experience sowed the seeds of my interest in travel and public health. In July 2003, I happily accompanied my husband to Dhaka for his new job as the information technology manager at the local United States Agency for International Development office. Dhaka in 2003 was a sprawling city of 12 million, barely recognizable as the place I had lived as a child. I had just completed my MPH from Emory University and knew that I wanted a career in public health research. Shortly after arriving, I met Rob Breiman, who was a CDC employee seconded to ICDDR,B (the International Centre for Diarrhoeal Disease Research, Bangladesh). Rob was the medical epidemiologist leading the newly formed Program on Infectious Disease and Vaccine Sciences (PIDVS) at ICDDR,B. Rob had been at ICDDR,B for 3 years and had a long and highly prolific career in epidemiologic research; he had served as the chief epidemiologist at the CDC's Respiratory Diseases Branch and as director of the U.S. National Vaccine Program Office. Some of his previous work had included investigating outbreaks of *Legionella* and the first hantavirus cases described in the United States. Given this experience, it was no surprise that he was routinely asked to lend his technical expertise to outbreaks occurring in Bangladesh. I told him that I was looking for work and that I was interested in research. By October 2003, I was working for Rob in PIDVS.

By November of 2007, I was the mother of two small children, aged 2½ years and 8 months, and referred to Dhaka as "home." I had been investigating outbreaks in Bangladesh for nearly 4 years. Our program worked closely with the Institute of Epidemiology, Disease Control and Research (IEDCR) at the Ministry of

Health and Family Welfare. This small group was officially responsible for all surveillance and outbreak investigations in Bangladesh—no small job in a country of 140 million people who face numerous health risks on a daily basis. Our interests naturally overlapped with theirs. They had a political mandate to solve outbreaks and take necessary public health action, but lacked adequate resources for the task. We had plenty of resources, academic interest, and expertise, but no formal mandate for action. Although the politics were sometimes tricky, our two groups managed to find opportunities to work together and, through the years, built a trusting, fruitful collaboration.

WHAT DOES THIS HAVE TO DO WITH THE PRICE OF RICE?

To comprehend the population density of Bangladesh, imagine that everyone in the United States living east of the Mississippi River was moved to the state of Wisconsin. Now, imagine that once per year, half of the land flooded. The monsoon rains come to Bangladesh every June or July and last through August or September. In 2007, the rains came and came and kept on coming. In August 2007, for example, more than half of the Sylhet District in northeastern Bangladesh was under water. The high population density meant that millions of people, who already live in poverty, lost their crops, lost their belongings, and were displaced.

At the same time, the entire world was reeling from increases in food prices. Bangladesh was no exception. Between October 2006 and October 2007, the loss of rice crops and global forces caused the retail price of rice in Bangladesh to increase by 38% (Figure 25-1).[1] Why is that important? Well, rice is consumed by almost every person in Bangladesh at almost every meal. They do not consider it to be a meal unless it includes rice. In addition, even in the best of times, approximately 46% of Bangladeshi children are undernourished (Bangladesh Demographic and Health Survey (BDHS), 2007) and households in Bangladesh spend approximately 70% of their income on food.[1] So, sudden increases in the price of rice mean that many people go hungry—even more than usual.

ONE OUTBREAK OR TWO?

On November 7, 2007, the director of IEDCR, Professor Mahmudur Rahman, called and invited me and the ICDDR,B outbreak investigation team to a meeting on

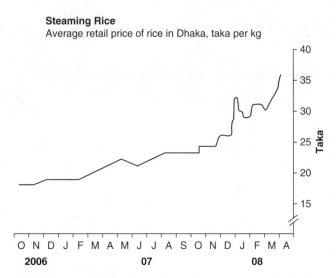

FIGURE 25-1 The rising price of rice in Bangladesh from 2006 to 2008, according to the Bangladesh Ministry of Agriculture. (Taka 70 ≈ US $1) Courtesy of the Bangladesh Ministry of Agriculture.

November 8 to review preliminary findings from a cluster of unusual deaths in Gowainghat Sub-district, Sylhet District, located within 5 km of the northeastern border with India. He had been notified about a suspicious cluster of deaths and had sent a team of medical epidemiologists to gather some additional information about this possible outbreak. The objective of the meeting was to hear about the preliminary findings from this team and to determine whether or not a more extensive investigation was required. Given the large numbers of suspected outbreaks reported to their office, only the most urgent receive more in-depth investigations or requests for support from ICDDR,B. My supervisor, Steve Luby, the CDC secondee to ICDDR,B since 2005 and epidemiologist extraordinaire (Figure 25-2), was out of town and I was in charge of the outbreak team. We met with IEDCR officials in their conference room, merely a 10-minute walk from our offices through rickshaws and pedestrian-clogged streets. Here's what we heard:

At 3:00 a.m. on November 4, a 6-year-old girl from the rural and impoverished village of Lathi became ill with vomiting and restlessness. She died at 5:00 a.m. at her home. Her mother, aged 26 years, and 3-year-old sister developed similar symptoms just after the girl's death and they were taken to the local government hospital, where they presented unconscious and died within a few hours. Relatives of the family reported that 3 young girls, cousins and neighbors of the index case, died in their home on November 4 from similar symptoms. On

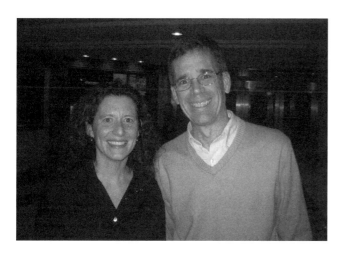

FIGURE 25-2 Photo of Emily Gurley and Steve Luby, American Society of Tropical Medicine and Hygiene Conference, Washington, DC, November 2009.

November 5, 6 more patients from the same village were admitted to the local health complex and referred to Sylhet Medical College Hospital, a tertiary care facility located about a 30-minute drive from the local hospital. These patients included three adult males, two adult females, and one child; one of the adult males was in a deep coma. Additional patients continued to arrive, including another mother and her four children from a village approximately 3–4 km away from Lathi.

The team returned with information regarding basic clinical signs and symptoms of patients and 11 acute blood samples. The defining features were rapid onset of vomiting with quick progression to unconsciousness in many cases. Remarkably, most patients were children. Because so many of the patients died before the initial team arrived, it was unclear if all of the blood specimens represented patients associated with the outbreak; although, at least one was from a patient who died with clinical signs and symptoms very similar to the index case.

Serious discussion ensued. Clearly, this merited closer investigation. Eight deaths had already been identified and patients were continuing to present to local hospitals. We all agreed on one point: given the rapid onset and progression of illness and absence of fever as a prominent feature of illness onset, this seemed to be related to a toxic exposure. The epidemiologic data also supported this—so far, patients were all from a specific geographic area and became sick within a few days of one another, suggesting a point source exposure. But what might the exposure be? Had patients been to a similar area or eaten the same meal? Information available suggested that they had not shared a meal or point source exposure. In 2007, H5N1 (bird flu) outbreaks were occurring all over Asia, including human cases. Despite rumors of poultry die-offs in Bangladesh, no outbreaks had yet been reported. However, bird flu was on everyone's mind and we were all somewhat relieved that these patients had no history of respiratory symptoms.

> *We all agreed on one point: given the rapid onset and progression of illness and absence of fever as a prominent feature of illness onset, this seemed to be related to a toxic exposure.*

As we finalized our plans to send additional investigators to the field, Prof. Rahman shared a second agenda item for our meeting. There was now a second outbreak being reported from Sylhet. Visits to Sylhet Medical College Hospital from the IEDCR team put them on high alert for identifying clusters of patients. On November 8, they reported a cluster of eight patients from Companyganj Sub-district currently hospitalized with what they described as meningo-encephalitis syndrome. They reported that five patients were hospitalized at the local Companyganj government hospital and that four patients had already died. The description of the illness from local physicians indicated that these patients were distinct from patients in Gowainghat—they reportedly had fever followed by altered mental status. Although unusual, the occurrence of two distinct outbreaks in one district at the same time was not impossible. We agreed to send two teams to Sylhet—one for the new Companyganj cluster and one for the Gowainghat cluster the following day (Figure 25-3).

Both teams consisted of ICDDR,B and IEDCR staff, including physicians, medical epidemiologists, and anthropologists. Although not standard practice in most settings, our outbreak investigation team had included anthropologists since 2004. Their expertise in gaining the trust of communities and in-depth interview techniques had proven invaluable in previous outbreaks. Specifically, their ability to illicit the "outbreak story" from affected communities was used to generate hypotheses about the cause of the outbreak. Their understanding of local terminology and case histories were tremendous assets when it came time to draft the epidemiologic questionnaire and identify proxy respondents. My role was to coordinate efforts from Dhaka and keep information flowing between organizations and with Steve, who was not due back in country for a few days. Following the meeting with IEDCR, I felt the absence of his expert counsel acutely.

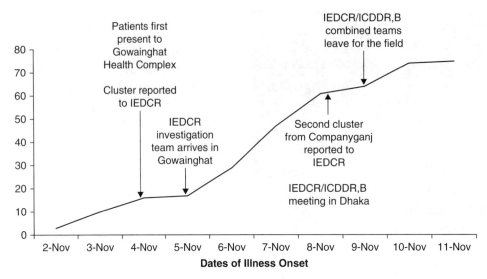

FIGURE 25-3 Timeline of initial outbreak events plotted with total cumulative case counts.

FINDING CASES AND GENERATING HYPOTHESES: WHERE TO FOCUS?

The team loaded up the minivans with specimen collection supplies, cold boxes, liquid nitrogen dewars (small containers used to carry liquid nitrogen for freezing specimens in the field), data collection forms, and packaged foods to eat on the road. It was a 6-hour drive to Sylhet Medical College Hospital, which was the first stop. By this time, patients from both Gowainghat and Companyganj were being referred there for treatment. By the end of the day on November 9, there were nearly 70 patients identified in hospital or reported to the team by case–patient family members. Liver function tests conducted on a subset of patients showed elevated liver enzymes, extremely elevated in some patients, which supported the hypothesis of a toxic exposure.

The hospital is typically the first visit we make in these investigations: you are sure to find patients there, you can more easily collect specimens than in the community setting, and patients are often accompanied by family members who can provide information about events leading up to the illness. After the first day in Sylhet Medical College Hospital, it became clear that the clusters from Gowainghat and Companyganj were the same outbreak. Initial reports from physicians about meningo-encephalitis syndrome were inaccurate because they relied heavily upon interpretation from family member reports rather than clinical signs and symptoms and because patients who had presented to this hospital with classic encephalitis, but were not associated with other cases, had been included in the "cluster" report. In particular, one patient with abnormal findings on a brain MRI drew the attention of local physicians who believed that they were seeing an outbreak of viral encephalitis. This conclusion was not without basis; there were patients admitted to this hospital who clearly exhibited symptoms consistent with viral encephalitis and a widely publicized outbreak of Japanese encephalitis had been raging in neighboring India since January 2007. There were three pieces of data from the outbreak, however, which did not support viral encephalitis as a cause of the outbreak and which supported that these were two presentations of the same outbreak. First, patients from the clusters reported that illness began with vomiting as opposed to fever. If the outbreak patients had presented with fever, we would have been more comfortable with a diagnosis of viral encephalitis. Second, outbreak patients progressed from illness onset to coma within only a few hours. Although some causes of viral encephalitis can progress quickly, such as the Nipah virus that causes outbreaks almost yearly in Bangladesh, they typically do not progress this quickly. Finally, the patient with the changes on MRI was from a different area of the district, from which there were no other illnesses reported, and his illness course was dissimilar to other clustered patients. The team settled on a case definition of vomiting followed by restlessness since November 2. Although opposition to our evolving hypothesis from some local physicians continued, we remained convinced that this outbreak was most likely due to some kind of toxic poisoning.

Physicians had constructed a makeshift isolation ward. All patients associated with the outbreak were hospitalized in one alcove of the ward, which was separated by the rest of the ward by a hanging sheet (Figure 25-4). Our team brought personal protective equipment for hospital staff, including latex gloves and N-95 (respirator) masks, which were typically unavailable in this hospital setting. While the physicians were busy collecting clinical data and organizing specimens, the anthropologists were interviewing family members, although they were not learning much. Most patients were accompanied by males because of local cultural constraints on women's movement outside the home. However, women were more likely to have been caregivers in the home and to have been present at the onset of illness. In order to hear their stories, and gain more insight into events leading up to the outbreak, the team had to go to the villages.

This was not an easy task. The team learned by firsthand experience that these villages were in remote areas, often a 3–4 kilometer walk from a paved road. After they reached the villages, they began to understand the depth of their poverty. Villagers told the team that severe 2007 monsoon floods had destroyed all rice and vegetable crops in the area. Most households earned income from providing daily labor services in either agriculture or small construction projects. However, because the crops were gone, so were the jobs. Some people had also been employed to collect small stones from a nearby river for use in making concrete, but a recent prohibition on collecting these stones was a further source of economic strain. Many families reported that they ate only two meals a day, which in Bangladesh is a sign of extreme poverty. They reported that they did not have enough money to buy food, so they relied heavily on uncultivated food sources in their communities, including small fish collected from ponds and ditches and wild plants. In addition to food scarcity, there were other exposures reported that might have been associated with the outbreak. As an example, I made the following notes about the index village after a telephone conversation with the field team on November 11:

> They usually drink tube well water (water from underground aquifers that is accessed by creating negative pressure through hand pumps attached to tubes tapped into the aquifers). However, during this season, the pump is dry, so they dug a hole along the back of the local river and use the water from that hole for drinking and all other household purposes.
>
> There are accounts of sick people and animals in the village in the weeks preceding the outbreak. One case had been suffering from jaundice and fever for 2 weeks and was taking multiple medications, including antibiotics and paracetemol. Three others from the index family (not cases) are still suffering from jaundice and they received allopathic and homeopathic remedies. One of the children who died had a history of vomiting with blood 2 years ago. The locals report that there were extensive poultry die-offs about 2 weeks before the illness and that 1–2 chickens in the village die every day. It's worth noting that dead animal carcasses are dumped in the same area of the riverbed where they retrieve drinking water.

Illness histories from community respondents were quite revealing, especially accounts from women who cared for patients and prepared their bodies for burial. They reported that patients first developed profuse and frequent vomiting. They reported that patients vomited blood, but it was not fresh blood; it was like reddish or blackish water. Afterwards, they developed a mild fever and many breathed rapidly. Then, they developed shivering and unconsciousness within a very short period of time, usually within hours. Some patients had frothing from their mouth and nose, even while their bodies were being cleaned for burial. Another interesting point was that they reported that the bodies had some reddish areas and some were blackish at burial, not the usual pale look that dead bodies have. The families involved in the outbreak had experienced stigma—they had a difficult time finding someone to prepare the bodies for burial and attend the funeral prayers. Many families sent their children away from the village to protect them from illness.

The field teams worked long hours and I spoke with them by cell phone each evening after 9:00 p.m. to discuss

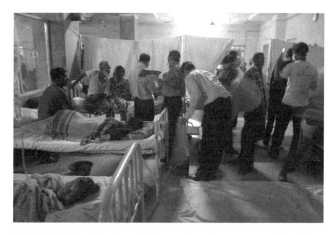

FIGURE 25-4 Outbreak investigation team collecting information and patient specimens in the make shift isolation ward at Sylhet Medical College Hospital.

findings from the day and make a plan for the next day's activities. The pressure was high because cases continued to arrive at the hospital and we still had no credible hypothesis about how they were being poisoned. We had identified cases from at least eight different villages, but the question remained: What common exposure did all of these people have? We reasoned that the toxin was either distributed through the area and brought into the case homes or came from a source common to all affected areas.

I asked the team to list all items that households with cases had purchased or brought into their homes in the week preceding the outbreak, the foods they had eaten in the 24 hours preceding illness, and where they had traveled in the days before the outbreak. Given the numerous health hazards already identified in these communities, there seemed to be limitless possibilities for toxic exposure. We were having a difficult time focusing our efforts.

Steve, who was still traveling at the time, forwarded our preliminary investigation report to friends and colleagues who were knowledgeable about Bangladesh and had expertise in outbreak investigations to assist us in generating hypotheses about the cause of the outbreak. One of these personal contacts, Dr. Yvan Hutin with the WHO in Delhi, directed us to papers published from India about outbreaks of hepatomyoencephalopathy in children associated with consuming toxic beans from wild plants.[2,3] Could the same thing be happening here? Our patients were also mostly children suffering from altered mental status with signs of liver damage. Were they eating a toxic plant? We focused our histories of foods consumed on uncultivated plant sources. Because we still did not have a hypothesis to test, we were asking open-ended questions to case families and community residents. We asked them questions like, "In the 24 hours before you (the case–patient) became ill, what plants did you (the case–patient) eat?"

The new focused line of questioning yielded quick results. Of the 33 cases interviewed in four villages, 31 reported that on the day before they became sick, they ate an uncultivated plant called *ghagra shak*. In addition, we had this story from the index household: In the evening before the illness, the index family ate *ghagra shak*. Their relatives (who also became cases) reported sharing in the meal. The *ghagra shak* gave the first family a stomach ache; they interpreted this illness as a result of the "evil eye" (meaning that others were jealous of their meal), so they decided that they should share the *ghagra shak* with their relatives to alleviate symptoms.

We did not know what *ghagra shak* was, but the team collected samples and took photos of the plant. With continuing pressure from affected communities and health authorities to find a culprit, we moved quickly to design an epidemiologic study to test whether or not consuming this plant was associated with illness.

Over the first few days of the investigation we tested patient blood and throat swab specimens for infectious causes at IEDCR: influenza, Nipah virus, malaria, Japanese encephalitis, and dengue fever tests were all negative. None of these were high on our suspicion list, but they represent the infectious causes that we had diagnostics for and they were useful to help us rule out those etiologies as causes of the outbreak.

COULD IT BE THE *GHAGRA SHAK*?

By November 11, there were 76 cases identified and 19 (25%) had died. Fifty-one cases (63%) were aged 16 years or younger and 70% were female (possibly because of their lower body weight). The most frequently cited signs and symptoms included vomiting (100%, per our case definition), history of fever (61%), and altered mental status (59%) which developed into coma for 38% of cases (Table 25-1A). Onset of mild fever was commonly reported by case–patients. After vomiting began, however, of the 63 case–patients who had their temperature taken during their illness, only 21% (16/63) had an elevated temperature between 99°F and 102°F. Patients had laboratory evidence of liver damage, evidenced by elevated alanine aminotransferase levels and prothrombin times (important for blood coagulation). Twelve patients (71%) of 17 tested had abnormal prothrombin times (>17 seconds) and 17 out of 23 (74%) experienced elevated ALT levels (>40 U/L); 5 of 19 (26%) tested had elevated serum bilirubin levels (Table 25-1B).

We had some choices to make about the design of our epidemiologic study. Do we use a case–control or a cohort approach? A challenge for all case–control studies is the issue of selecting controls—that is, do the cases and controls actually arise from the same underlying cohort? In this outbreak, cases tended to cluster within specific *paras*, or parts, of the village, suggesting that these *paras* represented the underlying cohort. Cases resided in nine different remote villages (Figure 25-5) and we knew that the logistics of finding all cases and selecting appropriate controls would be time-consuming for the field team. In addition, we also believed that

TABLE 25-1A Demographic characteristics and reported signs and symptoms of suspect and probable cases ($N = 76$)

Age in completed years (mean, range)	16.8, 1–55
	n(%)
Female	53(70)
Clinical signs and symptoms	
Vomiting*	76(100)
History of fever	46(61)
Altered mental status	45(59)
Unconsciousness†	29(38)
Fatigue/drowsiness	19(25)
Diarrhea	9(12)
Difficulty breathing	12(16)
Irritability	10(13)
Blood in vomitus	9(12)
Headache	8(11)
Frothy discharge from mouth	8(11)
Died	19(25)

*Per the case definition.
†Those with unconsciousness are a subset of those with altered mental status.

TABLE 25-1B Laboratory investigation findings from a subset of hospitalized patients‡

	n	mean; range
White blood cells	19	
Total count/cmm		13,074; 5900–25,000
Polymorphs (%)		73; 44–90
Lymphocytes (%)		20; 6–36
Platelets/cmm	17	263,000; 130,000–420,000
Serum electrolytes (μmol/L)	19	
Sodium		145; 129–149
Potassium		4.2; 3–5.5
Chloride		108; 90–116
Carbon dioxide		27; 18–37
Hemoglobin (gm/dl)	17	11.3; 9.1–13.1
Prothrombin time (seconds)	17	27; 12–69
Aspartate aminotransferase (U/L)	5	174; 111–336
Serum bilirubin (μmol/L)	19	1.2; 0.4–5.1
Alanine aminotransferase (U/L)	23	1871; 15–10,000

‡Laboratory testing was not performed for all cases; the number of cases tested is indicated by n.

Gurley ES, Rahman M, Hossain MJ, Nahar N, Faiz MA, Islam N, Sultana R, Akhtar S, Jasimuddin M, Haider MS, Islam MS, Rahman MW, Mondal UK, Luby SP. Fatal outbreak from consuming *Xanthium strumarium* seedlings during time of food scarcity in northeastern Bangladesh. PLoS ONE. 2010 Mar; 5(3): e9756. doi:10.1371/journal.pone.0009756.

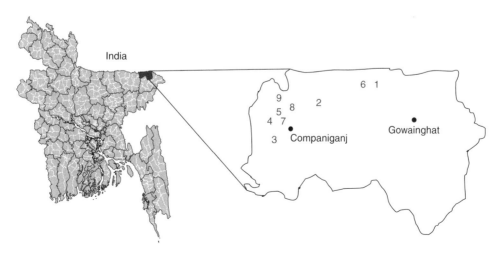

FIGURE 25-5 Approximate location of outbreak villages numbered by order in which illness occurred.

there were likely cases occurring in the community that we had not yet identified. There was also some debate about how to define a case in the community—would vomiting be specific enough? Should we use vomiting with unconsciousness, which might be more specific and easily reported by persons without medical training? Thus, we chose a cohort approach, where we would enroll everyone in two villages (where >50% of identified cases with vomiting and unconsciousness resided); we could streamline our field work, do more intensive case finding as part of the study, and conduct an analysis using both vomiting and vomiting with unconsciousness as outcomes. We accepted that all identified cases would not be in our study in exchange for completing the study more quickly and having greater flexibility in our case definition. (Note that this is not a true cohort study because all of the data were collected after the outcome. This study design has no formal name, as far as I know.)

In total, we interviewed 685 individuals residing in 131 households (86% of all residents in these villages). We asked about their exposures during the outbreak period, defined as the 2 days preceding the first death in the village through the day of the last death. We chose this time period because we believed deaths would be memorable to everyone in the village and would accurately reflect the outbreak period.

I remember receiving the study database late in the afternoon with great anticipation. I found 26 people who met our case definition of vomiting with unconsciousness. We identified only 15 such persons from these villages during our clinical case findings efforts, so it was clear that many cases occurring in the community had not sought care. The information on foods consumed by village residents was revealing. During the outbreak period, only two cases with vomiting and unconsciousness ate any kind of animal protein (eggs) and three ate getchu root, which is a food typically only considered appropriate for livestock (Table 25-2). We calculated odds ratios to investigate the association between each exposure and illness and we conducted the analysis twice, using both vomiting (as a relatively nonspecific case definition) and vomiting with unconsciousness (more specific) as our outcomes (the results of the second of these analyses are presented in Table 25-2). In the univariate analyses, eight exposures were associated with an increased risk of developing illness, including eating low-quality lentils, high-quality lentils, day-old rice with water, red spinach, cucumber, string beans, and *ghagra shak*. I included all of exposures with an associated p-value of 0.2 in a logistic regression model and used generalized estimating equations to account for household level clustering of outcomes; after all, household members do not eat the same meal just by chance. The results from the multivariate analysis confirmed our hypothesis and were similar in both analyses: people who consumed *ghagra shak* during the outbreak were 34 times more likely (95% CI 10.1–115.8, p-value <0.000) to develop illness than those who did not eat the plant. Eating *kheshuri* lentils (low-quality lentils) also remained significantly associated with disease in our multivariate model (OR 5.5, 95% CI 1.2–26.0, p-value=0.03). Despite this association, only 5 of the 26 persons (19%) in the study with vomiting and unconsciousness reported eating the lentils, which meant that it was unlikely to be the cause of their disease. Given all of the exposures we investigated in the study, it would be expected that at least one would be associated with disease by chance alone. This might explain the association between *kheshuri* lentils and disease.

WHAT IS *GHAGRA SHAK*?

Merely hours after completing my preliminary analysis, I shared the findings on *ghagra shak* with team members from IEDCR and ICDDR,B. Although we all shared the same satisfaction about finding an association, this quickly gave way to more questions, such as "What is *ghagra shak*?"

For immediate answers, we turned to the anthropologists who had interviewed villagers specifically about this plant. It grows wild near their homes and they frequently use the leaves and stalks of mature plants for medicinal purposes or to flavor curries. Some members of the investigation team recalled eating this plant in their childhood. If this plant is frequently eaten and consumed in these villages, however, why did it cause an outbreak now? We were still contemplating the possibilities.

Our epidemiologic findings raised another issue. If *ghagra shak* caused the outbreak, then why didn't all of the cases report eating it, especially when many of the same cases did report eating the plant during the in-depth interviews? Again, we turned to the anthropologists for insights. They explained that during the qualitative interviews, many families were reluctant to report that they had eaten the plant because they suspected the outbreak was caused by eating *ghagra shak* and did not want to be blamed for the deaths. These families were already facing stigmatization from their neighbors, as evidenced by their reluctance to be associated with their funerals, and they did not want to admit to doing something "wrong." The in-depth nature of

TABLE 25-2 Risk of experiencing vomiting with unconsciousness (N = 26) in two villages during the outbreak period by type of food consumed. The data in this table are based on the more specific case definition that included vomiting and unconsciousness.

Foods	Ate # Cases	Ate Total	Ate Attack rate %	Did not eat # Cases	Did not eat Total	Did not eat Attack rate %	Unadjusted Odds ratio	95% Confidence interval	P-value
Mashoor lentils (smaller, more expensive)	7	301	2	19	353	5	0.4	0.2–1.1	0.046*
Kheshari lentils (larger, the least expensive available)	5	13	38	21	641	3	18.5	4.3–69.7	<0.001*
Day-old rice with water, sometimes fermented (*panta bhat*)	3	20	15	23	634	4	4.7	0.8–17.9	0.011*
Wheat	0	17	0	26	637	4	0	—	—
Dried fish	8	180	4	18	474	4	1.2	0.4–2.9	0.705
Potato	7	197	4	19	457	4	0.9	0.3–2.2	0.717
Banana	3	41	12	23	613	4	2.0	0.4–7.2	0.258
Cucumber	2	9	22	24	645	4	7.4	0.7–41	0.005*
String beans (*borboti*)	7	62	11	19	592	3	3.8	1.3–10	0.002*
Red spinach	15	230	7	11	424	3	2.6	1.1–6.4	0.014*
Radish leaves	10	234	4	16	420	4	1.1	0.5–2.7	0.771
Chicken	0	43	0	26	611	4	0	—	—
Egg	2	67	3	24	587	4	0.7	0.1–3.0	0.661
Beef	0	4	0	26	650	4	0	—	—
Other meat	0	5	0	26	649	4	0	—	—
Uncultivated plants									
Gaghra shak (*Xanthium strumarium*)	12	36	33	14	618	2	21.6	8.1–55.9	<0.000*
Getchu root (*Apanogeton natans*)	3	29	10	23	625	4	3.0	0.6–11.0	0.073
Haincha shak (*Alternanthera sessilis*)	5	120	4	21	534	4	1.1	0.3–3.0	0.906
Ferns	2	17	12	24	637	4	3.4	0.4–16.0	0.096
Root of aram (*Colocasia esculenta*)	1	53	2	25	601	4	0.4	0.01–2.8	0.417
Small freshwater fish									
Gutum (*Lepidocephalus annandalei* or *guntea*)	13	238	5	13	416	3	1.8	0.8–4.3	0.141
Kailsha (*Colisa fasciatus*)	8	211	4	18	443	4	0.9	0.3–2.3	0.868
Punti (*Puntius puntio*)	16	419	4	10	235	4	0.9	0.4–2.2	0.784
Baim (*Mastacembelus armatus*)	7	154	5	19	500	4	1.2	0.4–3.1	0.679
Potka (A kind of puffer fish, species unknown)	0	12	0	26	642	4	0	—	—

*P-value statistically significant ≤0.05

Gurley ES, Rahman M, Hossain MJ, Nahar N, Faiz MA, Islam N, Sultana R, Akhtar S, Jasimuddin M, Haider MS, Islam MS, Rahman MW, Mondal UK, Luby SP. Fatal outbreak from consuming *Xanthium strumarium* seedlings during time of food scarcity in northeastern Bangladesh. PLoS ONE. 2010 Mar; 5(3): e9756. doi:10.1371/journal.pone.0009756.

qualitative interviews is much better at eliciting responses about stigmatized behavior than the structured questionnaires required for epidemiologic studies. Therefore, we accepted this underreporting as part of the limitations of our study methodology.

> As I drove home from work that evening through the congested Dhaka streets, I tried to imagine what it would be like to prepare a meal of weeds for my two young children to fill their stomachs because we had no food.

As I drove home from work that evening through the congested Dhaka streets, I tried to imagine what it would be like to prepare a meal of weeds for my two young children to fill their stomachs because we had no food. I was unable to imagine it.

COCKLEBUR SEEDLINGS—CAN WE MAKE A CASE FOR CAUSATION? IF SO, HOW MUCH IS TOO MUCH?

Internet searches for *ghagra shak* identified this plant as *Xanthium strumarium*, also known as common cocklebur (Figure 25-6). A botanist from Dhaka University confirmed this finding and we learned that this plant grows readily around the world. A primary limitation of the "after the fact" epidemiologic study we conducted is that these data alone are insufficient to show that *ghagra shak* was the cause of the outbreak. Some government officials and local researchers noted, and rightfully so, that we had not looked for or found the plant's toxin in patient specimens, nor had we actually tested the plants growing in the outbreak area to evaluate their toxicity. However, we employed the criteria suggested by Bradford Hill in 1965 to present evidence in favor of causality, even in the absence of such toxicologic analyses. First, *X. strumarium* was a biologically plausible cause of the outbreak because the plant's toxicity had been previously described. The toxic agent in the plant is carboxyatractyloside, which is present in the seeds and seedlings during the cotyledon stage, but is absent in plants with four or more leaves.[4] A study of rats given an intraperitoneal LD50 dose of carboxyatractoloside suggested that the chemical's cytotoxic and lethal effects are likely due to its active metabolite.[5] In fact, numerous outbreaks in livestock have been reported in association with consuming *X. strumarium* seedlings and seeds.[6–8] Second, the association we found with *ghagra shak* in our epidemiologic study was very strong and quite unlikely caused by chance alone ($p < 0.000$). Third, qualitative in-depth interviews were able to establish that exposure to *ghagra shak* had occurred before onset of illness, an assumption we could not make from our epidemiologic data. Finally, the clinical presentation of cases in this outbreak were quite similar to a case series published on *X. strumarium* seed poisoning in humans in Turkey.[9] Onset of symptoms began with nausea and vomiting and in some cases progressed quickly (within hours) to unconsciousness.[9] Liver enzymes were similarly elevated in patients who died in Turkey (ALT>7000 U/L) and in this outbreak (6795 and 10,000 U/L). In addition, our case fatality ratio was similar to the Turkish case series (33%) and the three deaths in Turkey occurred in children ≤10 years of age, which is the age group where most deaths occurred in this outbreak (13/19). A conclusion of causality was coherent with all of the data we collected and published about the plant.

We noted that people routinely ate *ghagra shak* without incident. Because other foods were not available after the floods and rising food prices in 2007, however, they changed their consumption practices. There are no published data on the toxic dose of cocklebur seedlings, but pigs that were fed seedlings at 0.75–3% of their body weight developed illness and death.[7] If we apply this dose to a child weighing 30 lbs, then the child would have to consume approximately a quarter of a pound (.23 lbs) to receive the same potentially lethal dose. There are quite likely differences between a lethal dose of seedlings for a pig and a human child. However, this calculation suggested to us that flavoring foods with cocklebur seedlings, although not advisable, was unlikely to be a major public health hazard. Rather, it was the practice of substituting seedlings for a meal that was to blame.

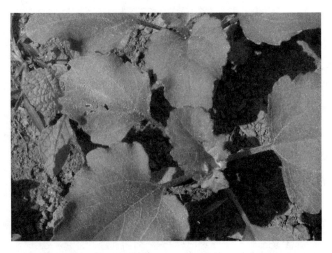

FIGURE 25-6 *Xanthium strumarium*, also known as cocklebur or *ghagra shak*.

DON'T EAT *GHAGRA*, BUT THAT'S REALLY NOT THE POINT

We concluded that the immediate cause of this outbreak was eating *ghagra shak* and we set about designing messages to communicate this to the general public. Our anthropology team returned to the outbreak villages to officially disseminate our findings to the villages that were affected by the outbreaks. Our team gathered villagers together at a predefined time and place to explain our study findings in plain language and answer questions. Specifically, we told them that we believed that consuming *ghagra shak* caused the outbreak and we asked them to refrain from eating it, especially small (immature) *ghagra shak*. One young boy from the index village wrote a special poem in honor of the occasion. Although it sounds much more eloquent in Bengali, I'll share the English translation here:

> "We will not eat *ghagra*.
> *Ghagra* is poisonous.
> People are dying by eating *ghagra*.
> Are you aware now?"

The villagers enthusiastically accepted our findings and encouraged us to share them with others in their area. A leading Bengali language daily newspaper ran a story about the investigation and published our prevention messages. Health education messages about *ghagra shak* were prepared for dissemination through government health channels.

> *As with every outbreak, certain circumstances aligned to cause this outbreak. Here, these circumstances included loss of income, death of household poultry, floods destroying crops, and rising food prices at the same time that cocklebur seedlings were sprouting.*

Still, this was not enough. The underlying cause of the outbreak, food insecurity, is an urgent global issue without easy solutions. As with every outbreak, certain circumstances aligned to cause this outbreak. Here, these circumstances included loss of income, death of household poultry, floods destroying crops, and rising food prices at the same time that cocklebur seedlings were sprouting.

Physicians working on the outbreak anecdotally reported seeing patients previously with *ghagra shak* poisoning, including an outbreak in 2001. This is not surprising; indeed, given that more than 34 million people in Bangladesh subsist on <1800 calories per day,[1] outbreaks associated with food scarcity are likely to continue. Until and unless people are able to feed themselves and their families with safe, nutritious food, they will be at risk for poor health outcomes beyond undernutrition (Figure 25-7a and 7b).

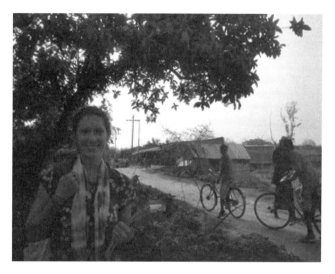

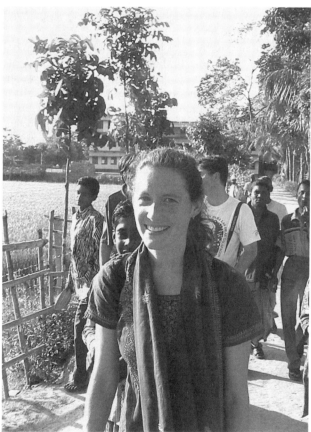

FIGURE 25-7A AND B A, The author, Emily Gurley, in a Bangladeshi village during an outbreak investigation. B, The author near a local school busy on an investigation.

LEARNING QUESTIONS

1. Early in this investigation, there was consideration that a second (meningo-encephalitis) outbreak was also occurring. What is meningo-encephalitis? Why did the investigators decide that many of these cases were more likely part of a single outbreak?
2. The investigation discovered several concerning behaviors and exposures that might predispose the villagers to risk for disease. These included the use of a hole dug along the side of a river for drinking water, exposure to ill animals, and poultry die-offs. What diseases should be considered, based on learning of these behaviors and exposures, and how well or how poorly do these diseases fit the outbreak disease?
3. The multivariate model analysis demonstrated that eating *kheshuri* lentils (low-quality lentils) was significantly associated with disease. In fact, persons who ate these lentils were more than 5 times more likely to be a case than persons who had not eaten the lentils and the results were statistically significant. Why is it not concluded that *kheshuri* lentils were responsible for this outbreak?
4. Often, during outbreak investigation epidemiologic studies, there are cases who do not report having the exposure associated with the outbreak. For example, during this investigation, only 45% of cases reported eating *ghagra shak*. What are some reasons why all cases may not report an exposure during an epidemiologic investigation? Why might this be a problem for an investigation?
5. Imagine that after conducting this investigation you are asked to present the findings to a group of physicians in Bangladesh. After completing your thorough and informative presentation, a gentleman in the first row stands and makes the following comment: "Thank you, for your excellent presentation. However, I do not believe that your findings are correct. Because you are a foreigner, you may not know that our people eat this plant all the time. And, many people are always suffering because of lack of food here. Despite this, we have never seen this kind of outbreak before. If this plant were really toxic, we would have seen this kind of outbreak happening all over the country. I kindly suggest that you continue to investigate to find the real cause of this outbreak." How would you respond to this critique of the investigation?
6. In what ways did collaboration with anthropologists augment the epidemiologic investigation?

REFERENCES

1. Food and Agricultural Organization (FAO). *Special Report: FAO/WFP Crop and Food Supply Assessment Mission to Bangladesh*. http://www.fao.org/docrep/011/ai472e/ai472e00.HTM#3. Published August 28, 2008. Accessed July 15, 2009.
2. Vashishtha VM, Kumar A, John TJ, Nayak NC. Cassia occidentalis poisoning as the probable cause of hepatomyoencephalopathy in children in western Uttar Pradesh. *Indian J Med Res*. 2007;125(6):756–762.
3. Vashishtha VM, Nayak NC, John TJ, Kumar A. Recurrent annual outbreaks of a hepato-myo-encephalopathy syndrome in children in western Uttar Pradesh, India. *Indian J Med Res*. 2007;125(4):523–533.
4. Cole RJ, Stuart BP, Lansden JA, Cox RH. Isolation and redefinition of the toxic agent from cocklebur (Xanthium strumarium). *J Agri Food Chem*. 1980;28(6):1330–1332.
5. Hatch RC, Jain AV, Weiss R, Clark JD. Toxicologic study of carboxyatractyloside (active principle in cocklebur—Xanthium strumarium) in rats treated with enzyme inducers and inhibitors and glutathione precursor and depletor. *Am J Vet Res*. 1982;43(1):111–116.
6. Mendez MC, dos Santos RC, Riet-Correa F. Intoxication by Xanthium cavanillesii in cattle and sheep in southern Brazil. *Vet Hum Toxicol*. 1998;40(3):144–147.
7. Stuart BP, Cole RJ, Gosser HS. Cocklebur (Xanthium strumarium, L. var. strumarium) intoxication in swine: review and redefinition of the toxic principle. *Vet Pathol*. 1981;18(3):368–383.
8. Witte ST, Osweiler GD, Stahr HM, Mobley G. Cocklebur toxicosis in cattle associated with the consumption of mature Xanthium strumarium. *J Vet Diagn Invest*. 1990;2(4):263–267.
9. Turgut M, Alhan CC, Gurgoze M, et al. Carboxyatractyloside poisoning in humans. *Ann Trop Paediatr*. 2005;25(2):125–134.

CHAPTER 26

Toxic Tryptophan? Investigating the Eosinophilia Myalgia Syndrome in Minnesota

Edward A. Belongia, MD
Minnesota, 1989

NEW MEXICO

It started in the summer and early fall of 1989. The first *Batman* film opened in theaters, the Berlin Wall crumbled, and *Seinfeld* made its debut on television. Hurricane Hugo struck South Carolina and a San Francisco earthquake disrupted the World Series. Across the United States, no one noticed the appearance of a painful and disabling new disease.

Bonnie Bishop was having trouble sleeping. Bonnie was an athletic 39-year-old graphic artist living in Santa Fe, New Mexico. She loved vigorous outdoor activities: triathlons, swimming, windsurfing, biking, and tennis.

> *At first is seemed like every insomniac's dream come true: reports of safe sleep-in-a-bottle. So hundreds of thousands of Americans started taking a nutritional supplement called L-tryptophan. Many got their good night's rest, but then something mysterious happened.*
>
> Bob Ehlert and Lewis Cope
> StarTribune, Minneapolis,
> July 22, 1990

Her doctor had recommended L-tryptophan as a natural over-the-counter treatment for insomnia. She started taking it in August 1989. Within days, Bonnie noticed pain with movement. At first it was mild, but it became more severe each day. Soon, she found it difficult to walk up a hill and she had to stop swimming because of the severe pain. Her family physician ran a blood count and was alarmed by the fact that eosinophils, a type of white blood cell, were extremely elevated in her blood. He suspected cancer and referred her to an oncologist.

Bonnie was shocked and frightened by her rapid deterioration. "I was sleeping sitting up because I was so uncomfortable lying down. I didn't realize that my lungs were filling with fluid." Her weakness was profound. She was a single mother with a 4-year-old son to care for, and none of the doctors seemed to know what was going on or how to treat it. She had exploratory abdominal surgery to look for a tumor, but none was found. A consulting rheumatologist, Dr. James Mayer, kept asking questions about her diet and lifestyle to get some clues about possible causes. Nothing jumped out as significant, but he kept coming back to the fact that she had recently started taking L-tryptophan.

Bonnie's oncologist, Dr. Bruce Greenfield, called Dr. Gerald Gleich at the Mayo Clinic for advice. Dr. Gleich was an immunologist and an international expert on eosinophilic diseases. He thought Bonnie might be suffering from hypereosinophilic syndrome, a disease of unknown cause. He recommended a high dose of prednisone to reduce inflammation. Bonnie credits the prednisone with saving her life, but she remained extremely weak. When she was discharged from the hospital after a month, she could barely walk across a room or even sit up in bed. Her weight was down to 90 pounds, and she was on home oxygen.

Eosinophils are specific types of white blood cells that normally reside in tissues, especially the epithelial surfaces of the lung and gastrointestinal tract (Figure 26-1). They serve several immunologic functions, including host defense against large multicellular parasites. For this reason, patients with trichinosis and other parasitic infections often have high eosinophil counts in the blood. Eosinophils contain toxic granule proteins that are released for defense against parasites, but these proteins are also toxic to human cells in normal tissue. Normal eosinophil counts in blood are less than about 350 cells per μL, but counts up to 1500 per μL sometimes occur with allergic rhinitis and asthma. Some types of cancer and other hematologic diseases are known to cause extreme eosinophilia, which led to the initial suspicion that Bonnie had a malignant tumor or leukemia.

A few days after consulting with Dr. Greenfield, Dr. Gleich received a second call from Dr. Phil Hertzman, a family physician in New Mexico. He was treating a woman who had been experiencing severe muscle and abdominal pain since September. She had an extraordinarily high eosinophil count, and her clinical presentation did not fit with any known autoimmune disease. She too had been taking L-tryptophan for insomnia.

This was starting to look suspicious, but the two cases could have been nothing more than an interesting coincidence. Dr. Gleich had never heard of any connection between eosinophilia and L-tryptophan. After all, L-tryptophan was an essential amino acid, so why would it be associated with a disease? Dr. Hertzman had called the New Mexico health department and learned that they were not aware of any other cases. Soon afterward, Dr. Hertzman spoke with another oncologist caring for Bonnie Bishop. The two physicians were struck by the fact that they had two patients with similar diseases, both had become ill around the same time, and both had taken L-tryptophan.

Two days later, Dr. Gleich received a third phone call from another doctor in Santa Fe. She had a patient with similar symptoms, and Bonnie's oncologist had suggested that she call Dr. Gleich. Her patient had an astronomical eosinophil count and she had taken L-tryptophan before becoming ill.

Dr. Gleich was alarmed. "Lightning might strike twice, but three times? No way!" He called Dr. Ed Kilbourne, Chief of the Health Studies Program in the National Center for Environmental Health at the Centers for Disease Control and Prevention (CDC) in Atlanta. Dr. Gleich knew Dr. Kilbourne because they had been involved in the investigation of another mysterious eosinophilic disease called toxic oil syndrome several years earlier in Spain. An alert was sent out to all the state health departments describing the New Mexico cases and the possible link with L-tryptophan. On November 9, the CDC and the Food and Drug Administration (FDA) sent a team to New Mexico to begin an investigation with the state health department. In the meantime, two more patients with a similar clinical picture were identified at the Mayo Clinic in Rochester. They too had taken L-tryptophan. It was now obvious that the problem extended beyond the borders of New Mexico.

MINNESOTA

In the fall of 1989, I was a second year Epidemic Intelligence Service (EIS) officer assigned to the Minnesota Department of Health (MDH). The EIS program was established by the CDC in 1951 as a 2-year training and service program in applied epidemiology. I entered the EIS program after completing a residency at the Univer-

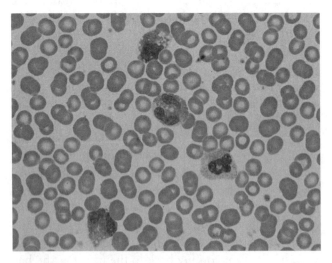

FIGURE 26-1 Blood smear with eosinophils. Photo courtesy of Dr. Gene Shaw, Marshfield Clinic.

EXHIBIT 26-1 Tryptophan Overview

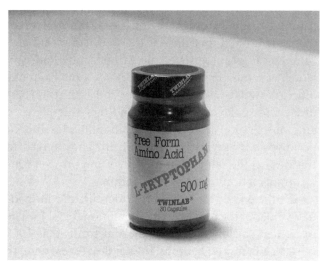

L-tryptophan is an essential amino acid that is metabolized in mammals to produce serotonin (a neurotransmitter) and other biologically active metabolites. It is found naturally in many types of food, especially protein-rich foods. Research in the 1970s and 1980s suggested that L-tryptophan might be useful for the treatment of depression. Other studies evaluated its therapeutic effect for treatment of conditions such as insomnia, premenstrual syndrome, and behavioral disorders. During the 1980s, articles in the popular media encouraged consumers to use L-tryptophan for these purposes. Multiple products containing L-tryptophan were sold in the United States and other countries, but all raw L-tryptophan powder was manufactured in Japan. L-tryptophan products were widely available in health food stores, department stores, and pharmacies, but the product labels made no therapeutic claims. L-tryptophan was classified as a dietary supplement rather than a drug, and it was not regulated or approved by the Food and Drug Administration.

---

sity of Wisconsin and working for a couple of years in emergency medicine. I enjoyed the adrenaline rush of emergency medicine and the opportunity to provide immediate help for people with urgent problems, but I was also interested in preventive medicine and public health. I had worked part-time in the fledgling HIV/AIDS program at the Wisconsin Division of Health after my residency, and I was impressed with the Wisconsin EIS officers and their stories of "shoe leather" epidemiology. I even attended the 1986 EIS conference in Atlanta where EIS officers presented their most important investigations from around the world to their colleagues and CDC staff. The presentations covered diverse topics such as outbreak investigations, AIDS, occupational health, international health, environmental health, enteric diseases, and several others. It was a potpourri of fascinating information for both seasoned and aspiring epidemiologists. It was all focused on improving public health, and I knew right away that I wanted to be a part of it.

Although the majority of EIS officers work at CDC headquarters in Atlanta, I was happy to be assigned to Minnesota, which was widely regarded as one of the best states for EIS officers. I was thrilled to be working with Minnesota State Epidemiologist Mike Osterholm and his well-known team of epidemiologists. Dr. Osterholm had a reputation for aggressively investigating public health problems and had published extensively in top-tier medical journals. He wasn't afraid to take on the lawyers and the politicians when the health of the public was at stake. I liked that approach.

In the fall of 1989, I was busy writing up an outbreak of herpes gladiatorum at a Minneapolis wrestling camp and wrapping up some other investigations. My EIS experience had been busy and productive so far, but I had no idea how much busier it was about to become. On Thursday November 9, I was in the office after back-to-back trips to Atlanta and North Dakota, and I was looking forward to the 3-day Veterans Day weekend. That afternoon, I received a call from Dr. Ed Kilbourne at the CDC regarding a developing public health problem in New Mexico and Minnesota.

I had not heard about the New Mexico cases, but he quickly brought me up to date. The new disease was being called eosinophilia-myalgia syndrome, or EMS. The CDC had just heard about two more suspected cases at the Mayo Clinic. Dr. Kilbourne asked me to drive down to Rochester and learn more about these cases and find out if the patients had taken L-tryptophan. The next day, I met with Dr. Joseph Duffy, a rheumatologist taking care of two patients who had been hospitalized in Rochester.

During our conversations, Dr. Duffy described a patient he had seen 3 years earlier with eosinophilic perimyositis, a syndrome that seemed to resemble the recent cases of EMS. He and other Mayo Clinic physicians had published a case report on her illness in the *Mayo Clinic Proceedings*.[1] One of the New Mexico physicians had come across this article and called Dr. Duffy for advice a few days earlier. We read through the case report carefully. It said that the patient had been taking some prescription medications with "numerous self-prescribed vitamin and mineral supplements." This sounded suspicious; we decided on the spur of the moment to call her, even though she last saw Dr. Duffy in 1986. We had no trouble reaching her at home. After inquiring about her present condition, Dr. Duffy asked her to list the specific dietary supplements that she was taking before her illness began. She mentioned several vitamins and minerals and a single amino acid: L-tryptophan. It now appeared that lightning had struck not only three times, but more like seven or eight times. Still, our knowledge was insufficient to implicate L-tryptophan as the cause of EMS, and we had not yet demonstrated an independent association between L-tryptophan consumption and EMS. Maybe L-tryptophan was just an innocent bystander, and EMS was being caused by something else entirely. Epidemiologists constantly worry about confounding in observational studies because it distorts the relationship between an exposure and a disease outcome. We knew we needed more evidence to confirm or refute the apparent link between EMS and L-tryptophan. And we needed it right away.

Confounding can lead to flawed conclusions regarding causal inferences. If we want to determine if exposure X (say, L-tryptophan) causes disease A (say, EMS), we need to consider potential confounders. Another exposure, exposure Y, would be a confounder if it is both associated with disease A and associated with exposure X. That is, people exposed to Y are more likely to be exposed to X. In this situation, exposure Y (the true risk factor) confounds the apparent association between exposure X and the disease. A straightforward example is the apparent association between alcohol consumption and lung cancer. Tobacco use is a major confounding factor in this analysis. People who drink excessively are more likely to be smokers, and nearly everyone on the planet knows that smoking is a strong risk factor for lung cancer. The association between alcohol consumption and lung cancer can be entirely explained by confounding.

Was there some unidentified exposure that triggered EMS and was also associated with L-tryptophan consumption? Because EMS was a newly recognized disease, we had no direct knowledge of potential confounders. However, it made sense that certain medications, dietary supplements, or known causes of eosinophilia (such as parasitic disease) might serve as confounders.

I returned to Minneapolis, eager to share this new information with Mike Osterholm and the team. We met back at the office on Friday evening and planned our next steps.

THE WEEKEND STUDY

We wasted no time. The top priority was to identify as many cases as possible and conduct a case–control study to evaluate not only L-tryptophan exposure, but also other potential exposures. How could we do that quickly? We contacted several rheumatologists at home on the weekend and learned that they had seen several cases of patients with unexplained eosinophilia accompanied by severe myalgia or muscle weakness. One of them mentioned that there was a weekend meeting of Minnesota pathologists at the Minneapolis Radisson Hotel, which happened to be one block away from our office. We walked over in blue jeans and T-shirts on Saturday and spoke to the group. Had they recently seen any muscle biopsies showing eosinophilic fasciitis or perimyositis? Several hands went up. They agreed to track down the samples immediately and provide contact information for our investigation.

By the end of the day, we had identified 12 individuals who met the tentative case definition for EMS. The case criteria included: eosinophil count greater than 1000 cells per μL, myalgia or muscle weakness severe enough to affect daily activities, and a muscle biopsy (if done) showing perimyositis, perivasculitis, or fasciitis. Our case definition differed slightly from the CDC case definition because we allowed muscle weakness to meet the symptom criteria in the presence of eosinophilia. We decided to exclude potential cases if the patient had another disease that was known to cause eosinophilia, although no exclusions were necessary for the 12 cases we identified.

We had decided to conduct a matched case–control study to avoid any potential confounding due to age and sex, particularly because many of the cases to date had been identified in women. It was certainly possible that sex or other individual characteristics might influence the risk of developing EMS, but our immediate and urgent hypothesis dealt with the suspected association with L-tryptophan use. We matched cases to controls on age group and sex with a 1:1 matching ratio. A 1:1 ratio allowed us to obtain results quickly and it provided sufficient power to detect the strong association that we expected to find. The selection of controls was straightforward and unbiased. We found the matched controls

---

EXHIBIT 26-2 CDC Case Definition for Eosinophilia-Myalgia Syndrome

An illness met the case definition for EMS if all of the following criteria were met:

1. peripheral eosinophil count greater than or equal to 1000 cells per µL;
2. generalized myalgia at some point during the illness severe enough to affect normal daily activities; and
3. absence of any infection or neoplasm that could account for the first and second features.

by dialing telephone numbers above and below the telephone number of the case until we found a household with someone in the required age group and sex.

I spent much of Saturday afternoon drafting and redrafting the interview form with frequent input from the investigation team. The interview was fairly extensive and it included a large number of environmental, dietary, and behavior factors. We asked EMS patients about use of L-tryptophan during the month before onset of illness and the matched controls were asked about L-tryptophan use during the same time period. We also asked the patients and controls about a variety of other exposures and conditions that might be associated with EMS. These included chronic medical conditions (such as asthma and allergies), use of prescription and nonprescription medications, and consumption of over-the-counter supplements before illness onset. We asked about undercooked pork and bear meat consumption because these are risk factors for trichinosis, a parasitic disease that is associated with eosinophilia.

The MDH office was a beehive of activity all day Saturday and Sunday as we finalized the 4- or 5-page interview form, conducted the telephone interviews, and entered the data into SAS (a statistical software application) for analysis. By midday Sunday, we were conducting our final analysis. All 12 patients who met the provisional case definition reported consuming L-tryptophan during the month before onset of illness. None of the matched controls had consumed L-tryptophan during similar periods (Figure 26-2). Because we had a zero in the denominator, the odds ratio was undefined, but the p-value was 0.0008—indicating a highly significant association between the exposure (L-tryptophan consumption) and the outcome (EMS). The only other significant finding was that 9 (75%) of the 12 case patients reported use of any prescription medication (as a category rather than a specific medication) compared to 4 (33%) controls, but this association was nonsignificant after adjusting for use of L-tryptophan. There was no single drug or class of drugs that was reported more often by EMS patients, providing further evidence that the association with prescription medication use was due to confounding.

Mike Osterholm has always been a big picture thinker on public health issues and he was several steps ahead of me in terms of understanding the regulatory implications of these findings. Our group met to review the results on Sunday afternoon. Mike decided to hold a press conference the same day to warn Minnesota consumers about the potential risk from L-tryptophan use. We faxed our initial results to the FDA and urged them

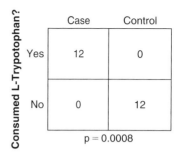

FIGURE 26-2 Results of first matched case-control study to assess the relationship between L-tryptophan consumption and EMS.

to take regulatory action to remove L-tryptophan products from retail shelves.

Our press conference was held in the early evening on Sunday, November 12, and the warning about L-tryptophan went statewide on the 10:00 p.m. local news broadcasts. This was the first coverage of EMS and L-tryptophan by the Minnesota news media—there had been no mention of the New Mexico cases or the suspected L-tryptophan link before our case–control study was completed. In front of the cameras, Mike urged Minnesota consumers to avoid taking L-tryptophan. He asked physicians to notify the MDH of suspected cases and he encouraged consumers to call the MDH if they were taking L-tryptophan. We knew we would need a comparison group of L-tryptophan users for the study that was coming next and the news coverage provided a great opportunity to reach many of those individuals quickly.

Jinx Engstrom did not watch the news that evening, but a friend called her and told her to watch the next local broadcast. There was some stunning news about L-tryptophan that Jinx needed to know. Jinx was very ill. Since August, she had been suffering from muscle aches, swelling in her legs, and extreme exhaustion. "I felt like I had the flu all the time." Her skin was so sensitive that even the touch of clothing was painful. Her family physician had run many different tests, but had no explanation. She had a high eosinophil count and she had an appointment to see a rheumatologist in a few days. In January, she had started taking L-tryptophan for insomnia on the recommendation of her gynecologist. When she became ill in August, there was no reason to suspect that L-tryptophan might be the cause. In fact, the sicker she got, the more she needed the L-tryptophan to help her sleep.

By Friday, November 17, the CDC had counted 287 cases of EMS, including one death. The woman who died had experienced severe neurologic damage, paralysis, and respiratory failure. EMS had become national news, with a headline in *The New York Times* reporting "Officials Investigating Drug's Role in Illness." The FDA issued a press release on November 17 to announce a voluntary recall of all products containing L-tryptophan in the United States. However, the recall only applied to products that contained at least 100 mg of L-tryptophan, and some products (such as infant formula and protein supplements) were exempt. The Minnesota results implicating L-tryptophan were published in the November 24, 1989 issue of the *Morbidity and Mortality Weekly Report* (*MMWR*) (Exhibit 26-3). The *MMWR* also reported similar findings from a case–control study in New Mexico that compared L-tryptophan exposure in patients meeting the EMS case definition and neighborhood controls.

We were not happy that it took 5 days for the FDA to issue this recall and we did not think they went far enough to limit access to all formulations of the product,

---

EXHIBIT 26-3   Epidemiologic Notes and Reports Eosinophilia-Myalgia Syndrome and L-Tryptophan-Containing Products—New Mexico, Minnesota, Oregon, and New York, 1989

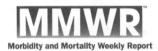

As of November 21, 360 cases of eosinophilia-myalgia syndrome (EMS) had been reported by state health departments to CDC. Studies examining an association of L-tryptophan-containing products (LTCPs) with the EMS epidemic (1) have been completed in New Mexico, Minnesota, and Oregon. In addition, a fatal case in New York has been reported.

New Mexico. In a New Mexico case-control study, EMS cases (N=12) were all persons for whom an eosinophil count of greater than or equal to 2000 cells/mm3 was recorded from May 1 through November 11, 1989, in nine laboratories in Albuquerque, Santa Fe, and Los Alamos and for whom incapacitating myalgia was documented, either in the medical record or by interview with the patient. Potential cases were excluded if eosinophilia could have been caused by any of a predetermined list of approximately 20 infectious, neoplastic, allergic, or other chronic diseases. EMS cases were compared with controls (two per case) who had been matched with case-patients by age (plus or minus 5 years), sex, and neighborhood of residence. Comparisons were made for factors such as the use of different vitamins, other health foods or raw food products, medications, and different water sources. All case-patients and two (8%) controls used LTCPs (odds ratio (OR) not calculable) (X((2))=20; p=6.9 x 10-6). There were no statistically significant differences between cases and controls on 32 other potential risk factors studied.

Minnesota. In Minnesota, potential cases for an initial case-control study of risk factors for EMS were identified by rheumatologists (who were asked by the Minnesota Department of Health to report patients recently diagnosed with eosinophilia and either severe myalgia or muscle weakness) and by clinical pathologists and a pediatric neurologist (who were asked to identify patients with muscle biopsies showing eosinophilic perimyositis or perivasculitis). Criteria necessary for these patients to be considered as cases were eosinophil count of greater than 1000 cells/mm3, myalgia or muscle weakness of severity sufficient to affect normal daily activities, and a muscle biopsy (if done) showing perimyositis, perivasculitis, or unspecified fasciitis. As in the New Mexico study, potential cases were excluded if EMS could have been caused by any of a predetermined list of diseases known to be associated with eosinophilia. Investigators had no prior knowledge of patients' use of LTCPs. Twelve cases were identified and compared with controls (one per case) matched by age, sex, and telephone exchange. All case-patients and no controls used LTCPs (OR not calculable) (p=8 x 10-4) during the month before onset of illness for case-patients and during a similar time period for matched controls. Nine (75%) case-patients and four (33%) controls were taking some type of prescription medication (not statistically significant after adjustment for use of LTCPs). Illness was not associated with consumption of vitamins and health-food products, wild game, undercooked meat or fish products, or nonprescription medications.

A follow-up study compared 30 EMS cases fitting the CDC surveillance case definition of EMS (1) with 36 asymptomatic users of LTCPs who responded to a public request and contacted the Minnesota Department of Health. Twenty (67%) case-patients reported using brands of LTCPs from one particular tablet manufacturer, compared with eight (22%) asymptomatic users (OR=7.0; 95% confidence interval (CI)=1.5-24.6 (p less than 0.0002)). Asymptomatic LTCP users were similar to case-patients for age, sex, and geographic areas of residence; additional population-based studies of LTCP use continue in Minnesota.

Oregon. The Oregon Health Division studied 29 EMS patients who conformed with the CDC case definition. All had eosinophilia and myalgia; four also reported respiratory signs or symptoms. These patients, all users of LTCPs, were compared with users of LTCPs identified by a random telephone survey of Oregon residents (control group A; N=32) and asymptomatic LT users who contacted the Oregon Health Division (control group B; N=24). Fourteen (48%) case-patients were exposed to LTCPs from a single lot of 4500 bottles, compared with two (6%) persons in control group A and two (8%) persons in control group B (ORs=14.0 (95% CI=2.5-103.0) and 10.3 (95% CI=1.8-76.8), respectively) who were so exposed. This association remains statistically significant when controlled for age, sex, or average daily LTCP consumption.

New York. In New York, a 58-year-old woman with EMS died September 17, 1989. The patient, who had become ill in July 1989 with myalgia, fatigue, and marked progressive weakness, had been taking 5-6 g of LT daily. She had leukocytosis (19,800 cells/mm3) with 18% eosinophils. Electron myelographic and nerve conduction studies were most consistent with axonal neuropathy. Studies considered to be within normal limits included: cerebrospinal fluid glucose, protein, and cell counts and celiac and renal arteriograms.

EXHIBIT 26-3 Continued

Serologic tests for a variety of autoimmune diseases were negative. The patient developed an ascending polyneuropathy with near-total quadriplegia and a bifacial hemiparesis. She failed to improve on corticosteroid and cyclophosphamide treatment and died following cardiorespiratory arrest. Reported by: M Eidson, DVM, R Voorhees, MD, M Tanuz, CM Sewell, DrPH, State Epidemiologist, New Mexico Health and Environment Dept. SL Glickstein, MD, WE Muth, MD, Park Nicollet Medical Center, Minneapolis; MT Osterholm, PhD, State Epidemiologist, Minnesota Dept of Health. DW Fleming, MD, LR Foster, MD, State Epidemiologist, Oregon Health Div, Oregon Dept of Human Resources. A Finn, Jr, MD, Univ Medical Center, Stonybrook; J Melius, MD, DL Morse, MD, State Epidemiologist, New York State Dept of Health. Div of Field Svcs, Epidemiology Program Office; Health Studies Br and Surveillance and Programs Br, Div of Environmental Hazards and Health Effects, Center for Environmental Health and Injury Control, CDC.

Editorial Note

Editorial Note: The case-control studies in New Mexico and Minnesota establish a statistically significant association between use of LTCPs and development of EMS. The strength of this association, the temporal relationship, the absence of apparent selection or data-ascertainment biases, and the failure of different potential confounders to account for this association support the potential causal relationship. In addition, of the 85 case-patients who initially called CDC before the full implementation of the state-based reporting system and for whom information on LTCP use was available, only one (1%) did not use LTCPs. However, the biologic mechanism for the development of EMS among LTCP users is unclear.

The report of an EMS-associated death in New York emphasizes the potential severity of this condition, and confirmatory data are being sought on other possible EMS-associated deaths. In the fatal case, the severe Guillain-Barre syndrome-like ascending polyneuropathy resembles clinical manifestations in patients with the intermediate and chronic phases of toxic-oil syndrome (TOS), a disease similar to EMS that was epidemic in Spain in 1981 (2-5). Frank vasculitis has been reported in some EMS cases. Physicians caring for patients with EMS should be alert to the possibility that such patients may develop clinical manifestations similar to those of chronic TOS, including peripheral neuropathy (mononeuritis multiplex), thromboembolic phenomena, sclerodermiform skin changes, joint contractures, and pulmonary hypertension (2-5). Case reports received at CDC suggest that, as with TOS, the clinical manifestations of EMS may not regress immediately on removal of LTCPs.

The findings of the lot and brand-name studies in Minnesota and Oregon, suggest multiple interpretations: some LTCPs could contain a contaminant that is causally associated with EMS; or host factors mediating the response to LT may be unique to patients who use a particular brand or set of brands associated with illness. Studies under way include identifying possible chemical or microbial contaminants in LTCPs, tracing the sources of individual brands and lots, identifying host factors related to clinical manifestations, and determining factors associated with use and purchase of LTCPs.

On November 17, the Food and Drug Administration (FDA) announced its intention to seek a nationwide recall of all LTCPs in which LT is the sole or major component; this reinforced a November 11 alert to the public to refrain from using LTCPs. FDA is attempting to trace suspect lots of LTCPs and is evaluating production procedures at the companies in Japan where LT is produced for eventual sale and consumption in the United States.

CDC's initial surveillance case definition for EMS required specific serologic testing or muscle biopsy to rule out trichinosis (1). It now appears the clinical presentation of some EMS patients may be sufficiently distinct from that of trichinosis patients that such specific laboratory tests are not warranted. Accordingly, the CDC surveillance definition of EMS no longer requires specific laboratory testing for trichinella. CDC now recommends defining EMS as an illness characterized by 1) eosinophil count of greater than or equal to 1000 cells per mm3, 2) generalized myalgia (at some point during the course of illness) of severity sufficient to affect a patient's ability to pursue his or her usual daily activities, and 3) absence of any infection or neoplasm that could account for 1 or 2 above. This change has been communicated to state health departments.

Epidemiologic investigations and research studies of EMS should be directed toward further defining a causal association between LTCPs and EMS and identifying specific etiologic factors and possible cofactors that may modify risk. Additional questions relate to the existence of a possible dose-response effect, the latent period between exposure and disease, establishment of the beginning of the epidemic, determination of the full spectrum of clinical manifestations, elucidation of pathogenetic mechanisms, and determination of prognosis and the response to specific therapies.

References

1. CDC. Eosinophilia-myalgia syndrome—New Mexico. MMWR 1989;38:765-7.
2. Grandjean P, Tarkowski S, eds. Toxic oil syndrome: mass food poisoning in Spain—report of a WHO meeting, Madrid 21-25 March 1983. Copenhagen: World Health Organization Regional Office for Europe, 1984.
3. Toxic Epidemic Syndrome Study Group. Toxic epidemic syndrome, Spain, 1981. Lancet 1982;2:697-702.
4. Kilbourne EM, Rigau-Perez JG, Heath CW JR, et al. Clinical epidemiology of toxic-oil syndrome: manifestations of a new illness. N Engl J Med 1983;309:1408-14.
5. Martinez Tello FJ, Navas Palacios JJ, Ricoy JR, et al. Pathology of a new toxic syndrome caused by ingestion of adulterated oil in Spain. Virchows Arch (A) 1982;397:261-85. *Includes persons reporting they currently had a cataract, had had surgery for a cataract, or had had a lens implant for a cataract. **Includes persons who reported they had ever had coronary heart disease, angina pectoris, myocardial infarction, or any other "heart attack."

given the severity of this illness and the strength of the association. *The New York Times* quoted Mike Osterholm on this point: "There is more than enough evidence to take L-tryptophan off the market, particularly because its benefits are limited and, in no case, life-saving." L-tryptophan was marketed as a dietary supplement. Therefore, it was not subject to the same regulatory requirements that apply to prescription drugs. The labels on L-tryptophan bottles contained no health claims or recommendations for therapeutic use, but it was widely regarded as an effective and safe therapy for insomnia, depression, and other conditions.

Despite the strength of the initial results, there were many aspects of the L-tryptophan and EMS association that were perplexing. L-tryptophan is an essential amino acid, and there was no obvious explanation as to how it might trigger EMS when taken as a dietary supplement. It had been available as an over-the-counter dietary supplement for several years without any apparent problems. Investigators around the country were discussing and debating two possibilities. The first possible explanation was that L-tryptophan itself caused EMS when consumed by susceptible individuals. A few years earlier, researchers at the National Institutes of Health published a case report of a scleroderma-like illness that developed in a patient who was treated with L-5 hydroxytryptophan for intention tremor.[2] Scleroderma is an autoimmune disease that causes tissue fibrosis. It has some similarities to EMS, but eosinophilia is not a characteristic finding. The patient in this case report had high levels of kynurenine, an intermediate metabolite of L-tryptophan, and the level remained high after the L-5 hydroxytryptophan was stopped. The researchers speculated that the patient had a disorder of L-tryptophan metabolism that was unmasked by the consumption of L-5 hydroxytryptophan. If such a disorder of L-tryptophan metabolism was common in the population, perhaps the epidemic had occurred because an increasing number of susceptible people had started taking L-tryptophan.

The other possible explanation was that EMS was somehow triggered by a contaminant in some L-tryptophan products rather than by L-tryptophan itself. CDC investigators quickly recognized the similarities between EMS and the toxic oil syndrome, which lent credence to the view that a contaminant might be responsible. The outbreak of toxic oil syndrome affected nearly 20,000 people in Spain during 1981.[3] Individuals affected by toxic oil syndrome had extremely high eosinophil levels, but they experienced more frequent and severe pulmonary disease compared to those with EMS. Epidemiologic investigations had found that the toxic oil syndrome was triggered by consumption of denatured rapeseed oil that was sold illegally as olive oil by street vendors. Spain allowed importation of rapeseed oil for industrial use, but the oil was made inedible by adding aniline. This was reportedly done to protect Spanish producers of cooking oils. The toxic oil products were illicitly refined to remove color and they were sold in plastic containers on the street. Studies implicated one refinery and a batch of imported oil that may have been the source of the toxic oil outbreak. However, the specific chemical that triggered toxic oil syndrome was never determined. The link between L-tryptophan consumption and toxic oil, if any, was a mystery to us.

There were many other related questions. Was EMS a new syndrome or merely a newly recognized syndrome? How did the occurrence of EMS relate to changes in the prevalence of L-tryptophan use? Why were most cases occurring in women? Were there environmental or individual cofactors that modified the risk of developing EMS when exposed to L-tryptophan?

LOOKING FOR EMS CASES AND L-TRYPTOPHAN USERS

We were inundated with calls on Monday morning after the press conference. Staff who normally worked in other units pitched in to help us deal with the intense public response. We quickly initiated active surveillance by requesting reports of suspected EMS cases through the news media and by mailing a letter to all rheumatologists, dermatologists, pathologists, primary care physicians, and chiropractors in Minnesota. In addition, we used television and newspaper coverage to encourage L-tryptophan users to contact their physician and MDH if they had muscle pain or weakness. As a result of this active case finding, we identified 63 individuals with EMS who became ill from September 1988 through November 1989 (Figure 26-3). All had consumed L-tryptophan before becoming ill.

The median age was 45 years, but the age range extended from 4 to 77 years. Fifty-five (87%) of the patients were female, raising the possibility that women were more susceptible or, alternatively, were exposed more often than men to L-tryptophan or the etiologic agent.

A striking pattern began to emerge as we collected information on the retail L-tryptophan products consumed by EMS patients and the healthy L-tryptophan users who contacted MDH. Individuals with EMS had consumed L-tryptophan from a variety of stores and

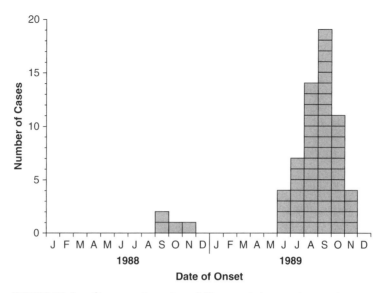

FIGURE 26-3 Cases of eosinophilia-myalgia syndrome in Minnesota according to date of symptom onset. Reprinted with permission from New England Journal of Medicine 1990; 323: 357–65. Copyright © 1990 Massachusetts Medical Society. All rights reserved.

retail brands, but some retail brands were used more often by patients with EMS. This seemed unusual and it supported the hypothesis that not all L-tryptophan products were associated with EMS.

We had many people manning the phone lines during those early weeks and we kept a list of all L-tryptophan users who called. We collected basic data on demographic characteristics (age and sex), the presence or absence of specific symptoms, duration of L-tryptophan use, and retail brand/purchase location. Individuals with symptoms were referred to their physicians for evaluation, and the asymptomatic L-tryptophan users were told that MDH staff might contact them later for more information. In the meantime, all L-tryptophan users were asked to hang onto their L-tryptophan bottles with any remaining tablets or pills. We immediately began picking up the L-tryptophan containers from any individuals with EMS who still had the original container for L-tryptophan that was taken before onset of illness. In several cases, those containers still had leftover tablets, which proved to be critical for the contaminant analyses that would occur in the upcoming months. We also picked up L-tryptophan containers from the "asymptomatic L-tryptophan users" who contacted the MDH but reported no illness.

EMS was a new syndrome and we knew very little about the spectrum of illness—we couldn't be sure that the asymptomatic L-tryptophan users did not have a milder or preclinical form of EMS. Because the healthy L-tryptophan users would serve as a control group in the second case–control study, inclusion of subclinical EMS cases in the control group would lead to misclassification of case status. If this misclassification were nondifferential (i.e., not associated with the brand or manufacturer of L-tryptophan), it would bias the results toward the null.

We evaluated this potential source of misclassification by inviting a group of asymptomatic L-tryptophan users to provide blood samples for eosinophil counts. If we didn't find any abnormal eosinophil counts or eosinophilic proteins in these asymptomatic L-tryptophan users, we could be reasonably certain that they did not have subclinical or undetected EMS. With the help of Dr. Jerry Gleich, the Mayo Clinic eosinophil expert, we also evaluated these blood samples for other immune system markers for eosinophilic disease, including an eosinophilic granule protein.

We successfully recruited 18 asymptomatic L-tryptophan users to provide blood samples. They had been taking various doses of L-tryptophan daily until the week of November 12 when the news media announced the link with EMS. The eosinophil count was normal in all of them. Jerry Gleich and his immunology team confirmed that these individuals had normal levels of eosinophilic granule protein, supporting the absence of subclinical or undetected EMS.

We were now confident that our asymptomatic L-tryptophan users did not have EMS, but we had yet to tackle the issue of representativeness. After all, these asymptomatic L-tryptophan users had called MDH after the initial press release; they were not representative of all the other L-tryptophan users who did not call the health department. Selection bias was an important concern with this group. Perhaps these individuals took higher doses or used L-tryptophan for longer periods compared to other L-tryptophan users. Selection of an appropriate control group is critical in a case–control study and this group had some issues because they were self-referred. On the other hand, it might be difficult or impossible to identify a true random sample of L-tryptophan users. The manufacturing source of L-tryptophan was not evident to consumers purchasing retail products, so it was unlikely that bias would occur with regard to manufacturer even when self-referred controls were used for comparison. Nevertheless, we had concerns about relying on self-referred controls and we considered alternative strategies to recruit control L-tryptophan users.

CLINICAL AND PATHOLOGIC FEATURES OF EMS

In addition to myalgia, we found that the most commonly reported early symptoms were joint pain, weakness, fatigue, cough, shortness of breath, rash, edema, fever, and paresthesias. A normal eosinophil count is typically less than 350 cells per μL. According to the national case definition, all patients had an eosinophil count in excess of 1,000 cells per μL. The eosinophil count was generally in the range of 4,000 to 6,000 cells per μL, far higher than the level expected with asthma or allergies. Biopsies showed inflammation in the dermis, fascia, and muscle tissue with perivascular infiltrates and damage to small blood vessels. There was often thickening of the fascia with infiltrates of mononuclear cells and eosinophils. The biopsy findings were similar to those of eosinophilic fasciitis, a rare disease that is similar to scleroderma. Lung biopsies in some patients showed a perivasculitis and chronic interstitial pneumonitis. High doses of corticosteroids were recommended to reduce the inflammation associated with EMS, and there was some evidence that they helped during the acute phase of illness.[4] However, it was clear that corticosteroids did not cure EMS and they did not prevent chronic complications.

COMMUNITY SURVEY OF L-TRYPTOPHAN USE

We suspected that L-tryptophan use had increased a great deal in recent years. Could this explain the dramatic increase in EMS cases in 1989? Perhaps EMS had always been associated with L-tryptophan use and we were just detecting it for the first time because L-tryptophan use had increased to a level where we could detect it. We designed a community survey to find out.

We contacted Dr. Phyllis Pirie in the School of Public Health at the University of Minnesota to help us. She directed the Health Survey Research Center at the University and had special expertise in survey design and analysis. We decided that the best option would be a telephone survey of Minneapolis and St. Paul (Twin Cities) households to estimate the prevalence of L-tryptophan use over time. We developed a series of questions about L-tryptophan use during each year going back to 1980. Interviewers at the University of Minnesota used a list-assisted random digit dialing method to call residential telephone numbers, with up to 20 attempts per number. This was still in the pre-cell phone era and nearly all households in the Twin Cities had a land line, so we were confident that we could obtain valid information on L-tryptophan use patterns. The interviewer asked to speak with an adult female, who then served as a proxy respondent for all household members. An adult male was an acceptable respondent if an adult female was not available.

The survey took more than 3 months to complete, but it provided critical knowledge to answer the question posed previously. More than 2,000 households were successfully contacted during the survey and 93% agreed to participate. In four percent of households, at least one person had consumed L-tryptophan since 1980 and 2% of all household members had used L-tryptophan from 1980 to 1989. We were not surprised to see that the prevalence of use had increased during the 1980s. The most striking finding, however, was the discrepancy in L-tryptophan use between men and women, and the dramatic increase in L-tryptophan use among women from 1988 to 1989 (Figure 26-4).

We used the estimated prevalence of L-tryptophan use along with Minnesota census data to estimate the number of men and women who used L-tryptophan products in 1988 and 1989. We then calculated the EMS attack rate among L-tryptophan users. In 1988 and 1989, there were an estimated 7,400 and 16,400 women, respectively, who used L-tryptophan in the Minneapolis–St. Paul area. In 1988, four EMS cases occurred in

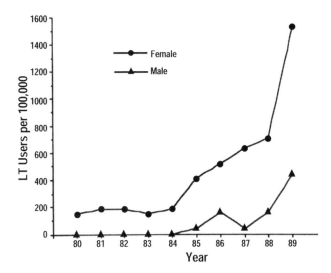

FIGURE 26-4 Prevalence of L-tryptophan use among male (shown as triangles) and female (shown as circles) members of 2012 randomly selected households in metropolitan Minneapolis-St. Paul.
Reprinted with permission from New England Journal of Medicine 1990; 323:357–65. Copyright © 1990 Massachusetts Medical Society. All rights reserved.

women in the Twin Cities area, yielding an estimated attack rate of 54 cases per 100,000 female L-tryptophan users (4/7400 × 100,000). In 1989 there were 44 cases, yielding an estimated attack rate of 268 cases per 100,000. These findings indicated a 5-fold increase in the EMS attack rate among female L-tryptophan users from 1988 to 1989. The estimated EMS attack rate also increased among male L-tryptophan users, from 0 in 1988 to 144 cases per 100,000 in 1989. Clearly, the EMS epidemic could not be entirely attributed to increasing rates of L-tryptophan use. Something had changed from 1988 to 1989, but what?

L-TRYPTOPHAN TRACEBACKS

We noticed right away that many EMS patients had purchased L-tryptophan from a particular retailer in the Twin Cities. Craig Hedberg naturally took on the role of product traceback expert. Craig had a master's degree in Environmental Health from the University of Minnesota and he supervised the Foodborne, Vectorborne, and Zoonotic Disease Unit at the MDH. Craig discovered that the L-tryptophan consumed by many of the EMS patients had been manufactured into tablets by P. Leiner Nutritional Products, one of the largest manufacturers of food supplements and herbs for department stores, drugstores, supermarkets, and other retailers.

Mike Osterholm engaged the assistance of the company's president, who agreed to provide full support for our investigation. He assigned several of his staff members to assist us and the company funded the community survey that was conducted by Dr. Pirie and staff at the University of Minnesota.

We quickly embarked on a crash course to learn about L-tryptophan manufacturing and distribution. There were six manufacturers of raw L-tryptophan powder in the world and all were located in Japan. Each was reported to use a unique manufacturing process, but we did not know the details. There were numerous manufacturers of tablets, capsules, and other types of products containing L-tryptophan, but all of the raw material came from Japan. One company in particular seemed to have the lion's share of the market: Showa Denko K.K. All of the L-tryptophan tablets that were manufactured and distributed by P. Leiner Nutritional Products and consumed by EMS patients had been made from Showa Denko L-tryptophan powder.

Craig Hedberg dove into the traceback effort using phone and fax. We knew that the Food and Drug Administration was tracing L-tryptophan products for a study in New Mexico, but Craig Hedberg and Mike Osterholm were confident that we could get faster results by directly contacting distributors and importers to determine the source for each retail brand and lot number. This was a time-consuming and detail-oriented task. The first step was to obtain the brand name of the L-tryptophan product from a study participant (EMS patient or healthy L-tryptophan user) and find out where it was purchased. Some individuals gave us the actual bottles, and others reported the retail lot number and expiration date. They wanted to keep their bottles in case they were needed for litigation. Craig then called the retailer to find out which company manufactured the tablets. The next step was to contact the tablet manufacturer to determine which company manufactured the raw L-tryptophan powder that was used in the tablet-making process.

The number of completed tracebacks grew steadily in late 1989 and early 1990. EMS patients had consumed many different retail products containing L-tryptophan before becoming ill, but all of our tracebacks were identifying Showa Denko as the original powder manufacturer. The FDA traceback process was going much more slowly. An FDA inspector had to be dispatched to each location to physically examine documents of interest, starting with the retail outlet and working back to the tablet manufacturer and importer. When the traceback process led to another part of the country, all the documents had to be transferred to another FDA office and a different FDA employee became responsible. This was a cumbersome and slow process and our traceback effort was proceeding on a much faster timeline. We shared our results with the CDC and the FDA as the investigation progressed, but we didn't mind when we uncovered some new information before they did. There was a bit of healthy competition going on to see who could solve this first.

The web of L-tryptophan manufacturing and distribution was complex. We discovered that a single retail lot of tablets could be comprised of one or two lots of granular L-tryptophan. The granular lots, in turn, might contain raw L-tryptophan from multiple powder lots from a Japanese manufacturer. A single manufacturing (powder) lot could end up in multiple retail lots and a single retail lot might include L-tryptophan from several manufacturing dates.

TESTING FOR CONTAMINANTS

In the early stages of the investigation, Dr. Jerry Gleich was invited to a meeting in Atlanta. He was surprised to see that he was the only nongovernment employee in attendance. CDC investigators described a variety of technologies that were being tried to identify contaminants in lots of L-tryptophan from different sources. One promising technology was high-performance liquid chromatography, or HPLC. The HPLC unit has a column filled with tiny particles and the test sample is pumped through the column. A detector shines ultraviolet light through the fluid coming off the column, generating signals that appear as peaks on a graph. The chemical components in the sample pass through the detector at different time points. This retention time varies for different molecules and the peaks on a retention time graph represent different chemical substances that are present in the test sample. The size of each peak corresponds roughly to the concentration of each substance. When applied to L-tryptophan, HPLC could theoretically detect multiple contaminants, including those present in low concentrations. HPLC would not identify the chemical structure of contaminants, but the CDC researchers thought it might still yield useful new information for this investigation.

When Jerry heard this, he thought, "Gee, this is a no-brainer." He had a postdoctoral fellow, Arthur Mayeno, who had experience using HPLC. Jerry hurried back to Rochester and outlined the urgent new mission for their group. "Arthur is an extraordinary person and he demanded a degree of perfection that was perfect for this investigation," recalled Jerry. Arthur began testing tablets and retail lots of L-tryptophan that had been submitted to them by distributors and manufacturers outside Minnesota, but most of the L-tryptophan they received did not have a well-defined epidemiologic link to EMS cases. There was no way to distinguish *case* L-tryptophan from *control* L-tryptophan in samples that arrived with little or no epidemiologic information. In fact, we weren't even sure if control L-tryptophan existed; some researchers still argued that EMS might represent a disorder of L-tryptophan metabolism rather than the toxic effects of a contaminant.

We could learn much more from testing the samples obtained from EMS patients in Minneapolis–St. Paul and the asymptomatic L-tryptophan users. This allowed us to identify implicated and nonimplicated lots of L-tryptophan, and Jerry's lab had the capacity to test the tablets from these lots for trace contaminants. We started our own courier service to get the samples to Jerry and Arthur as quickly as possible. Mike Osterholm drove down with a box of L-tryptophan bottles from EMS patients and asymptomatic L-tryptophan users, and Jerry offered to meet him at a truck stop in Cannon Falls, a convenient halfway meeting point. Their first attempt to meet failed because freezing rain caused Jerry to turn back. Subsequent transfers were successful and we had a regular pipeline of "hot" and "cold" L-tryptophan that was sent down to Mayo via the truck stop meeting point.

We continued to collect retail bottles and detailed information on L-tryptophan use from all the Minnesota EMS patients and asymptomatic L-tryptophan users, and we were in the process of obtaining blood samples from some of the latter group to verify that they did not have any evidence of subclinical EMS. We had a mountain of epidemiologic data that would be essential to help us interpret the HPLC results that were being generated by Jerry and Arthur. The MDH team and the Mayo laboratory groups forged a strong collaboration, and within a few weeks Jerry was referring to us as the "Minnesota Mafia." I have no idea how he came up with that.

Arthur Mayeno quickly discovered that all L-tryptophan products contained many trace contaminants, although the overall purity of L-tryptophan was high. According to the United States Pharmacopeia (USP), the reference standard for L-tryptophan purity was 98.5%, and the products tested by Arthur met that standard. USP is a nongovernment organization that establishes independent standards for purity, strength, and consistency both for medications and for dietary supplements. Despite the overall high level of purity, Arthur pointed out a curious finding: the L-tryptophan from each manufacturer had a characteristic HPLC pattern or "fingerprint" that represented the presence of trace contaminants. These patterns were so distinct and consistent that Arthur could identify the manufacturer of the L-tryptophan based on the HPLC fingerprint alone. After that meeting, Mike Osterholm turned to him and said, "Arthur, you are going to solve this." He was right: Arthur's work on HPLC would prove critical for our analysis of implicated lots of L-tryptophan.

CASE–CONTROL STUDY II

The second case–control study was restricted to L-tryptophan users and our goal was to determine if EMS was associated with a single manufacturer or distributor, which would suggest that EMS was triggered by a byproduct or contaminant rather than L-tryptophan itself. On the other hand, if EMS was due to abnormal L-tryptophan metabolism in susceptible individuals, we would expect to see no association with any manufacturer or distributor. We were also interested in investigating cofactors that might modify the effects of L-tryptophan consumption on EMS. In particular, we were interested in determining if there was a dose–response relationship between L-tryptophan consumption and EMS. In other words, was the risk of EMS influenced by the dose and duration of L-tryptophan use?

For the second case–control study, we excluded 11 of 63 EMS patients in Minnesota because they either lived outside the Twin Cities area ($n = 7$) or because they became ill before June 1, 1989 ($n = 4$). The latter four individuals were excluded because we wanted to focus on the etiology of the outbreak that occurred in late 1989 and we recognized the possibility that sporadic cases of EMS had occurred at a low incidence before 1989. If these earlier cases had a different etiology, they could bias the results if included in the case–control analysis of the outbreak. Patients outside the Twin Cities were excluded because all of the controls lived in the Twin Cities and we wanted to avoid any potential bias based on area of residence, particularly regarding access to L-tryptophan products in urban versus rural areas of the state.

We used two separate control groups for this study: the asymptomatic L-tryptophan users who contacted the MDH after the initial press conference in November (self-referred controls), and the healthy L-tryptophan users who were identified in the random digit dialing telephone survey of L-tryptophan (random controls).

The latter control group was very important because we knew the self-referred controls might differ from other L-tryptophan users in important ways. L-tryptophan users identified in the community telephone survey were more representative of all L-tryptophan users in the Twin Cities, but fewer of them still had the L-tryptophan bottles that were needed for product traceback to identify the manufacturer. Many of them had discarded those bottles by the time they were contacted for the telephone survey. Each control group had different limitations and we decided to use both in the case–control analysis. If consistent associations were found with each control group, our confidence in the findings would be greater.

We identified the random controls by reinterviewing the primary L-tryptophan users in 34 households who reported L-tryptophan use after May 31, 1989 in the community telephone survey. We excluded 10 potential controls who had consumed L-tryptophan only once or had symptoms possibly related to EMS, leaving 24 random controls to be included in the analysis. The self-referred control group included 33 people who were selected based on absence of symptoms and use of L-tryptophan between June 1 and November 15.

We developed a standard interview form to collect detailed information from EMS patients, self-referred controls, and random controls. The interview included potential risk factors and the frequency, duration, and daily dose of L-tryptophan used before onset of illness (cases) or during the period of August 1 to November 15, 1989 (for controls). We assessed consumption of antibiotics, oral contraceptives, asthma medication, antidepressants, and several other prescription and over the counter medications. We included questions about specific vitamins and food supplements that might modify the risk or severity of illness. We also asked questions regarding potential chemical exposures that we hypothesized might be effect modifiers: painting, ceramic work, film developing, as well as exposure to pesticides, anesthetic agents, or industrial chemicals.

We initially compared the demographic characteristics of the EMS patients and each of the control groups. The gender distribution was similar: 86% of the EMS patients, 83% of the random controls and 79% of the self-referred controls were female. The EMS patients were significantly older than the random controls, but not the self-referred controls. The median age was 45 years for EMS patients, 39 years for random controls, and 43 years for self-referred controls. The youngest patient with EMS was 4 years old and the oldest was 72 years old.

EMS patients had consumed much higher doses of L-tryptophan for a shorter period of time, compared to either of the control groups. The median amount consumed per month was 40.5 grams for case patients, 6.0 grams for random controls, and 15.0 grams for self-referred controls. At the same time, the overall duration of L-tryptophan use was shorter for the EMS patients. The median duration of use was 7 months for case patients, 14 months for random controls, and 41 months for self-referred controls.

Throughout this investigation, we had seen that certain L-tryptophan products were used more often by patients with EMS and the product tracebacks pointed to Showa Denko as the manufacturing source. For some EMS patients and controls, the manufacturing source of L-tryptophan could not be determined because they did not keep the bottles with retail lot numbers. We were able to determine the L-tryptophan powder manufacturer for 30 (58%) of 52 EMS patients, 9 (38%) of 24 random controls, and 26 (79%) of 33 self-referred controls.

All but one of the EMS patients with traceable retail lots had consumed L-tryptophan manufactured by Showa Denko. When cases were compared with each control group, there was a strong association with consumption of L-tryptophan made by Showa Denko (Table 26-1). There was no association between EMS and the U.S. distributor or retail brand of L-tryptophan. There was one EMS patient who consumed L-tryptophan that was traced back to another company: Mitsui Toatsu Chemicals, Inc. This person had purchased only one bottle of L-tryptophan tablets before becoming ill, and she had taken 20 pills from that bottle over a 2 month period. Our results strongly implicated Showa Denko L-tryptophan as the source of the EMS epidemic in 1989, and yet we had a well-documented case that occurred after exposure to L-tryptophan from a different manufacturer. This was troubling and puzzling. If EMS was triggered by some event in the manufacturing process at Showa Denko, why would L-tryptophan from a different company cause the same illness? We had verified the accuracy of the retail lot traceback, and the patient had a well-defined and limited exposure to L-tryptophan. The laboratory analyses of L-tryptophan would later provide the key to unraveling this mystery.

We also examined a large number of potential cofactors that might influence the risk of EMS among people who were exposed to Showa Denko L-tryptophan. Other than age, we did not find any evidence that host factors contributed to the risk of EMS. Our EMS patients were significantly older than the random controls after adjusting for the amount of L-tryptophan consumed per month. This was consistent with another study of L-tryptophan users in South Carolina where the risk of EMS increased with age after controlling for dose.[5] In our case–control analysis of L-tryptophan users, we found no association with pre-existing illnesses, asthma, smoking, alcohol consumption, or specific dietary supplements. We also found no association with use of nonsteroidal anti-inflammatory drugs, tricyclic antidepressants, benzodiazepines, or pyridoxine.

SHOWA DENKO MANUFACTURING PROCESS

After it became clear that L-tryptophan manufactured by Showa Denko K.K. was strongly associated with EMS, we wanted to learn more about their manufacturing processes and any changes that could have introduced higher levels of trace contaminants. We had been in communication with the company through a U.S. law firm and they agreed to a private meeting with our investiga-

TABLE 26-1 Manufacturer of L-tryptophan consumed by patients with eosinophilia-myalgia syndrome prior to illness onset and controls from June 1 to November 15, 1989. The odds ratio represents the odds of consuming Showa Denko L-tryptophan among case patients compared to each control group. Individuals with an unknown L-tryptophan manufacturer were excluded from the odds ratio calculation.

	L-tryptophan manufacturer						
	Showa Denko	Other company	Unknown	Total	Odds ratio	95% CI	P Value
Case patients	29	1	22	52	—	—	—
Random controls	5	4	15	24	23.2	1.6–1179.6	0.007
Self-referred controls	16	10	7	33	18.1	2.1–812.9	0.001
Combined control groups	21	14	22	57	19.3	2.5–844.9	<0.001

Reprinted with permission from *New England Journal of Medicine* 1990; 323:357–365. Copyright © 1990 Massachusetts Medical Society. All rights reserved.

tion team to review our preliminary results. The meeting was attended by several production engineers from Japan, their translator, and Washington counsel. Up until that point, they had been operating under the assumption that all L-tryptophan was linked to EMS and their product was showing up more often just because they had greater market share. They were astonished to see our L-tryptophan traceback results for EMS patients and the two control groups.

They immediately pledged to cooperate with our investigation. Within two weeks, I received a thick book that described details about their L-tryptophan manufacturing procedures and changes that had occurred in late 1988 and early 1989. The company used a fermentation process involving a bacteria, *Bacillus amyloliquefaciens*. This bacteria was used to synthesize L-tryptophan from precursor molecules in a bioreactor. Following fermentation, the L-tryptophan was extracted from the broth and purified using a series of filtration, crystallization, and separation processes.

In December 1988, Showa Denko introduced a new strain of *B. amyloliquefaciens* (Strain V) that had been genetically modified to increase the synthesis of intermediates in the L-tryptophan biosynthetic pathway. Showa Denko reported that the biochemical and physiologic characteristics of *B. amyloliquefaciens* (Strain V) did not differ from earlier strains, and yet there had to be some differences if the new strain boosted production of L-tryptophan precursors.

There was more. In early 1989, Showa Denko reduced the amount of powdered activated carbon from at least 20 kg to 10 kg in one of the purification steps. From October 1988 through June 1989, some fermentation batches bypassed a filtration step that used a reverse osmosis membrane filter to remove impurities. The company had conducted tests of L-tryptophan purity, and they said that these changes did not alter the purity of the final product, which was reported to be at least 99.6% pure L-tryptophan. When we examined the manufacturing dates for Showa Denko L-tryptophan consumed by EMS patients and controls, we saw a cluster of manufacturing dates in early 1989 for the cases and not for the controls (Figure 26-5). The differences in manufacturing dates between cases and controls suggested that these changes in manufacturing processes might be important.

This led us to conduct additional analyses of Showa Denko L-tryptophan consumed by EMS patients and controls. Our hypothesis was that implicated lots of L-tryptophan were associated with particular manufacturing changes that occurred in late 1988 and 1989. In this analysis, powder lots were the unit of analysis

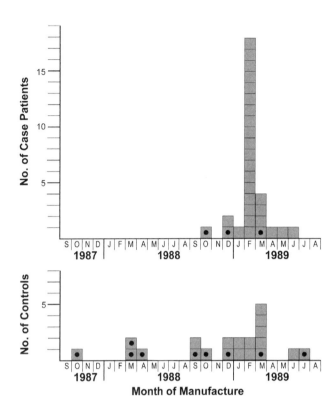

FIGURE 26-5 Month of L-tryptophan manufacture by Showa Denko for use in products consumed by EMS patients (during the month before illness onset) and controls. The period of use for controls was June 1 through Nov 15, 1989. Each box represents the L-tryptophan product consumed by one person. The most recent month of manufacture is shown for persons who consumed L-tryptophan products manufactured during different months (boxes with bullets). One control consumed L-tryptophan manufactured by Showa Denko in 1986 (not shown). Reprinted with permission from New England Journal of Medicine 1990; 323:357–65. Copyright © 1990 Massachusetts Medical Society. All rights reserved.

rather than study participants. We compared "case lots" of Showa Denko L-tryptophan with "control lots" also made by Showa Denko. The case lots were consumed before illness onset by EMS patients and the control lots were consumed only by healthy controls. Our analysis showed that both a reduction in the amount of powdered activated carbon and the use of the genetically modified bacteria (Strain V) were significantly associated with case lots. Nine of 12 case lots were manufactured with the reduced amount of activated carbon, compared with 3 of 12 control lots (odds ratio 9.0; 95% confidence interval 1.1 to 84.6; P=0.014). Similarly, 9 of 12 case lots and 4 of 12 control lots were manufactured using *B. amyloliquefaciens* Strain V (OR 6.0; 95% CI 0.8

to 51.8; P=0.04). Bypass of the reverse osmosis membrane filter was not significantly associated with the case lots.

We were unable to assess the independent effects of introducing bacterial Strain V and reducing the amount of activated carbon because there was a very high correlation between these two manufacturing changes (r = 0.78; P<.001). We concluded that a contaminant was introduced into retail L-tryptophan products as a result of increased synthesis by the recombinant strain of bacteria, or by ineffective removal of impurities during the separation and purification processes. It is also quite possible that both factors contributed, but we will never know for sure.

PEAK E

By February, Arthur Mayeno had made a great deal of progress with HPLC testing of L-tryptophan tablets in Jerry Gleich's lab. He had completed HPLC testing on dozens of L-tryptophan powder lots that were manufactured by Showa Denko. The company had also provided us with 45 bulk samples of L-tryptophan that were manufactured between September 1986 and July 1989. These samples represented nearly all of the retail lots that were consumed by EMS patients and controls in the Minneapolis–St. Paul area.

All the samples had the characteristic Showa Denko HPLC fingerprint with five signature peaks that were present in all L-tryptophan manufactured by that company. Each peak represented a chemical byproduct of the manufacturing process that was present in a low concentration. There were many other peaks as well, and we were able to identify a total of 33 trace chemical constituents other than L-tryptophan. Arthur spent a great deal of time visually inspecting the HPLC patterns and comparing the distribution of peaks in "case" and "control" lots of L-tryptophan powder. He noticed that one minor peak kept showing up in case lots but rarely in control lots.

He faxed us several of the chromatograms so we could perform our own visual comparison. The case and control lots appeared to be identical, with the exception of a single peak that represented a trace chemical constituent with a retention time (i.e., the time required to pass through the HPLC column) of 24.6 to 24.9 minutes (Figure 26-6). Arthur and Jerry decided to call it *peak E* for *eosinophil*. We had found the first evidence of a trace contaminant that was present more often in case lots than in control lots, although we later learned that peak E was not the only trace contaminant that was associated with the case lots.

For the analysis of HPLC chromatograms, we defined a case lot as a powder lot of Showa Denko L-tryptophan that was consumed by one or more EMS patients before onset of illness. A control lot was defined as a retail lot containing Showa Denko L-tryptophan that was consumed by healthy (control) L-tryptophan users and not by any patients with EMS. Peak E was present in

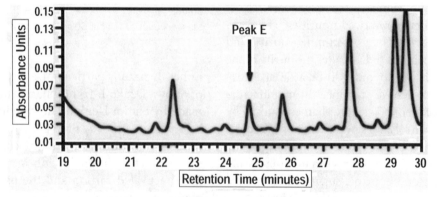

FIGURE 26-6 High performance liquid chromatography (HPLC) chromatogram for L-tryptophan manufactured by Showa Denko. Trace chemical constituents with retention times between 19 and 30 minutes are shown. Peak E represents a chemical constituent that was associated with implicated lots of L-tryptophan. Reprinted with permission from New England Journal of Medicine 1990; 323:357–65. Copyright © 1990 Massachusetts Medical Society. All rights reserved.

9 (75%) of 12 case lots of L-tryptophan and 3 (27%) of 11 control lots of L-tryptophan (odds ratio 8.0; 95% CI 0.9–76.6; P=0.02).

We then looked at the relationship between manufacturing conditions and peak E. Our hypothesis was that the presence of peak E was associated with manufacturing changes in late 1988 and 1989. For this analysis, we used the 45 bulk lots of raw L-tryptophan powder, each with a different manufacturing date. We found a significant association between the presence of peak E and the use of *B. amyloliquefaciens* Strain V, the use of 10 kg of powdered carbon per batch, and partial bypass of the reverse osmosis membrane filter. When these variables were included in a multiple logistic regression model, the only manufacturing variable that was independently associated with peak E was the genetically modified strain of *B. amyloliquefaciens*. However, there was a high correlation between the different manufacturing changes (multicollinearity), and we could not be certain that the bacterial strain was the only factor that contributed.

It was satisfying to discover that the investigation was pointing toward a clear explanation for the EMS outbreak, even though we did not know whether peak E was the actual trigger for EMS or merely a surrogate marker for another, as yet undiscovered, trace chemical that triggered eosinophilia. However, there was one puzzling observation that did not fit with our hypothesis that manufacturing changes by Showa Denko led to the presence of a trace chemical constituent in certain lots of L-tryptophan that triggered EMS.

Previously, I mentioned that the traceback process identified one patient with EMS who consumed L-tryptophan that was manufactured by Mitsui Toatsu Chemicals rather than Showa Denko. Arthur Mayeno tested the remaining L-tryptophan tablets from the retail bottle that she used, and the HPLC pattern matched the characteristic fingerprint of Showa Denko L-tryptophan, including the presence of peak E. The HPLC fingerprint of this L-tryptophan was distinct from the characteristic pattern that he saw in all other lots of L-tryptophan manufactured by Mitsui Toatsu. The discrepancy between the retail lot traceback and the HPLC fingerprint was never resolved, but there was no doubt that this patient had consumed L-tryptophan that was manufactured by Showa Denko.

The chemical structure of peak E was determined to be 1,1'-ethylidenebis(tryptophan), a tryptophan dimer that we called EBT for short. Further studies of case–lots and control–lots demonstrated that both EBT and another contaminant, 3-(phenylamino)alanine (PAA) were present in higher concentrations in case–lots.[6] The concentration of both PAA and EBT was approximately three-fold higher in the case retail lots relative to the control-lots. We estimated that EMS patients ingested approximately 10 to 15 times greater amounts of PAA and EBT than control L-tryptophan users. Investigators in the environmental health laboratory at the CDC performed extensive testing of case–lots and control-associated lots of Showa Denko L-tryptophan, and they reported the presence of more than 60 minor contaminants in the L-tryptophan powder, including EBT or peak E (they called it peak 97).[7] Six of those contaminants, including EBT and PAA, were associated with EMS in their analysis.

Peak E, or EBT, may or may not have been the trigger for EMS, but it was a strong marker for L-tryptophan powder that contained the etiologic agent. Animals exposed to EBT did not develop eosinophilia, and efforts to replicate the syndrome in animals were unsuccessful in general. The identification of PAA in implicated lots of L-tryptophan provided an important clue regarding connections between the EMS outbreak and the 1981 toxic oil syndrome epidemic in Spain. PAA is structurally similar to another compound that was isolated from samples of implicated toxic oil, and later work by Arthur Mayeno proved that a component of toxic oil could be metabolized into PAA by human liver cells.[8] This raised the possibility that PAA was the common etiologic trigger for both diseases.

Unfortunately, progress ground to a halt at that point. The absence of an animal model has made it impossible to determine if EBT, PAA, or another contaminant was the chemical trigger for a cascade of events leading to EMS. PAA remains the most likely suspect due to the connection with the toxic oil syndrome, but we may never know for certain. Whatever the cause, we know it was an extremely potent biologically active agent that was present in very low concentrations.

OTHER STUDIES

Our investigation results were publicly reported at a meeting of L-tryptophan investigators in Los Alamos in June 1990, and they were published later in the summer.[9] There were several other teams working simultaneously on this problem in other regions of the United States, and many of them also reported findings at the Los Alamos meeting. New Mexico investigators played a key role by simultaneously confirming our initial implication of L-tryptophan consumption as a major risk factor for EMS.[10] Other studies confirmed that exposure to Showa Denko L-tryptophan was nearly universal among EMS patients and relatively uncommon among controls. In South Carolina, a study of patients receiving L-tryptophan from a psychiatrist demonstrated that the risk of EMS was 28-fold higher for users of brand A (manufactured by Showa Denko) compared to users of brands manufactured by other companies.[5] Among users of Showa Denko L-tryptophan, the daily dose was the single most important predictor of EMS. A case–control study of L-tryptophan users with and without EMS in Oregon demonstrated that there was no association with any importer, wholesaler, tablet maker, or distributor. There was, however a very strong association with Showa Denko as the manufacturing source.[11] In a New York study, EMS was strongly associated with consumption of Showa Denko L-tryptophan that was manufactured after December 1, 1988.[12] In another study at a New York City medical clinic, a case–control analysis was conducted among patients who purchased L-tryptophan that was manufactured by Showa Denko.[13] The overall attack rate was about 2%, and EMS was strongly associated with exposure to a particular lot that had a higher concentration of EBT (peak E) compared to other lots consumed by patients who were not ill.

National surveillance identified more than 1500 EMS cases by July 1990, including 27 patients who died from the condition.[14] More than 90% reported onset of symptoms after April 1989, with the peak onset occurring in October 1989. The number of new cases fell dramatically after widespread publicity and recall of L-tryptophan products in November 1989. Many patients continued to suffer the effects of EMS for years after discontinuing use of L-tryptophan. The severe myalgia, pulmonary symptoms, rash, and edema improved over the course of several months in many patients, but most individuals have suffered long-term disabilities.[4,15,16] These mainly involve musculoskeletal and neurological problems such as cramps, joint pain, weakness, peripheral neuropathy, and memory or concentration difficulties.

ASSOCIATION AND CAUSATION

In 1965, Sir Austin Bradford Hill, the renowned British statistician who first identified a link between cigarette smoking and lung cancer, described nine criteria to distinguish causal and noncausal associations.[17] These included strength and consistency of the association, specificity, temporality (exposure precedes disease), and biologic gradient (dose–response effect), among others. Hill recognized that no single criterion provides indisputable evidence of cause and effect, and no single criterion is essential (except temporal relationship). Despite these qualifications, his criteria have been criticized for their limitations and exceptions.[18] In 1991, Mervyn Susser, Professor Emeritus at Columbia University and former editor of the *American Journal of Public Health*, reviewed the history of causal inference in epidemiology and proposed five pragmatic criteria that are most useful for distinguishing causal and noncausal associations.[19] The first is *strength* of the association, which is determined by the magnitude of elevated risk. The second is *specificity* in cause and effect. In the ideal situation, a given effect has a unique cause and a given cause has a unique effect. The third is *consistency*, defined by the persistence of an association in multiple assessments. The fourth is *predictive performance*, demonstrated by the ability to predict an unknown fact from the causal hypothesis. The last property is *coherence*, or the extent to which a proposed causal association is consistent with existing knowledge. He describes four types of coherence, including biologic, factual, theoretic, and statistical. Statistical coherence requires compatibility with a model that explains the distribution of cause and effect, such as a dose–response relationship.

We can apply these criteria to the EMS investigations to see if the evidence is supportive of a causal relationship. When considered as a group, the EMS investigations satisfy all of Susser's criteria for a causal association (Table 26-2). The evidence that EMS was triggered by a biologically active substance in certain lots of Showa Denko L-tryptophan is compelling, but these findings do not rule out the possibility that other factors may have modified the risk of EMS. For example, our study and two other studies found that increased age was associated with EMS among L-tryptophan users.[5,9,12] Another study suggested that chromium or pyridoxine use increased the risk of EMS among users of Showa Denko L-tryptophan,[13] but these exposures were not evaluated in other studies. It is also possible that exposure to high doses of L-tryptophan itself somehow contributed to the pathogenesis of EMS among individuals exposed to the etiologic trigger, particularly because a dose–response relationship was observed. We don't know if the dose–response effect was determined by ingestion of the etiologic trigger, ingestion of higher L-tryptophan doses, or a combination of both.

It is important to recognize that these investigations focused on the 1989 epidemic, but some cases of EMS were found to occur before and after this period. The

TABLE 26-2 Application of Susser's criteria for causation[19] to eosinophilia-myalgia syndrome (EMS) epidemic investigations

Criteria	Association between any L-tryptophan use and EMS epidemic	Association between Showa Denko L-tryptophan use and EMS epidemic
Strength of association	• Matched case–control studies in Minnesota and New Mexico found strong associations between EMS and L-tryptophan consumption.[10,24] Odds ratios were not reported because 100% of cases ($n = 12$ and $n = 11$, respectively) were exposed in each study. Each study was small but associations were very strong.	• High odds ratio (≥ 18) for consumption of Showa Denko L-tryptophan in cases versus control L-tryptophan users in Minneapolis–St. Paul area. Similar or higher risk associated with Showa Denko L-tryptophan consumption in case–control studies in Oregon and New York, and in a South Carolina cohort.
Specificity in cause and effect	• Only 1 variable (L-tryptophan use) was independently associated with EMS in each study. Use of any prescription medication (in 9/12 cases and 4/12 controls) was associated with EMS in Minnesota, but no single drug or class of drugs was associated. Ingestion of homemade pork sausage (in 2/11 cases and 0/22 controls) was associated with EMS in New Mexico. These associations were likely due to confounding (prescription medications) or chance (pork sausage).	• Consumption of Showa Denko L-tryptophan predicted the subsequent occurrence of EMS, and no other important exposures were identified among L-tryptophan users. All studies of manufacturer found that a given effect (EMS) had a unique cause (consumption of Showa Denko L-tryptophan).
Consistency	• Case–control studies in two different states found consistent associations, although the number of cases in each study was small.	• Studies by different investigators in Minnesota, Oregon, South Carolina, and New York all implicated Showa Denko L-tryptophan.
Predictive performance	• The primary causal hypothesis predicted that the incidence of EMS epidemic would decline after withdrawal of L-tryptophan from the U.S. market. This was observed.[14]	• The hypothesis predicted that particular manufacturing conditions would be associated with implicated L-tryptophan made by Showa Denko. This was found to be the case in the Minnesota investigation.
Coherence	• These studies are coherent in the sense that later studies implicated a particular manufacturer of L-tryptophan. If the initial studies in Minnesota and New Mexico had been spurious, later studies of L-tryptophan manufacturers would have shown no association with EMS. The manufacturing sources would have been randomly distributed among cases and controls.	• Biologic coherence was suggested by the observation that implicated L-tryptophan contained trace contaminants that were similar to chemicals found in Spanish toxic oil samples. One study demonstrated that human liver cells could metabolize one of the trace contaminants of implicated L-tryptophan into a chemical that was present in toxic oil. Statistical coherence was shown by a dose–response relationship that was detected in three different studies.

existence of cases outside the epidemic period does not diminish the strength of the epidemiologic evidence. It is likely that sporadic cases of EMS occurred before (and after) the EMS epidemic at a very low incidence, possibly caused by exposure to the chemical trigger from other sources, or an unrelated cause. The epidemiologic investigations explained the sudden increase during 1989, but their relevance for sporadic EMS cases occurring in other time periods is uncertain.

LITIGATION, ETHICS, AND SCIENTIFIC DEBATE

A class action lawsuit was filed against Showa Denko by people who developed EMS, and the company eventually reached a settlement agreement for an undisclosed amount. While litigation was ongoing, the U.S. law firm representing Showa Denko hired four individuals to serve as expert consultants. In 1995 and 1996, they published three articles (each with one to three authors) in peer-reviewed medical journals. The articles contained strongly worded critiques of the published studies on the cause of the EMS epidemic.[20–22] Each article contained a disclaimer that the author(s) served as expert consultants for attorneys representing Showa Denko. The first published commentary stated that "the authors have received no compensation from attorneys for the preparation of this manuscript, nor were attorneys permitted to review this manuscript prior to submission for publication."[20] One of the authors was a member of the editorial consultants board for the journal that accepted the article for publication.[20] The second article stated that "no support was provided in preparation of this manuscript."[22] The authors of the third article made no statement regarding compensation for preparation of the manuscript, and the citation list included many references to legal depositions that were given by EMS investigators (including myself).[21] It is unusual that a reference list in a medical journal would include legal depositions that are not publicly available. Indeed, the whole process for determining "truth" is quite different in the scientific world and the legal world, but that's a separate issue.

Their interpretation of the scientific evidence was stated unequivocally in the final sentence of each abstract: "The cause of the eosinophilia-myalgia syndrome remains unknown."[20] "The questionable validity of these studies considerably weakens the claim that LT [L-tryptophan] or a contaminant caused EMS."[22] "The search for the cause of EMS should continue without the underlying assumption that LT or some contaminant is responsible."[21] Astonishingly, they even expressed doubt that the EMS epidemic was real.[20]

A primary criticism of our first case–control study was based on the fact that it was published in the *MMWR* (a CDC publication) rather than a peer-reviewed journal, and therefore it did not (in the opinion of the author) meet acceptable standards for scientific evidence.[22] A different standard for scientific evidence was applied in the concluding paragraph where the author stated, "In conclusion, clinical observations have raised the suspicion but have not proved that LT may cause EMS…To the contrary, unpublished data from a key study suggest that EMS may be an unusual manifestation of an allergic state."

The author of this critique accused us of misrepresenting a critical element of the study: the enrollment of cases and controls without prior knowledge of L-tryptophan use. This is a basic concept in epidemiology—cases and controls must be ascertained independent of exposure status. According to the consultant, "The investigators contacted rheumatologists, pathologists, and a pediatric neurologist from November 9 to 12, 1989; yet by November 7 the putative association between LT and EMS had already received nationwide publicity." He asserted that we broadcast the hypothesis with "maximum publicity" by (1) soliciting cases at the meeting of clinical pathologists, (2) sending a letter to physicians requesting reporting of cases with unexplained eosinophilia and myalgia, and (3) announcing through the news media that individuals who used L-tryptophan should contact a physician if they had muscle pain. We did indeed solicit cases at the meeting of clinical pathologists, but the pathologists had no knowledge of L-tryptophan use by the patients who had characteristic biopsy findings. We also sent a letter to physicians and made announcements through the news media, but these occurred *after* the case–control study was completed. Active case finding is an important element of an outbreak investigation, and these surveillance measures were appropriate after the initial study results were compiled.

The allegation that the association between L-tryptophan and EMS had received nationwide publicity by November 7 is false. A search of news media archives confirmed that there was no mention of EMS in the Minnesota news media until we held a press conference on November 12, announcing the results of the first case–control study. All of our cases were identified over a 2-day period (Friday and Saturday), and the physicians had no opportunity to contact the patients beforehand to ascertain L-tryptophan exposure.

Another criticism was that our case definition was nonspecific because it included either severe myalgia or muscle weakness as symptoms.[22] In contrast, the CDC case definition required myalgia and did not mention muscle weakness. In the early stages of an epidemic, case definitions are based on limited information and may be nonspecific, particularly when facing a new disease entity. In retrospect, the EMS case definition we used was valid. Although the author criticized our inclusion of patients with eosinophilia and muscle weakness, we ultimately found that 63% of EMS patients in Minnesota experienced muscle weakness. It was a real and common manifestation of this syndrome.

The specificity of our EMS case definition was enhanced by the inclusion of an objective and extreme laboratory abnormality (eosinophil count >1000 per μL). This level of eosinophilia greatly reduced or eliminated any misclassification due to nonspecific symptoms. Although asthma and allergies can cause eosinophilia, they rarely cause such extreme eosinophil counts. In addition, many of the patients had muscle biopsies that demonstrated characteristic pathologic abnormalities of EMS. The concerns about a nonspecific case definition were not credible, given this evidence.

The author of this critique argued that our use of a nonspecific case definition increased the potential for finding a spurious association through selection bias. This was a surprising claim because nondifferential misclassification of the outcome (EMS) would bias results toward the null (i.e., no association). However, the logic of the consultant was as follows: "In the face of publicity, and of the knowledge that the patient had used LT [L-tryptophan], the reporting physician, patient, or interviewer could easily have perceived incapacitating weakness if the patient had been exposed to LT." There are three errors in this statement that deserve mention. The first is that there was no publicity regarding EMS and L-tryptophan in Minnesota before or during the first case–control study, as described previously. The second is that the physician and interviewer did not know if the patient took L-tryptophan when he or she was identified and contacted for the study. The third is that the patients and controls were not aware of the study hypothesis, and they would have no way of knowing that L-tryptophan use was the main exposure of interest. The question about L-tryptophan use was buried in the middle of many other questions about drugs, dietary supplements, diet, and environmental exposures.

Another criticism of the first case–control study was that we did not consider confounding caused by prescription drug use.[22] In the *MMWR* publication, we reported that prescription medications were used by 9 of 12 case patients and 4 of 12 controls. According to the consultant, the relevant question was "whether such use could have partly or wholly accounted for the association between LT and EMS. Data were insufficient to examine that question, either by exclusion (which would have left only 3 cases) or multivariate adjustment." It is a relevant question, but the answer is no; it is not plausible that use of prescription medication could have accounted for the association between L-tryptophan and EMS, and multivariate analysis is not needed to reach that conclusion. To serve as a confounder, prescription medication use would have to be associated with both L-tryptophan use and EMS. It is not plausible that multiple unrelated prescription drugs were all associated with EMS. This would have been a potential source of confounding only if we had found that a single drug or class of drugs accounted for most of the prescription medications used by EMS patients, but that was not the case.

In one of the other articles, the authors criticized our study by suggesting that the results were invalid due to confounding by indication.[20] This is a situation that arises when there is an observed association between a medication or other therapeutic intervention and a disease outcome, but the association is confounded by the underlying condition that led to the therapeutic intervention. Confounding by indication is important to consider in observational studies of medications, but it's hard to see how it applies in this circumstance. Their logic was based on the knowledge that common indications for L-tryptophan use included insomnia and depression, and these symptoms might also be manifestations of fibromyalgia, a syndrome of unknown etiology causing widespread pain, fatigue, sleep disturbance, and joint stiffness. They acknowledged that fibromyalgia and depression are not typically associated with eosinophilia, but they nevertheless argued that the symptoms of fibromyalgia might account for part or all of the EMS symptoms rather than L-tryptophan. They rationalized this by suggesting that perhaps the eosinophilia was caused by L-tryptophan, but not the symptoms.

After interviewing a number of patients who developed EMS, I am confident that confounding by indication was not responsible for the association between

L-tryptophan and EMS. These individuals developed severe and incapacitating symptoms that were not present before taking L-tryptophan. Even if you accept the unlikely premise that the eosinophilia and symptoms had different causes, a dietary supplement causing extreme eosinophilia with unusual pathologic findings represents a serious and urgent public health problem.

These articles contained additional criticisms of the studies implicating Showa Denko L-tryptophan, but they did not acknowledge that the association between EMS and the manufacturer would be implausible if the initial case–control studies of L-tryptophan use and EMS were flawed. If the association between EMS and L-tryptophan use was due to bias or confounding in our first case–control study, we would expect to find no association between EMS and the L-tryptophan manufacturer among L-tryptophan users. The manufacturing sources would be randomly distributed among cases and controls, and the odds ratio would approximate one.

We responded to these and other criticisms raised by the Showa Denko consultants in an editorial that was published in the *Journal of Rheumatology*.[23] The views expressed by the consultants were far outside the mainstream thinking on EMS epidemiology, and they included implausible or factually incorrect criticisms of the EMS studies. Individuals who read those commentaries may well have concluded that the evidence implicating L-tryptophan was weak unless they had detailed knowledge of the investigations. This raises several issues regarding the intersection of science, public health, and the judicial system. Is it appropriate for expert legal consultants to publish commentaries in peer reviewed medical journals on topics that may influence the outcome of litigation? Are financial disclosures sufficient to address ethical concerns regarding conflict of interest in this circumstance? These are important questions for future investigations that may involve product liability. In the meantime, Mike Osterholm still has a vintage bottle of 1989 L-tryptophan in his office, and I don't think he's going to be taking any the next time he has trouble sleeping.

EPILOGUE

I spoke to Bonnie Bishop in New Mexico and Jinx Engstrom in Minnesota many years after they developed EMS. Bonnie was determined to recover from EMS, and she pushed herself hard over the first couple of years. She slowly regained her strength and flexibility, but it was a painful process. She was able to engage in part-time work after a year. Twenty years later, she still suffers from chronic pain, cramping, tremors, and insomnia. Jinx Engstrom went back to work within a year of developing EMS, but she experienced constant and severe pain from sitting in an office. She switched to a different job that involved more movement. For the next 20 years she continued to experience body aches and muscle spasms, worse on some days than others. She was treated with immunosuppressive drugs, which helped her function better and allowed her to work. After several years of treatment, she developed multiple cancers and decided to stop taking the immunosuppressive drugs. Since then, her symptoms have gradually worsened and she has experienced increasing muscle spasms.

Was the EMS epidemic preventable? It is obvious that there was no regulatory oversight of companies that manufactured amino acids and other food supplements. L-tryptophan was widely promoted and used for its pharmacologic effects, even though the product labels made no therapeutic claims. The Dietary Supplement Health and Education Act (DSHEA) was signed into law in 1994, but it did little to ensure that amino acids and other dietary supplements met minimum standards for safety and quality. The DSHEA allowed dietary supplement manufacturers to make certain health claims without an FDA petition. More importantly, it shifted the burden of proving safety from the manufacturer to the FDA. This made it more difficult for the FDA to remove dietary supplements from the market. More than a decade passed before the FDA implemented standards for good manufacturing practices of dietary supplements. Since 2008, dietary supplement manufacturers and distributors have been required to monitor and document the production process for quality assurance, and perform laboratory analysis of raw materials and finished products to document product purity and the absence of contaminants.

This is a meaningful step forward, but it does not guarantee another EMS-like epidemic will not occur. The number and variety of dietary supplements or "nutraceuticals" is enormous, and the burden of evaluating safety and efficacy still falls on the consumer. Many of these products contain biologically active substances, and they are consumed in much higher concentrations compared to normal dietary intake. Some of these, such as omega-3 fatty acids, have been extensively studied, but many others have not. Surveillance and adverse event reporting systems are essential for early detection of outbreaks. But if another EMS-like epidemic occurs, it will most likely be detected first by astute clinicians, just like those in New Mexico in 1989.

LEARNING QUESTIONS

1. L-tryptophan is an essential amino acid in the human body. Why should this fact not lead to the dismissal of the hypothesis that it could have been responsible for this outbreak?
2. The Minnesota investigators did not use the same case definition as the CDC. How was their case definition different? Consider what might be the reasoning behind this choice and its implications. What was included in the case definition to increase its specificity?
3. Why did the investigators include matching in their first case–control study and what characteristics did they use to match?
4. After the initial case–control study, the FDA issued a voluntary recall of some, but not all L-tryptophan products. Dr. Michael Osterholm argued that all products containing L-tryptophan should be taken off the market. Discuss the merits and concerns with these different levels of public health action.
5. What was the toxic oil syndrome and how was it relevant to this eosinophilia-myalgia syndrome investigation?
6. Did peak E cause eosinophilia-myalgia syndrome? Respond based on the information provided in the investigation and your knowledge of the strengths and limitations of epidemiologic methods.
7. What were the criteria suggested by Mervyn Susser for delineating causal and noncausal associations? Apply these criteria to the findings of this investigation.
8. A primary criticism of the first case–control study was that the results were published in the *MMWR* (a CDC publication) rather than a peer-reviewed journal. Is there any merit to the argument that publication in the *MMWR* is not the same as publication in a peer-reviewed journal and therefore "does not meet acceptable standards for scientific evidence"?
9. What constitutes a conflict of interest when epidemiologists serve as paid consultants for parties in litigation? Is disclosure of financial relationships sufficient to eliminate concerns regarding conflict of interest? To what extent should they participate in scientific debate regarding epidemiologic evidence?
10. What is confounding by indication? What was the argument against the eosinophilia-myalgia syndrome investigation regarding this indication and what is your opinion about the investigation if there was such confounding?

ACKNOWLEDGMENTS

I would like to thank Dr. Michael Osterholm, Dr. Gerald Gleich, Dr. Joseph Duffy, Dr. Craig Hedberg, and Dr. Mary Kamb for reviewing the manuscript and helping me recall details of the investigation. Dr. Laura Coleman, Dr. Steve Waring, and Dr. Robert Greenlee provided additional helpful comments and suggestions. Finally, I would like to extend a special thanks to Bonnie Bishop and Jinx Engstrom for sharing their stories and helping me understand how EMS impacted their lives.

REFERENCES

1. Lakhanpal S, Duffy J, Engel AG. Eosinophilia associated with perimyositis and pneumonitis. *Mayo Clin Proc*. 1988;63(1):37–41.
2. Sternberg EM, Van Woert MH, Young SN, et al. Development of a scleroderma-like illness during therapy with L-5-hydroxytryptophan and carbidopa. *N Engl J Med*. 1980;303(14):782–787.
3. Kilbourne EM, Rigau-Perez JG, Heath CW Jr, et al. Clinical epidemiology of toxic-oil syndrome. Manifestations of a new illness. *N Engl J Med*. 1983;309(23):1408–1414.
4. Hertzman PA, Clauw DJ, Kaufman LD, et al. The eosinophilia-myalgia syndrome: status of 205 patients and results of treatment 2 years after onset. *Ann Intern Med*. 1995;122(11):851–855.
5. Kamb ML, Murphy JJ, Jones JL, et al. Eosinophilia-myalgia syndrome in L-tryptophan-exposed patients. *JAMA*. 1992;267(1):77–82.
6. Mayeno AN, Belongia EA, Lin F, Lundy SK, Gleich GJ. 3-(Phenylamino)alanine, a novel aniline-derived amino acid associated with the eosinophilia-myalgia syndrome: a link to the toxic oil syndrome? *Mayo Clin Proc*. 1992;67(12):1134–1139.
7. Hill RH Jr, Caudill SP, Philen RM, et al. Contaminants in L-tryptophan associated with eosinophilia myalgia syndrome. *Arch Environ Contam Toxicol*. 1993;25(1):134–142.
8. Mayeno AN, Benson LM, Naylor S, Colberg-Beers M, Puchalski JT, Gleich GJ. Biotransformation of 3-(phenylamino)-1,2-propanediol to 3-(phenylamino)alanine: a chemical link between toxic oil syndrome and eosinophilia-myalgia syndrome. *Chem Res Toxicol*. 1995;8(7):911–916.
9. Belongia EA, Hedberg CW, Gleich GJ, et al. An investigation of the cause of the eosinophilia-myalgia syndrome associated with tryptophan use. *N Engl J Med*. 1990;323(6):357–365.
10. Eidson M, Philen RM, Sewell CM, Voorhees R, Kilbourne EM. L-tryptophan and eosinophilia-myalgia syndrome in New Mexico. *Lancet*. 1990;335(8690):645–648.
11. Slutsker L, Hoesly FC, Miller L, Williams LP, Watson JC, Fleming DW. Eosinophilia-myalgia syndrome associated with exposure to tryptophan from a single manufacturer. *JAMA*. 1990;264(2):213–217.
12. Back EE, Henning KJ, Kallenbach LR, Brix KA, Gunn RA, Melius JM. Risk factors for developing eosinophilia myalgia syndrome among L-tryptophan users in New York. *J Rheumatol*. 1993;20(4):666–672.
13. Henning KJ, Jean-Baptiste E, Singh T, Hill RH, Friedman SM. Eosinophilia-myalgia syndrome in patients ingesting a single source of L-tryptophan. *J Rheumatol*. 1993;20(2):273–278.

14. Swygert LA, Maes EF, Sewell LE, Miller L, Falk H, Kilbourne EM. Eosinophilia-myalgia syndrome. Results of national surveillance. *JAMA*. 1990;264(13):1698–1703.
15. Campbell DS, Morris PD, Silver RM. Eosinophilia-myalgia syndrome: a long-term follow-up study. *South Med J*. 1995;88(9):953–958.
16. Pincus T. Eosinophilia-myalgia syndrome: patient status 2–4 years after onset. *J Rheumatol Suppl*. 1996;46:19–24; discussion 24–25.
17. Hill AB. The environment and disease: association or causation? *Proc R Soc Med*. 1965;58:295–300.
18. Rothman KJ, Greenland S, Lash TL. *Modern Epidemiology*. 3rd ed. Philadelphia, PA: Lippincott Williams & Wilkins; 2008.
19. Susser M. What is a cause and how do we know one? A grammar for pragmatic epidemiology. *Am J Epidemiol*. 1991;133(7):635–648.
20. Daniels SR, Hudson JI, Horwitz RI. Epidemiology of potential association between L-tryptophan ingestion and eosinophilia-myalgia syndrome. *J Clin Epidemiol*. 1995;48(12):1413–1427; discussion 1429–1440.
21. Horwitz RI, Daniels SR. Bias or biology: evaluating the epidemiologic studies of L-tryptophan and the eosinophilia-myalgia syndrome. *J Rheumatol Suppl*. 1996;46:60–72.
22. Shapiro S. Epidemiologic studies of the association of L-tryptophan with the eosinophilia-myalgia syndrome: a critique. *J Rheumatol Suppl*. 1996;46:44–58; discussion 58–59.
23. Belongia EA, Gleich GJ. The eosinophilia-myalgia syndrome revisited. *J Rheumatol*. 1996;23(10):1682–1685.
24. Centers for Disease Control. Eosinophilia-myalgia syndrome and L-tryptophan-containing products—New Mexico, Minnesota, Oregon, and New York, 1989. *MMWR*. 1989;38:785–788.

CHAPTER 27

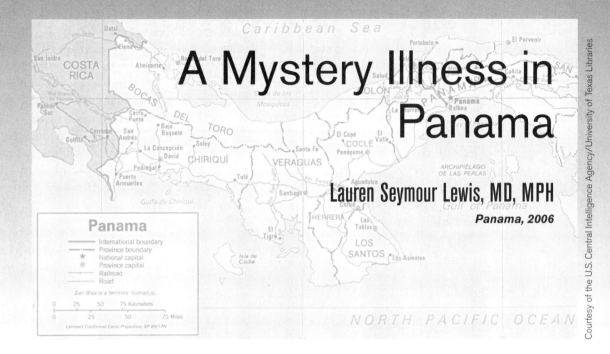

A Mystery Illness in Panama

Lauren Seymour Lewis, MD, MPH

Panama, 2006

THE CALL

Our division at the Centers for Disease Control and Prevention (CDC) had recently instituted a new policy that allowed staff to telecommute one day per week. I was quite content working from home in my pajamas and answering emails from my couch when I got a call from Dr. Carol Rubin, my branch chief. Carol needed me to come into the office immediately for a meeting. She said that there was an emergency situation in Panama and our branch, the Health Studies Branch (HSB) in the National Center for Environmental Health (NCEH) at the CDC, would be leading the response. She told me that I would be on the response team and needed to be prepared to leave for Panama as soon as the CDC could arrange our travel. She had more people to contact and could not discuss specifics over the phone. I would have to learn more at the meeting—so much for the pajamas!

The first thing I needed to do, however (even before changing clothes), was to warn my husband that he was about to be a single parent for the next 2 to 4 weeks. As a mom whose 12-year-old son had a busy sports schedule, sudden, unexpected travel was a challenge for the whole family. My family and I had learned to adapt to this aspect of my job since I left my career as an internal medicine clinician to pursue a public health career at the CDC.

My interest in public health began in medical school. My dream of a career in public health became a reality when I became an Epidemic Intelligence Service (EIS) officer at the CDC's National Center for Injury Prevention and Control. I then pursued further public health training through the CDC's Preventive Medicine Residency program receiving my MPH in Epidemiology and medical specialty board certification in Public Health. When it was finally time to grow up and get a job, I joined the staff at HSB.

On my way to the office, I thought about the possible public health threat I could be facing in the next few days. What could be happening in Panama? For HSB, an emergency situation could mean just about anything. HSB responds to a wide range of environmental public health threats, from extreme weather events to mass poisonings. In the three years I had been with the branch, we had responded to hurricanes and heat waves, and we had investigated mercury poisonings, intentional arsenic poisonings, aflatoxicosis outbreaks in Kenya, and a large multistate outbreak of pruritus. Switching gears and quickly becoming experts on some new or emerging environmental issue was simply a part of life at HSB and it was futile to try to guess what was happening in Panama.

I did, however, have one clue as to what we were dealing with. Carol usually asked staff if they were available to deploy when putting together an outbreak team, but this time she firmly told me that I would be deploying. Immediate supervisors and spouses typically had the luxury of weighing in when a deployment created a hardship or conflict with important family or work obligations. The definitive nature of Carol's tone indicated that this outbreak investigation was not routine. Whatever was happening in Panama was particularly urgent. It took priority over any other obligations and Carol needed to act quickly and efficiently.

THE PREPARATION

Carol had assembled several branch toxicologists and epidemiologists for the meeting. We crowded around the small table in Carol's office. My pride in how readily I responded from working at home (3 miles away) was quickly overshadowed by the sight of one of our branch epidemiologists, Eduardo Azziz Baumgartner. About 10 pounds lighter, with dark circles under his eyes, Eduardo had arrived only hours earlier from the Ivory Coast where, for the past 3 weeks, he had helped the World Health Organization (WHO) investigate a chemical contamination of the public drinking water system. His dedication and enthusiasm was unparalleled.

Everyone settled down, and Carol began to share the information she had received so far. An astute physician in Panama had noticed that he was seeing an unusual number of patients with unexplained acute renal failure that was often accompanied by some type of neurologic deficit (such as cranial nerve palsies, extremity weakness, or paralysis). He had reported this to the Panama Ministry of Health (MOH). Subsequently, the MOH Epidemiology Unit initiated a preliminary investigation and confirmed a cluster of 21 case–patients of primarily older men (mean age = 62 years). Twelve of the 21 cases had died (case fatality rate = 57%) despite treatment, which included hemodialysis. This was a remarkable fatality rate that made the need for urgent action to identify and stop the cause of this outbreak immediately clear. All of the reports of case–patients were from the Caja del Seguro (CSS) hospital system. The MOH had conducted an extensive investigation for bacterial and viral causes of the outbreak. All laboratory results were negative.

It is typical for HSB to be consulted at this point in the investigation. When an outbreak of a mysterious or unknown illness occurs, a potential toxin exposure usually is considered only after every possible infectious cause has been excluded. This tends to be especially true in developing countries, where the public health infrastructure is focused on infectious disease control and little toxicology awareness or expertise is available. Sometimes toxicologists in our branch served a purely consultative role, or the toxicologists in the NCEH's Division of Laboratory Services provided assistance with the laboratory analysis. However, this outbreak was large, fatal, and the case numbers were rapidly climbing, so even though the Panama MOH had considerable epidemiology capacity, the request to HSB was for immediate and comprehensive (epidemiologic, toxicologic, and laboratory) assistance to investigate and control this outbreak. The objectives of the investigation were clear—to rapidly determine the cause of unexplained renal failure and identify the route of exposure to the toxin so that control measures could be initiated (Exhibit 27-1).

> *However, this outbreak was large, fatal, and the case numbers were rapidly climbing, so even though the Panama MOH had considerable epidemiology capacity, the request to HSB was for immediate and comprehensive (epidemiologic, toxicologic, and laboratory) assistance to investigate and control this outbreak.*

An intense discussion of the possible causes of acute renal failure and neurologic deficits ensued. Some aspects of the clinical presentation were consistent with a toxin exposure, in particular the absence of fever. The presence or absence of fever is a key feature that distinguishes an infectious process from a toxin poisoning. Among the long list of toxins that can cause acute renal failure, the clinical presentation of renal failure combined with neurotoxicity was most consistent with diethylene glycol (DEG) poisoning.

> *The presence or absence of fever is a key feature that distinguishes an infectious process from a toxin poisoning.*

> **EXHIBIT 27-1** The presenting problem and objectives during an investigation of unexplained illness and death in Panama
>
> **Presenting Problem**
> - Unexplained acute renal failure with or without
>   - neurologic deficit
>   - cranial nerve palsies
>   - extremity weakness
>   - paralysis
> - Objectives of the investigation
>   - Rapidly determine the cause of unexplained renal failure.
>   - Identify the route of exposure to the toxin so that control measures could be initiated.

DEG is commonly used in commercial products (such as antifreeze) and is highly toxic to humans.

Outbreaks of DEG poisoning have been known to occur when DEG is substituted for the more expensive pharmaceutical grade glycerin that is used in the production of liquid medications. As a result of this illegal practice, outbreaks of DEG poisoning have recurred worldwide. The first and largest outbreak (which resulted in 105 deaths) occurred in the United States in 1937.[1] This historically significant event led to the Federal Food, Drug, and Cosmetic Act that requires proof of safety before drugs are introduced into the marketplace. Liquid medications are generally produced for the pediatric population, and the more recent outbreaks of DEG poisoning have occurred among infants and children in developing countries. For example, in 1998, DEG-contaminated medicine resulted in the deaths of 33 children (out of 36 case–patients) in India. In 1996, HSB responded to a DEG outbreak in Haiti that resulted in the deaths of 88 children out of 105 case–patients.[2]

Although the clinical presentation in Panama fit the picture of DEG poisoning, the case–patient demographics (older adults, with a preponderance of men) simply did not fit a DEG poisoning outbreak. The etiology of this outbreak remained unclear.

As chief of Health Studies, Carol had been directing environmental health responses for many years and knew exactly what combination of skills would be needed to identify the etiology of illness and the source of exposure. The initial team would include Dr. Joshua (Josh) Schier, a medical toxicologist and emergency physician in HSB. He would provide the toxicologic expertise that was always critical when a toxin exposure was suspected but the specific toxin was unknown. Dr. Danielle Rentz, a PhD epidemiologist who recently started as an EIS officer at HSB, was also on the team. Danielle and the other branch EIS officers were gaining experience in outbreak investigations and other aspects of public health through the CDC's applied epidemiology training program. Danielle came to EIS and to Health Studies specifically for this kind of experience—to utilize her epidemiologic skills in outbreak investigations. Her strong analytic skills would prove valuable in rapidly producing the epidemiologic data needed to determine how people were being exposed to the presumed toxin. However, this would be the first outbreak investigation for both Danielle and Josh. Carol knew that in an event of this magnitude, she needed some experience on the team. That was my role. I had been investigating outbreaks since coming to the CDC as an EIS officer 7 years ago and was confident in a response role. Other members of the branch were asked to be on standby and prepare to join the team if needed as the investigation progressed. In addition, Carol knew that laboratory testing would likely play a major role in this investigation, as it often does. In environmental investigations, analyses of urine, serum, and or blood samples to measure human exposure to a toxin (biomarkers of exposure) and analysis of environmental samples (such as food, water, and soil) are often conducted. At Carol's request, the Division of Laboratory Services sent Jacob (Jay) Wamsley, a laboratorian, as part of the initial team to oversee the laboratory specimen collection.

The next stop for the initial team was to meet with Dr. Michael (Mike) McGeehin, director of NCEH's Division of Environmental Hazards and Health Effects, and then pack and prepare to leave for Panama the following day. Carol, Danielle, Josh, and I sat around the large table in a conference room adjacent to Mike's office. Mike joined us and began to share some of his insight and experience. We discussed our hypothesis and he agreed that this appeared to be a toxin exposure that was clinically consistent with DEG. However, he cautioned us against concentrating on DEG or any one hypothesis this early. Approaching an investigation with preconceived ideas was a fatal mistake that could cause us to overlook the true etiology of the outbreak. Mike emphasized the importance of keeping an open mind and casting a wide net. We discussed the clues provided by the preliminary case demographics.

> *Approaching an investigation with preconceived ideas was a fatal mistake that could cause us to overlook the true etiology of the outbreak.*

The age range was not consistent with DEG poisoning, which had almost always occurred in infants and young children. And, why were 90% of the cases men? He explained that if men were involved, it could complicate our investigation because we could not discount bizarre and unexpected explanations. He said, "Above all else, please remember that men do really stupid things." Armed with those final words of wisdom, Mike sent us off to conquer the outbreak.

On the plane, Danielle and I plowed through copies of toxicology textbook chapters and renal disease articles in order to become the subject matter experts that the MOH expected us to be when the plane landed in Panama. We discussed potential epidemiologic approaches and started developing some standard questions. We thought a case–control study would likely be the most appropriate next step. However, any next step would need to build on the information learned from the initial descriptive investigation and would usually be limited by logistic factors, such as available resources and infrastructure. We could not make any real decisions until we arrived, assessed the situation, and conferred with our Panamanian colleagues.

I took a break from thinking about the investigation when I noticed that the other passengers on the plane were unusually social. People were milling about in the aisle, greeting and talking to each other as if they were all friends. I wondered if a large tour group was on the plane traveling together and tried to eavesdrop to find out, but everyone was talking in Spanish. I asked Josh, the only Spanish speaker on our team, to find out what was going on. Based on the conversations he overheard, there was no tour group. It all just seemed to be casual, friendly conversation. Over the next few weeks, I would learn that this unusually warm social behavior was typical of Panamanian culture.

THE ARRIVAL

It was night when our plane began its descent toward the Tocumen International Airport in Panama City. We could see the lights outlining the city skyline, indicative of the cosmopolitan nature of the nation's capital. Panama is a small Central American country that occupies 30,193 sq. miles of land between Columbia and Costa Rica. Its culture, customs, and language are predominantly Caribbean Spanish. The population is more than 3 million, with half the people living in Panama City. Panama is perhaps best known for the Panama Canal, an engineering marvel that is central to Panama's economy and is critical to world trade and commerce.[3]

We were met at the gate by an official from the Panama MOH and Dr Jorge Motta, director of the Gorgas Memorial Institute (a large, prestigious medical institution in Panama). We were led directly to a private VIP lounge in the airport. The lounge, which had several seating areas, was completely empty except for us. Dr. Motta, one of the leads of the MOH investigation, led us to a group of sofas. After brief introductions and pleasantries, he updated us on the status of the outbreak and informed us that more cases had occurred. We were also cautioned that the MOH was overwhelmed with epidemiologists wanting to help with the investigation. There happened to be an abundance of World Health Organization (WHO) and Pan American Health Organization (PAHO) epidemiologists in the country at that time who were attending an epidemiologic workshop being held in Panama City. The MOH did identify two conference participants who would be valuable additions to the investigation—Miguel Cruz, a health services officer with NCEH's emergency preparedness and response group and Oscar Mujica, an epidemiologist at PAHO and alumni of the Field Epidemiology Training Program (FETP) in Peru. The FETP is a CDC program in other countries that offers applied epidemiology training equivalent to the EIS program. While we talked in the VIP lounge, a government official had shepherded our baggage and passports through customs and immigration. After we finished our meeting, we were guided out of the airport through a private exit, bypassing customs and baggage claim. The exit led directly to a car where our bags had been loaded and a driver was waiting to take us to our hotel.

When we arrived at a relatively new Country Inn and Suites, an American chain of hotels, the familiar surroundings were both comforting and reassuring. When on international government travel, it is often difficult to predict the type of accommodations. Sometimes, for security reasons or because of a prearranged federal rate, we may stay in an opulent, luxury hotel. Other times, the only option may be accommodations without running water or electricity. By contrast, domestic government travel is very predictable and this was just the type of hotel that we typically use when on government travel in the United States.

When we approached the front desk to check in, the receptionist asked if we were the group from the CDC and told us that the Panama Minister of Health had been alerted to our arrival and was on his way to meet us. At this point, it was almost 11:00 p.m. There had to be a mistake. I asked, "Are you sure the Minister is coming here to our hotel now?" We proceeded to check in, assuming that the message had been some miscommunication, when the charismatic Minister of Health for Panama entered the hotel lobby. Even though we had never seen the Minister, we sensed who he was when he walked in the door. He had an imposing stature, firm handshake, and the powerful, yet congenial, manner of a politician. After introductions, we found a comfortable place to sit in the lobby and had a few minutes of discussion about some of the political and media issues as well as the itinerary for the following day. He asked if we had any additional recommendations and Josh requested that we go to the hospital in order to examine some of the case–patients and review their medical records. The minister agreed to arrange this, thanked us for coming to Panama so quickly, and left as promptly as he had arrived. We were left wondering why this discussion could not wait until the next morning. I had the distinct impression that he really just wanted to know who the CDC was sending and he did not want any surprises. I wondered whether we met his expectations.

First the airport and now this, it was definitely not a typical arrival. I had never received this level of official attention. It emphasized the urgency of this outbreak and the high expectations of the Panama MOH.

THE INVESTIGATION

Our first day began by meeting with the Minister of Health, all the MOH officials, and other stakeholders involved in the investigation. At this meeting, the MOH Epidemiology Unit presented the results of the investigation to date. The case count was rapidly climbing. It had almost doubled from the 21 original cases. As the number of cases increased, the male to female ratio had evened out and was almost one-to-one. It was likely that the preponderance of men among the original cases was purely chance or perhaps a reporting issue. The preliminary data we had reviewed was based on a small number of cases and was not to be completely trusted. It was good for hypothesis generation, but its ability to represent the whole picture (in this case the whole picture of the distribution based on sex) was unreliable. Based on the current data, males and females were now equally likely to develop the illness. However, other demographic factors remained unchanged—the cases were primarily older patients who receive their care from the CSS hospital or other facilities in the CSS system. The team also reported that there was no family clustering of cases. This made a foodborne or waterborne toxin exposure less likely and heightened concern about more individualized routes of exposure, such as personal care products or pharmaceuticals. In addition, clinicians recognized that several of the affected patients had hypertension and were being treated with lisinopril (an angiotensin-converting enzyme [ACE] inhibitor). Lisinopril had been recently added to the CSS hospital formulary as a first-line treatment for hypertension. There was growing concern among physicians that this change was the cause of the outbreak. However, the epidemiologic evidence to date was not compelling. The descriptive data showed that approximately 35% of the cases were taking lisinopril. The fact that the majority of cases did not report taking lisinopril weakened that hypothesis. In addition, as a first-line antihypertensive, lisinopril was a very common medication, especially among older people receiving care at the CSS; thus, we did not know if 35% was higher than expected.

The Minister of Health was in a difficult position and under increasing pressure to take some kind of action, despite the fact that he had little information to act upon at this point. Ministry officials were divided over whether to recall the lisinopril. A heated debate ensued during the meeting. The Minister needed to make a decision within the hour in order to prepare an announcement for an evening press conference. The debate was not slowing down and it was obvious that consensus would not occur in time. The Minister turned to Josh and asked, "Dr. Schier, what do you recommend?" The entire room became quiet and everyone turned to Josh and awaited his answer. Josh looked stunned; which amused the Minister whose laughter broke the silence and softened the tension in the room. He was not asking Josh's personal opinion. He wanted expert advice from the CDC. Josh knew this and carefully crafted his response. The descriptive data available at this point did not clearly support lisinopril as the etiology. However, it also did not completely rule it out either. Josh explained to the Minister that there was simply not enough data at this point to use for public health decisions like this one. We would send samples of lisinopril to the U.S. Food and Drug Administration (FDA) to test for purity; however, the immediate decision about whether to recall the lisinopril could not be based on the current available data. The Minister adjourned the meeting so that he could confer with his closest advisors. Later that evening, we watched as he announced a national recall of lisinopril.

Our investigation continued at the CSS hospital. Until this point, all the information we had about the cases was from other sources. We were eager to review charts and examine the patients for ourselves. Dr. James (Jim) Sejvar, the CDC's only neuroepidemiologist was joining the team. Prior to this, Jim had worked on many important public health investigations, including the emergence of West Nile virus in the United States and the emergence of Nipah virus. He had just arrived in Panama and met us at the hospital with our other new team members, Oscar and Miguel. The CSS hospital was a large, busy municipal hospital. It was utilitarian and basic with current facilities. The emergency department appeared full. Patients lined the halls waiting to been seen.

Dr. Nestor Sosa met us at the hospital entrance with his team of Internal Medicine residents. Dr. Sosa and his team were managing the clinical care of the case–patients and had compiled a database of the clinical features. After a brief tour of the hospital, they took us to the bedsides of some of the case–patients. The patients were severely ill and some were medically unstable, needing close monitoring in the intensive care unit. The outbreak was beginning to overwhelm the hospital capacity, particularly the hemodialysis unit.

Upon entering the first case–patient's room, I was struck by the dramatic neurologic impairments. He had the appearance of someone who had a recently suffered a massive stroke with a resultant facial paralysis. With the help of medical residents, we attempted to review case–patients' charts that were in Spanish. Seeing firsthand the severity of this illness magnified my anxiety level; however, it did not put us any closer to identifying the cause.

While Josh helped Jim complete some neurologic tests on the case–patients, Dr. Sosa, Danielle, and I went to a nearby café and discussed our next steps over coffee. Clinical findings seemed most consistent with DEG poisoning, but little was known about DEG poisoning in adults. In addition, there were no readily available diagnostic tests at the CDC or in Panama to measure DEG in people (through serum or urine) in order to confirm that diagnosis. However, tests were available to detect DEG in pharmaceuticals and other products. These tests are widely used for consumer product safety purposes. Agencies that regulate consumer products, such as the U.S. Food and Drug Administration (FDA) have the capacity to test for DEG in products. The CDC laboratory also had this capacity and had used it in previous outbreaks to confirm suspected DEG poisonings.[4] In order to get to that point however, we needed to narrow the possible routes of exposure and shorten the list of potentially contaminated products to test for DEG.

This highlights a common issue related to laboratory confirmation of toxicologic emergencies. The more definitive means of confirming a poisoning is to measure the toxin in a person using human biomarkers of exposure (such as urine and serum tests). However, human biomarkers do not tell us how a person was exposed to the toxin (the route of exposure), which is the critical information needed for interventions to prevent exposures and stop the outbreak.

> Human biomarkers do not tell us how a person was exposed to the toxin (the route of exposure), which is the critical information needed for interventions to prevent exposures and stop the outbreak.

Some biologic and environmental samples from case–patients (including the lisinopril) were en route to the CDC laboratory and FDA for testing. Dr. Sosa agreed to document and obtain samples of any medications, nutrition supplements, and other personal consumables (particularly those in liquid form) from case–patients. In terms of the next step for the epidemiologic investigation, everyone had agreed at the morning meeting with the MOH that the most efficient and appropriate next step was a case–control study. A case–control study design was favored because it could be conducted relatively quickly and multiple exposures could be explored.

The study would be hospital-based at the CSS because all of the case–patients were severely ill, requiring inpatient care, and the majority of cases had received care from this one hospital. Cases were defined as patients who were admitted to the CSS hospital on or after August 15 (one week before the outbreak) with acute

> *Cases were defined as patients who were admitted to the CSS hospital on or after August 15 (one week before the outbreak) with acute renal failure of unknown etiology, characterized by oliguria or anuria and a serum creatinine level ≥ 2mg/dl or with an acute worsening of preexisting chronic renal disease with or without neurologic deficits.*

renal failure of unknown etiology, characterized by oliguria or anuria and a serum creatinine level ≥ 2mg/dl or with an acute worsening of preexisting chronic renal disease with or without neurologic deficits. Neurologic symptoms were not required because the neurologic deficits were often late manifestations that occurred after the initial presentation. Controls were defined as those admitted to the CSS hospital for any cause other than renal failure. For every case–patient, we attempted to enroll, five controls who matched to the case on age (+ 5 years) and date of admission (up to 2 days prior to the case admit date). We chose to match on date of admission so that cases and their matched controls would share the same timeframe and potential for exposure. We administered a questionnaire designed to capture demographic, health, and exposure data. Blood and urine samples from cases and controls were analyzed for a variety of toxic exposures that had potential nephrotoxic and neurotoxic effects.[5]

To do this quickly would require a massive effort. Dr. Sosa secured hospital space and support. An entire first-year medical class had their studies temporarily suspended in order to help interview patients. As we prepared to wrap up the day and return to the hotel, Dr. Sosa expressed his frustration about having so many unanswered questions as people were continuing to die. One of the case–patients was a particular mystery that he could not explain. This patient appeared to have developed the illness while in the hospital. He had multiple chronic medical problems and had been hospitalized for several weeks. Upon admission, he had completely normal renal function, but developed acute renal failure and neurologic dysfunction during his second week in the hospital. Although he had multiple medical problems, none could adequately explain the sudden onset of renal failure or the neurologic disease. A hospital is a controlled environment. How could he possibly be exposed to the toxin causing this outbreak in the hospital? Perhaps he was not a case. After all, his baseline medical status was poor to begin with and there were likely multiple reasons for him to develop additional medical problems. Overwhelmed by all the information we had received over the past 24 hours and the daunting task ahead, my brain did not have room for one more mystery to consider, one more problem to solve.

THE CASE–CONTROL STUDY

After a night of refining, translating, and copying questionnaires and pouring over hospital log sheets to find matched controls among the recent hospital admissions, we arrived at the CSS hospital to begin the case–control investigation. We were now using the delivery entrance at the back of the hospital in order to avoid the press. Media relations had become a major issue with international attention beginning to turn to Panama, prompting a request for high-level CDC assistance. Jana Telfer, associate director for Communication Science for NCEH and the Agency for Toxic Substances and Disease Registry had arrived in Panama to assist the MOH. All media responses would be handled by the MOH and we had been instructed not to answer questions from the press. Nonetheless, reporters often waited for us outside the hospital entrances, so we had to find creative ways to enter without being seen.

A large classroom in the hospital had been converted to a study staging area. The medical students and hospital staff who were going to collect the data were already there, being trained on the study procedures and data collection. At one end of the room, Jay was going over laboratory data collection procedures with the hospital phlebotomists who would be collecting blood samples. At the other end, Danielle and Oscar were reviewing the questionnaire with a group of about 30 bright young medical students. Danielle, Oscar, and I affectionately called them "the kids." They were smart, energetic, and volunteered to do just about anything, from the emotionally challenging (interviewing family members of deceased patients) to the mundane (data entry). We did not know whether their enthusiasm stemmed from the opportunity to be a part of something important or whether they just wanted to prolong their temporary reprieve from the rigors of medical school. Danielle and I suspected that it was probably a little of both.

At this point, we had narrowed our focus to potential exposures that were (a) common to older adults, (b) individualized and not shared household exposures, and (c) potential vehicles for a toxin. However, this still represented a broad range of potential exposures such as medications, personal care products, herbal or folk remedies, and nutrition supplements. Although we had narrowed the scope, ideally we would have more specific hypotheses about the route of exposure to test with the case–control study. It was not optimal, but in reality we did not have other options.

As the teams assembled to begin interviews, I received a call from Dr. Sosa. His residents had just admitted two new case–patients who met the case definition. He noticed that each patient had a bottle of sugar-free cough syrup that they had received from the CSS hospital pharmacy. The medications were identical and even shared the same lot number.

This was the first promising clue. A contaminated cough syrup would fit with DEG exposure. The fact that it was sugar-free would explain the age range and lack of pediatric cases. That it was made by the CSS hospital pharmacy would explain why this hospital system was the focus of the outbreak and even how a hospitalized patient could become exposed.

Jay made arrangements to get the cough syrup and other specimens prepared for shipment to the CDC lab in Atlanta to test for DEG and other contaminants. Josh worked with Carol and Mike in Atlanta to convince the agency to release the CDC plane (which was only used under the most critical circumstances) to fly to Panama to retrieve the samples and carry them back to Atlanta immediately (Figure 27-1).

Danielle, Oscar, and I ran after "the kids" to stop them before they started the interviews and ushered them back to the staging area. They helped with the tedious task of adding some questions by hand to the questionnaires to specifically tease out exposure to cough syrup. The questions included a direct dichotomous (yes/no) question about whether or not the patient consumed prescription cough syrup. We instructed "the kids" not to lead the patients to answers and not to let them know that we suspected the cough syrup. We now had a plausible hypothesis for the exposure and needed objective, unbiased data to either prove or disprove that hypothesis.

THE RESULTS

While we were working around the clock on the case–control study (collecting and analyzing interview data), the CDC laboratory was working around the clock to analyze the cough syrup, other medication samples, and biologic samples from both case–patients and controls that had arrived on the special flight.

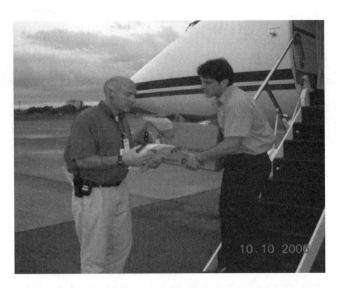

FIGURE 27-1 Team laboratorian, Jay Wamsley and EIS Officer Eduardo Azziz-Baumgartner loading samples onto the CDC plane to ship back to Atlanta for laboratory analysis.

We were entering data when I got a call from Carol on my cell phone. "Hi Lauren, are you somewhere private where we can talk? I have some very important news to share but you have to keep it quiet for now." I rushed to find an isolated corridor that seemed to have little traffic. I sat on the concrete floor, leaning against the wall. I took a deep breath and told Carol, "Go ahead, I am ready."

I listened intently as she explained, "We have some initial laboratory results. The FDA tested the lisinopril for purity. Their analysis confirmed that there were no production errors; the formula was within the expected pharmaceutical parameters and it contained no contaminants. However, test results for the sugar-free cough syrup showed high levels of DEG. In addition, the NCEH lab had been developing a method to detect DEG in people's urine. It also confirmed DEG exposure in the cases."

The Panamanian officials were also being notified, and an official announcement was being planned. I was under strict orders not to share this information with anyone, including "the kids" and my own team members until the official announcement was made. We now had the information needed to interrupt this outbreak and it felt as if the weight of the world had been lifted.

It was impossible to hide my relief, and the tense, worried demeanor I had displayed all week melted away. But, I tempered my joy by reminding myself that this outbreak and the previous DEG poisonings were all completely preventable; and yet they continue to recur.

This was the 11th known mass poisoning from exposure to DEG-contaminated pharmaceuticals and unfortunately it would not be the last (Table 27-1).[2]

Our job still was not complete. We needed results from the case–control study to help identify other risk factors (in addition to consuming the sugar-free cough syrup) that might help guide interventions. When Danielle produced the initial, crude results from the preliminary data analysis, we were all relieved to see that they confirmed the laboratory results. Consuming cough syrup was strongly associated (odds ratio =15.75) with becoming a case. The odds ratio changed a little after additional data cleaning, but was still very high. The final results are presented in Tables 27-2 and 27-3.

Josh communicated these results to Mike and Carol by emailing them a picture of Danielle holding a piece of paper with the number 15.75 (Figure 27-2). It is rare to get such dramatic, definitive results from epidemiologic data produced during an outbreak investigation because of small numbers and other limitations associated with outbreak response.

Epidemiologic data also showed a predominance of older case patients with preexisting renal insufficiency and/or chronic conditions that undermine kidney function, such as hypertension and diabetes. It is plau-

TABLE 27-1 Known mass poisonings from exposure to pharmaceuticals contaminated with diethylene glycol (DEG)

Year	Country	Implicated product	Reported deaths
1937	United States	Sulfanilamide	105
1969	South Africa	Sedatives	7
1985	Spain	Silver sulfadiazine	5
1986	India	Glycerine	21
1990	Nigeria	Acetaminophen	47
1990–1992	Bangladesh	Acetaminophen	236
1992	Argentina	Propolis	29
1996	Haiti	Acetaminophen	88
1998	India	Cough expectorant	33
1998	India	Acetaminophen	8
2006	Panama	Cough syrup	78
2006	China	Armillarisin-A	12
2008	Nigeria	Teething medication	84

TABLE 27-2 Final results of open-ended question asking patients to list prescription medications taken within the past 3 months and the odds ratio for being a case and including cough syrup on the list of medications was calculated.[5]

Response	Cases (N = 42) n (%)	Controls (N = 140) n (%)	Crude odds ratio (95% CI)
Yes = cough syrup included among list of medications	17 (40.5)	4 (2.9)	13.1 (3.92–43.6)
No = cough syrup not included among list of medications	25 (59.5)	136 (97.1)	Referent

TABLE 27-3 Final results of the dichotomous (yes/no) question were added by hand when patients were directly asked whether or not they had consumed prescription cough syrup within the past 3 months and the odds ratio of being a case and consuming prescription cough syrup was calculated.[5]

Response	Cases (N = 42) n (%)	Controls (N = 140) n (%)	Crude odds ratio (95% CI)
Yes = consumed prescription cough syrup	37 (90.2)	29 (20.9)	37.3 (8.82–158)
No = did not consume prescription cough syrup	4 (7.3)	110 (79.1)	Referent

sible that these individuals, who likely had some underlying kidney damage, were more susceptible to the nephrotoxic effects of DEG and, thus, were more likely to become a case. They were also more likely to be prescribed the sugar-free formulation of cough syrup implicated in the outbreak. The data also showed an association between taking lisinopril and becoming a case. This can be explained by the fact that lisinopril was a first-line treatment for hypertension on the CSS medication formulary; thus, it was commonly prescribed to hypertensive patients receiving care at the CSS. It was also specifically indicated to treat hypertension in people at risk for renal disease. Thus, the susceptible persons at risk of becoming a case were also those most likely to be prescribed lisinopril. In addition, lisinopril is known to cause a dry cough. It is likely that the same persons who filled their lisinopril prescriptions at the CSS pharmacy would be prescribed the implicated cough medicine as well.[5]

THE IMPACT

In response to our findings, the Panama MOH immediately initiated a comprehensive effort to interrupt exposure to the contaminated cough syrup and to identify and treat those potentially exposed. The actions taken by the MOH included a recall of more than 60,000 bottles of presumably contaminated cough syrup, an intensive nationwide awareness campaign, and widespread renal function screening for potentially exposed persons.

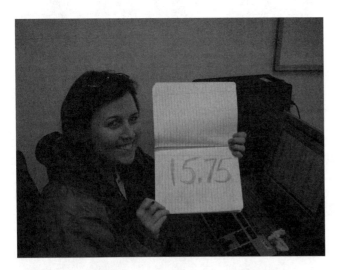

FIGURE 27-2 The photograph of Danielle Rentz holding up the odds ratio of 15.75. This was an exciting moment!

Carol sent several additional epidemiologists from HSB to help the MOH initiate surveillance for new cases. Surveillance data would be needed in order to monitor the status of the outbreak, evaluate the effectiveness of interventions, and allocate resources. FDA officials conducted a traceback investigation and found the source of the DEG. The product, imported from China, had been mislabeled as glycerin and used to make the implicated cough syrup.

In addition to the public health impact, this investigation had a profound personal impact on me as well. Having the opportunity to apply my skills and training in response to a true public health emergency, and contribute to an effort that directly saved lives was exactly why I chose this career path. I already had served in a response capacity for more than 7 amazing years at the CDC; however, this was, without question, the most rewarding experience of my career. As I recalled the picture of Danielle holding up that huge odds ratio, I wondered how starting a career like this must feel. I also worried about how this experience may influence her expectations for the remainder of her training as an EIS officer. Although much of this investigation would mirror others, there were many aspects (like that odds ratio) that she may never see again.

> *In addition to the public health impact, this investigation had a profound personal impact on me as well. Having the opportunity to apply my skills and training in response to a true public health emergency, and contribute to an effort that directly saved lives was exactly why I chose this career path.*

THE EXIT

We had finished our reports to the MOH and supervisors in Atlanta, so the team had nothing left to do but relax and enjoy each others company. We sat by the hotel pool trying to figure out how we could possibly attend all the farewell events to which we had been invited. We had received social invitations from everyone, from "the kids" and the CSS hospital staff to the Minister of Health (further evidence of the gracious Panamanian culture). We were particularly excited about the official government reception that was being planned. We were told that the President of Panama might make an appearance to personally thank us for our assistance. It would be my first time meeting a president.

Back in my hotel room, I turned on the television and caught a glimpse of myself on Spanish CNN. I had never seen myself on television and called my family to share the excitement. They were not impressed. My son had even more exciting news to share. His baseball team had won their game that day and would be playing in the championship game of the local park league on Friday. He asked if I would be there and I told him that I would try. The reception with the President was on Friday and I was scheduled to leave on Saturday. I could easily change my flight to leave earlier and make the game, but it would mean missing the reception and I may never get the opportunity to meet a president again. In the end, I changed my flight and missed the reception, but made it home in time for the championship game. My son's team won the championship and I was happy to be there to see them do it.

LEARNING QUESTIONS

1. Review the information in reference 1 and describe the 1937 mass poisoning from diethylene glycol. Explain why this outbreak was so historically significant.
2. During the outbreak, an antihypertensive medication, lisinopril, was suspected as being the cause of the unexplained illnesses and deaths. Review the adverse effects information for lisinopril (just as the Ministry of Health official had likely done) (Exhibit 27-2). Then, consider the information you would want to have in front of you if you were responsible for deciding if there should be a recall of lisinopril. Keep in mind that if a recall had turned out to be unwarranted, it could have caused adverse economic and health consequences, and could have ultimately led to one or more lawsuits against the Ministry of Health.
3. Why was lisinopril suspected as the cause of the outbreak early on? Why did the investigators decide this was not a strong hypothesis?
4. The laboratory investigation conducted in response to this outbreak included analysis of human biomarkers of exposure (urine and serum tests) and analysis of environmental samples (including analysis of lisinopril and cough syrup). Discuss the roles and limitations of both approaches in laboratory confirmation of toxicologic emergencies.
5. Exposure to cough syrup was captured by two questions: (a) an open-ended question asking patients to list prescription medications taken within the past 3 months; and (b) a dichotomous (yes/no) question added by hand when patients were directly asked whether or not they had consumed prescription cough syrup within the past 3 months. Review and compare the data in Tables 27-2 and 27-3. Compare the results for each question and interpret the difference in the odds ratio between the two sets of results. Describe the potential factors driving this difference.

REFERENCES

1. Wax PM. Elixirs, diluents, and the passage of the 1938 Federal Food, Drug and Cosmetic Act. *Ann Intern Med*. 1995; 122(6):456–461. http://www.annals.org/content/122/6/456.long. Accessed January 17, 2010.
2. Schep LJ, Slaughter RJ, Temple WA, Beasley DM. Diethylene glycol poisoning. *Clin Toxicol*. 2009;47(6):525–535.
3. US Department of State. Background note: Panama. US Department of State Web site. http://www.state.gov/r/pa/ei/bgn/2030.htm#. Updated December 30, 2009. Accessed January 17, 2010.
4. Barr DB, Barr JR, Weerasekera G, et al. Identification and quantification of diethylene glycol in pharmaceuticals implicated in poisoning epidemics: an historical laboratory perspective. *J Anal Toxicol*. 2007;31(6):295–303.
5. Rentz ED, Lewis L, Mujica OJ, et al. Outbreak of acute renal failure in Panama in 2006: a case–control study. *Bull World Health Organ*. 2008;86(10):737–816.

CHAPTER 28

"We're Prepared to Believe You"—Investigating Cancer Cluster Reports

Tim E. Aldrich, PhD, MPH

INVESTIGATING CANCER CLUSTERS—BACKGROUND AND HISTORY

I am now one of the old hands, but when I began, there were already some old hands. Cancer clusters appeared in people's imagination perhaps a decade after World War II. It is noteworthy that this was a period of proliferation of chemical technology, as well as the emergence of cancer from behind a veil of secrecy. Yes, for years people spoke of cancer in hushed tones and sawmill whispers. The disease terrified the U.S. public, in part because cancer risk was associated with survivors of the atomic bombing in Japan. It terrified people because the prognosis was so dire, and it was not unusual for people to die within weeks of their diagnosis. Finally, part of the horror associated with cancer was the common phrase "the cancer had eaten them up." Such grotesque vernacular conjured horrific images, and the dismal prognosis hardened one's mind toward the disease.

Percivall Pott was a British physician in the late 18th century. He investigated a famous cluster of testicular cancer among chimney sweeps in London, but the earliest reports of cancer clusters in recent times appeared in the late 1950's (Appendix 1). Those early reports tended to focus on leukemia and children. Another urban legend of that period was the concept of *cancer houses*. That is where a series of successive residents contracted cancer. The renowned Dr. Abraham Lilienfeld of Johns Hopkins wrote one of the first books on cancer epidemiology, and he spoke of both of these attributes for cancer clusters.[1]

More cluster reports came to light in the early 1960's. In 1965, the National Cancer Institute convened a national conference to consider space–time clusters of cancer.[2] Legendary epidemiologist Dr. Alexander Langmuir of the CDC was one of the speakers. He made two quips that I believe are indicative of the conventional wisdom in those times.

> While I don't play poker often, I do know that four-of-a-kind can be beaten by a straight flush. But, when I draw four-of-a-kind, I am going to bet on it.

The constructive approach to this situation, in my opinion is not to develop highly refined statistical techniques to determine whether or not a certain cluster might have resulted by chance alone. But, rather to investigate each cluster as it is reported and see if additional associations of possible interest can be found. If none turn up, there is obviously a cold trail, and any good hunting dog will abandon it and go look for a better one. If the scent strengthens, then hot pursuit is in order.

It was on the heels of those remarks in the 1960s that Dr. Langmuir established the first *cluster busters* at the CDC. Drs. Clark Heath and Glenn Caldwell were the premier investigators of cancer cluster reports that made their way to the national center. In their 1976 paper, Caldwell and Heath discussed several of their earliest investigations.[3] From a U.S. perspective, the investigation of cancer clusters began in Niles Illinois, in 1963, with a series of leukemia cases in a parochial school. Similar pediatric leukemia clusters were reported a year later in England.

Over the next decade, many things happened that promoted the public concern about cancer clusters. One of these was the publication of Rachel Carson's novel, *Silent Spring*.[4] It spoke of the devastating effects of chlorinated hydrocarbon pesticides on eggshell formation for birds, leading to fewer surviving birds to sing the joys of new birth in the spring. It gripped many American's imaginations. Another milestone was the national visibility given to the toxic contamination at Love Canal, New York.[5] Other clusters of historic renown were reported from Woburn, Massachusetts[a] and Triana, Alabama. A common culprit of these sensational episodes were "chemicals" and the biologic plausibility of hydrocarbon-based carcinogens left the door wide open for public speculation and rising fears.

The pattern of federal legislation in these years reflects the priority concerns of the American people: 1969–Environmental Protection Act, 1970–Occupational Safety and Health Act, and 1971–War on Cancer Act.[6] I came onto the scene in 1972, as the Comprehensive Cancer Center at the University of Alabama, Birmingham (UAB) was established in February 1972. Each of these first 10 nationally designated cancer centers included an epidemiology service in their core structure. At UAB, this assignment came to my mentor, Dr. Herman Lehman. He had one funded "position," which was designated for a graduate assistant—fortune brought that inaugural designation to me. Dr. Lehman knew of my fascination with cancer. It was a driving force in my career aspirations, primarily because of my father's death from lung cancer when I was 4 years old in 1955, and my hearing of the illusive "cure for cancer" for years. These cancer centers were tasked to train new cancer epidemiologists because a national assessment of these "disease detective" specialists, conducted by the imminent Dr. Lilienfeld, reported that there were only 12 such professionals in the United States.

I experienced my first cancer cluster investigation in 1973. It involved three sisters (close next-door neighbors in a very rural area of northeastern Alabama), who each died of liver cancer. A familial predisposition was not without possibility, yet the technology of those days did not support an investigation of genetic traits as today's technology might. So, we turned our attention to environmental factors; that was the prevailing "theory" for cancer clusters in those days. This experience fixed in my mind two sentinel attributes associated with cancer clusters: a minimum of three cases, and a rare disease (Exhibit 28-1). It was in these years that I first learned of Clark Heath and Glenn Caldwell, and their amazing 23-year thrill ride across the nation in search of that illusive "strengthening scent" that Langmuir had iconized. My imagination was captured and my own 35-year pilgrimage as a "cluster buster" began. I wrote my MPH thesis on the topic: "A Search for Cancer Clusters." My fascination with cancer clusters also figured intensely with my doctoral studies. By 1982–1985, I had performed some 120 cancer cluster investigations; I had published a bit, and had decided that Dr. Langmuir was wrong. Statistical methods were, in fact, the key to investigating cancer clusters, and to ferreting out those gems of nature that had meaning. I believe that Dr. Langmuir might have viewed statistical evaluation of cancer clusters differently if he had experienced the exposure

---

EXHIBIT 28-1 Suggested criteria for suspecting a cancer cluster report is meaningful

The following criteria might suggest that a cancer cluster report is meaningful:[15,26]

- at least three cases of the same type
- cases of a very rare cancer (e.g., incidence less than 10/100,000)
- a literature-based suspected risk of 5-fold
- occurrence in a short period of time (e.g., 5 years or less)
- a credible, proposed environmental hazard

---

[a] In 1998, the story of the Woburn cancer cluster was made into a movie titled *A Civil Action* starring John Travolta. The scene of the lake catching on fire was a true event and spectacular in legend.

to statistical methods that were published in years subsequent to his earlier remarks, and if he had computer technology and geographic information systems (GIS) used in public health today.

Fast forward to the early 1990's. I was nearing 200 cancer cluster investigations now, only two or three of which I regarded as *bona fide*, or meaningful.[7,8] But, I was about to begin an amazing series. In the next decade, I would have the occasion to investigate clusters of birth defects, cystic fibrosis, multiple sclerosis, lupus, amyotrophic lateral sclerosis (ALS), and even one small cluster of leprosy. Cancer is not the only disease suspected of clustering, and sometimes "cluster busters" have skills that private citizens seek when they find no other place to report their concern. In the early 1990's, there were no geographic information systems used with public health; there were only two or three statistical software packages for testing case-clustering, and only 19 population-based cancer registries in the United States. I will relate three cancer cluster reports to draw you along to the emergence of the current state-of-the-art cancer cluster studies.

A FAIR CLUSTER INVESTIGATION

In 1990, I was working at an Atlantic Coast Conference college. A cancer cluster call came to the state cancer registry and then it made its way to my desk. When I spoke with the woman who placed the call, I was prepared with paper and pen to record her comments. She began by explaining that she lived in a community some 90 miles to the northeast of my location, near the neighboring state border. She said she was concerned by the number of brain cancers that she was hearing about, and that her husband was recently diagnosed with this type of tumor. I took details of dates and directions to various locations. I asked her what she thought might be a risk factor in common for these cancers.

"It's the chicken shit," she said. I suppressed my laughter, but smiled to myself.

"Excuse me," I said, expecting my smile was in my voice, "but did you say 'chicken shit'?"

"Yep! There are chicken houses all around here, and the folks just pile the chicken shit in big stacks all around. I expect it runs into the water; most of us out here are on wells. And when it dries, it blows around in clouds, and it stinks to high heaven." Clearly she was a bit agitated.

"Do you have a chicken farm near your home?" I inquired.

"Yes," her voice was rising, distress apparent. "It's right next door. Their chicken shit mound is next to our fence. We had to move the clothes line, and the flies drive us crazy!"

I explained that I understood. I had learned the lesson about laughing at far-fetched ideas related to cancer clusters from just such a character-building sort of *faux pas* in my Florida years (12 years earlier) when I scoffed at the idea of electromagnetic fields (power lines) and cancer risk. On that occasion, I rapidly found evidence in the professional literature that this was at least being researched.[9]

I explained to the caller that in our state, the cluster investigation protocol would involve my sending her a letter to confirm that her cluster report was received and would be investigated. I also explained that cluster reports were studied in the order received, so it might be a few months until we could begin our investigation. I indicated that when we began, I would be pleased to visit the community to talk with folks about what we would do, and then when the investigation was completed, she would receive a written report of the findings. At that latter time, if the community wished, I would return and discuss our work and results with them. She seemed satisfied with this arrangement. I said that in the meantime, I would mail her a dozen questionnaires. It would be a great help to our efforts if she could distribute these to the families of the brain cancer cases, and have them completed and returned to me. I emphasized that the forms included a part that asked permission to review medical records, and that signing the form was completely optional; the person could complete the form, and leave anything blank that they did not want to answer. The process was all voluntary, and we were required to keep all information we received confidential within the state's cancer cluster advisory committee. She said she understood.

About confidentiality with regard to cancer clusters or other cluster investigations, note that in these years (the early 1990's), there was no Health Insurance Portability and Accountability Act (HIPAA), nor as much apprehension about internal review board (IRB) procedures. These sorts of considerations would arise in later years, and many states have their cancer cluster protocol reviewed and approved by an IRB. However, in those days, because I was working as a designated state health department investigator, I was "covered" by the state laws indicating that the health department should investigate health hazards. And, my collection data was "covered" by the state's disease reporting law that said the health department could define which diseases were reportable. Today, many state-based cancer cluster busters are similarly "covered" by their state laws regarding patient privacy; HIPAA specifically has an exemption for public health investigations.

Let me say that this cluster investigation was an absolute prototype experience of that time period. There was a system in place, the community was cooperative, and the process seemed to go without a flaw. I mailed the letter and the forms, after recording the cluster report in the state's log of cluster reports. At this point, our state did not have a full-time cluster buster, but that would change in a few years. I was whittling along on my teaching and research for about 5 months, from April to December, before this cluster came up for investigation. In that elapsed time, two interesting things had happened.

First, our state was assigned a CDC Epidemic Intelligence Service (EIS) officer.[10] The EIS was established by Dr. Alex Langmuir and it became the principal training ground for state epidemiologists for decades. The program accepted mainly persons with professional degrees, especially male physicians in the early years. Then a few veterinarians began to come through the annual class of 30 or so positions (now grown to at least twice that number). Today, about half the class are PhDs (There are many colleges of public health now; when EIS began, there were only a handful.); and about half of EIS appointees are now women. Each EIS officer receives a summer training curriculum. Then, the officer is sent to (1) a state, large city, county, or territorial health department or (2) a federal program for a 2-year training experience in applied field epidemiology. In these 2 years, the EIS officers have a set of prescribed tasks to perform, using the local resources. Among these tasks is the performance of an evaluation of a surveillance system and the performance of an epidemiologic investigation and data analysis. Our young man was also using a brain cancer cluster report for his required assignment. The geographic area for his study was one for which hospitals serving the region were performing exceptionally well in submitting incidence data to the new cancer registry, and it did have a "generally" elevated rate of brain cancer, about 1.8-fold the state's rate. He would do a very fine job. For me, this meant that there was someone handy to discuss brain cancer and to relate to for the period of the chicken investigation.

The second event was a sobering phone call. The call was from a basic science researcher at a highly prestigious, medical research center nearby. This scientist was studying viruses and brain cancer. He said that he had heard that we were going to investigate the cluster in the county the woman had called from. I affirmed this intention. He said that he just wanted to be sure that I didn't scoff at the implication of the avian (chicken) risk factor. He pointed out that his laboratory research used mammalian systems (probably rats or mice, I thought; it turned out to be dogs), as compared to tissue cultures or cloned cell lines. He explained to me that in order to induce brain tumors in their test animals, they infected them with Rous avian sarcoma virus. That was enough to get my attention. I knew a bit about that virus. He explained that this virus, in mammalian systems, produces brain tumors. For his research, they then tried experimental treatments to reduce the animals' tumors.

> *He explained to me that in order to induce brain tumors in their test animals, they infected them with Rous avian sarcoma virus. That was enough to get my attention.*

I sat for a moment, looking out my window. A group of pigeons were perched on a nearby rooftop. My mind returned to a lecture years earlier, when I was in graduate school and learning cancer epidemiology. The topic had been immunology; we were being instructed about the body's defense systems, specifically white blood cells. At that time, a dramatic breakthrough had been published describing T and B cells. Their distinct functions in the body's defense were incredible, and convinced me (one of many times as I studied cancer epidemiology) that a Divine mind must have guided the construction of human anatomy and physiology. As the lecture unfolded, our professor described a pivotal discovery in the progression of research. This discovery was made in chickens, and it was a gland called the bursa of Fabricius. The bursa was analogous to the thymus in humans; it was one of the three critical tissues that "seeds" the immature immune system with progenitor white blood cells. The appendix and tonsils are the other two tissues that serve this role in humans. After this developmental function, these tissues are vestigial (that is, they just hang around with no apparent use). For the appendix and tonsils, we know that they butt their way into infections and often have to be removed.

In chickens, the bursa is located near their cloacae (anus). The avian researcher, Rous, discovered the enlargement of the bursa (literally sack) in chickens with sarcomas (soft tissue masses) that were infected with a specific virus. His study of the virus and its effect on chickens was a fundamental depiction of immunologic function that informed human studies for decades. I was later to learn that there is no record of avian sarcoma virus ever jumping species to mammals. This information reached me from the poultry industry during our brain cancer cluster investigation. This industry is keenly aware of the virus and monitors its distribution in commercial flocks in the United States and most developed countries. During this cluster investigation, I learned more about the U.S. poultry industry than I really preferred.

When the time came for us to begin the cluster investigation (that is, it came up on our list as the next report to study), I pulled out the file. I had not recalled, but the questionnaires were completed and returned. There were eight of them; one case family declined to respond. I looked at a computer printout of brain cancer cases from our cancer registry and saw that this county had a total of 16 brain cancers, including seven others during the 5-year period of the nine questionnaire reports (all of the reports were in the cancer registry files). Hmmm, a quick calculation showed that the county should have had about seven cases if the statewide, expected rate had occurred in this community. That is 2.3 times the expected number; without these extra nine cases, the other seven observed cases would have been right on the expected number.

Generally speaking, in cancer cluster investigations, besides the magic number of three tumors of the same type, we prefer to see risk values in the 5.0 or higher magnitude. Measured risk values between 1.0 (no risk) and 2.5 are considered small and are generally viewed with skepticism. From 2.5 to 5.0, we say it's a judgment call. Things the cluster buster takes into account are the type of cancer (rare, common, exotic), the population involved (e.g., old, young, one gender), and the presence of a credible postulated risk exposure. I was going to investigate the cluster report in any case, but the amount of time and effort I would invest was influenced by these sorts of considerations.

In the letter sent to me with the questionnaires was a request that I speak to the community residents before the investigation began. I called the local health department (a standard procedure), described the information I had, and asked about meeting locations. The health department director was a wonderful woman; she had heard of the cluster report (it was a small, rural community after all) and she volunteered their meeting room. As it turned out, this was a newly constructed health department building, and it proved to be a splendid setting for this session. The director and I settled on a day and time (a week-day, and early evening is usual for community meetings). I called the woman who had first reported the cluster and told her of the plans. She said she would contact the local newspaper with the announcement, and contact each of the brain cancer case families. I pointed out that there were more than the cases she knew about, and agreed that the newspaper was a good idea. We hung-up, both satisfied that the ball was rolling.

The appointed time was 3 weeks later. I took my mother with me to the meeting. I often used these trips to spend time with her or my children. It was a lovely day, and I enjoyed the rural, farm scenery. Crops were mid-size and brilliantly green. I noted the high voltage power lines as we approached the health department—a particular interest of mine. We arrived about an hour early and set up the 35mm projector and screen. I arrayed educational materials the state health department had developed about cancer clusters, and pamphlets about brain cancers from both the American Cancer Society and the National Cancer Institute. When I left, I was amused that every single document was taken by the attendees.

About 30 folks attended; nearly all were adults. The health director introduced me, and I rose and gave my spiel. My prepared remarks took about 15 minutes, by design. I spoke about cancer clusters in general and about cancer in broad terms. I described the steps we would take, and the projected time course of 1 to 3 months before we would report back. Then, I lifted a notepad and asked for questions or comments. There were several of each. I made notes, most to be ignored, but when one older gentleman began to rant about the chicken guano, I realized the community was sensitized to this factor. Another kindly older man spoke up in my defense and called the speaker by name, "Let the boy finish his work before you get all riled up." I was amused about being called a boy, and I later learned my defender was the only MD in the county.

We began our work, which included mapping. Geographic information systems were still 3 to 4 years from bursting onto the scene, but I had several colleagues at the university who were topflight spatial statisticians. We needed a basis for describing the population distribution to evaluate the grouping of all 16 cases' residences. At this time, it was between population censuses, and the county was virtually all sparsely populated. We settled on using election districts, and voter registrations for weighting the districts. One of my colleagues, Roger Grimson, was the developer of a splendid analytic method for determining the random occupancy of the units by cancer cases in a series of contiguous spatial units (24 election districts in our case).[11] The analytic method was not automated yet, but with only 24 spatial units and 16 cases, the calculations only took us about 3 hours and a six-pack to do. We then assigned the "repeat of the calculation" task to a pair of industrious graduate students, as we waited to see if the intricate, repetitious computations would show the same result. To the delight of myself and my friend, it did!

I then applied another half dozen other cluster analysis solutions; this was not the same day…the beer was gone. In a week, I had five of six statistical tests that said this clustering of up to nine of the 16 total cases was not random. In order to obtain a distance metric for the spatial analyses, I copied a grid onto my map using a drafting, cross-hatched page. Some of the statistical methods utilized the distances between cases for analysis.[12,13] Another used the case characteristics, including race (all white), gender (about evenly split), age (one child), and space and time.[14]

The whole investigation took about 1 month of actual personal effort, but with teaching classes, the end of the school year, and a family vacation, a total of 5 months or so had elapsed. I had read the medical records of the cases who gave me permission to do so. I had a limited amount of very useful information on all 16 cases from the cancer registry. It was my decision to include all of the brain tumors, and not simply those shown to be malignant. Our registry was one of very few that collected benign brain tumors.

The dispute regarding studying only malignant versus including benign tumors was a thorny one. Some folks argued that including nonmalignant tumors with a "cancer" study would compromise the biologic integrity of the research; that is, benign tumors are technically not regarded as malignant neoplasms, that is, cancer. Others argued that benign brain masses were just as fatal and as difficult to treat as the malignant ones. The clinching point for me was that very often brain tumors were rapidly fatal and it was common to have a person decline rapidly after the diagnosis, and die before treatment could have any benefit. This meant that for many poor and "conservative" families, their loved one would die before a determination was made of malignant or benign. Conservatism plays in because they would not permit an autopsy. I didn't quibble. I took all the cases; 12 were deceased. My final justification for using all cancers was that the citizens reporting the cluster had not made a distinction of malignant versus benign or unspecified. In instances where cancer cases are found to be misclassified, e.g., the citizen regards the cancer as "lung" when, in fact, the lung disease is metastatic and the primary site is the colon, I would correct that misunderstanding.

The findings were impressive. The nine "cluster" cases were part of a tightly grouped aggregate, residing in two adjacent election districts (Figure 28-1). To my analytic judgment, the nine cluster cases were comprised of two expected cases and seven "extra" ones. The remaining cases were dispersed across the county, with no more than two brain cancers in any election district. When I mapped the power lines, industries, and chicken farms, the intercept was compelling. The high voltage power lines did run through the two election districts, but they also ran across the county. There was no industry nearby *per se*. The two large factories were near the interstate and the river, on the western edge of the county. But the chicken farms—well that was another matter. There were nine chicken farms in the county—seven in these two election districts; the other two were not far away (Figure 28-2).

Summer came, and I took vacation in June. Then, when I called the woman who had made the cancer cluster report, she asked me to delay the second community meeting until "after the harvest." I did not tell her my findings or interpretation. But, I did speak with the health director and local physician about them. I sent both of them my preliminary report that would only be finalized after the town meeting. I had discussed the findings with our cancer cluster advisory committee. No one laughed at the chicken guano hypothesis, and their directions to me were unanimous.

I am proud of this cluster investigation, and what followed. My only regret is that I was over an hour late for the fall meeting. I was delayed leaving, and called the woman and the health director to alert them I would be 15–30 minutes late. On the way, traffic snarls unexpectedly impeded driving time as well; I called again to change my delay to 45 minutes to an hour and asked if the folks would like to reschedule. The health department director called back and said everyone was "just fine, come on." Finally, when we got close to the health department (my mother and one of my sons were with me), I missed my turn and became thoroughly lost. I was 75 minutes behind the scheduled start time. As I walked in, the room was full. No one sniped or called to me, they just waited.

I began to organize things, as my son set up the projector and screen. I showed 10 slides, four that were from the analysis. My concluding statement was, "My friends, this observation of excess brain cancer cases is a genuine cluster." No sounds. I went on, "However, in

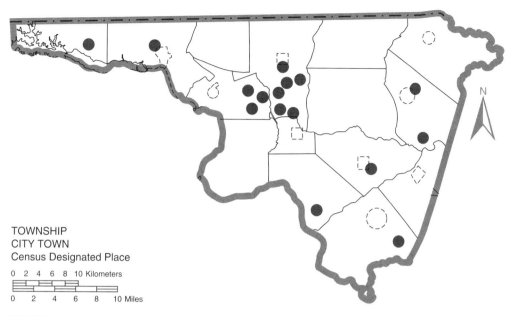

FIGURE 28-1 Map of the brain cancer cases, and the election districts used for analysis. The dotted-line figures signify towns.

this rural area, with so few cases, I cannot properly investigate the risks that are implied for this cluster." It is the standard form with such a finding to move to a different location, which has not already been studied as a result of a cluster report, and to conduct a case–control study. I explained a bit about what was involved with a case–control study, including a sample size of 80–100 cases and a duration of 1–2 years.

I had explored possibly doing blood testing for the Rous virus in the chickens and/or residents. The cost of the analyses was exorbitant, and even the friendly researcher could not lower his cost much. A representative of the American Poultry Association had explained to me that they did routine sampling of flocks, including these. While they would not provide me with the results of their tests, they indicated that like virtually every flock in the world, these were positive for the virus, and they gave me the specific substrains that they had found. But, the poultry industry continually monitors their workforce, especially for "related" diseases. The workers handle much more than just the guano of the birds; they handle blood, feathers, and residual tissues after slaughter. They clearly have the greatest exposure to potential virus infections. So far, no elevated rates of cancer, specifically of sarcomas, or any other disease had been noted. This was all in my report, but I spoke very little of it to the community because I believed these sorts of consideration were the ones I was expressly responsible for evaluating and, unless I believed they were relevant to the report cluster, they might simply confuse the community. In our written report, I did speak to the paucity of sarcomas in the community as part of my reasoning of the biologic plausibility of the cluster report.

There were no questions. I was dismayed. However, after the close of things, several folks came up to shake my hand, thank me for the investigation, and say they had not minded waiting at all because my talk was well

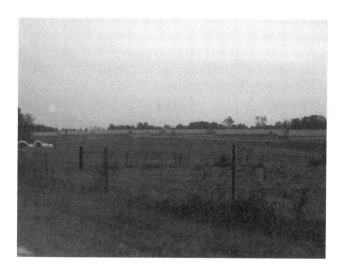

FIGURE 28-2 Photograph of a chicken farm surrounded by barbed wire.

> However, after the close of things, several folks came up to shake my hand, thank me for the investigation, and say they had not minded waiting at all because my talk was well worth the wait. I was always a proponent of the service owed to private citizens by the public health profession, but this response humbled me deeply.

worth the wait. I was always a proponent of the service owed to private citizens by the public health profession, but this response humbled me deeply.

Only about half of the copies of the report I had brought along were taken. I have never heard from this community again. It was nearly 2 years before I was able to conduct the promised case–control study, but the report from that study (which is described later in this chapter), including the eventually published journal article, was sent to the woman who asked for the cluster investigation, to the local physician, and to the county health department.

This sort of follow-up to a cancer cluster is one of only two recourses for a "meaningful" cancer cluster (Figure 28-3).[15,16] Most cluster reports (about 80%) are "dead ends." About 15–17% of cluster reports are found to be "real" (that is, there is an excess of cancer cases, and/or evidence of clustering), but no real implications of what might explain it are found.[17] These sorts of "real" cluster reports are generally kept under ongoing surveillance (that is, the occurrence of cancer in the community is studied again, each year, for 2–5 years) to see if the "elevated" pattern of cancer risk continues (Figure 28-4). This process is highly productive for identifying the random statistical phenomena that often prompt cluster reports. But, it is that tiny residual of 2–5% of cluster reports that are "real" (statistically credible) and meaningful (they lead to a biologically plausible association) that lead to follow-up studies as this one did.

A VERY GOOD CANCER CLUSTER INVESTIGATION

The phone rang; it was a colleague whose office was down the hall from mine. He was with a doctoral student who wanted to work with a cancer cluster for his field experience requirement, and he asked whether he could send him down to talk with me. I replied affirmatively, and the young man showed up at my door shortly. David was a redhead covered in freckles. He was in our DrPH program (that is, Doctor of Public Health); this is a practice-based degree that requires students to perform professional activities in the field as part of their course of study. The DrPH is contrasted to the PhD degree that is given in a public health discipline, like statistics or epidemiology. The PhD degree is generally awarded to individuals who wish to do research or teach for their career. For completeness, let me say that Public Health curricula also have two versions of the master's degree as well, the M.P.H., and the M.S.P.H. Essentially, these degrees have the same professional connotation as their doctorate versions; one is practice oriented and the other is science-directed. I spoke with David about the current cluster investigation at what was called the Watts Retreat; we made plans to visit the community in a week's time.

The Watts Retreat is a federal superfund site. The Comprehensive Environmental Response, Compensation, and Liability Act of 1980 (also known as CERCLA or "Superfund") specified that companies handling hazardous materials were required to pay for the cleanup of those sites. A fund was created for "orphaned" sites, and this was the basis for the term. The listing of a waste site as "superfund" meant that the Environmental Protection Agency or the Agency for Toxic Substances and Disease Registry had done an assessment of the site (the involved agency depends if the assessment was completed before or after 1987).[18] The publicly available assessment described the site and its contents (they used corporate purchasing and manufacturing manifests for this purpose), and presented information regarding surrounding communities and the potential (or description of) migration of the contamination off the site. I had read the health assessment before I met with David; it was one of the things that I had given him to read before our trip.

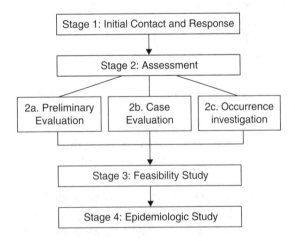

FIGURE 28-3 CDC protocol for investigating clusters of adverse health.

■ A Very Good Cancer Cluster Investigation 357

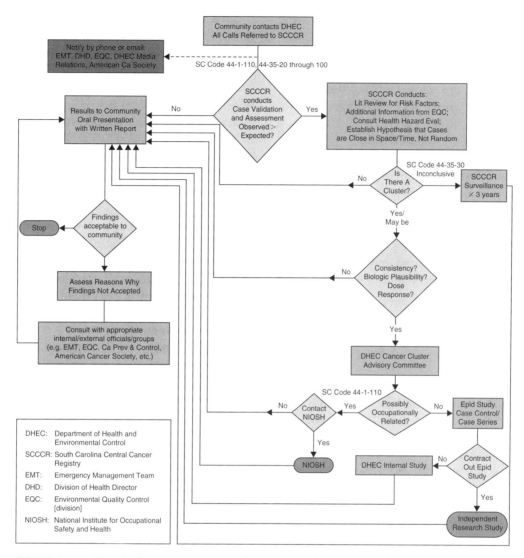

FIGURE 28-4 South Carolina protocol for cancer cluster investigations. Prepared by: SC Central Cancer Registry, Office of Public Health Statistics & Information Services, Department of Environmental Health and Control (DHEC), 7/19/2000

Watts Retreat is an old home place (that is, it contained an abandoned residence) in the foothills of the Appalachian Mountains. The son of the former landholders was a physician. As a profit-making venture, the good doctor began to purchase medical and chemical waste (and purportedly radioactive waste, but this was not verified) from hospitals that needed to dispose of the waste, but could not send it to public dumps. Dr. Watt's actions in the late 1960's occurred long before there were regulations concerning hazardous waste disposal or reporting the handling of hazardous waste. The Resource Conservation and Recovery Act of 1976 had begun the process of tracking hazardous waste in the United States, but two more federal bills were needed in 1980 and 1986 to actually get the process going. The Watts Retreat site was the oldest of the identified waste disposal sites in our state. The citizenry had learned of the site eventually (it was rather secluded), and with the rising population over time, someone eventually registered concern about it when he or she became sensitized to the number of cancers among the neighbors.

The Watts Retreat cancer cluster report was a longstanding one. Investigation of the Watts Farm site had predated my arrival at this community by a couple of years. The community had been visited by a state health department epidemiologist a few years earlier; the gentleman managed to thoroughly infuriate the local residents. Their voicing of umbrage to elected officials and the governor was acerbic because of their affront at his brusque and elitist manner. He also managed to berate and frustrate the local health department leaders, who also registered their outrage. Regrettably, this was not an unusual experience for cancer cluster follow-ups in many states before there was a systematic protocol for responding to cluster reports, and before there was broadly distributed public health training on responding to citizens. It is likely unnecessary to say that this fellow and I were not comfortable in each other's company, because I saw the "public" as an accountable audience for our profession and I was requested to "clean up" his mess.

I had spoken in advance to the local health department administrator, who said that I absolutely should come prepared for anger and poor regard, and he would not defend me if the citizens responded that way; he had caught too much gruff for the previous visit "by the state." I explained that I understood the situation and that I would endeavor to soothe the ruffled citizenry, and would keep him copied on all activities and actions. He calmed down a bit, and said he would not attend the public meeting, but would send one of his staff. I thanked him for his time.

I spoke with the person who had made the original cluster report; she was quite hostile, but accepted my apology and promise to do better by their concerns. Before she convened another community meeting, she insisted that she wanted to meet with me and a few select citizens. I agreed. It was this meeting that our doctoral student, David, and I would attend at her home.

David and I drove up to the lovely mountain home at 10:00 a.m., as invited. We were greeted by the home owner, ushered into the living room, and introduced to four folks already present. These were simple people, all middle age or older; they were clearly skeptical of us, being from the state health department. They were reserved and quiet, and sat in furniture placed across from the sofa where David and I were directed to sit. What I am about to describe to you about this meeting has a relationship to the designation, "cluster buster." The nickname "cluster buster" was first given after the movie *Ghostbusters* (with Bill Murray and Dan Ackroyd) was popularized in 1984. The movie's slogan was "We're prepared to believe you." Cluster busters was a derogative term applied to folks like me, who offered to believe what citizens told them about cancer clustering in communities. After receiving a glass of tea, showing our identification, and describing ourselves a bit, I asked our hostess to tell me about her concerns for a cancer risk from the Watts Retreat site. David and I had brought notepads and I had alerted him that we needed to be prepared to listen to these people for a good while. She started…

It was nearly 1:00 p.m. before David and I left her home. Besides the hostess, everyone there had spoken to us at some length. Then, the host and hostess took us downstairs to their basement, where they had an office. The walls were lined with maps, pictures, and lists that were part of their own investigation of the Watts Retreat site. I was quite amazed. It was crude, but evidenced much effort, long hours, and a great attention to detail. I praised the couple for their efforts, and commented on the high quality of the materials. I then asked for two things: one was a few maps of the site; the other was someone to guide us there. With one map, I asked the citizens to mark and initial where they thought the cancer cases were clustered in relation to the site. All six of them did so, and the consensus was that the risk was downstream from the site, along a small river that flowed below the hill on which the old home site was located. I wrote my name and the date on the map, and gave it back to our hostess. I took an identical map, and signed and dated again. I told them I would return this second map, with our results on it.

Time was passing; our hostess served us a lunch of sandwiches upstairs, as the other citizens discussed our plans in the basement. Shortly, the folks joined us at the kitchen table and indicated that one of their group would ride with us to the site. Further, they had decided to accept our offer to hold a town meeting before we began work. They selected a date in 2 weeks time. They would notify us of the exact location and time.

Our guide was an older gentleman who told us a variety of stories as we drove through the scenic valleys and along back roads. Mainly, he recounted the population growth in the community, and when the highway came through, he disparaged all the newcomers and the congestion they made in restaurants and stores. Before our departure, the hostess had called the local health department's office of Environmental Health and asked for one of their staff to meet us with keys to get onto the site. After a short time, we were driving beside a shallow river, about 30 feet wide, with its rocky bottom visible to us. We were directed across a bridge and climbed a slight incline. On our right was a large home place, with well tended grass, but a clearly unoccupied white house. There were fruit trees in rows with cattle grazing underneath, and an outbuilding was visible at the rear of the orchard. Our guide directed us to turn up the driveway and drive past the house. There sat an official looking truck, with a fellow standing beside it.

Now, I could see the outbuilding was a sheet-metal construction, surrounded by a 10-foot fence with barbed wire running along its top. This was the Watts Retreat federal hazardous waste site. The Environmental Health official greeted our guide by name, but examined and recorded our identifying documents. He declined my request to take some photographs, as he opened a padlock upon an enormous chain that was twined around the fence gate.

Inside, I would say that the enclosed area was about an acre. To the left was a grass-covered mound, with half-a-dozen monitoring wells visible. Seeing my glance, the environmental officer commented that there were monitoring wells in tiers, descending to the river, and along the river. He said they were checked after each "big rain" and/or monthly. A monitoring well is just a large pipe, pushed into the earth to a specific depth. The buried end of the pipe has holes bored into it so that water can collect in the pipe from the specific depth. The pipes are capped and locked. When sampling is to be done, water is drawn from the pipe and tested. It is a very clever strategy, really.

The sanitarian moved to unlock the padlocked sliding door of the sheet-metal building. As the lock was removed, he shoved the door aside and waved us inside. The building was about 50 square feet, with dozens of metal barrels (I would estimate that they were 100-gallon barrels) that were arrayed along the walls and stacked nearly as high as the 20-foot ceiling, which had a translucent panel to light the area. In the middle of the building stood an old rusted device—it was a furnace with a chimney flue and a large chamber. Flanking the chamber were roller panels, also rusted, about 2 feet wide and 8 feet long. I tried to move the rollers; they squeaked terribly, but still rolled. I asked the obvious question. "What's this?"

"Dr. Watts hired truck drivers from the surrounding states to bring in the waste that he was paid by hospitals to dispose of," began the environmental officer. "They came in with tankers, tractor–trailer trucks, and even pickups. The waste was "logged" by hospital and date, but not much else. Then, the waste was pitched, shoveled, poured, or rolled into the furnace. If things didn't burn up, or periodically when they would clean the furnace, the residue was thrown into that big pit outside, that is now capped." He was very sober. I wondered at his disposition toward the community concerns.

At my inquiry, he said the pit was 90 feet deep. It had been dug "around" and lined with clay. Durable plastic sheeting was lining the clay "cap." The clay cap, in principle, is the top and the sides of the burial site. When a sanitary landfill is made, its bottom is also lined (or capped), but the man did not indicate why the pit contents simply had not been hauled away. The site remediation (cleanup) was in the early 1980's, before his time as an environmental sanitarian. I expected there was a cost explanation for the cleanup and suspected that the minimum required was done because no company was readily identified to bear the cost. Also, the opinion of the remediation team was likely that the site was isolated from residential areas, so less thorough cleanup would be acceptable. I was told that the fence was built to federal hazardous waste site specifications. I asked about the rumor of radioactive waste. The environmental sanitarian who was our guide to the site said he knew nothing about that, but said he had seen no mention of radioactive isotopes among the monitored residue.

After this, the older man (our guide to the location) began to recount the days when the site was operating. You could see the furnace fires from the road he said, and late at night it would make silhouettes of the trees along the ridge rim, for home sites nearby. The smoke would climb high into the sky, and folks told him the smell of the raw waste as it was trucked in was terrible if you were downwind from the site. Odors are often revealing because they may signify the presence of "aromatic" hydrocarbon chemicals. Also, odors may signify that particulate matter is travelling some distance from the incineration site. I asked as we drove away, and he replied that he'd lived in the vicinity for more than 60 years. The Watts Retreat fires were active only from about 1950–1960. The old Dr. Watts was supposed to be a millionaire, but no one seemed to know where his surviving family was or how the cleanup was paid for. When David asked when the cleanup had occurred, the old man said the cleanup took place about 10 years ago, so it must have been done by the EPA.

> *Odors are often revealing because they may signify the presence of "aromatic" hydrocarbon chemicals. Also, odors may signify that particulate matter is travelling some distance from the incineration site.*

We dropped the old gentleman off at his home, and immediately drove back to the site. We parked on the bridge over the river, and consulted our map from the citizens. Then, we drove up and down the roads to become familiar with the residential areas nearby, and the lay of the valleys. We stopped for supper on the way back to the campus. David was quite excited about our plans, and wanted to be part of "all of it." I smiled and welcomed his youthful energy.

Two weeks later, we were back to meet with citizens at a local church. I gave my usual spiel and waited for questions and comments. There were surprisingly few. Then, I described our plan to collect information about cancer cases in the community by going door-to-door and contacting former residents (cancer cases among persons who had recently moved away from the community were a particular concern for the citizens). The citizens wanted to be sure that several cancer patients who had recently moved away from the community, just before their diagnoses, would be considered part of the local incidence. I said that we would ask for cancer-related information over the last 10 years, and then focus our analysis on the last 5 years. Everyone agreed to the plan, and most said they would help us with the canvassing planned for 2 weeks later. The church representative offered their facility as the focal point of the field operations. David and I would come to the community to conduct training sessions on Friday and Saturday night. Then, door-to-door visits would be made (with a maximum of two calls per house) for an area about 5 square miles around the Watts Retreat site. Advertisements about the plan would be published in the local paper twice a week until the survey weekend.

I asked the folks present what cancers they specifically wanted us to focus on during our investigation. I explained that breast, lung, colon, and prostate cancers were not good candidates for cluster studies because they were "common" diseases and so many risk factors were already debated for each. I further explained that the principle constituents of the Watts Retreat's pit were solvents and chemicals. I explained that with radioactive exposure, bone cancer and leukemia would be possible outcomes. They chose leukemia, lymphoma, brain, bone, kidney, and liver cancers, with some counseling from me that "common" cancers (such as lung, breast, and prostate) would not be prudent sites to include. As the meeting broke up, the people milled about a bit as David and I gathered our projector, screen, and leftover handouts. David headed out before me because I stopped to talk with a couple who were waiting at my car.

They were the parents of a young man who had died a few years before of bone cancer. They appealed to me to include all pediatric cancers in our analysis as well. I assured them that we would do so. Then, they asked me about bone cancer, why it struck young children, and why it was so fatal. I described to them the differences of cancer types between adults and children, and said bone cancer was the third or fourth most common cancer among children. Because of the marrow in the bones, the cancerous cells can be swept away readily and the metastases were usually the cause of death. The woman wept openly as I spoke; people came by to pat her or the man's shoulders as they filed out of the building. Soon the only cars left were theirs, the host couple's, and mine. The woman who hosted the meeting came over and embraced the woman whose son had died and led her away to their car. In a husky voice, the weeping woman's husband thanked me for coming and for talking with them. Then, he followed his wife.

As I opened my car door, the local host told me, "Their boy was a sad loss for these people." He speculated that much of the local concern was from friends of that couple or fellow church members. I didn't ask then, nor did they ever volunteer, why he and his wife were so vehement about the potential of a cancer cluster. Both wished me a safe drive, and I headed home.

David and I prepared a two-page questionnaire for the survey, which included the details of cancer cases, the anatomic site, where they were treated, a physician contact, and other information. We would use the survey to find cases, but we would verify any diagnosis by reviewing medical records. I explained to David, as he stacked materials for the survey, that this approach had been used effectively at the Woburn, Massachusetts cluster.[19] Many people criticized using private citizens for data collection, but we had no money and our new cancer registry was not complete enough for us to rely on it having all of the cases, particularly for the earlier years that were the concern for these people. We gave the surveyors a letter of introduction from the local health department to give to anyone they surveyed. The letter explained the purpose of the survey and gave local contact numbers for questions. We provided an "assent" page stating that responding to the questionnaire was voluntary and informing them that the surveyors had envelopes that the respondents could put the questionnaires into and seal, if they wished only us to see their replies. Our questionnaire asked about any other diseases that they believed might be relevant; and we asked if cancer was identified in any of their pets that had died. No one used the envelopes. No disease besides cancer was reported. Only two pet deaths were reported. Only one pet death was caused by a cancer.

The Friday night training drew two dozen folks and nearly all were there the next day. We started at 10:00 a.m. and went to 6:00 p.m. Soft drinks, pizza, and snacks were provided by the church. Each survey team (always two people) was given an assigned road, and a series of five to six addresses to call on. The stack of completed forms mounted, and the day passed. The Saturday evening training drew only five folks. My mother, youngest son, and I attended church the next day at this location. The minister recognized me and encouraged people to "help out." There were fewer teams on Sunday, and fewer forms were completed, but many of the "no answer" homes were visited a second time.

Finally, it was over. Fifty-four (non-duplicate) forms were sorted into date-of-diagnosis order. Another 40 duplicate forms were kept for reference. Only one cancer case had more than two reports. That one case was reported in five separate responses. David and I began to contact the hospitals and physicians identified; we made these contacts under the authority I mentioned earlier, from the state's laws regarding public health investigations. Only 45 of the cancers were verified, 33 occurred in the last 5 years. Several of the cancers turned out to be different sites than reported by the survey form, mostly metastatic sites mistaken for primary ones. We calculated expected rates, performed several cancer cluster analyses, and prepared our report (Table 28-1). We scheduled a town meeting almost exactly 2 months after the first one.

The report contained a map with the selected cancer sites marked, but this map was without roads, an indication of the type of cancer, or the date of occurrence. This way, we hoped to prevent the identification of specific cases too easily. Our findings were daunting. The five lymphoma cases produced a rate four-fold the expected. The two kidney cancers and five brain cancers were eleven times higher than expected. There was only one pediatric cancer, the case of bone cancer. This was a small community; we placed this population at 1000 at a maximum, more likely 750–800. In such a small community, even a few cases can give high "excess" rates. In a simple example, if 0.01 cases are expected and one case occurs, this represents 100-fold risk

I had to explain these numeric issues and the map to the people. I had transcribed our findings onto the map given to us by the citizens. Our map was posted on the wall at the church entrance with the one that the local folks had signed weeks before. The two maps did not agree, the pattern of cancer cases was not along the river below the Watts Retreat site, nor were they "downstream." There was no aggregation *per se*. I knew this because I knew which cases were which. There was only one pattern of note, a "string" of the four brain cancers, in the opposite direction of the citizen's concern. I did not divulge that observation to the citizens; it simply was not part of the agreement we had made with the community leaders (1) when we acknowledged their map, and (2) when they picked their cancer sites for study. There were six cancer cases among persons who had recently moved away from the area; none of these

TABLE 28-1 Observed cancer cases for the Watts Retreat Farm cancer cluster[22]

Site of cancer	1980	1981	1982	1983	1984	1985	1986	1987	1988	1989	Total	SIR*
Lung	1	1		1		2	2	2			9	**2.7**
Colon				1	1	1	1	1		1	6	2.2
Breast	2	1			1			1			5	1.2
Prostate			1					2	1		4	
Leukemia	1					1					2	
Lymphoma	1						1	1	1	1	5	**4.4**
Stomach						2					2	
Liver								1			1	
Pancreas								1		1	2	4.3
Melanoma			1	1		2					4	
Brain				1	1	1	1		1		5	**11.8**
Kidney			1	1							2	
All Others	1	2					2	1	1		7	
Total	6	4	3	5	3	9	7	10	4	3	54	2.3

*Standardized Incidence Ratio: selected sites only, age-adjusted to the 1970 U.S. census population and compared to national data.

cancers were of cancer sites that figured into the elevated rate findings. The community had higher overall cancer rates than expected, and I committed to ongoing surveillance by the state's new cancer registry for at least 3 years to see if these high rates would continue. The rationale for such continued surveillance is based on the relatively slow course of cancer (e.g., it is not like an infectious disease that may wax-and-wane in a few days). Cancer latency is generally considered in decades or several years at the least. Further, a finding of an overall "elevated" rate is a simple statistical probability, so unless the excess was very large or involved a single type of cancer, conventional wisdom was to rule out a simple, periodic, up-and-down "swing" in rates, and to consider that the local concerns and the advent of the statewide cancer registry might accentuate case-finding in this region. The annual updates would be mailed to addresses left on a sign-in pad.

When I asked if there were any questions, there was not a single one. I thanked our surveyors and our lead group who had met with us on our first visit. I commended the health department administration, and left my business card for any thoughts that might occur later. Only two of my cards were taken, and only four addresses were on the list to receive the annual updates. I never heard from anyone in that community again. This is the nature of cancer cluster investigations and defusing emotionally charged situations. A community may be outraged, but if you give them attention, show respect, and are forthright with them, no matter the findings, they usually will be satisfied that they were "heard." The annual updates from the successive years diluted all impressions of "high rates" of cancer except for the brain cancer rate, but that is another story that follows shortly.

As I left the community, it was early evening, and still light during daylight savings time. I drove toward the "string" of brain cancer cases, checking roads on my map. Coming to the top of a rise, I parked and stepped from my car. In the valley below spread dozens of homes, new developments it appeared. In the near distance were the distinct metal towers of high voltage power lines, and I recognized two chicken farm buildings at least. I did not know the exact locations of the brain cancer cases, but I resolved to myself that the promised case–control study would begin soon.

Follow-up Case-Control Study

This chapter is about cancer cluster investigations, but I will digress briefly to tell you a bit about the follow-up case–control study mentioned in the previous two accounts. We elected to conduct the study in a four-county area south of both the chicken farm cluster and the Watts Retreat, and nearly a hundred miles from each. This area included one county that our EIS officer had studied in his project that found no significantly elevated disease rates.

The rationale for conducting an "in-depth" study to evaluate findings from a cancer cluster investigation mainly has to do with what is called the "Texas sharpshooter" criticism of cluster investigations. A Texas sharpshooter is described as one who fires a series of shots at a wall, then draws his target around the bullet holes to show how they are concentrated in the bull's-eye. Similarly, to conduct an in-depth study in a community where a cluster was already found is regarded in the manner of the Texas sharpshooter; one may argue that the elevated cancer rates were already known before the in-depth study was performed. The idea is that if the implication of the cancer cluster finding has *bona fide* biologic meaning, then reason says that the finding should appear elsewhere among cases of the same type.

In the mid-1990's, GIS technology was surging, but was still pretty rudimentary compared to today. We had to purchase some 40 different topographic pages for mapping the brain cancer cases and controls onto. The cancer registry's cluster buster was an urbane young man named Julius Lindsey. Our sample size was 240 persons, with 120 in each group; it took us nearly a year to map all of these cases. Our field work was funded by a local cancer center. We literally looked up each address and marked it on these 3 ft by 3 ft topographical maps, using a black "X" for a case and a red "X" for a control. We took these maps back to our GIS folks who had digitized the maps (pretty easy for them because they were designed for use with land surveys), and then they simply had to point an electronically-linked pen at each case or control "X" to get the exact coordinates. Digitizing the data permitted us to associate a denominator to various aggregates of cases that stood out. This sort of search for maxima emulates the software package SaTScan that is widely used today. Clustering was evident! Simple odds ratios were sufficiently robust for the analysis. This underlies the rationale for performing a case–control study as an assessment of a finding from a series of promising cluster investigations. One selects an area different from the earlier cluster investigations, and (necessarily) where more cases may be used to achieve greater precision.

I will not expand this digression, but I will say two things. First, the chicken farm hypothesis failed! There was no statistically significant association with being a brain cancer case and living near a chicken farm. But, the relationship based on proximity to power lines was tantalizingly strong. Second, this brain cancer case and control data set was applied to maps of the power lines provided by Duke Power (so that we had some detail of the power line's transmission characteristics). We collaborated with a physicist from Michigan and another graduate student (not David) to examine an exceptionally complex and subtle risk relationship of the brain cancer cases to the power lines. Just to allay your frustration at this brief discussion, we incorporated factors like the power lines' elevation, and their relative alignment to the case or control's home and to the earth's natural magnetic poles. We had to include measures of the earth's magnetic field strength, which was a function of underlying mineral layers. Amazingly enough, the requisite data was already available in GIS files. We applied the physicist's formula of eight factors to estimate electromagnetic fields at distances progressing from the power lines to the case or control subject's home. We later published our findings.[20] For completeness, let me mention that David wrote a very nice manuscript from the Watts Retreat investigation that was also published.[21]

To conclude this digression, let me mention that Julius and I had noticed as we were mapping the cases, that the "brain cancer case" residence was not always the closest one to the power lines. Also, the complex theoretical measure based on the physicist's theories produced an analysis where only brain cancer cases were in the "exposure" window; that is, only the brain cancer cases resided in that distance from the power lines. No control subjects resided at that distance from these power lines. I sent copies of the article to both of the communities where I had previously conducted investigations, but I never received a reply. Now, let's return to cancer cluster investigations.

AN OUTSTANDING CANCER CLUSTER INVESTIGATION

Dr. Ken Rothman, the keynote speaker at the 1989 conference, Investigation of Clusters of Adverse Health Outcomes, offered a plea for more cancer registries.[22] These databases are invaluable resources for responding to cancer cluster reports. In the previous episode, the state cancer registry was brand-new; it would be 2 years before they had complete coverage of the state's incidence. The years of the brain cancer case–control study were just inside their leading edge of complete data collection. In 1992, the federal government would pass the Cancer Registries Amendment Act, requiring all states to operate population-based, statewide cancer registries.[23] In some of the lobbying effort for that Act, cancer clusters were prominently discussed.[24] This proliferation of cancer registries was an incredible boon to cancer cluster investigations. This final story is illustrative of the impact on cancer cluster investigations from what I regard as good cancer registries.

Seven years had passed since the Watts Retreat study, almost 10 years since the chicken farm one. I was working as director of Chronic Disease Epidemiology in South Carolina in 1999. Their new cancer registry was a splendid system. As they got up and running, their first cluster buster, a young lady named Laura Cave, asked me for a consultation regarding a lung cancer cluster report she had received from residents of a coastal community. I have mentioned before that lung cancer is too common to be studied productively in a cluster report. However, a specific type of lung cancer had caught Laura's attention: mesothelioma. Mesothelioma is technically a sarcoma of the lining of the lungs, not actually a cancer of the lung itself. Mesothelioma has a protracted history for its association with durable fibers, especially asbestos. The biologic mechanism for this cancer is generally regarded as resulting from the body's own defenses trying to destroy the irritating fiber lodged between the lungs and the pleura (slippery tissue surface over which the lungs move during respiration). Mesotheliomas occur about 1/10,000th as often as lung cancer, so it is regarded as rare.

To indicate the awesome advances with cancer-related technology in these intervening years, Laura had mapped all of the cases reported by the community as well as others from the cancer registry; she did this at her desk. She was able to calculate observed and expected age-adjusted, site-specific, race- and gender-specific disease rates using the SEER*Stat Software (SEER stands for Surveillance Epidemiology and End Results program) from the National Cancer Institute.[25] This software incorporated the denominators from the recent 2000 census, and permitted Laura to do standardized incidence ratios (SIRs) and standardized mortality ratios (SMRs). There are several merits to considering both measures (new cases as well as deaths), but a simple one is that citizen reports of cancer clusters are often oriented to the deceased cases because those represent greater emotional impact. Sometimes, you may have a different appreciation for what a community is describing if you can look at the data a bit from their perspective.

Laura also had access to a CDC distributed software package for performing several statistical cluster analyses; this is where she most wanted my assistance.[26] Being the bright capable professional that she is, Laura had sliced the data a variety of ways—by younger ages, by race/gender groups, and by different subtypes of cancer. In this process, she had found a startling cluster in the community reporting the cluster. As we prepared the report, meticulously preparing maps and performing various statistical tests, the finding was clear. This was a very statistically "strong" cluster, immense biologic plausibility, and a nearby environmental source that could be suspected of producing the hazardous exposure. We treaded lightly.

Cancer clusters can evoke awesome media coverage. Having a credible environmental source necessitates notification of regulatory agencies, local officials, and the potential representatives of the suspected point source. This sort of scale with agencies and media, as well as so robust a finding so early after the beginning of the new cancer registry's operation, was daunting. I agreed to assist with composing the narrative report. Exceptional maps and figures were produced [Figures 28-5–28-8]. In subsequent years this experience would be presented as a model cluster investigation at national meetings.[27]

The type of lung cancer that produced such an impressive clustering was mesothelioma. The proximal, suspect environmental source was a naval shipyard. As soon as we had enough information to present, we called for a town meeting. The meeting drew a variety of elected officials and representatives from federal agencies. It was a packed house. I opened with part of my traditional spiel, but cut to the chase and presented the findings and the substantiating evidence. When I concluded, I disappeared from the "limelight" and the Navy representatives spoke up about their plans for providing assistance to the residents and compensation for medical care. The local medical college described the opening of a new respiratory disease clinic, and recruitment of a distinguished respiratory specialist (who was present). No angry words were spoken, much less shouted. People immediately moved on to planning cleanup and

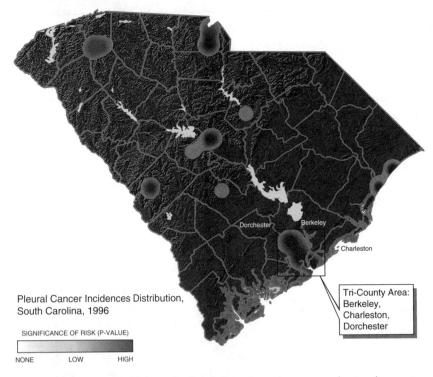

FIGURE 28-5 The initial analysis of the pleural cancer cluster in South Carolina. Exceptional GIS technology produced this figure and Figures 28-5 and 28-7. Here, the statistical significance of the observed-to-expected case ratio was the basis for shading. The reported cluster along the coast is clearly a distinctive pattern from other areas of the state, including heavily industrialized areas as Greenville and Spartanburg [to the north]

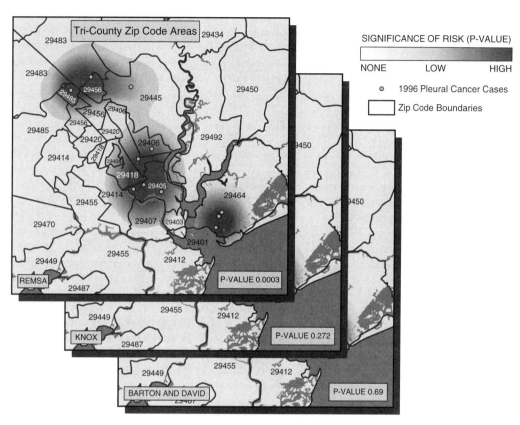

FIGURE 28-6   Three analyses of pleural cancer (mesothelioma) case clustering in 'space and time'. Statistical significance is reported from only one test, the failure for the other two analytic procedures may reflect the considerably large geographic area that was involved. This one statistically significant result with those from the 'temporal' analyses provides a consistency of finding that is one of the premises that is recommended for 'verifying' bona fide case clustering [26]. See reference 26.

community mobilizations. I nearly cried—this sort of acceptance of a cluster report was unique to my (now more than 450) cluster investigations.

I sat quietly in the back and contemplated the impact of analytic sophistication, complete case information, and the openness for discussing cancer risk. Some 30 years had elapsed since the descriptions that I gave in my opening remarks in this chapter. So much progress had come with cancer treatment and detection, it is no longer a terrifying, whispered fear. The rapidity of the cluster report response (about 2 weeks) was incredible. This was not the new cancer registry's first investigation; it was about their twelfth. However, none of the others had been "productive" or had produced so much notoriety. One of the aspects for national recognition of this investigation was the splendid cooperation of so many diverse partners and agencies.

I consulted with the Toms River cluster study in New Jersey.[28] That investigation of childhood brain cancer was my first experience seeing the awesome, contemporary mapping technology and analysis resources applied with faultless data. That study (the Toms River cluster) cost tens of thousands of dollars (it was 3–4 years before this episode) and had taken a year. In some respects, this mesothelioma investigation didn't cost any new money, because all the processes and activities were ongoing agency programs. This was a good example of an investment in public health paying off. Today, the public health infrastructure is really primed for cancer cluster investigations of this ilk. The National Environmental Public Health Tracking Network (NEPHT) is designed specifically to benefit investigations of disease risk from environmental factors, similar to what Laura had for her work.[29] The South Carolina data was already automated, so keying data from paper was not required for the disease, the population, or the environmental factors. Agencies cooperated, talked to one another, and saw the public as their customers. The state of the art is

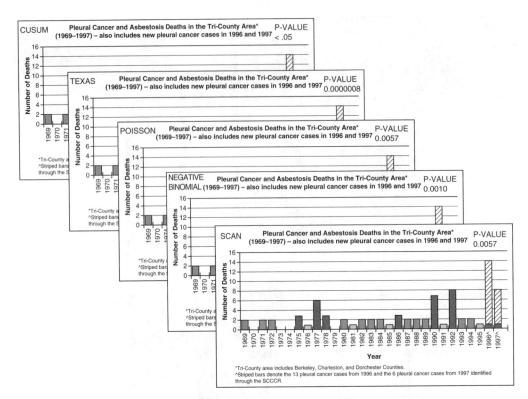

FIGURE 28-7 Five analyses of case clustering in 'time.' Again, as in Figure 28-5, the figures are each identical, only the methods of statistical analysis varied, and the respective results; each name and finding is reported along the top of the series of figures. Note that all indicate statistical significance, the varying levels of the p-values reflects differences in the analytic procedures, yet the consistency of finding is the premise that is recommended for 'verifying' bona fide case clustering.[26] See reference 26.

a far cry from copying square grids onto a map to approximate distance. The capacity of contemporary data analysis software is amazing to behold.[30] The linkage of databases and the automation of analysis procedures (as envisioned with the NEPHT) make the recognition of statistically suspicious findings (not solely cancer) much simpler, so that even less-experienced investigation staff may access these useful data. The ideal position to be in today involves the prospect of finding a cancer cluster as it emerges; that is, to do so prospectively, and to do so from the data side—not like the "old days" when we were relying on lay citizens to report disease pattern anomalies after many persons had been stricken. Yet, of course, reports of cancer clusters still occur! Good luck to you.

LEARNING QUESTIONS

1. What are considered the sentinel attributes of cancer clusters?
2. How are the magnitudes of potential risk values viewed in cancer cluster investigations (such as a twofold increased risk of cancer from a certain potential exposure)?
3. In the Watts Retreat investigation, the investigators only noted one pattern, a string of four brain cancers in the opposite direction of the citizens' concern. The investigators did not divulge that observation to the citizens. Do you agree with the investigators about discussing this observation with the citizens? Why or why not?
4. What is the "Texas sharpshooter" criticism and how is it relevant to cancer cluster investigation?

REFERENCES

1. Lilienfeld AM, Pederson E, Dowd JE. *Cancer Epidemiology: Methods of Study*. Baltimore, MD: The Johns Hopkins Press; 1967.
2. Langmuir AD. Formal discussion of: epidemiology of cancer: spatial-temporal aggregation. *Cancer Res.* 1965;25(8):1384–1386.
3. Caldwell GG, Heath CW Jr. Case clustering in cancer. *South Med J.* 1976;69(12):1598–1602.

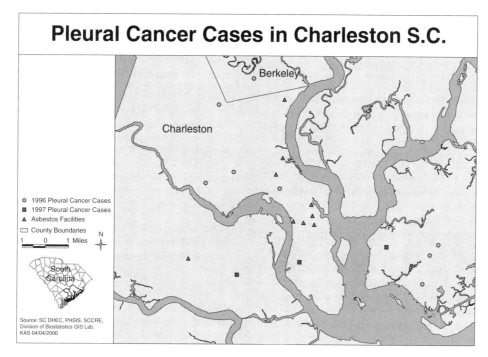

FIGURE 28-8 Illustrative example of case mapping for presentation to citizens. Note the absence of roads or streets, to obfuscate the exact location of cases and hazardous exposure sites that are candidates for connection with the case cluster, but are not interpreted to be related.

4. Carson RL. *Silent Spring*. Boston, MA: Houghton Mifflin Company; 1962.
5. Janerich DT, Burnett WS, Feck G, et al. Cancer incidence in the Love Canal area. *Science*. 1981;212(4501):1404–1407.
6. National Cancer Institute. President Nixon's war on cancer. National Cancer Institute Web site. http://dtp.nci.nih.gov/timeline/noflash/milestones/M4_Nixon.htm. Accessed September 12, 2009.
7. Aldrich TE, Garcia N, Zeichner S, Berger S. Cancer clusters: a myth or a method. *Med Hypotheses*. 1983;12(1):41–52.
8. Aldrich TE, Glorieux A, Castro S. Florida cluster of five children with endodermal sinus tumors. *Oncology*. 1984;41(4):233–238.
9. Wertheimer N, Leeper E. Electrical wiring configurations and childhood cancer. *Am J Epidemiol*. 1979;109(3):273–284.
10. Centers for Disease Control and Prevention. Epidemic Intelligence Service (EIS). Centers for Disease Control and Prevention Web site. http://www.cdc.gov/eis/index.html. Accessed September 12, 2009.
11. Grimson RC, Wang KC, Johnson PW. Searching for hierarchical clusters of disease: spatial patterns of sudden infant death syndrome. *Soc Sci Med*. 1981;15(2):287–293.
12. Knox EG. The detection of space-time interactions. *Appl Statistics*. 1964;13:25–29.
13. Barton DE, David FN, Merrington M. A criterion for testing contagion in time and space. *Ann Hum Genet*. 1965;29:97–103.
14. Aldrich TE. Detecting space–time aggregation of rare events [Abstract]. *Am J Epidemiol*. 1984;120:464.
15. Aldrich TE, Griffith JR. *Environmental Epidemiology and Risk Assessment*. New York, NY: Van Norstrand Reinhold; 1993.
16. Centers for Disease Control and Prevention. Guidelines for investigating clusters of health events. *MMWR*. 1990;39(RR-11);1–16.
17. Aldrich TE, Sinks T. What to know and do about cancer clusters. *Cancer Investigation*. 2002;20:810–816.
18. FEMA. Superfund Amendments and Reauthorization Act (SARA), Title III. FEMA Website. http://www.fema.gov/government/grant/sara.shtm. Accessed September 12, 2009.
19. Lagakos SW, Wessen BJ, Zelen M. An analysis of contaminated well water and health effects in Woburn, Massachusetts. *J Am Stat Assoc*. 1986;81(395):583–596.
20. Aldrich TE, Andrews KW, Liboff AR. Brain cancer risk and electromagnetic fields (EMFs): assessing the geomagnetic component. *Arch Environ Health*. 2001;56(4):314–319.
21. Graber DR, Aldrich TE. Working with community organizations to evaluate potential disease clusters. *Soci Sci Med*. 1993;37(8):1079–1085.
22. Rothman, KJ. A sobering start for the cluster busters' conference. *Am J Epidemiol*. 1990;132(1 Suppl):S6–S13.
23. Centers for Disease Control and Prevention. *A National Program of Cancer Registries: At a Glance, 1994–1995*. Atlanta, GA: U.S. Department of Health and Human Services; 1995.

24. Healey JH. The cancer weapon America needs most. *Reader's Digest.* 1992;June:69–72.
25. Surveillance Epidemiology and End Results. SEER*Stat Software. National Cancer Institute Web site. http://seer.cancer.gov/seerstat/. Accessed September 12, 2009.
26. Aldrich TE, Drane JW. *CLUSTER: User's Manual for Software to Assist with Investigation of Rare Health Events.* Atlanta, GA: Agency for Toxic Substances and Disease Registry; 1991.
27. Cave LA, Bolick-Aldrich SW, Aldrich TE, et al. Fire the weapon: the sequel. Presented at: North American Assoc. Central Cancer Registries Annual Conference; April, 2000; New Orleans, LA.
28. ATSDR. Health officials investigate childhood cancer cluster. *Hazardous Subst Public Health.* 1996;6(3):149–153.
29. Centers for Disease Control and prevention. National Environmental Public Health Tracking Program. http://www.cdc.gov/nceh/tracking/. Accessed September 12, 2009.
30. SaTScan. SaTScan Web site. http://www.satscan.org/. Accessed September 12, 2009.

APPENDIX A: SELECTED CHRONOLOGY OF CANCER CLUSTER REPORTS

1775—Report of scrotal cancer among young chimney sweeps of London
1959—Childhood leukemia in Buffalo, NY
1963—Childhood leukemia in Niles, Illinois
1964—Childhood leukemia in Northumberland and Durham, England / Knox Method
1965—NCI Conference on Space-Time Aggregation of Cancer Cases
   Rachel Carson published *Silent Spring*
   Leukemia and lymphoma in Connecticut
1967—Burkitt's lymphoma in Uganda
1969—National Environmental Policy Act passed
1971—"War on Cancer" declared by President Nixon
   Diethylstilbestrol (DES) and clear cell cancer of the vagina in Boston, MA
1972—Hodgkin's disease cluster in high school students in Albany, NY
1974—Angiosarcoma of the liver cluster in Louisville, KY.
1975—NCI publishes first atlas of cancer
1976—Resource Conservation and Recovery Act passed
1977—Birth defects in Alsea, OR from aerial spraying of 2,4,5-T
   Infertility among California vineyard workers from DBCP
1979—Birth defect among residents of Love Canal, NY
   Soil contamination with PCBs in Times Beach, MO
   Radiation Leak in reactor at Three Mile Island, PA
   Childhood cancer and electromagnetic fields
1980—Comprehensive Environmental Response, Compensation, and Liability Act establishes Agency for Toxic Substances and Disease Registry
   Leukemia and Hodgkin's disease in Rutherford, NJ
   Scan statistic for temporal clusters
1986—Nuclear reactor fire in Chernobyl, USSR
   Childhood leukemia in Woburn, MA
   Superfund Amendments and Reauthorization Act (implemented ATSDR)
1987—NIOSH reports of 61 occupational cluster investigations
1988—Birth defects around Hanford Nuclear Reservation, WA
   National inventory of state-based cancer cluster protocols
   Spatial studies of childhood leukemia near Seascale Power Plant, UK
1989—CDC/ATSDR conference about investigating clusters of adverse health events
1990—CDC guidelines for investigating clusters of health events
1991—ATSDR distributes CLUSTER computer software
1992—SARA Title III—Community Right-to-Know Act, Toxic Chemical Release Inventory (TRI)
   Cancer Registries Amendment Act establishes National Program of Cancer Registries
1996—Childhood brain cancer in Toms River, NJ
1997—Council of State and Territorial Epidemiologists Cancer Cluster Seminar
1998—International Congress on GIS and Public Health
   Kulldorff spatial scan statistic developed at NCI
2000—*Erin Brockovich* draws national attention to cancer clusters in California
2001—Birth defects and hazardous waste landfills, UK
2006—Childhood acute lymphoblastic leukemia cluster in Fallon, NV

APPENDIX B: ADDITIONAL RECOMMENDED READING ON THE STATISTICAL METHODS FOR INVESTIGATING CLUSTERS OF CANCER

Pearson K. On the appearance of multiple cases of disease in the same house. *Biometrika.* 1912;8(3/4):404–412.
Pinkel D, Nefzger D. Some epidemiological features of childhood leukemia in the Buffalo, N. Y. area. *Cancer.* 1959;12(2):351–358.
Woodward RH, Goldsmith PL. *Cumulative Sum Techniques.* Edinburgh: Oliver & Boyd; 1964.
Knox EG. The detection of space-time interactions. *Appl Statistics.* 1964;13(1):25–30.
Ederer F, Myers MH, Mantel N. A statistical problem in space and time: do leukemia cases come in clusters? *Biometrics.* 1964;20(3):626–638.
Barton DE, David FN, Merrington M. A criterion for testing contagion in time and space. *Ann Hum Genet.* 1965;29:97–103.
Naus JI. Some probabilities, expectations, and variances for the size of largest clusters and smallest intervals. *J Am Stat Assoc.* 1966;61(316):1191–1199.
Mantel N. The detection of disease clustering and a generalized regression approach. *Cancer Res.* 1967;27(2):209–220.

Pike MC, Smith PG. Disease clustering: a generalization of Knox's approach to the detection of space-time interactions. *Biometrics*. 1968;24(3):541–556.

Bailar JC, Eisenberg H, Mantel N. Time between pairs of leukemia cases. *Cancer*. 1970;25(6):1301–1303.

Klauber MR. Two-sample randomization tests for space-time clustering. *Biometrics*. 1971;27:129–142.

Lloyd S, Roberts CJ. A test for space clustering and its application to congenital limb defects. *Br J Prev Soc Med*. 1973;27(3):188–191.

Pike MC, Smith PG. Case-control approach to examine diseases for evidence of contagion, including diseases with long latent periods. *Biometrics*. 1974;30(2):263–279.

Chen R. A surveillance system for congenital malformations. *J Am Stat Assoc*. 1978;73(362):323–327.

Ohno Y, Aoki K, Aoki N. A test of significance for geographic clusters of disease. *Int J Epidemiol*. 1979;8(3):273–280.

Wallenstein S. A test for detection of clustering over time. *Am J Epidemiol*. 1980;111(3):367–372.

Weinstock MA. A generalized scan statistic test for the detection of clusters. *Int J Epidemiol*. 1981;10(3):289–293.

Grimson RC, Wang KC, Johnson PW. Searching for hierarchical clusters of disease: spatial patterns of sudden infant death syndrome. *Soc Sci Med*. 1981;15(2):287–293.

Tango T. The detection of disease clustering in time. *Biometrics*. 1984;40(1):15–26.

Whittemore AS, Friend N, Brown BW Jr, Holly EA. A test to detect clusters of disease. *Biometrika*. 1987;74(3):631–635.

Shulte PA, Ehrenberg RL, Singal M. Investigation of occupational cancer clusters: theory and practice. *Am J Public Health*. 1987;77(1):52–56.

Frumkin H, Kantrowitz W. Cancer clusters in the workplace: an approach to investigation. *J Occup Med*. 1987;29(12):949–952.

Sever LE, Hessol NA, Gilbert ES, McIntyre JM. The prevalence at birth of congenital malformations in communities near the Hanford site. *Am J Epidemiol*. 1988;127(2):243–254.

Warner SC Aldrich TE. The status of cancer cluster investigations undertaken by state health departments. *Am J Public Health*. 1988;78(3):306–307.

Openshaw S, Craft AW, Charlton M, Birch JM. Investigation of leukaemia clusters by use of a geographical analysis machine. *Lancet*. 1988;1(8580):272–273.

Stroup DF, Williamson GD, Herndon JL, Karon JM. Detection of aberrations in the occurrence of notifiable diseases surveillance data. *Stat Med*. 1989;8(3):331–332.

Griffith J, Duncan RC, Riggan WB, Pellom AC. Cancer mortality in US counties with hazardous waste sites and ground water pollution. *Arch Environ Health*.1989;44(2):69–74.

Hardy RJ, Schroeder GD, Cooper SP, Buffler PA, Prichard HM, Crane M. A surveillance system for assessing health effects from hazardous exposures. Am J Epidemiol. 1990;132(1 Suppl):S32–S42.

Grimson RC, Aldrich TE, Drane JW. Clustering in sparse data and an analysis of rhabdomyosarcoma incidence. *Stat Med*. 1992;11(6):761–768.

Kulldorff M. A spatial scan statistic. *Commun Statistics: Theory Methods*. 1997;26(6):1481–1496.

Elliott P, et al. Spatial epidemiology. *Brit Med J*. 2001;323:363–368.

Kulldorff M. Prospective time period geographical disease surveillance using a scan statistic. *J Royal Stat Soc*. 2001;164:61–72.

In addition—Several teaching exercises for investigating cancer clusters (compiled by Heath CW Jr, NIOSH, and myself) are available from the author. Aldrich@etsu.edu

PART IV

Cases in Environmental and Occupational Health

CHAPTER 29

Fine Wines and Cohorts Take Time: The History of a Cohort Study of Workers Exposed to Ethylene Oxide

Leslie T. Stayner, PhD[a] and Kyle Steenland, PhD[b]

United States, 1980s to 1990s

BACKGROUND

Ethylene oxide (EtO) is a colorless gas that is highly reactive at room temperature and can be explosive when heated. It has a sweet odor, but it has a very high odor threshold and one cannot generally smell it at the levels encountered in today's workplaces or general environment.[1] It is a major industrial chemical that had a worldwide consumption of 18 million metric tons in 2006.[2] Its greatest use is as a chemical intermediate in the production of textiles, detergents, polyurethane foam, antifreeze, solvents, medicinals, adhesives, and other products. It is also used as a fumigant, a sterilant for food (spices) and cosmetics, and in hospital and commercial sterilization of medical devices that cannot be sterilized by steam. The National Institute for Occupational Safety and Health (NIOSH) has estimated that approximately 270,000 people were exposed in the United States in the 1980s, principally in hospitals (96,000) and commercial sterilization (21,000).[3]

In 1979, an international group of scientists met at the International Agency for Research on Cancer (IARC) in Lyon, France to review the evidence that EtO causes cancer in humans.[4] The IARC is a part of the World Health Organization (WHO), and this meeting was one of many that have been organized by the IARC's Monographs Program to review the evidence that environmental factors are associated with cancer. Since 1971, more than 900 agents have been evaluated, of which approximately 400 have been found to be carcinogenic to humans. The IARC had previously reviewed EtO in 1976. At that time, there were no human studies available and very limited evidence from animal studies that EtO caused cancer in humans.[5] By 1979, at the time of the second IARC monograph meeting, there were experimental and a few epidemiologic studies raising concerns about the carcinogenic hazards associated with exposure to EtO. Inhalation of EtO had been shown to increase the

---
[a] Professor and director, Division of Epidemiology and Biostatistics, University of Illinois at Chicago, School of Public Health, Chicago, Illinois.

[b] Professor, Department of Occupational and Environmental Health, Rollins School of Public Health, Atlanta, Georgia.

incidence of mononuclear leukemia and peritoneal mesothelioma in rats in an industry-sponsored study.[6] An excess of leukemia among workers was reported in two Swedish cohort studies.[7,8] However, these studies were small and workers at these facilities were exposed to other chemicals in addition to EtO. At the 1979 monograph meeting, it was concluded that the epidemiologic evidence for a cancer hazard in humans from exposure to EtO was limited, and that EtO was only possibly (IARC category 2b) carcinogenic to humans.[4]

This was the state of the science on the carcinogenicity of EtO when one of us (LS) received a call in the summer of 1981 from Dr. John Paul Jones,[c] who was an occupational physician who worked at the headquarters of Johnson & Johnson (J&J) in New Jersey. At the time, both of us (LS and KS) had just recently begun working in the Industry Wide Studies Branch (IWSB) at the NIOSH in Cincinnati, Ohio. Both of us had also recently earned our Masters degrees in Epidemiology.[d] J&J had sponsored a cytogenetic investigation of workers at their facilities who were exposed to ethylene oxide.[9] A dose-related increase in sister chromatid exchange (SCE) rates in lymphocytes of workers exposed to ethylene oxide was observed in this study.[e] Dr. Jones was concerned about the possible health consequences of the findings from the cytogenetic study, and encouraged us to consider conducting a study of cancer risk among workers exposed to ethylene oxide in the medical devices industry. J&J had already lowered their internal standard from a 10 ppm to a 1 ppm 8-hour time-weighted average (TWA) of EtO in air, which was soon to become the Occupational Safety and Health Administration (OSHA)[f] standard.

PRELIMINARY FEASIBILITY STUDY

Before conducting a study, it is generally necessary to conduct preliminary studies to convince oneself and others that the study is feasible. The first step for us was to conduct a review of the scientific literature on the health effects of EtO. Our review of the literature on EtO suggested to us that the medical supply industry might indeed be an excellent setting for an epidemiologic cohort study of workers exposed to ethylene oxide. The industry employed a relatively large number of workers with potential exposures to EtO, and there were reports of very high exposures occurring in this industry prior to the first reports of a possible leukemia risk in 1979. There also appeared to be little evidence of exposure to other potential confounding exposures for leukemia (e.g., benzene or radiation) in this industry.

We developed a preliminary proposal for a retrospective cohort mortality study in the medical supply industry. This proposal called for a feasibility study that would include two phases: (1) a mail and telephone survey, and (2) walkthrough surveys at selected plants. The methods used and the findings from these surveys are described in detail in a previous publication[10] and in a more abbreviated form in this chapter.

Based on existing literature, we identified approximately 200 facilities that had potentially used EtO for the sterilization of medical supplies or spices. After contacting these facilities by phone, we identified 75 companies that had definitely used EtO for sterilization of products. These companies were sent a letter requesting more detailed information on the number of workers exposed to EtO, as well as the dates and volume of EtO use. Remarkably, the response to our letters was nearly 100%. It is likely that the statutory authority of NIOSH to acquire this data was helpful in obtaining this high response rate. Under the Occupational Safety and Health Act, NIOSH has the legal authority to subpoena company records for the purposes of research (Public Law 91-596, 91st Congress, December 21, 1970). Based on data from these questionnaires, we were able to crudely estimate the number of person-years, the expected number of leukemia deaths of exposed workers, and the statistical power of the study. We estimated that the study would have 116,000 person-years of observation, which would provide the study with sufficient statistical power (>80%) to detect a relative risk of 2.7 for leukemia.

ENLISTING THE SUPPORT OF THE MEDICAL DEVICE MANUFACTURING INDUSTRY

Our initial probe into the possibility of conducting a study quickly revealed that not all of the companies involved in the health supply manufacturing industry shared J&J's enthusiasm for a cohort study of their EtO-exposed workers.

---

[c] Dr. John Paul Jones is deceased.

[d] At that time, Kyle Steenland had a doctorate in history from the University of New York at Buffalo, and later received his doctorate in epidemiology from the University of Pennsylvania in 1985. Leslie Stayner received his doctorate in epidemiology from the University of North Carolina in 1989.

[e] Sister chromatid exchange is the exchange of genetic materials between two sister chromatids.

[f] OSHA and NIOSH were both created by the same Occupational Safety and Health Act of 1970. OSHA's primary function is to develop and enforce standards to protect workers from hazards in the workplace. NIOSH's primary function is to conduct research and provide information about workplace hazards.

> We tried to convince the industry that the best study could be performed with their involvement, but that we nevertheless could use the NIOSH authority to obtain records if needed.

As mentioned earlier, NIOSH has the legal authority to obtain company records for the purpose of research. When NIOSH has used this authority, they are occasionally challenged in court. Although the courts recognize the NIOSH legal authority, these legal challenges are resource- and time-consuming. Thus, we hoped to enlist the voluntary support of the industry to minimize resources devoted to legal challenges. We tried to convince the industry that the best study could be performed with their involvement, but that we nevertheless could use the NIOSH authority to obtain records if needed.

We were fortunate that most of the companies were members of a trade organization called the Health Industry Manufacturers Association (HIMA). Most of the workers in this industry were not unionized. We first contacted HIMA in a phone call and letter that was sent in December of 1981. The letter was written by Dr. William Halperin,[g] who was, at the time, the chief of IWSB at NIOSH to the senior vice president for Scientific Affairs of HIMA. The letter introduced our concept for the study and requested a meeting with HIMA and their interested member companies. The meeting was held in late February 1982 in Washington, DC. Representatives from 13 of HIMA's member companies attended this meeting, and it's fair to say that they were not all enthusiastic about our study plans. Following this meeting, in early March, we sent HIMA a memorandum summarizing our plans to conduct a feasibility study and requested that they circulate this proposal to their member companies for review. On April 16, 1982, we received a response from HIMA that they would be conducting their own feasibility study. We objected to their plans to conduct a feasibility study for us, which led to a long series of correspondence and meetings between NIOSH and HIMA. These meetings ultimately resulted in the signing of a memo of understanding (MOU) in 1984. Under this agreement, NIOSH formed a Scientific Advisory Board that would review the study. The board consisted of Drs. Brian MacMahon and Tom Smith from the Harvard School of Public Health, Dr. Howard Rockette from the University of Pittsburgh Graduate School of Public Health, and Dr. Henry Anderson from the Wisconsin Division of Public Health. Drs. MacMahon, Rockette, and Anderson had expertise in epidemiology and Dr. Smith's expertise was in exposure assessment. We had meetings of the Scientific Advisory Board in which HIMA, labor unions, and company representatives were also invited to participate in 1983, 1984, and 1986. Our MOU also included an agreement to provide HIMA's consultant, Dr. Otto Wong, who worked for Environmental Health Associates, with a copy of a computer tape of identifiable data of the entire cohort at the end of the study, and to allow him to sample 5% of the personnel and other records we acquired from the companies for quality control purposes after the cohort was assembled but before follow-up began. Dr. Wong would be provided with the full cohort computer tape only

> In 1984, approximately 3 years after our first proposal to HIMA, a final protocol for the study was approved by NIOSH. Thus, after 3 years of extensive negotiations with HIMA and extensive reviews by our Scientific Advisory Board, we were finally ready to conduct our study.

after we had completed our own analysis and published our final report on the study. The companies also provided Dr. Wong with copies of all of the files that we would microfilm at their facilities and he was able to construct his own study files using this information. Although this agreement was somewhat burdensome, we had maintained our right to do the study and eventually to publish our findings.

In 1984, approximately 3 years after our first proposal to HIMA, a final protocol for the study was approved by NIOSH. Thus, after 3 years of extensive negotiations with HIMA and extensive reviews by our Scientific Advisory Board, we were finally ready to conduct our study. The protocol identified 39 companies with the largest number of potential person-years for further feasibility assessment.

Around that time, we received funding of approximately $500,000 from the National Cancer Institute (NCI) for the study. The NCI had a program to support funding of collaborative studies with NIOSH. This is not a lot of money in today's terms, but it was a lot back then. Dr. Richard Hayes[h] from NCI was the project officer and a collaborator with us on this study.

---

[g] Dr. Halperin is currently chairman of the Department of Prevention Medicine and Community Health at the New Jersey Medical School.

[h] Dr. Hayes has recently retired from the NCI and is currently director of the Division of Epidemiology, Department of Environmental Medicine, and associate director for Population Sciences at the New York University (NYU) Cancer Institute.

WALKTHROUGH SURVEYS

The first step in our study was to perform walkthrough surveys to determine the suitability of inclusion of the facilities in the study. Walkthrough surveys of a plant facility, as the term implies, involved members of our research team literally walking through areas of the facilities that had potential for exposure to EtO and areas of the facility with key records systems (i.e., personnel and industrial hygiene records). The criteria for inclusion that were established, based on our experience from the mail and phone survey, were (1) the plant must provide at least 400 person-years to the study, (2) the plant must have adequate records to identify past and present workers with potential exposure to ethylene oxide, and (3) workers at the plant must not have potential confounding exposures to other known or suspected leukemogens (e.g., radiation or benzene). The first restriction (> 400 person-years) was purely a pragmatic choice because we wanted to concentrate our efforts on plants that would contribute substantial numbers of workers and person-time to our study. The second criterion (adequate records) was necessary because we could not include workers from plants that did not have adequate records to identify workers. The third criterion was necessary to ensure that the study findings were not confounded by exposures to other agents known to cause leukemia.

The study was also restricted to the inclusion of workers who had experienced at least 3 months of exposure to EtO prior to 1978. This restriction was imposed to eliminate workers with short-term exposures and inadequate latency (time since first exposure). We were anticipating that follow-up would continue until 1984, which would mean that workers first exposed prior to 1978 would have a minimum of 7 years of latency. It was expected that this might be a sufficiently long time because leukemia induced by exposure to benzene and radiation has been found to have a relatively short latency period (e.g., approximately 5 to 10 years). An additional advantage of the 1978 cutoff was that workers employed prior to 1979 were expected to have relatively high exposures because most companies began installing engineering controls to limit exposures to EtO in 1978.[11]

> *Leukemia induced by exposure to benzene and radiation has been found to have a relatively short latency period (e.g., approximately 5 to 10 years).*

The walkthroughs were conducted by a team that generally included one epidemiologist (LS or KS), and one industrial hygienist. The NIOSH industrial hygienists who participated in these surveys were Dr. Alice Greife,[i] Larry Elliott,[j] John Morawetz,[k] and Virginia Ringenburg.[l] Each survey was initiated by an opening conference with key personnel at the plant. We discussed the purpose of our study, the history of EtO usage at the plant, and the availability of industrial hygiene, personnel, and other records. Following the opening conference, we went on a plant tour of areas in the facility where EtO exposures were believed to have occurred. After the tour, the NIOSH industrial hygienist reviewed the plant's EtO sampling records and the epidemiologist reviewed its personnel records. At the end of the survey, a preliminary decision was made in consultation with plant and union personnel about which job categories were likely to be exposed to EtO.

Determining the adequacy of the personnel records was a key objective of the study because these records form the basis of the cohort enumeration. The personnel records were considered to be adequate if they included the name, social security number, date of birth, and a sufficiently detailed work history to determine where they had worked over time. The job and department titles or codes used in the personnel record needed to be sufficiently specific to identify areas of the plant that had potential for exposure to EtO. Information on gender and race was also desirable, but we could obtain this information from the Social Security Administration.

In order to be included in the study, the plant's personnel records also had to be relatively complete. An inventory was conducted of the completeness of records for both current and former employees. Records for terminated employees were frequently arranged by year and we checked to see if any years were missing. We also checked record systems that were alphabetic for whether they included all of the common letters of the alphabet. Finally, the completeness of personnel records was checked against alternative lists, including IRS payroll and union membership records where available. When we discovered that a plant was missing a significant number of records, it was excluded from the study.

---

[i] Currently dean of the College of Science & Technology, University of Central Missouri.
[j] Currently an associate director of NIOSH.
[k] Currently director of the International Chemical Workers Union Center for Workers Health & Safety.
[l] Retired from the Industrial Hygiene Section of IWSB, NIOSH.

A 5% random sample of all personnel records was copied in order to estimate the number of EtO-exposed workers and the person-years that the facility would contribute to the study. Based on this sample, we estimated the percentage of the current and former workforce that was exposed and extrapolated that to the entire workforce at the plant. Using the average year of first exposure to EtO, we could then estimate the average and total number of person-years that the plant would contribute to the study. Using the average age of the cohort at the midpoint of follow-up (1975), we estimated the expected number of leukemia and other lymphatic-hematopoietic neoplasms by applying the person-years to the corresponding rates in the U.S. population for that age group.

We started our investigation with a visit to five of the identified potential study facilities as an initial test of our assumption that this industry would be suitable for study and to further test and develop our survey methodology. We found that these plants would contribute more person-years than expected, based on our estimates from our initial mail survey. Exposure records indicated that, in many cases, not only were the workers involved directly in the sterilization of medical supplies or spices exposed to EtO, but also that a large number of workers were incidentally exposed at these facilities because of the migration of EtO gas from the sterilizer areas to other areas of the plant. In fact, it was not uncommon to find that the entire plant personnel were significantly exposed, including the plant management. These five plants were also found to be suitable for study because they had adequate personnel records and few exposures to other carcinogens.

In total, we visited 35 of the 39 plants that were initially identified and 14 of them were selected for inclusion in our study. Approximately one half of the 39 plants were found to be ineligible because they had missing records, inadequate numbers of exposed workers, or records that were inadequate to identify EtO-exposed workers. In addition, four plants were eliminated because they totally lacked any industrial hygiene records that could be used for estimating the level of EtO exposure. Based on our walkthrough surveys, we estimated that the 14 plants selected for inclusion in the study would contribute approximately 19,000 workers and 261,000 person-years of observation to the study. Based on 1975 U.S. mortality rates for leukemia for age 40-44 years (all gender and race groups combined), we estimated that we would expect to observe 8.6 cases of leukemia and 20 cases of all types of lymphatic-hematopoietic neoplasms. It is noteworthy that after we completed our study we found that these estimates were somewhat low. In our first publication on this study in 1991, we reported that the study included 13 cases of leukemia, and 36 deaths from all lymphatic and hematopoietic neoplasms.[12] The difference between our observed and expected numbers occurred because our feasibility study used the mortality rates for age 40-44 years, which was the estimated average age in our sample at the midpoint of the follow-up period. Leukemia rates increase exponentially with age, and our analysis did not give sufficient weight to the person-time from older age groups, which resulted in an underestimate of the expected deaths for these older workers.

Based on the predicted number of deaths and a standard formula for estimating power in cohort studies,[13] we estimated that our study would have adequate power (80%) to detect a relative risk of 2.0 for leukemia and 1.7 for all lymphatic and hematopoietic neoplasms. This was considered adequate power and data collection was initiated for the full study.

An important side benefit of these walkthrough surveys was that we were able to establish a personal relationship with local plant management, unions and workers at these facilities. Many of these facilities had never worked with people from NIOSH. Some would confuse us with OSHA, which is generally not a positive association for the company management. Building a positive personal relationship with local company personnel and union representatives was an important step in convincing the companies and their workers to cooperate with our investigation. It seemed to work because we generally received very good cooperation from the companies when we moved to the next phase of the study.

COHORT CONSTRUCTION

NIOSH staff visited and microfilmed personnel records for all workers employed at the 14 study facilities in 12 states. Alternative record systems were used to validate the completeness of the personnel records. At two plants, we used Social Security Administration payroll records; at six plants, we used payroll lists for the validation. We found that 90-99% of the workers listed on the alternative record systems were also located in the personnel records. At the plant with the lowest percentage (90%) of congruence, the alternative record system lacked social security numbers, which likely resulted in a large number of mismatches caused by differences in the spelling of names.

NIOSH industrial hygienists worked with knowledgeable plant personnel to identify areas of the plant in which workers were potentially exposed to EtO based on their knowledge of the industrial process or actual exposure measurements. Because EtO is a gas that migrates freely in the air, workers from areas of the plant that shared the air with either the sterilization area or areas containing recently sterilized products were considered to be exposed. Workers who were never exposed and workers with less than 3 months of exposure to EtO were excluded from the cohort. Detailed coding of the demographic and work histories was conducted for eligible workers and a computer master file was created for the study.

Characteristics of the study population are summarized in Table 29-1. A total of 18,254 workers contributing 286,787 person-years were included in the study. Approximately 20% of the workers were employed as sterilizers or in the sterilizing area where the exposures to EtO were the highest. Eighty-six percent of the workers were employed prior to 1978 and were eligible for the study. A slight majority of these workers were female (55%) and the vast majority were white (79%).

VITAL STATUS ASCERTAINMENT

Initially, the cohort was followed for vital ascertainment until December 31, 1987 using a variety of resources, including data from the Social Security Administration, the National Death Index (NDI), the Internal Revenue Service, and the U.S. Postal Service. If a worker was determined to be alive on January 1, 1979 (when the NDI began) and was not found in a search of the NDI, they were assumed to be alive at the end of follow-up (December 31, 1987). Using these methods, we were able to successfully trace more than 95% of the cohort (Table 29-1). Through this follow-up, we identified a total of 1177 deaths. We were able to locate the death certificate for 1137 (97%) of these deaths by contacting the states in which they died.

EXPOSURE ASSESSMENT

Estimating historic exposure levels is generally one of the most challenging aspects of conducting retrospective studies of occupational exposures. This study was no exception. The problem is a general lack of data on exposure concentrations experienced by individual workers, particularly during the earlier time periods of the study.

TABLE 29-1 Characteristics of the study population

No. of workers	18,254
Job category-no. (%)*	
Sterilizer operator	1,222 (7)
In sterilizer area, not operator	2,301 (13)
Maintenance	1,937 (11)
Production	14,965 (82)
Laboratory	484 (3)
Warehouse	1,937 (11)
Employed before 1/1/78	15,750 (86)
No. of person-years at risk	
Total	286,787
With >7 years of exposure and >20 years latency	12,734
With >7 years of exposure and >10 years latency	46,350
Sex (% of cohort)	
Male	45
Female	55
Race (% of cohort)	
White	79
Black	16
Other	5
Vital status as of 12/31/87-no. (%)	
Alive	16,242 (89.1)
Dead	
Death certificate received	1,137 (6.2)
Death certificate not received	40 (0.2)
Untraceable, vital status unknown	820 (4.5)
Average length of exposure (yr)	4.9
Average length of follow-up (yr)	16.1

*Workers are included in all categories in which they ever worked.

We were fortunate in this study that industrial hygiene sampling data for EtO was available from most of the study facilities. However, exposure data were generally available only after the late 1970's, when the companies

> *Estimating historic exposure levels is generally one of the most challenging aspects of conducting retrospective studies of occupational exposures.*

first became aware of the potential carcinogenic hazards of EtO.

One approach that has been commonly used is to assign historic exposure levels based on the subjective opinions of the investigators or knowledgeable plant personnel about the work processes and changes in these processes over time that would affect exposures. This study was one of the first occupational studies to employ an alternative approach of developing a statistical model of the existing exposure data that would be used to predict exposure levels for periods of time and operations where data was absent.

The approach that we used for developing the statistical model for predicting retrospective exposure to EtO for the study was the result of very intense, and at times even tense, interactions among the industrial hygienists, epidemiologists, and statisticians involved in the study. The methods used to develop and evaluate the accuracy and bias of this model are fully described in two papers[14,15] and briefly described in the following sections.

The industrial hygiene team collected some samples, but, by and large, we relied on historic samples taken by the companies to develop the exposure model. At one site, we had a crisis when a team visited a Chicago facility to take industrial hygiene measurements. Exposure concentrations at this facility were extraordinarily high and were not likely to have changed much over time. Because of the relatively high EtO levels, one of our industrial hygienists, John Morawetz, decided to wear a respirator to protect him while monitoring exposures in the sterilization area. When one of the sterilizer operators asked Mr. Morawetz why he was wearing a mask, he explained that NIOSH was doing a study of the possible association between exposure to EtO and cancer risk as a possible long-term effect. The operator asked about more immediate health effects and Mr. Morawetz explained that the current study would not examine these effects, but NIOSH did conduct Health Hazard Evaluations that could be targeted toward more acute effects.

After NIOSH left the facility, the operator went to the plant management, wanting to know more about EtO health effects and what could be done to offer the workers better protection. The company called NIOSH, voiced their extreme displeasure concerning what Mr. Morawetz had said, and demanded that Mr. Morawetz not return to the plant. Believing that there was no need to return to the facility, NIOSH agreed that Mr. Morawetz would not return to the facility. When the team decided that additional exposure samples were needed, a second site survey was planned. Because of a last-minute staffing change, Mr. Morawetz was asked to return to the site, although he was not aware of management's position or the NIOSH agreement to keep him away from the facility. When the team arrived at the site, the management representatives said they didn't want Mr. Morawetz there, and that if they had a gun they would have pulled it to order NIOSH off their property. They also called the team's lead industrial hygienist, Larry Elliott, a communist for insisting on NIOSH's right of entry. The team was finally allowed to remain on site and collect samples with certain restrictions on John Morawetz's access to the high exposure areas of the plant.

The dependent variable for the development of our statistical model was the mean of the log-transformed mean of all EtO measurements taken for a given job and/or location within each plant for a given year. A log-transformed mean was necessary because the exposure data were highly skewed and not normally (but rather log normally) distributed. The sampling data used were based on personal samples taken using a charcoal tube method. We excluded area samples and samples taken using a passive monitor because of concerns about the reliability of these measurement methods. Personal exposure data were available from 18 of the facilities that were included in the walk-through surveys, even though not all of these plants were eventually included in the study. Data from six randomly selected plants (approximately 20% of the data) were reserved for subsequent model validation exercise. This left 205 annual arithmetic means based upon 2,350 full-shift charcoal tube measurements from 12 different plants for model development.

A weighted[m] multiple linear regression model was fitted to these data. A number of variables that we believed, based on our experience, might be potential predictors of exposure were evaluated for inclusion in the model. Exposure category and product type were forced into all of the models because they were believed to have a high probability of impact on EtO exposure levels (see Table 29-2). Of the 17 engineering, administrative, and process control variables considered for inclusion in the model, only aeration of the product after sterilization and use of a powered rear exhaust valve in

---

[m] The weights used were a function of the inverse of the coefficient of variation and the sample size (n) of the means.

TABLE 29-2 Exposure categories and product types used in retrospective exposure model

	Exposure categories		Product types
1	Laboratory	1	Spore strips
2	Sterilizer area (except operator)	2	Plastic
3	Warehouse	3	Gauze
4	Production area	4	Spices
5	Clean room	5	Glass or metal
6	Quarantine room		
7	Sterilizer operator		
8	Maintenance		

TABLE 29-3 Weighted multiple regression model for estimation of retrospective exposure to ethylene oxide

Exposure factor	dL	F test	p value
Exposure category	7	3.40	0.002
Product type	4	17.41	<0.01
Age of product	1	68.31	<0.01
Year	1	124.02	<0.01
(Year)^2	1	31.91	<0.01
Exhaust	1	4.02	0.046
Aeration	1	2.71	0.404
Cubic feet	1	77.35	<0.01
(Cubic feet)^3	1	55.71	<0.01
Error	186		

$R^2 = 0.85$

the sterilizer unit provided statistically significant reductions in EtO levels.

EtO exposure levels were found to significantly decrease with increasing calendar years. We assumed that calendar year was acting as a surrogate for some changes that were made in the process to reduce exposures to EtO that was not accounted for by the other covariates, and thus decided to include it in the final model. Predictions of EtO concentrations from this model were the highest in 1978. Because we had little exposure data prior to that year, we assumed that the levels predicted for 1978 applied to prior years in the study. Our final EtO exposure prediction model is presented in Table 29-3.

The final EtO prediction model, remarkably, explained 85% of the variation in the model development data. Comparing the predictions from this model with the actual measured values from the validation data set yielded an estimate of bias of −1.13 ppm and a precision of 3.66 ppm. As a further evaluation of the model, we had a panel of 11 industrial hygienists estimate the EtO exposure levels for the 46 measurements that were included in the model validation dataset. We found that the model predictions resulted in lower bias than 9 out of 11, and better precision than all 11 of the industrial hygienists.

After our model validation procedure convinced us that we had a reliable model, we used the model to predict annual EtO exposure levels for each worker in our study. We noticed that the predicted exposure levels were relatively high for workers in the warehouse under certain conditions. Because of this, we carefully reviewed the original 205 records that were used for the model development. It was found that 8 records that were previously coded, as "Office" or "Supervisor" should have actually been assigned to warehouse locations. The data were corrected and the model refitted. This illustrates how careful checking of model predictions for an exposure matrix is very important.

TEN YEARS LATER, FINALLY SOME RESULTS!

Approximately 10 years after our initial exploration into the feasibility of the study, the initial findings were published in the *New England Journal of Medicine* (*NEJM*) on May 16, 1991.[12] Publication in the *NEJM*, which is one of the premier biomedical journals, was a significant event for our study team. A number of papers have been published since this initial paper, and we present the following brief summary of the findings from each of the papers in chronologic order.

This first paper presented the findings from a life table analysis of the cohort using the NIOSH life table program.[15] This program groups the observed deaths into many categories and computes expected numbers of deaths for these categories by multiplying the age, calendar time, gender- and race-specific mortality rates from the standard population (in this case the United States) by the corresponding person-years distribution from the study population. The ratio of the observed to expected number of deaths is called the standardized mortality ratio (SMR). A summary of the findings from the NIOSH life table analysis is presented in Table 29-4.

TABLE 4 Mortality According to Cause of Death for All Plants Combined

Cause of Death	Deaths Observed	Expected	SMR	95% CI
All causes	1177	1454.3	0.81	0.76–0.86
All cancers	343	380.3	0.90	0.81–1.00
All hematopoietic cancers**	36	33.8	1.06	0.75–1.47
Lymphosarcoma-reticulosarcoma	8	5.3	1.52	0.65–3.00
Hodgkin's disease	4	3.5	1.14	0.31–2.92
Leukemia—aleukemia	13	13.5	0.97	0.52–1.67
Others	11	11.7	0.93	0.47–1.68
Non-Hodgkin's lymphoma	8	6.7	1.20	0.57–2.37
Myeloma	3	5.1	0.59	0.12–1.73
Brain—nervous system cancer	6	11.6	0.52	0.19–1.13
All digestive cancers	80	85.6	0.93	0.74–1.16
Stomach	11	11.6	0.95	0.45–1.70
Esophagus	8	7.7	1.04	0.44–2.06
Pancreas	16	16.9	0.95	0.54–1.53
Respiratory system cancer	96	101.7	0.94	0.76–1.15
Breast cancer	42	49.6	0.85	0.61–1.14
Urinary-organ cancer	17	12.4	1.37	0.80–2.19
Kidney	13	7.2	1.80	0.96–3.08
Bladder	4	5.2	0.77	0.21–1.96
Heart disease	358	430.0	0.83	0.75–0.92
Nonmalignant respiratory disease	61	76.4	0.80	0.61–1.03
Nonmalignant digestive disease	48	79.4	0.60	0.44–0.80
Nonmalignant genitourinary disease	12	18.8	0.64	0.33–1.12

*SMR denotes standardized mortality ration, CI confidence interval, and SMR 1978 the SMR for workers first exposed to ethylene oxide before January 1, 1978 (86 percent of the cohort).
**Includes the following diseases designated by the codes indicated in the *International Classification of Diseases*, 9th revision: lymphosarcoma-reticulosarcoma (200), Hodgkin's disease (201), leukemia (204-208), & other hematopoietic cancers (202, 203), divided in this table into non-Hodgkin's lymphoma (202) & myeloma (203).

Results are also presented in this table for workers first employed prior to 1978 when EtO exposures were presumed to be higher. Overall mortality for our cohort was significantly less than expected (SMR=0.81, 95% Confidence Interval [CI] = 0.76-0.86), which is not unusual for a working population that is generally healthier on average than the general population (i.e., the healthy worker effect). There was no statistically significant evidence of an excess in any specific cause of death, including mortality from all lymphatic and hematopoietic neoplasms (SMR=1.06, 95% CI = 0.75-1.47) and leukemia (SMR=0.97, 95% CI = 0.52-1.67), which were the sites of primary concern based on previous studies. However, there were some findings of a positive association in subgroup analyses of the cohort. A significant increase in mortality from all lymphatic and hematopoietic neoplasms (SMR=1.55) was observed among men. The excess of lymphatic and hematopoietic neoplasms was even more pronounced (SMR=2.63, 95% CI = 1.05-5.42) among men in the longest duration of exposure and time since first exposure group. The effect modification by gender might be a reflection of the fact that, for the most part, males worked in the sterilization and other areas of the plants with the highest exposures to EtO. However, there was little evidence of higher mortality among workers employed as sterilizer operators or in other high-exposure job categories. Mortality from lymphatic and hematopoietic neoplasms was also not observed to increase with duration of exposure to EtO, but a significant trend ($p = 0.03$) with time since first exposure (sometimes referred to as latency) was observed.

Our first paper concluded that, "Although our study is the largest to date of workers exposed to ethylene oxide, the results for the relatively rare cancers of a priori interest are still limited by the small number of cases and perhaps limited by the short follow-up. Our findings are therefore not conclusive." Having such inconclusive findings was somewhat disappointing to us. After 10 years of performing this study we hoped for a clearer signal one way or the other.

Stronger evidence of an association between EtO and hematopoietic neoplasms was observed in our second paper, which examined whether there was evidence for an exposure-response relationship.[17] In this study, we utilized prediction of exposure from the statistical model that was previously described[14,15] to estimate exposure measures for each worker in the study, including their average exposure (ppm), maximum exposure (ppm), and cumulative exposure (i.e., duration*average exposure to EtO). Exposure-response analyses using these exposure measures were conducted both with the NIOSH life table analysis system (LTAS) and with a Cox proportional hazards model. The Cox model included variables to control for the effects of calendar time, age at risk, gender and race. The analyses were limited to workers from 13 of the 14 study facilities that had exposure information for estimating historical exposures. Analyses were conducted for cancers of the kidney (International Classification of Diseases, Ninth Revision (ICD-9), codes 189.0-189.2), stomach (ICD-9 code 151), pancreas (ICD-9 code 157), all hematopoietic neoplasms (ICD-9 codes 200-208), all leukemias (ICD-9 codes 204-208), non-Hodgkin's lymphoma (ICD-9 codes 200 and 202) and all other hematopoietic neoplasm (ICD-9 codes 201 and 203). In addition, the Cox model was fitted using a combined category of non-Hodgkin's lymphoma (ICD-9 codes 200 and 202) and lymphocytic leukemia (ICD-9 code 204) that was referred to as "lymphoid" tumors. It has been suggested that these cancers are etiologically related and should be combined for epidemiologic purposes.[18]

Results from the life table analyses for cumulative EtO exposure are presented in Table 29-5. There was weak evidence of a trend ($p = 0.32$) of increasing mortality from all hematopoietic neoplasms and cumulative exposure to EtO, which was somewhat stronger for males ($p = 0.19$), and a significant excess was observed among males in the highest exposure group (SMR=1.96, 95% CI = 1.10-3.43). Stronger evidence for an exposure-response relationship was observed in the findings using the Cox proportional hazards model for all lymphatic and hematopoietic neoplasms combined (10 year lag,[n] (χ^2=4.96, $p = 0.03$), non-Hodgkin's lymphoma (10 year lag, Chi-square ((χ^2)=3.98, $p = 0.05$), and particularly for lymphoid tumors (5 year lag, (χ^2=8.44, $p = 0.004$) when a lag period[o] was assumed. This is a useful example of the increase in statistical power that can be obtained by performing regression analyses in which the exposure is treated as a continuous variable rather than as a categorical variable as they are in life table analyses.

THE INDUSTRY CONSULTANTS ETO STUDY

As mentioned earlier, NIOSH agreed in its MOU with HIMA to provide their consultant with a study computer tape that they could use to verify our coding of the data. We also anticipated that they would use these tapes to confirm the results from our analysis. However, under our MOU, they would not receive this data tape until our analysis was completed and published. Their consultant was also receiving copies of all of the records that we microfilmed from the companies. Using these records, they were able to create their own study files, and to conduct their own follow-up and vital status ascertainment for the cohort.

In 1992, their consultants, Dr. Otto Wong and a colleague (Lisa Trent), published a paper that presented

---

[n] In using a lag period, one assumes that exposure prior to some period of time (e.g., 10 years) is not relevant to disease occurrence and, thus, is not counted in estimating exposures.

[o] A lag period is a period of time prior to the occurrence of disease or the time at risk when exposures are discounted.

TABLE 5 Observed numbers of deaths and standardized mortality ratios for mortality due to all cancers and cancer at selected major sites, by cumulative exposure to ethylene oxide: US workers followed to December 31, 1987

Cancer site (ICD-9 code(s))	Cumulative exposure to ethylene oxide (ppm-days)												Total			Trend test	
	<1,200			1,200–8,500			>8,500										
	Obs	SMR	95% CI	Obs	SMR	95% CI	Obs	SMR	95% CI				Obs	SMR	95% CI	x2	p
All cancers	100	94	76–114	120	90	74–107	108	86	70–104				328	90	80–100	0.10	0.66
Stomach (151)	5	174	57–407	4	124	29–260	1	23	1–132				10	90	43–166	4.32	0.04
Pancreas (157)	3	69	14–203	10	170	81–312	3	50	10–147				16	98	57–161	0.76	0.38
Brain (191 and 192)	0	0	0–102	4	99	27–253	2	59	7–212				6	54	20–118	0.63	0.43
Kidney (189.0–189.2)	1	52	1–292	8	322	139–635	3	122	25–357				12	175	90–306	0.01	0.98
All hematopoietic cancers (200–208)	8	79	34–157	12	101	52–177	13	124	66–213				33	102	71–144	0.97	0.32
Leukemia/aleukemia (204–208)	4	99	27–252	4	85	23–219	3	75	15–218				11	86	43–154	0.13	0.72
Non-Hodgkin's lymphoma (200 and 202)	4	117	32–298	4	96	26–246	7	192	77–395				15	133	75–220	1.04	0.31
Other hematopoietic cancers (201 and 203)	0	0	0–147	4	134	36–343	3	111	23–325				7	85	34–176	1.26	0.26

the findings from a life table analysis of their own computer file for the ethylene oxide cohort.[19] We were surprised that neither Dr. Wong nor HIMA had alerted us that they were publishing this paper, and even more surprised that this paper did not even refer to our paper that was published just 2 years earlier! To pretend that they had conducted an independent study, and to not even reveal that a previous study of virtually the same study population had been published seemed to us to be a serious ethical lapse. We wrote a letter to the editors of *BJIM* to alert them and their readership to this issue.[20] Drs. Wong and Trent responded that theirs was an independent study in which they had collected records directly from the HIMA companies that were included in our study and performed their own follow-up of the cohort for ascertainment of vital status.[21] They included some records that we had apparently missed and not microfilmed. Unbeknownst to us, they had presented the findings from their study to HIMA in 1990 and sent a final report in 1991 to HIMA. They acknowledged in their letter that they regretted "the oversight of not citing the NIOSH study," but maintained that their study was an independent investigation.

It was reassuring that the results from the analyses in the Wong and Trent paper were very similar to those found in our life table analysis[12] Of course, this was not surprising, given that their study population was nearly identical to ours. Their study included 18,278 workers and ours included 18,254 workers exposed to EtO. The difference appears to be largely due to the fact that, as mentioned previously, they had access to some company records that we did not have. As with our study, they found an excess of non-Hodgkin's lymphoma among the men in the study. They observed that the excess of non-Hodgkin's lymphoma among men did not increase with duration of employment or latency. Based on the lack of dose-response and the inconsistency of the findings for the sexes, the authors concluded, "the increase in non-Hodgkin's lymphoma among the men did not seem to be related to exposure to EtO." Their conclusion was more conservative than ours, which was that the evidence was "not conclusive."[12] However, a limitation of their study was that they did not use detailed work histories (as we did) and were, thus, not able to examine trends with duration of exposure or cumulative exposure to EtO as we did in our study. Furthermore, their analysis of latency was not based on time since first exposure, but rather on time since first employment.

FURTHER UPDATES AND STUDIES OF THE NIOSH COHORT

Two additional studies[12,17] of the NIOSH EtO cohort study have been conducted since the publication of our first reports in 1991 and 1992. In one of these studies,[22] follow-up for vital status ascertainment was extended from 1987 to 1998. It is common for NIOSH to continue follow-up on their major cohort study populations, particularly for studies with relatively young populations like our EtO cohort. In fact, many of these cohort studies can provide valuable information for many years, and may even outlive the original investigators. Updating mortality for these cohorts has become relatively simple because the National Death Index (NDI) can be searched for deaths occurring after 1978. Social Security Administration (SSA) records and Internal Revenue Service (IRS) records were also used in this study to update vital status, primarily because it is cheaper to search these databases than it is to search the NDI (which charges a fee). The additional follow-up of this cohort more than doubled the number of deaths available for the study from 1,177 to 2,852. Qualitatively, the findings in this update were very similar to those from the prior studies[12,17] A significant exposure-response was observed among males between cumulative EtO exposure (lagged 15 years) for all lymphatic and hematopoietic neoplasms, which was primarily explained by an even stronger exposure-response for "lymphoid" tumors (ICD-9 codes 200, 202, and 204). These trends were weaker than those observed in the previous studies, and there was no evidence of an exposure-relationship for the post-1987 data (i.e., from the period of additional follow-up). The lack of a trend may be accounted for by the fact that exposures to EtO were dramatically decreased in this industry during this time period due to concerns that had already been raised about its safety. It might also reflect a relatively short latency period for lymphatic and hematopoietic neoplasms, and that the study had passed the peak of the epidemic curve for this population. It is not uncommon in occupational epidemiology to see a drop in the effect of exposure with continued follow-up.[23] This is probably because after the maximum latency period has been passed, the cohort would not be at increased risk of disease; thus, the addition of person-time from the follow-up would just dilute the overall association.

The second paper was a study of breast cancer incidence in our EtO cohort.[24] An excess in the incidence of breast cancer had been reported in two studies of women exposed to EtO.[25,26] An increased incidence of breast tumors had also been reported in a study of mice exposed to EtO.[27] An increased incidence of breast cancer was not observed in two small studies of women exposed to EtO.[28,29] Breast cancer mortality was also not found to be elevated in our previous studies[12,22] or in another small study of women exposed to EtO.[30] In our most recent follow-up of the NIOSH cohort, the SMR for all exposed women was very close to one and had a relatively tight confidence interval (SMR=0.99, 95% CI = 0.81-1.20).[22] However, evidence of an exposure-response relationship between cumulative exposure to EtO and breast cancer mortality was observed. A statistically significant excess risk of breast cancer mortality (OR=3.1, 95% CI = 1.4-6.9) was observed in the highest cumulative EtO exposure group.

Breast cancer incidence for our cohort was ascertained via questionnaires, death certificates, cancer registries (for states that had them), and medical records. Cancer registries were available in nine of the 11 states in which our plants were located, but generally for just a limited period of the study time. The questionnaires were administered using both mailed and phone interviews. In the end, questionnaires were completed for only 68% of the study subjects. This response rate is lower than we hoped, but not lower than what most epidemiologists would consider acceptable. Medical record confirmation was sought for all cases identified from the questionnaires or death certificates.

One of the challenging aspects of conducting this study was that the contents of the questionnaire had to be first approved by the Office of Management and Budget (OMB). The OMB claims the authority to review survey questionnaires under the authority of the Paperwork Reduction Act (PL 104-13). In April of 1995, the questionnaire and other study materials were sent to the OMB for clearance. In the Federal Register, the OMB published a request for comments on the proposal, and they received comments from HIMA objecting to the study. In July of 1995, the OMB gave NIOSH tentative approval on the conditions that NIOSH (1) perform a pretest of the questionnaire in 30 women, (2) form a Scientific Advisory Board (SAB) to review the protocol, and (3) report the results from the SAB to the OMB. From August to December of 1995, NIOSH conducted the pretest of the questionnaire, formed a SAB, and had held a public meeting in the District of Columbia. The OMB finally approved the study in April of 1996.

The breast cancer incidence study was restricted to women in our EtO cohort who had been employed for at least one year (72% of the original cohort). The one-year requirement was imposed to limit the cost of the study, because a smaller group of women would need to be interviewed and followed for vital status. It is generally also very difficult to locate women with short-term employment in occupational cohort studies because of name changes.

It was anticipated that this study would under-ascertain breast cancer incidence, given the low response rate for the questionnaires and the limited coverage of the cancer registries. Our findings were consistent with our expectations. In the entire cohort, there were 319 incident breast cancer cases observed, which was significantly lower than the number expected based on life table analyses using SEER[p] as the referent (standardized incidence ratio (SIR) =0.87, 95% CI = 0.77-0.97). However, there was significant ($p = 0.002$) evidence of a positive exposure-response trend in internal analysis using standardized incidence ratios (15 year lag). A statistically significant increase in risk was also observed in the highest exposure (lagged 15 years) quintile (OR=1.74, 95% CI = 1.16-2.65).

A nested case-control study was also conducted in which incident breast cancer cases and controls were selected from the cohort. The study was limited to those women with interviews (i.e., complete ascertainment). Using a conditional logistic model to analyze these data, a positive and highly statistically significant ($p = 0.0005$) exposure-response relationship was observed. There was also evidence for an exposure-response in categorical models using quintiles of cumulative exposure, with the highest risk being observed for the top quintile (OR=1.87, 95% CI = 1.12-3.10). However, there were some inconsistencies in the exposure-response trend that raise questions about whether this association was causal. First, the relationship between breast cancer and cumulative exposure of EtO was not stronger than the relationship with duration of exposure of EtO. One would expect a stronger relationship with cumulative exposure than duration of exposure if EtO were causally related to breast cancer. Of course, this might not be the case if there were large errors in the estimation of EtO. However, as previously noted, our methods for exposure assessment were validated using external data. Another issue with the exposure-response findings was that there appeared to be a downturn of the exposure-response at

---

[p] The Surveillance, Epidemiology and End Results (SEER) Program is a NCI program that provides cancer incidence and survival data from population based cancer registries that cover 26% of the U.S. population.

high levels of cumulative EtO exposure. Downturns and leveling off of the exposure-response relationship are frequent occurrences in occupational cohort studies.[31]

The findings from this study lent support to the hypothesis that EtO may be associated with an increased risk of breast cancer in women. However, we felt that a causal interpretation of these findings was weakened by "some inconsistencies in exposure-response trends and possible biases due to nonresponse and incomplete cancer ascertainment."

EPILOGUE

As noted earlier, it took us more than 10 years of work to get to point where we could publish the first findings from this study. This is an unusually long period of time for an occupational cohort study. Typically, occupational cohorts may take 3 to 5 years to complete. This study took longer, in part, because of delays related to the extensive negotiations we had to undertake to convince HIMA and the companies involved to cooperate with the study. It was also because this was an unusually complicated study that involved the inclusion of workers from numerous facilities. Most occupational cohort studies involve one plant or just a few plants.

In addition to time, this study required innumerable person-years of effort on our part and on the part of our entire study team. In going through historical records to write this chapter, we discovered that there were more than a dozen file drawers containing the memos, letters, and other documents that were written concerning this study. These were all written before the time when personal computers and email were available to facilitate communications. During the first few years of the study, each of us travelled several times per month to more than 30 study locations across the country.

Both of us are now employed in academia and it is interesting to note how difficult (if not impossible) it would be to conduct a similar study in our present positions. First, as noted earlier, without the NIOSH right of entry, this study would not have been possible. Just getting funding for the study would be very difficult, because NIH or NIOSH will generally not fund a study that would last 10 years. In addition, this study required virtually 100% of our time for at least the first 2-3 years, and it's difficult to imagine how we could perform the other responsibilities for teaching and service that we have in an academic setting. This study is just one of many examples of how critically important NIOSH is to research workers' health and safety.

In retrospect, one can't help but ask whether this study was worth the effort. Thus far, it has resulted in the publication of seven peer reviewed journal articles, several of which have been in very good journals (e.g., the *New England Journal of Medicine* and the *American Journal of Epidemiology*). According to Google Scholar, collectively these papers have been cited more than 200 times in the peer review literature. Therefore, many people have thought our work was important enough to at least mention it in their work. We also received the Alice Hamilton Award at NIOSH for two of our papers, which is an award for the best NIOSH scientific publication of the year.

Clearly, our work made an impact on the scientific community. More importantly, did it also positively impact the public, and particularly, workers' health? We like to think the answer to this question is yes, but it is difficult to measure the impact of one study on the public's health. In 1984, OSHA revised its permissible exposure limit on EtO to 1 ppm, and, in 1988, they added a 5 ppm short-term exposure limit. These standards were promulgated before our study was completed, so we can't claim any responsibility for these changes. Nonetheless, we believe our findings have supported the OSHA revised standards for EtO and have been useful to OSHA in its continual needs to evaluate and justify its standards.[32]

IARC recently performed a reassessment of the evidence for the carcinogenicity of ethylene oxide.[33] One of us (LS) chaired this monograph meeting. In this assessment, IARC reaffirmed its position from a prior review in 1994 that EtO was a known cause of cancer in humans (Group IA). Our study was cited as a key study in the IARC review, but, as in previous meetings, the human data was not judged to be sufficient to establish causality in humans. Instead, the classification was justified on the basis of sufficient evidence in experimental animals and the combination of limited data in humans with strong support from mechanistic studies. Nonetheless, we believe our findings were influential on the IARC decision.

Our study is one of the only epidemiologic studies that provides exposure-response data that could be used in a risk assessment. Risk assessment is a systematic approach to the evaluation of the hazardous properties of substances, the extent of human exposure to them, and the characterization of the resulting risk for EtO.[34] Exposure-response data is an essential element for the characterization of risk. Risk assessment has become a requirement for setting exposure limits and other standards by OSHA, EPA, and most other U.S. regulatory agencies. A risk assessment using the findings from our study has already been published.[35] This assessment resulted in estimates of risk that were orders of magnitude lower than those from previous EPA and OSHA risk assessments that were based on animal data. The EPA is currently working on a revised risk assessment for environmental exposure to EtO. They are conducting additional analyses of our data, and one of us (KS) has been retained as a consultant in that effort. A draft of the proposed EPA risk assessment has been published for review online (http://cfpub.epa.gov/ncea/cfm/recordisplay.cfm?deid=157664). This risk assessment utilizes data from the NIOSH studies for estimating risk for lymphatic and hematopoietic neoplasms in males and breast cancer in females. It also reports risk estimates from analysis of studies of three rodent bioassay studies. The risk estimates from the analysis of the NIOSH study were about an order of magnitude higher than those based on the rodent studies.

In closing, we do believe this study was worth the effort and we probably would do it again if it weren't for our age and current responsibilities in academia. We like to think that this study has served workers, people in the community exposed to EtO, and even the medical devices industry and other industries using EtO. We hope our experiences are useful to you and other readers of this chapter who may be embarking on a similar study in the future. We also hope that new investigators in this field will not be discouraged by this story, and will instead view this story as a lesson in how important it is to think big and how with perseverance you can succeed (Figure 29-1). Like good French wines, cohorts do take time, but in the end it is worth the wait!

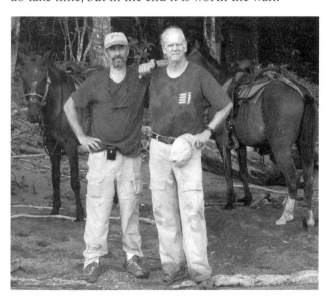

FIGURE 29-1 Leslie and Kyle horseback riding on the beach in Corcovado, Costa Rica in June of 2008.

LEARNING QUESTIONS

1. What steps did the authors take to assess the feasibility of the study? Were these steps adequate? Can you think of any other steps that should have been taken to establish feasibility?
2. How was the cohort followed to determine vital status, cause of death, and incident cases of disease? Was the ascertainment of mortality and incident cases of disease adequate?
3. How was the exposure to EtO estimated for this cohort for the early period of the study when exposure measurements were not available? Were these estimates of exposure likely to be unbiased and have minimal errors?

ACKNOWLEDGMENTS

The authors would first like to recognize the many contributions of our former NIOSH colleagues, including Bill Halperin, Alice Greife, Rick Hornung, Larry Elliott, and Virginia Ringenburg. We are also indebted to Dr. Richard Hayes and the support we received from the National Cancer Institute for the study. This study would never have happened if not for the support, guidance, and diplomatic skills of Dr. William Halperin, who supported our work and skillfully guided us through innumerable difficult minefields in our negotiations with the industry. Finally, we would like to dedicate this paper to the memory of the late Dr. John Paul Jones from Johnson & Johnson, who encouraged us to conduct this study.

Disclaimer This work does not, in any way, represent the views or positions of the National Institute for Occupational Safety and Health.

REFERENCES

1. Amoore JE, Hautala E. Odor as an aid to chemical safety: odor thresholds compared with threshold limit values and volatilities for 214 industrial chemicals in air and water dilution. *J Appl Toxicol.* 1983;3(6):272–290.
2. SRI Consulting. *Chemical Economics Handbook (CEH)*. SRI Consulting web site. http://www.sriconsulting.com/CEH. Accessed May 21, 2010.
3. National Institute for Occupational Safety and Health. *National Occupational Exposure Survey: Sampling Methodology*. Cincinnati, OH: US Department of Health and Human Services; 1989. DHHS (NIOSH) Publication No.89–102.
4. Althouse R, Huff J, Tomatis L, Wilbourn J. *Chemicals and Industrial Processes Associated with Cancer in Humans*. Supplement No. 1. Lyon, France: IARC Monographs Program; 1979. IARC Monographs Volumes 1–20.
5. IARC. *Cadmium, Nickel, Some Epoxides, Miscellaneous Industrial Chemicals and General Considerations on Volatile*

Anaesthetics. Lyon, France: IARC Monographs Program; 1976. *IARC Monographs on the Evaluation of Carcinogenic Risk of Chemicals to Man;* vol. 11: 157-167.
6. Snellings WM, Weil CS, Maronpot RR. A two-year inhalation study of the carcinogenic potential of ethylene oxide in Fischer 344 rats. *Toxicol Appl Pharmacol.* 1984;75(1):105–117.
7. Hogstedt C, Malmqvist N, Wadman B. Leukemia in workers exposed to ethylene oxide. *JAMA.* 1979;241(11):1132–1133.
8. Hogstedt C, Rohlen O, Berndtsson B, Axelson O, Ehrenberg L. A cohort study of mortality and cancer incidence in ethylene oxide production workers. *Br J Ind Med.* 1979;36(4):276–280.
9. Stolley PD, Soper KA, Galloway SM, Nichols WW, Norman SA, Wolman SR. Sister-chromatid exchanges in association with occupational exposure to ethylene oxide. *Mutat Res.* 1984;129(1);89–102.
10. Steenland K, Stayner L, Greife A. Assessing the feasibility of retrospective cohort studies. *Am J Ind Med.* 1987;12(4):419–430.
11. JRB Associates. Economic and environmental impact of study of ethylene oxide. Washington, DC: Occupational Safety and Health Administration; 1983.
12. Steenland K, Stayner L, Greife A, et al. Mortality among workers exposed to ethylene oxide. *New Engl J Med.* 1991;324(20):1402–1407.
13. Beaumont JJ, Breslow NE. Power considerations in epidemiologic studies of vinyl chloride workers. *Am J Epidemiol.* 1981;114(5):725–734.
14. Greife AL, Hornung, RW, Stayner LG, Steenland KN. Development of a model for use in estimating exposure to ethylene oxide in a retrospective cohort mortality study. *Scand J Work Env Health.* 1988;l4(Suppl 1);29–30.
15. Hornung RW, Greife AL, Stayner LT, et al. Statistical model for prediction of retrospective exposure to ethylene oxide in an occupational mortality study. *Am J Ind Med.* 1994;25(6):825–836.
16. Steenland K, Spaeth S, Cassinelli R 2nd, Laber P, Chang L, Koch K. NIOSH life table program for personal computers. *Am J Ind Med.* 1998;34(5):517–518.
17. Stayner L, Steenland K, Greife A, et al. Exposure-response analysis of cancer mortality in a cohort of workers exposed to ethylene oxide. *Am J of Epidemiol.* 1993;138(10):787–798.
18. Heath CW. Leukemia. In: Schottenfeld D, Fraumeni JF Jr, eds. *Cancer Epidemiology and Prevention.* Philadelphia, PA: WB Saunders Company; 1982:728–738.
19. Wong O, Trent LS. An epidemiological study of workers potentially exposed to ethylene oxide. *Br J Ind Med.* 1993;50(4):308–316.
20. Steenland K, Stayner L. Correspondence regarding: An epidemiological study of workers potentially exposed to ethylene oxide. *Br J Ind Med.* 1993;50;1125–1127.
21. Wong O, Trent LS. Reply to correspondence. *Br J Ind Med.*1993;50:1125–1127.
22. Steenland K, Stayner L, Deddens J. Mortality analyses in a cohort of 18 235 ethylene oxide exposed workers: follow up extended from 1987 to 1998. *Occup Environ Med.* 2004;61(1):2–7.
23. Silver SR, Rinsky RA, Cooper SP, Hornung RW, Lai D. Effect of follow-up time on risk estimates: a longitudinal examination of the relative risks of leukemia and multiple myeloma in a rubber hydrochloride cohort. *Am J Ind Med.* 2002;42(6):481–489.
24. Steenland K, Whelan E, Deddens J, Stayner L, Ward E. Ethylene oxide and breast cancer incidence in a cohort study of 7576 women (United States). *Cancer Causes Control.* 2003;14(6):531–539.
25. Norman SA, Berlin JA, Soper KA, Middendorf BE, Stolley PD. Cancer incidence in a group of workers potentially exposed to ethylene oxide. *Int J Epidemiol.* 1995;24(2):276–284.
26. Tompa A, Major J, Jakab MG. Is breast cancer cluster influenced by environmental and occupational factors among hospital nurses in Hungary? *Pathol Oncol Res.* 1999;5(2):117–121.
27. IARC. *Some Industrial Chemicals.* Lyon, France: IARC Monographs Program; 1979. *IARC Monographs;* vol 60.
28. Hagmar L, Welinder H, Linden K, Attewell R, Osterman-Golkar S, Tomqvist M. An epidemiological study of cancer risk among workers exposed to ethylene oxide using hemoglobin adducts to validate environmental exposure assessments. *Int Arch Occup Environ Health.* 1991;63(4):271–277.
29. Gardner MJ, Coggon D, Pannett B, Harris EC. Workers exposed to ethylene oxide: a follow-up study. *Brit J Ind Med.* 1989;46(12):860-865.
30. Hogstedt C, Aringer L, Gustavsson A. Epidemiologic support for ethylene oxide as a cancer-causing agent. *JAMA.* 1986;255(12):1575–1578.
31. Stayner L, Steenland K, Dosemeci M, Hertz-Picciotto I. Attenuation of exposure-response curves in occupational cohort studies at high exposures. *Scand J Work Environ Health.* 2003;29(4):317–324.
32. OSHA. Regulatory review of the occupational safety and health administration's ethylene oxide standard [29 CFR 1910.1047]. US Department of Labor Web site. http://www.osha.gov/dea/lookback/ethylene_oxide_lookback.html. Accessed May 22, 2010.
33. Grosse Y, Baan R, Straif K, et al. Carcinogenicity of 1,3-butadiene, ethylene oxide, vinyl chloride, vinyl fluoride, and vinyl bromide. *Lancet Oncol.* 2007;8(8):679–680.
34. Committee on Risk Assessments of Hazardous Air Pollutants; Board on Environmental Studies and Toxicology; Commission on Life Sciences; National Research Council. *Science and Judgment in Risk Assessment.* Washington, DC: National Academy Press; 1994.
35. Teta MJ, Sielken RL Jr, Valdez-Flores C. Ethylene oxide cancer risk assessment based on epidemiological data: application of revised regulatory guidelines. 1999;19(6):1135–1155.

CHAPTER 30

Why Have the Children of Chernivtsi Lost All of Their Hair?

Daniel Hryhorczuk, MD, MPH

Ukraine, 1988

INTRODUCTION

Many years ago, I was reading a Ukrainian newspaper that featured an inspiring photo. What struck me about the photo was the reassuring look in the mother's eyes. She was hugging her 2-year-old daughter, who was smiling, beautiful, and bald. Though her daughter was suffering from the "Chernivtsi illness," the mother seemed to know that her child was going to recover. The newspaper article said that in the fall of 1988, several hundred children in the Ukrainian city of Chernivtsi were stricken with a mysterious illness. The clinical features included total alopecia, upper respiratory symptoms, and night terrors. The Soviet and Ukrainian Ministries of Health had launched independent investigations searching for the cause. Both investigations concluded that the illness was most likely caused by a chemical toxin. According to the article, the identity and source of the toxin continued to elude the public health authorities.

I had good reasons to be interested in the story. As an assistant professor of Epidemiology and Environmental and Occupational Health Sciences at the University of Illinois at Chicago School of Public Health, I was teaching a course in environmental epidemiology. My favorite topic was outbreak investigation. I was also the chief of Clinical Toxicology at Cook County Hospital. A story about a mysterious environmental outbreak due to an as yet unknown toxin—what better reading for a public health detective? What fascinated me most about this story was the location. I am a first–generation Ukrainian American, and my parents had both been born within 100 kilometers of Chernivtsi.

My parents had immigrated to the United States shortly after the Second World War. Before the war broke out, my father was in the seminary and my mother was studying medicine. As members of the intelligentsia, they were forced to flee the advancing Soviet army to avoid arrest, exile to Siberia, or worse. They met in a Displaced Persons camp in Germany, married, and completed their university studies in Munich. After the war, America greeted my parents with open arms. They settled in Urbana-Champaign where my father took a job as research assistant at the University. Shortly after I was born, my mother was accepted for a residency in obstetrics and gynecology, and we moved to join the vibrant Ukrainian émigré community in Chicago. After retiring from private practice, my mother took a position in Maternal and Child Health at the Chicago Board of Health, which is how I first became interested in public health. My father managed to become president of every organization he joined. He started and ran several businesses before being elected president of the Ukrainian National Credit Union Association of North America. He helped to revive the cooperative movement in newly independent Ukraine and was honored by both the White House and the president of Ukraine for his nation-building efforts. Needless to say, Ukrainian was the only language spoken at home. Though I was born in the heart of the U.S. Midwest, I learned to how to speak English in the first grade. The story in the newspaper was bringing me back full circle.

A HYPOTHESIS AND AN INVITATION TO INVESTIGATE

My first guess after reading the article was that the children were suffering from thallium poisoning. When a clinical toxicologist encounters a toxidrome (a constellation of signs and symptoms that is specific for a poison or a group of poisons) that includes rapid onset alopecia, thallium leads the list of usual suspects. I later learned that in April 1989, the World Health Organization had sent two experts on thallium poisoning to Ukraine to assist in the investigation. After a review of the official Ministry reports and review of a sample of 24 pediatric cases (9 who had had alopecia totalis and 15 with patchy alopecia), the experts concluded that the illness was not thallium poisoning. The bioassays of blood and urine conducted by Soviet laboratories had not detected thallium. In addition, their review of the medical records did not reveal any cases of peripheral neuropathy, which is a key feature of severe thallium poisoning. They agreed with the official consensus that it was a chemical illness, but did not offer an alternative diagnosis.

The incidence of cases of total alopecia peaked in late October and early November and had totally disappeared by the end of November. Many families took their children and fled the city to live with relatives. Traffic was banned in the center of the city. The military hosed down roofs and streets and tilled the soil in certain parts of the city. Leaf burning was banned. Anger at the government's failure to identify the cause continued to grow, even after the worst of the outbreak was over. Each new case of alopecia, whether due to alopecia areata or tinea capitis (a form of alopecia that may be caused by autoimmunity or fungal infection), was viewed as a recurrence of this mysterious illness. Officially, the government was promoting a policy of *glasnost*, or openness in communication, especially after the public outrage over their secrecy in the aftermath of the Chernobyl accident less than 2 years before. In April 1986, a nuclear reactor accident at Chernobyl, Ukraine had released a radioactive cloud that contaminated much of Ukraine, Belarus and parts of Europe. Residual radiation from radiocesium still contaminated various parts of Ukraine, including the area around Chernivtsi. The residents of Chernivtsi remained skeptical about the government's failure to find the cause and viewed the official announcements as the same, old-style Soviet propaganda.

The Ukrainian president's representative in Chernivtsi was a young, charismatic politician who was also a distant relative of the prime minister of Canada. He was trying to establish his city, which is strategically located at the intersection of trade routes to Turkey, Moldova, and southeastern Europe, as an economic free zone and tourist destination. The mysterious illness was bad for business. On his own initiative, he sent a delegation to Canada to seek international assistance. The delegation was greeted by the Ukrainian Medical Association of North America, which put out an appeal to its members to see if anyone could help. Not surprisingly, only one of the Association's members happened to be both an environmental epidemiologist and clinical toxicologist. I flew to Toronto to see what I could do.

The Ukrainian delegation consisted of two people: the city's chief public health physician and a member of the city council. They did not bring any official documents to review because the Ministry reports were still highly classified. They said that I would need to travel to Chernivtsi, where they would give me full access to the files. They also wanted me to physically examine a sample of children who were registered as victims of the "Chernivtsi illness." Because the outbreak appeared to be over, we agreed that I would travel to Chernivtsi in July, after I had finished teaching my spring semester classes. I still had family in Ukraine. I had not seen them since 1979, when I first visited Ukraine on a trip with St. Ignatius

High School. My memories from my last visit were not especially pleasant. I remembered a place of oppressive grayness, riddled with red communist slogans.

THE INVESTIGATION

When I arrived at Borispol Airport in Kyiv, I was pleasantly surprised. The airport was still run-down and the security checks were as long as ever, but the immigration officers were uncharacteristically friendly, as if they were actually happy to have foreigners visiting their country. There was optimism in the air that had not been there before. My uncle and cousin picked me up in their old Volga, and we drove the 300 kilometers to the city of Ternopil in western Ukraine. At the halfway point, we pulled over to picnic on the hood of the car. We ate rye bread, sausage, cheese, tomatoes, and homemade pickles. My cousin proudly pulled out a small bottle of reagent grade ethanol, which he had taken from the lab where he operated an electron micrograph, and we toasted to our family reunion. My visit with family in Ternopil was emotional but brief, and after a few days, my cousin drove me the rest of the way to Chernivtsi.

Chernivtsi is unlike any other city in Ukraine. While central and eastern Ukraine are known for their Byzantine architecture and gold-domed churches, Chernivtsi is a remnant of the glory days of the Austro-Hungarian empire. Bukovyna, the "land of beech trees," changed rulers multiple times over the centuries. The population is cosmopolitan. In addition to ethnic Ukrainians, the residents included Romanians, Moldovans, Armenians, and Jews. Italian tourists were paying high prices to hunt bear in the nearby Carpathian Mountains. Chernivtsi was also famous for its art, music, and culture. It was the birthplace of Volodymyr Ivasiuk, the popular young Ukrainian songwriter who had been tortured and killed in 1979, allegedly by Soviet security forces.

When I arrived at the City Hall, I was greeted by the president's representative and his deputy, who also happened to be a popular local poet, and the chief public health physician I had met in Toronto a few months earlier. I was treated to an official luncheon "forshet" with every sort of local delicacy that was complete with local wine, Ukrainian vodka, and Armenian cognac. Toasting is an obligatory art in Ukraine. The politician-poet managed to craft a toast in my honor that began with seemingly disparate threads of compliments that he wove into a tapestry of praise. I could see why he was so valuable on these kinds of occasions. After lunch, the poet gave me a tour of the city that included a visit to the graves of famous Ukrainian writers, many of whom I had actually read during my 11 years attending "Uki School" on Saturdays in Chicago. The mayor paid for my room at the 4-star Cheremosh hotel that had been built only a few years before my visit. The elevators to the guest rooms were guarded by security personnel with machine guns who would stop anyone who wasn't a guest or a hotel-sanctioned prostitute.

My work on the outbreak began in earnest the following morning. I was taken to the local Institute of Medico-Ecologic Problems to meet with the director, Dr. Mukola Prodanchuk. Dr. Prodanchuk was a dynamic, politically savvy, young physician who had worked his way up through the Communist Party and was aspiring to climb to the top of Ukrainian medicine. We became good friends over the years (Figure 30-1). In 2008, he reached his goal and became the Deputy Minister of Health of Ukraine. He launched a much-needed measles vaccination campaign that was endorsed by the World Health Organization (WHO) and the United Nations Children's Fund (UNICEF). Unfortunately, when a child died in Donetstk after receiving the vaccine, the Party of Regions turned on him and politicized the incident. Dr. Prodanchuk had to resign his post to protect the minister. While meeting with the WHO, he was arrested and charged with complicity in the death of the child because the Indian vaccine, though used widely around the world, had not undergone clinical testing and certification in Ukraine. His case is still pending in court.

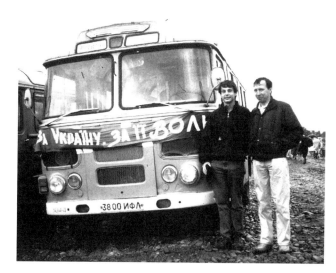

FIGURE 30-1 The author (left) with Dr. Mukola Prodanchuk. The sign on the bus reads "Freedom for Ukraine."

The Institute of Medico-Ecologic Problems was a two-story, well-preserved building with ample space for the director and modest environmental chemistry laboratories. It was an "All-Union" institute, meaning that it served not only the Ukrainian Soviet Socialist Republic, but the entire Soviet Union as well. Given the Chernivtsi outbreak, it was in the right place at the right time. The Institute was planning a conference on "Medico-Ecologic Problems of Women and Children," which would bring together the many Ukrainian and Russian academicians who were working on the Chernivtsi illness. Mukola and I agreed to join forces and work on the outbreak investigation together.

My first request was to tour the city. I especially wanted to visit the homes of children who had been ill. I climbed on the roof of the city hospital to get a better perspective of the topography. The city was built at the convergence of two rivers in the foothills of the Carpathian Mountains. The old center of the city was surrounded by new high-rise developments that the local population called "Krushovky," because they were constructed during the rule of Nikita Kruschov (Figure 30-2). The industrial base of the city was a densely packed conglomeration of factories in the northwest sector. Several factories in the city had been part of the Soviet military industrial complex. These modern factories were off-limits to visitors and were located in the outskirts of the city. The highest buildings were the churches and local hospital. The highest structures were the chimneys from the power plant and the city's three brick kilns. The homes of affected children did not seem to have any factor in common, other than their proximity to playgrounds.

While my official hosts were accommodating, the most tangible cooperation came from the pediatricians at Pediatric Clinic Number 2. This clinic had been the clinical epicenter of the outbreak. The clinic had the largest number of registered cases and was designated by the City Council as the lead clinic for the disease. The director of the Clinic pledged his full cooperation. He was especially eager to have his patients examined by an outside expert. We agreed that I would see patients in the mornings and work on the epidemiologic investigation in the afternoon. I asked him to provide me with an assistant who could help me review the medical records. He assigned an enthusiastic pediatric resident who turned out to be a natural-born epidemiologist. I don't recall his name, but let's call him Vasyl. He had his own theories about the illness that he was eager to share. Given his status, no one was taking his views seriously, even though he had more direct clinical experience with

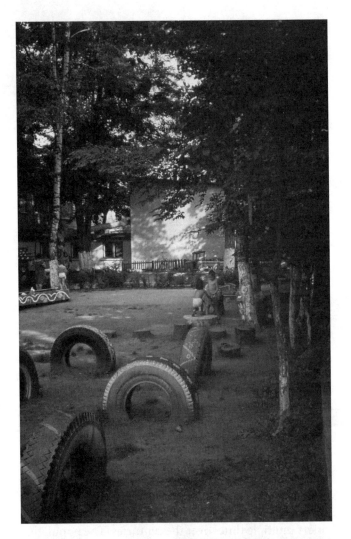

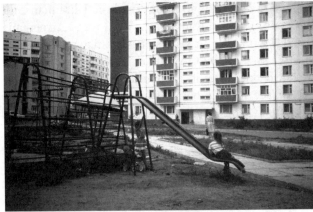

FIGURE 30-2 Playground adjacent to a housing complex that had a large cluster of cases.

the cases than any of the experts who had come from Kyiv, Moscow, and Geneva. Over my many subsequent years working in Ukraine, I came to see how bright, original ideas can be quickly stifled by expert opinion.

Fortunately, I chose to forego my ego and made this young pediatric resident my intellectual partner in the investigation.

We decided to base our outbreak investigation on the cases that were registered in the clinic. I explained to Vasyl how we needed to characterize the outbreak in terms of person, place, and time. I asked him to abstract key elements from the medical records, including age, gender, date of onset, address of residence, and clinical features. I showed him how we could put the information on the edges of index cards, which would allow rapid sorting to do frequency counts. Vasyl jumped to the task. Over the next 2 weeks, he was meticulous and abstracted these data from the medical records. He would prepare his graphs and charts using multi-colored pencils. It was years later that I received a grant from the NIH Fogarty Center for "International Training and Research in Environmental and Occupational Health." If I had this grant back in 1989, I would definitely have recruited Vasyl as a Fogarty Fellow.

We decided that the case definition would include all children with sudden onset of alopecia totalis who presented to the Pediatric Clinic Number 2 between July and December 1988. The pediatricians treating the cases believed that this was the true duration of the outbreak. I decided on alopecia totalis to avoid misclassification with other types of alopecia. During my examinations of children in Pediatric Clinic Number 2, I saw cases of patchy alopecia that could easily have been attributed to fungal infections or autoimmune disease. While alopecia totalis can also be a manifestation of alopecia areata, and some degree of misclassification was inevitable, at least it would be minimized. I also decided to limit our chart reviews to the patients from Pediatric Clinic Number 2, because it had been designated as the official referral center for all pediatric cases of "Chernivtsi illness."

A review of the registry and medical records identified 110 children who met this case definition. The outbreak curve for these total alopecia cases is presented in Figure 30-3.

The earliest case began on July 20, the outbreak peaked in late October and early November, and there were no new cases after November

> The earliest case began on July 20, the outbreak peaked in late October and early November, and there were no new cases after November 25. Ninety-two percent of the cases were between 1 and 5 years of age.

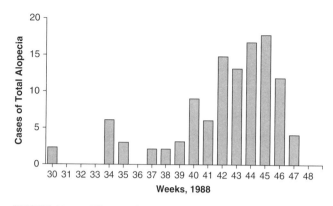

FIGURE 30-3   The outbreak curve.

25. Ninety-two percent of the cases were between 1 and 5 years of age. Boys and girls were equally affected. The clinical signs and symptoms for the 110 cases are shown (in the original Ukrainian version prepared by Vasyl) in Figure 30-4.

One hundred percent had alopecia totalis because that was how we defined a case. Eighty-nine percent had upper respiratory symptoms, 60% had sleep disturbances, and 58% had behavioral changes. I asked Vasyl to prepare a spot map of the cases by place of residence (Figure 30-5). The cases clustered in the old part of the city with an interesting cluster near one of the more modern industrial plants that was designated as off-limits to the investigation.

My mornings were spent conducting clinical examinations. Parents would accompany their children and were truly grateful that I made the effort to interview them and examine their children. The children who had had total alopecia had completely regrown their hair. Only one of the two dozen children that I examined had

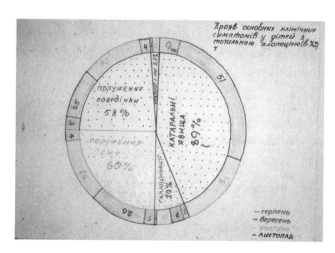

FIGURE 30-4   Frequencies of signs and symptoms (Ukrainian original).

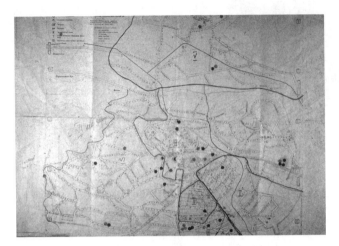

FIGURE 30-5 Spot map of cases. Different color dots show month of onset of illness.

evidence of a mild peripheral neuropathy. For almost all the cases, the symptoms had completely resolved. I also saw several cases of alopecia areata, tinea capitis, and even trichotillomania. These had not been part of the original cases, but their parents feared that this was a reemergence of the original illness. My interviews with the families did not reveal any common factors that would provide clues as to the cause of the outbreak.

The chief public health physician was the gatekeeper for my access to the official government documents that resulted from the outbreak investigations conducted by the Soviet and Ukrainian Ministries of Health. Each document was stamped and signed. There were no Xeroxed copies. The documents included reports generated by scores of different research institutes. The investigation into the cause of the outbreak eventually involved 57 different research institutes and more than 200 experts from various disciplines. What struck me in reviewing these documents was that I was probably only one of a handful of people who had actually seen, let alone read, the full set of papers. There appeared to be little sharing of information or collaboration among the experts from the various research institutes. Each viewed the problem from their own narrow perspective and only carried out the orders they received from the center.

THEORIES, RUMORS, AND HYPOTHESES

There were several theories as to the cause of the outbreak. Some were noted in official records. Others, I heard from my unofficial collaborators. It was difficult to separate fact from fiction, information from deliberate misinformation. As Mukola Prodanchuk aptly said,

"Every theory has a right to life until it is disproven by fact." While I was given unprecedented access to secret government documents and allowed to freely conduct my clinical and epidemiologic investigation, the chief public health physician made it clear that, for security reasons, I could not request any information related to the activities of the soviet military–industrial complex.

The infectious disease experts concluded that the illness was not due to an infectious agent. While some families had more than one child affected, there was little evidence of person-to-person spread. There were no localized outbreaks in schools or kindergartens. Despite the fact that a respiratory illness preceded the onset of alopecia by about 2 weeks, cultures and serology did not identify a common infectious agent. A mycologist at the local university believed that the illness was caused by a new fungus, which she christened "Zalmonella." She even sent hair and scalp skin scrapings to the U.S. Centers for Disease Control and Prevention in Atlanta to help identify the new fungus. The CDC identified the fungus as a common saprophyte, which is not known to cause alopecia.

The radiation medicine experts concluded that the illness was not caused by radiation. In 1986, the Chernobyl cloud had passed through southwestern Ukraine on its westward drift to Europe. Precipitation deposited a patchwork of cesium-137 throughout the city and surrounding countryside. Health physicists had measured and mapped the soil contamination. While alopecia can be a symptom of acute radiation poisoning, the radiation doses were simply not high enough to cause an outbreak of alopecia totalis.

Environmental toxicologists ruled out water and diet as the sources of exposure. The city of Chernivtsi receives its drinking water from two different rivers. Both rivers have different sources in the Carpathian Mountains, and the cases did not appear to be associated with the source of water. The dietary histories obtained from the parents of affected children did not reveal any suspect food source. Environmental and bioassays for pesticides were negative. One institute even tested for dioxin, which was not an easy thing to do in 1988.

An important piece of the puzzle was one question: why were children the most affected? There were sporadic reports of alopecia among adults, but rapid onset

> *While alopecia can be a symptom of acute radiation poisoning, the radiation doses were simply not high enough to cause an outbreak of alopecia totalis.*

> *From an environmental toxicologist's perspective, the high attack rate in children was not surprising. Children are often the highest risk group for environmental poisonings.*

> *Children are not little adults. A child's central nervous system is still developing and the blood–brain barrier is not fully developed. A child breathes more and has a higher skin surface area relative to body weight than an adult, which provides greater exposure to toxins.*

alopecia totalis seemed to be specific to children. From an environmental toxicologist's perspective, the high attack rate in children was not surprising. Children are often the highest risk group for environmental poisonings. Children were disproportionately affected in several of the major environmental disasters of the past 50 years, including Seveso in 1976, when a chemical plant in Italy discharged a dioxin-contaminated cloud onto the local countryside, and Chernobyl in 1986. Children are not little adults. A child's central nervous system is still developing and the blood–brain barrier is not fully developed. A child breathes more and has a higher skin surface area relative to body weight than an adult, which provides greater exposure to toxins. Because of their differences in body weight, a set amount of toxin results in a much higher milligram per kilogram body weight dose in a child than in an adult. Children have much more hand-to-mouth behavior, which leads to greater ingestion of toxins in contaminated environments. Children also do not make their own risk management decisions. The age distribution of the cases of Chernivtsi illness looked similar to the age distribution of lead poisoning cases in the United States. Lead poisoning affects primarily young children who live in contaminated housing and exhibit high hand-to-mouth behavior. If the toxin fell from the air and contaminated streets and playgrounds, we would expect this type of age distribution. Acting on this possibility, the military had hosed down the roofs and streets, tilled the soil in certain parts of the city, and prohibited leaf burning.

While I was in Chernivtsi, one of the rumors I heard was that in the summer of 1988, there was a major accident at a chemical plant in Romania about 50 km from Chernivtsi. The wind direction was blowing from the southeast, which would have brought a chemical plume over the city. Ukrainian public health experts asked for access to the plant and were reportedly denied. Another rumor was that in August, a truck carrying an SS-40 rocket was in an accident resulting in the spillage of SS-40 rocket fuel. The Soviet military was decommissioning SS-40 rockets somewhere nearby in the mountains. While I could not get my local contacts to give me information about the composition of their rocket fuel, I later learned that they might contain hydrazine compounds. These could be on a list of suspect chemical agents, but would have dispersed too quickly to result in an outbreak lasting several months. Moreover, the cases were not clustered near the site of the spill.

Ukrainian toxicologists supported my view that the illness was caused by thallium, despite the negative findings of the WHO experts. I disagreed with the WHO experts on several points. First, they relied on the results of bioassays conducted by Soviet institutes and did not conduct any bioassays themselves. Second, they reviewed the case histories of only 9 children who had alopecia totalis. Third, while peripheral neuropathy is clearly a manifestation of thallium poisoning, I believed that lower doses could produce alopecia without necessarily producing neuropathy. One of the children I examined did have clinical evidence of a mild peripheral neuropathy.

The leading local theory was that the illness was caused by exposure to a mixture of thallium, aluminum, and boron. All three elements were reportedly found in soil core samples taken from different points in the city. In the results I reviewed, the sampling method involved vertical mixing of the core sample, which would have diluted elements that were concentrated in the top few centimeters of soil. Finding even trace amounts of thallium in the soil was an important finding.

One popular rumor that I heard around this time was that local cab drivers were illicitly adding organic thallium antiknock compounds to their gasoline. The theory seemed plausible. Gasoline was generally scarce and of poor quality. Taxi drivers would load their trunks with gasoline canisters to keep from running out. I heard that a local taxi driver had been arrested for questioning. I never learned his fate. Dr. Prodanchuk favored this theory. He believed that children were more affected because they were closer to the ground and more easily inhaled the noxious fumes generated by these vehicles. Acting on this theory, during the height of the outbreak, authorities had banned all traffic in the old part of the city.

When the local population learned that I was helping in the investigation of this mysterious illness, I was visited by all sorts of people. The Soviet Union was near the point of collapse, and Ukrainian nationalism was on the rise. One young man gave me a drawing of his proposal for a military uniform for the new republic. This drawing was removed from my luggage by the chief public health physician prior to my departure. He said he went through my things for my own safety. Another woman was convinced that the illness was caused by extraterrestrials. I don't know how many of these encounters were spontaneous and how many were contrived.

My third and final week in Chernivtsi was coming to an end. I presented the chief public health physician with our outbreak analysis, my clinical opinion that we were dealing with low-dose thallium poisoning, my belief that it was most likely airborne, and my suspicion that the children were exposed through both inhalation and hand-to-mouth spread from contaminated soil and contaminated objects. At this point in an outbreak investigation, the next logical step is to do a case control study. I explained to Dr. Prodanchuk that we should take the 110 cases that met our case definition of alopecia totalis and compare them to a random sample of children who did not have the illness. The most practical source of controls would be age and gender matched children from Pediatric Clinic Number 2 who did not have the disease.

My advice to do a case control study was not taken. Instead, they opted to do continuing medical surveillance (ongoing physical examinations) of the tens of thousands of children living in Chernivtsi. I found this decision perplexing. This approach smacked of Soviet "gigantism," (why study a few when we can study all?). It could have been their unfamiliarity with analytic observational study designs. In 1993, I conducted a critical review of Ukrainian environmental epidemiology studies as a consultant to the World Bank Environmental Mission to Ukraine. I discovered that while cross-sectional and ecologic designs were common, case control studies were not. Another possibility is that the authorities were deliberately trying to obfuscate the investigation. I clearly remember what one mother told me when I explained how I was trying to help. She said, "We don't need another epidemiologist, we need a prosecutor." She was implying, "How could the authorities not know what happened?" Somebody knew, but powerful interests were trying to hide the truth.

> *"We don't need another epidemiologist, we need a prosecutor."*

I returned to Chernivtsi the following summer, again at the invitation of the president's representative to help confirm that indeed the worst was over. He asked me to examine pediatric cases of patchy alopecia that had continued to occur sporadically since the end of December 1988. There had been no new cases of alopecia totalis. While the incidence of other forms of partial alopecia in children in Chernivtsi was higher than in other parts of Ukraine, this could be attributed to increased surveillance. Because I suspected that the illness had been the result of an air pollution event, I brought along two outstanding air pollution experts from the University of Illinois: Dr. Rick Wadden and Dr. Peter Scheff. Our goal was to conduct air pollution measurements using proton-induced X-ray emission spectroscopy and use their statistical receptor modeling method to identify potential sources. Receptor modeling is a statistical method for analyzing air pollution measurements and apportioning them to specific sources. I also convinced the Outokumpu Corporation from Finland to send a team of their scientists to look for thallium in the soil. They had developed a portable X-ray diffraction instrument, which, when hooked up to a portable computer and the right software, could provide real–time analysis of surface soil samples. Because thallium is an element, it is indestructible, and we should still be able to detect some traces of the metal that had not been blown away by wind, washed away by rain, or buried by tilling. Our air pollution modeling did not detect any current thallium hazard and the X-ray diffraction found only traces of thallium remaining in the top layers of soil.

Much to my surprise, and somewhat to my trepidation, I was asked to meet with military toxicologists who were conducting feeding experiments in rats. Ukraine had recently become an independent state and was no longer under Soviet control. Dr. Bilous, a Ukrainian military toxicologist, showed me photos of how he and his colleagues were able to induce alopecia in rats by feeding them micro-doses of thallium, aluminum, and boron (Figure 30-6). The theory that toxicity is caused by mixtures of micro-doses of toxins is prevalent in Soviet toxicology. At the time, I was happy to hear that he supported my belief that we were dealing with thallium poisoning.

AN IMPORTANT DISCOVERY AND LESSONS LEARNED

The real break (at least to the public's knowledge) in the investigation came from bioassays conducted by Professor Fitin from Moscow. He collected hair, nail, blood, and urine samples from affected children and from controls; he was able to demonstrate significantly higher

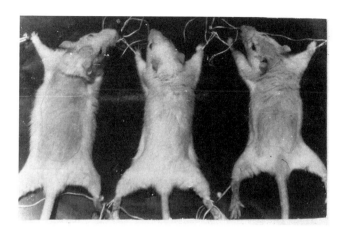

FIGURE 30-6 Results of experimental toxicology studies by Ukrainian military toxicologists. Showing hair loss in rats fed a mixture of thallium, aluminum, and boron.

concentrations of thallium in the bioassays from affected children. Why was this not discovered earlier? Perhaps the government research institutes did not have the proper equipment. Perhaps the blood and urine samples were collected weeks after the children were poisoned. Thallium has a fairly short half-life and would not be detectable in blood and urine samples more than 2 weeks after a poisoning. The hair and nail samples, however, will retain the thallium until they are cut and discarded.

So where did the thallium come from? Why did it need to be such a well-kept secret? It turns out that the answer was known back in November of 1988. What first appeared to be incompetence on the part of the Soviet and Ukrainian commissions, turned out to be suppression of the truth. Their official reports, which were labeled as "top secret," have now been declassified. Here is what they knew, and how they knew it.

In a top-secret report submitted to the Central Committee of the Communist Party of Ukraine, the Praesidium of the Ukrainian Congress, and the Cabinet of Ministers on December 5, 1988, the experts on the commissions concluded that "the most likely cause of the illness among children in Chernivtsi is intoxication with thallium compounds in combination with salts of other heavy metals." The commissions based their conclusions on (1) the clinical picture was consistent with thallium poisoning (including six cases of peripheral neuropathy); (2) electron micrographs of the hair of the victims showed structural changes consistent with thallium poisoning; (3) soil sampling had revealed thallium concentrations in the upper layers of soil that were six times higher than background. In addition, thallium had been identified in the air and wastewater emissions from five factories in Chernivtsi. Needless to say, these were the factories that, for security reasons, were off-limits to outside investigators. This report and other declassified documents now show that in parts of the city, thallium soil concentrations were 13–60 times higher than background. Unsafe concentrations of thallium were detected in locally grown foods, such as cabbage, onions, beets, and carrots. In 89 children who were tested, 57 showed thallium in the urine at concentrations that ranged from 1.5 to 96 times normal.

To this day, the exact source of the thallium that contaminated Chernivtsi has not been disclosed. The following version has not been proven. It is, however, the version that best meets the facts, and no one has actually denied it. The five factories in Chernivtsi that were named in the top-secret report were part of the Soviet military–industrial complex. Thallium is used in the manufacture of some types of military equipment, such as high-performance optical devices and night vision glasses. The unofficial story purports that these factories were initially disposing of their wastes in landfills. After the landfills were full, or perhaps in response to local complaints, these factories began burning their wastes in the city's three brick kilns. Meteorologic conditions during the late summer and fall favored inversions and prevented dispersion of air pollutants. Air pollution monitoring data collected by the local public health station showed that in March 1988, dust concentrations averaged 2.28 mg/m^3 (Ukrainian air pollution standard for dust was 0.15 mg/m^3). Hydromet, the "official" government meteorology and environmental protection agency, reported average dust levels of only 0.3 mg/m^3 for that same period. Air pollution monitoring data from the months of October and November 1988 is missing for both agencies. If these factories were indeed burning their wastes in the city's brick kilns, the emissions could have easily contaminated the streets, playgrounds, and local vegetable gardens. In addition to breathing in these pollutants, children could have ingested them from contaminated food and soil.

If the whole city was contaminated with thallium over a period of several months, why did only 110 of the 60,000 children living in the city become ill? This is a clear example of the "iceberg effect" in environmental epidemiology. Not all children are equally susceptible, because of differences in characteristics such as age, hand-to-mouth behavior, and health status. Not all children receive the same dose. There is likely to be a wide distribution in doses caused by factors such as patchy deposition of toxicants (e.g., "hot spots"), location of residence, time spent outdoors, and diet. As a result, the children who are most highly exposed and most susceptible become clinically ill; they are the "tip of the iceberg." In addition to these most severe cases, there were probably hundreds or even thousands of children and adults who were overexposed, but not to the point of developing clinical illness that required medical attention.

What began as curiosity over a story in a Ukrainian newspaper quickly grew into a passion for global environmental health. With a start-up grant from the Ukrainian National Credit Union Association, I initiated the "Ukrainian Environmental Health Project" at the University of Illinois at Chicago. I recruited Americans and Ukrainians alike to join the effort. We convinced the Minister of Health to enroll Ukraine into the European Longitudinal Study of Pregnancy and Childhood. This study, which is being conducted in Kyiv, Mariupol, and Dniprodzerzhinsk, continues to the present day and has helped train more than a dozen U.S. and Ukrainian epidemiologists. We established a data management center in Kyiv to support our studies. I was elected as an international member of the Ukrainian Academy of Medical Sciences. My epidemiology research has since spanned the globe, from studying mercury poisoning in Yanomami Indians in the Amazon basin to dioxin poisoning in chemical workers in Bashkortostan in the Russian Federation. I have had the opportunity to work with the Pan American Health Organization, the World Health Organization, and the World Bank.

On a more personal note, I have been lucky enough to witness Ukrainian independence, the Orange Revolution, and the ups and downs of the land of my parents with my own eyes. The "downs," such as my disillusionment with the politicization of public health issues, are balanced by the "ups" of believing that, in some small ways, I have made a difference. It's an uneasy equilibrium.

What lessons can I share from my work in Chernivtsi?

1. **Diseases occur in communities.** An understanding of the community, its politics, language, and culture, is invaluable in an outbreak investigation. I have a very difficult name in English, and a very easy name in Ukrainian. In many ways, in those early days, I felt more at home in Chernivtsi than I did in the United States. I was neither an outsider nor an insider, but a denizen of that "no man's land" between both cultures. It's a convenient role for an observational scientist.

2. **Get as close to the data as you can.** My most productive work on the outbreak was conducted where the patients were: in Pediatric Clinic Number 2. I knew that data was real and reliable. Whatever hypotheses emerged, and there were many, they had to reconcile with the clinical and epidemiologic reality of these patients.

3. **Be wary of the opinions of experts.** While I appreciate expertise when I see it, I also know that experts can be misleading, or as in the case of the WHO investigators, they can be deliberately misled. Rather than relying on expert opinion, talk to the patients and to the people who have actually been involved in the day to day management of the outbreak.

4. **An outbreak can be solved through disciplines other than epidemiology.** While outbreak investigation is a tried and true method, don't be surprised if the answer comes from an unexpected direction. You might get a call from a clinician, a lab scientist, or a bystander who provides the clue that solves the outbreak. Outbreak investigation is not a competition. It's a group race to find the cause to prevent others from getting sick. The winners are the population you are trying to serve.

5. **Sometimes you need a prosecutor, and not an epidemiologist.** History has shown that with many outbreaks of environmental illness, someone knows what happened; they are just not saying. They may be trying to hide an accident (Chernobyl), an unwanted byproduct in a commercial product (dioxin in trichlorophenol), or an attempt to profit by cutting corners (melamine in baby formula). If the perpetrators don't confess, a prosecutor can pursue lines of inquiry that might not be open to an epidemiologist. P.S. Also be wary of prosecutors. As Ukrainian President Yushchenko said, "the system corrupts people faster than we can reform it."

LEARNING QUESTIONS

1. Why are children often disproportionately more affected by environmental disasters?
2. What is the "iceberg effect" in environmental epidemiology?
3. When investigating outbreaks of environmental illness, some "stakeholders" may have reasons to keep you from discovering the truth. What steps can you take to ensure that the data you are collecting is reliable?

4. One of the hypothesis for this alopecia outbreak was that it was caused by an infectious agent. Why did the investigator decide that was not likely?

REFERENCES

1. Hryhorczuk DO. Thallium intoxication. *J Ukr Med Assoc (North America)*. 1989;2(120):94–99.
2. Hryhorczuk DO, Prodanchuk M. *A Pediatric Outbreak of Thallium-like Illness in Chernivtsi, Ukraine.* Tampa, FL: Abstract presented at the Annual Scientific Meeting of American Academy of Clinical Toxicology (AACT), American Association of Poison Control Centers(AAPCC), and American Board of Medical Toxicology (ABMT); 1992.
3. Scheff PA, Wadden RA, Levenberg K, Hryhorczuk DO, Prodanchuk MG. *Evaluation of Toxic Air Pollutants in Chernivtsi, Ukraine.* Pittsburg, PA: Proceedings of the 9th World Clean Air Congress; 1992.
4. Hryhorczuk DO. Environmental health in Ukraine. Report to the World Bank. Washington, DC: World Bank; 1992.
5. Hryhorczuk DO, Forowycz A, Wiebel V. Environmental and occupational health in Ukraine: a critical review of selected Ukrainian studies. Report to the World Bank. Washington, DC: World Bank; 1993.
6. Scheff PA, Wadden RA, Ticho KL, Nakonechniy JJ, Prodanchuk M, Hryhorczuk DO. Toxic air pollutants in Chernivtsi, Ukraine. *Environ Int*. 1997;23(3);273–290.
7. Bilous VI, Bilous VV. Thallotoxicosis: Chernivtsi Chemical Syndrome. Publishing House Mistro. Chernivtsi, Ukraine; 2002.
8. Zerbino DD, Serdiuk AM. Chernivtsi Chemical Illness. Lviv. Missioner, Lviv; 1998.

CHAPTER 31

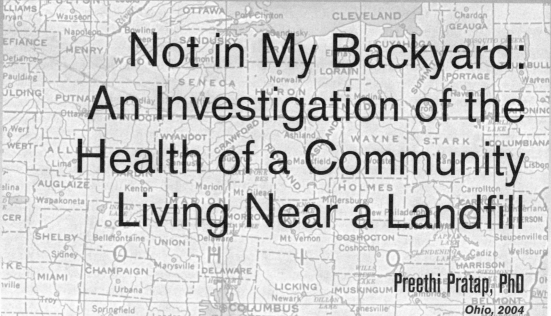

Not in My Backyard: An Investigation of the Health of a Community Living Near a Landfill

Preethi Pratap, PhD

Ohio, 2004

INTRODUCTION

Not every investigation begins with the buzz of a pager or a phone call at 4:00 a.m., and neither does every investigation take you to the deep jungles of the Congo in search of a virus. Some roads less traveled take you to Warren, Ohio, and this is my story.

I arrived in the United States as a graduate student in the fall of 1999. It was a very long flight from my hometown in India and I knew I wasn't going to wake up to the sounds of my Mom's kitchen for a very long time. My parents always thought I would be a physician and I knew I wanted to be called "Dr. Rao," like my father, but I did not want to go to medical school. I was interested in health, but also in the environment. I was always asked by people—what is this "environmental science"? What are you going to do with that degree? My answers somehow did not appeal to my peers, who never thought beyond a degree in engineering or medicine. Honestly, there were days when I myself did not know the answer, and that only strengthened my resolve. So, armed with a bachelor's degree in Environmental Sciences and a master's degree in Biological Sciences, I pursued my doctorate in Environmental Health at the University of Cincinnati. Prior to this, my only exposure to epidemiology had been when I became one of the thousands of cases of the *Plasmodium falciparum* malarial epidemic in the small coastal town of Mangalore in the mid-90's and, of course, reading Robin Cook's fascinating tale about the hunt for the Ebola virus in *Outbreak*.

Hope is a very powerful emotion. By July 2001, I completed two pilot projects in India funded by the National Institute for Occupational Safety and Health (NIOSH) Education and Research Center (ERC). The projects aimed at identifying unsafe pesticide use and storage practices among farm workers in rural India that led to unintentional poisonings among the workers and their children. I travelled on dusty roads at the peak of the Indian summer to remote farms and villages that I had never seen, even when I lived in India. It also gave me this wonderful opportunity to partner with community health workers and physicians at a rural hospital that routinely treated cases of pesticide poisonings, most often with fatal outcomes. Together, we created some safety messages for the farm worker families that could be shared during health campaigns. No brochures or Web sites were used; the community workers were the messengers. The messages were as simple as "do not eat on the fields after you have sprayed it with pesticides" or "do not let your children play with empty pesticide cans." This work led to an internship at NIOSH where I worked with researchers on a take-home pesticide study among rural farm worker families in Iowa. The setting was different, but the problems were very similar.

The summer of 2002 brought big changes in my life. I read *Level 4: Virus Hunters of the CDC* in two nights and finally accessed the Epidemic Intelligence Service (EIS) program Web site and requested an application package. What I loved most about my experiences in the doctoral program at the University of Cincinnati was that I had the opportunity to actually go out into the field and use my skills in identifying problems and finding simple solutions that could help people. The selling point of the EIS program—"shoe leather epidemiology"—is romanticized on glossy paper and in novels, but the essence of it was that I loved the one-on-one interaction with people, the challenge of being in places unknown, and the work that could make a community safer or healthier. I wanted to belong to this elite class that did it all. I briefly mentioned this to my advisor, Dr. Carol Rice. She told me that years ago she was accepted into the EIS program fresh from graduate school, but she chose not to join the program and instead came to Cincinnati to be an academician. She said, "I think you should do it. Just get your dissertation done." This was a sign from above. Dr. Rice was not only my advisor, but my mentor and philosopher, and if she said I could do it—then I could.

I applied to the EIS program and interviewed in the fall of 2002. This meant that I had to defend my dissertation in order to join the program the following summer, so I doubled the hours I worked on my dissertation. I hoped somewhere deep in my heart that these long hours would pay off. I was accepted into the EIS program in December 2002, about 4 months before I defended my doctoral dissertation. I knew my life would never be the same again—this was my calling. It was also about the time I found out that I was assigned as an officer to the Agency for Toxic Substances and Disease Registry (ATSDR) Health Investigations branch in Atlanta. I was a little apprehensive about my assignment because ATSDR is not a typical agency to house an EIS officer, but Alden Henderson, who was assigned as my supervisor, was very determined to change that. Alden, an EIS graduate ('92) from the CDC's National Center for Environmental Health (NCEH), was recently appointed chief of the ATSDR's Health Investigations branch. Alden had years of experience supervising EIS officers at NCEH, and had led many local and international environmental investigations (including an investigation of lead poisoning among children in Bangladesh). He had this positive energy about him and always worked toward making things happen. I credit the richness of my EIS experience to Alden's efforts, for he made every opportunity available, providing a great learning environment.

All through the humid summer bioterrorism training in Alabama, the class of '03 buzzed with stories of investigations past and the glory of EIS. Events such as 9/11 and the anthrax scare had brought us EIS officers to the front line, at least by the media. We walked around with pagers on our belts and waited with bated breath for that "phone call." By the winter of 2003, my classmates had investigated outbreaks from El Salvador to Russia, and at the Executive Park campus of the ATSDR in Atlanta, my supervisor and Lynn Wilder, a senior environmental scientist, were working on making an EPI-AID happen. You see, an "EPI-AID" was not the traditional way the ATSDR conducted a community health investigation. In the branches of the CDC where influenza, hepatitis, or foodborne outbreaks are investigated, a request for acute epidemiologic aid from the CDC is not uncommon. However, for the kinds of matters that the ATSDR investigated, it was unusual for the phone to ring with a request to hurry up and go somewhere because many of the effects of toxic substances are much more chronic and insidious in nature.

The ATSDR is part of the Public Health Service in the U.S. Department of Health and Human Services and a federal public health agency. Although the ATSDR is not a regulatory agency like the U.S. Environmental Protection Agency (EPA), it was created by Superfund legislation in 1980 to prevent exposure and adverse human health effects and diminished quality of life associated with exposure to hazardous substances from waste sites, unplanned releases, and other sources of pollution present in the environment (http://www.atsdr.cdc.gov/). Through its regional offices and programs across the 50 states—including surveillance, registries, health studies, environmental health education, and applied substance-specific research—and its work with other federal, state, and local government agencies, the ATSDR acts to protect public health.

A typical public health assessment process at the ATSDR primarily involves two components—*the exposure evaluation* and *the health effects investigation*. These two components lead to making conclusions and recommendations as well as identifying specific and appropriate public health actions to prevent and respond to harmful exposures in our community. What this means is—we don't pack our bags and wait for that "phone call." We work to make that "phone call" happen that will give us the information or invitation we may act upon!

THE PROBLEM

Construction and demolition debris (C&D) landfills are considered non-hazardous, unlike the more popular municipal solid waste and hazardous waste landfills that are federally regulated. The EPA does not regulate these landfills, so they are under the purview of state or local health agencies. Most states do not have guidelines or requirements because these landfills usually collect inert material, such as gypsum board, asphalt, glass, roofing material, and drywall.

Warren Recycling Incorporated (WRI), located in Warren, Trumbull County, Ohio was authorized to operate by the Ohio Environmental Protection Agency (Ohio EPA) in 1994. The property encompassed approximately 200 acres of land and contained a construction and demolition debris landfill. Residential and commercial properties surrounded the WRI site. Some homes were within 100 feet of the WRI property line, and many residential yards abutted facility boundaries. Approximately 9,500 residents lived within one mile of the facility and approximately 1,600 students attended three neighborhood schools that were located within a mile of the landfill.

> *Some homes were within 100 feet of the WRI property line, and many residential yards abutted facility boundaries. Approximately 9,500 residents lived within one mile of the facility and approximately 1,600 students attended three neighborhood schools that were located within a mile of the landfill.*

Since February 2002, the Ohio EPA had received more than 800 odor complaints from people living in more than 100 different homes near the WRI landfill. Complaints were phoned in to the city, township, county, or Ohio EPA odor hotline, or were faxed to the Ohio EPA. These 24-hour toll-free hotlines allow people to anonymously report nonemergency environmental violations, such as smoke or strong odors from industrial facilities, to the federal government for response. Reportable problems may also include any tampering with waste treatment control systems; improper treatment, storage, or disposal of hazardous wastes; any unpermitted industrial activity; and late-night dumping.

The local schools reported that children complained of "pink eye" symptoms that usually resolved when they went home (away from the landfill). A citizens' group, Our Lives Count (OLC), was formed in early 2002, because of concerns about adverse health effects they attributed to living or working near the landfill. In April 2002, the local school board petitioned the ATSDR to evaluate ambient air hydrogen sulfide levels in the Warren Township, Ohio community. The petition noted exposure of children attending schools and residents living in close proximity to Warren Recycling, Inc. as a special concern. Self-reported health effects included fatigue, nausea, headaches, eye irritation, and exacerbation of preexisting respiratory illness. In response, the ATSDR visited the community and reviewed the available information, including hydrogen sulfide (H_2S) monitoring data collected in spring 2002 by an environmental consultant hired by the LaBrae Local School District and Warren Township Board of Trustees. The ATSDR recommended additional air monitoring for hydrogen sulfide exposure, with proper quality assurance, inside and outside homes near the landfill.

From November 14, 2002 to March 8, 2003, the ATSDR conducted an exposure investigation that involved air monitoring for hydrogen sulfide at six residential locations around the landfill.[1] The ATSDR conducted indoor and outdoor sampling for hydrogen sulfide at six homes using continuous real-time ambient air monitors commonly known as "tapemeters." These devices use chemically treated tapes with a compound-specific (for hydrogen sulfide in this case) electronic chip to provide information related to detection range, sample time, and alarm levels. The tapemeters were capable of monitoring hydrogen sulfide at three different ranges (low: 2 parts per billion (ppb) to 90 ppb, mid-level: 50 ppb to 1500 ppb, and high: 1.1 parts per million (ppm) to 15 ppm). Low-level tapemeters were used inside the homes and mid-level tapemeters were placed at all but one outdoor location. The outdoor location closest to the landfill (which was the home that had the most odor complaints) had a high-level tapemeter. The ATSDR concluded that the levels of hydrogen sulfide, along with conditions at the landfill, posed an "urgent public health hazard." This category is used in the ATSDR's public health assessments for sites "where short-term exposures (less than 1 year) to hazardous substances or conditions could result in harmful health effects that require rapid intervention." Following this, the Ohio EPA began to work with the landfill owners to reduce hydrogen sulfide emissions, although they did not have the authority to enforce it.

Hydrogen sulfide (H_2S), commonly known as sewer gas, is a colorless, flammable gas with a characteristic odor of rotten eggs. Paper mills, tanneries, waste water treatment facilities, and landfills are some of the major industrial sources of hydrogen sulfide emissions. Hydrogen sulfide is the second leading cause of toxin-related death in the workplace, after carbon monoxide.[2]

The spectrum of illness depends on the concentration and duration of exposure to hydrogen sulfide. Accidental exposures of 500–800 ppm in industrial settings have resulted in neurologic and pulmonary symptoms and death.[3]

You can smell hydrogen sulfide at levels as low as 2 ppb. Chronic low-level exposures may primarily cause irritation to mucous membranes and the respiratory system as well as memory and mood changes.[4] Hydrogen sulfide is not currently classified as a hazardous air pollutant by the EPA; it is primarily a local and minor regional concern, and there is limited toxicity data available for low-level chronic exposures. Information concerning the toxicity of low-level chronic exposure is important for evaluating the health risks of hydrogen sulfide exposure among populations living near a hydrogen sulfide source. Therefore, investigation of this Ohio complaint could be useful in better understanding this poorly researched subject area.

The Warren City Health Department renewed the WRI landfill's license shortly after the ATSDR submitted the exposure investigation report in November 2003. But then, in early April 2004, residents of Warren reported adverse respiratory health effects, fatigue, nausea, headache, and eye irritation after a large release of hydrogen sulfide into the air from the nearby WRI construction and demolition debris landfill. After this event, the lack of any response from the landfill owners to contain the hydrogen sulfide emissions (despite the Ohio EPA's intervention), and many, many phone calls, the Ohio Department of Health requested that the ATSDR conduct a health investigation. The primary objective of this investigation was to determine whether there was an association between hydrogen sulfide and adverse health effects.

The EPI-AID was sanctioned on June 2, 2004. Three days later, Lynn and I drove 13 hours from Atlanta to Warren. We broke our journey at Lynn's sister-in-law's home shortly after we entered Ohio. This journey also marked many other firsts for me in the United States—my first EPI-AID as a lead investigator, my longest car ride, my introduction to *Mustang Sally* (Lynn and her sister-in-law's favorite song from the 60's that made them giggle like little girls), and my first five-egg omelet for breakfast the next day at a family diner. The long drive and introduction to Lynn's family was a welcome distraction from all that was in my head. Lynn had more than a decade of experience with the ATSDR and this was my first investigation. I was glad she was with me. It wasn't the investigation that worried me. It was this whole new ATSDR process that I really wanted to get right. If this went well, then it would open the door for officers to come because I was the branch's first EIS officer in many, many years. Don't ask me how many, because nobody at the ATSDR remembered.

THE INVESTIGATION

Keeping with the ATSDR tradition, a public meeting was convened on June 9, 2004, to inform the residents of Warren, Ohio about the purpose of the investigation. The meeting was organized at the Johnson Community Center with the assistance of Warren Township Trustees and members of Our Lives Count. Officials from the Ohio Department of Health, local departments of health, and the Ohio EPA were also present at this meeting. A team of scientists including Alden Henderson (my supervisor), Dan Middleton (senior medical epidemiologist), Sharon Saydah (a very pregnant fellow EIS officer from the CDC's National Center for Health Statistics (CDC/NCHS), and co-lead on this investigation), and an ATSDR media person flew down to represent the CDC/ATSDR at this meeting. I tried to remember every single thing I was told during the media-training class I attended a few months earlier. This was for real—I just hoped I would not freeze in front of a television news camera, because I expected our arrival would be considered local news. Alden had this tremendous faith in my ability and stood across from me while I interacted with the media, like he said he would. Completing the first interview was like catching my breath after a very deep dive, the second one was a breeze, and after 4 weeks at Warren, I wasn't camera shy any more. I do not remember every single word of my SOCO (the single overriding communication objective) or the message map we created, but I do remember saying this in a hundred different ways—"We (CDC/ATSDR) are here in response to the community's request and we need all of you to enroll in this health investigation and participate for the next 4 weeks. This will help us answer the questions about health effects from exposure to hydrogen sulfide gas from the landfill." We knew that the community meeting would not reach out to all residents of Warren; so, in order to increase awareness about the health investigation and promote participation, we also distributed fact sheets and placed announcements in local newspapers and on the local television news stations inviting families to participate in the investigation.

To be eligible to participate, study volunteers had to

1. be 6 years of age or older;
2. live, work, or attend school within 1 mile of the landfill;
3. agree to remain in the Warren area during the 4-week study period; and
4. give written consent/parental consent/assent.

Recruiting began bright and early on June 10, 2004, at the Warren Township building, which is adjacent to the landfill. We set up stations (A–E) in the room to help with the flow of participants. Figure 31-1 outlines the various tasks participants completed at each station during the enrollment process. Prior to consenting, participants were briefed about the study objectives and eligibility criteria. We used a map (Figure 31-2) to help participants point out if they lived, worked, or went to school within a mile of the landfill boundaries. Figure 31-3 outlines the different activities that were performed, over the 4–week study period, by the enrolled participants based on their responses to the respiratory symptoms screener.

At station B, participants provided responses to a validated, nine-question respiratory prescreen survey to identify individuals with asthma-like respiratory

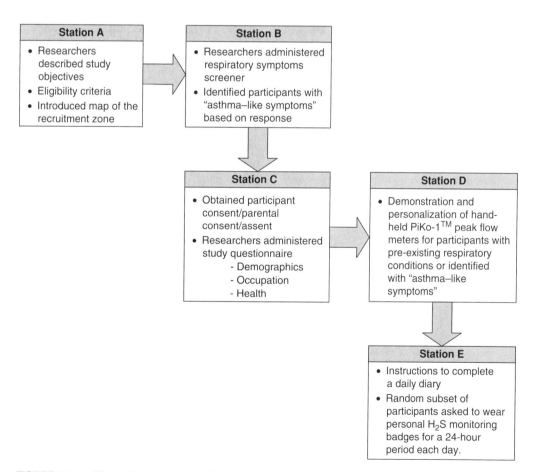

FIGURE 31-1 Flowchart depicts the tasks that participants completed at each of the stations (A-E) during the study enrollment process.

406 CHAPTER 31 ■ Not in My Backyard: An Investigation of the Health of a Community Livng Near a Landfill

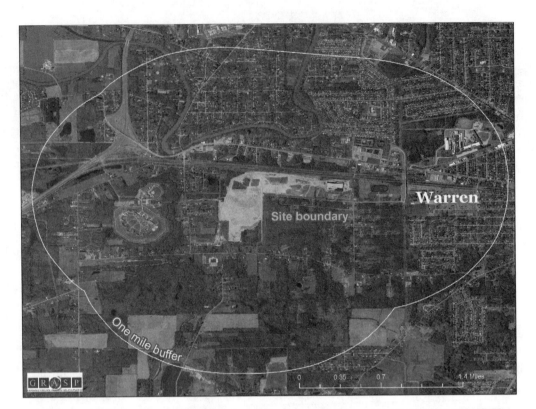

FIGURE 31-2 This map outlines the boundaries of the construction and demolition debris landfill site in Warren, Ohio, and the one mile radius participant recruitment zone. Courtesy: Geospatial Research, Analysis, and Services Program (GRASP), Division of Health Studies (DHS), Agency for Toxic Substances and Disease Registry (ATSDR), Centers for Disease Control and Prevention, Atlanta GA.

symptoms.[5] This prescreening survey is routinely used in occupational and environmental settings and has been validated in previous studies. People who responded positively (yes) to two or more questions were considered to have *asthma-like respiratory symptoms*. These individuals were candidates for recording peak flow readings.

Consent, assent, or parental permission was obtained prior to administering a more thorough questionnaire at station C to obtain respiratory and cardiovascular histories, demographic information, and residential and occupational histories.

Prescreened participants with asthma-like symptoms or participants who had been previously diagnosed

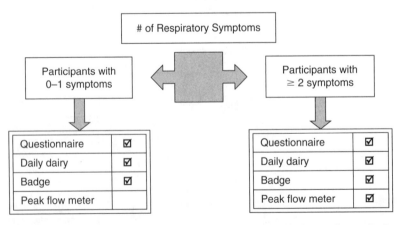

FIGURE 31-3 Activities performed, over the 4 week study period, by enrolled participants based on their responses to the respiratory symptoms screener.

with asthma were then directed to station D, where Dan Middleton gave them a demonstration of a peak flow meter, a handheld expiratory flow meter designed to monitor respiratory conditions such as those found in asthma. It measures the forced expiratory volume in the first second of expiration (FEV1), and then displays and stores the test results. It is intended for a single patient use and also evaluates the blow quality to notify the patient to repeat the test in case of a cough or any suspect blow. FEV1 is the maximum observed volume of air that can be exhaled in the first second after a deep breath. FEV1 is considered by many asthma specialists to be a reliable indicator of an impending asthma attack or respiratory distress. These participants were asked to take FEV1 (forced expiratory volume) readings twice a day, preferably at the same time every morning after waking and every night before bed. We used forced expiratory volume (FEV1) as a measure of pulmonary function. The predicted FEV1 was calculated using equations based on an analysis of data from the National Health Interview Survey (NHIS) and equations from Hankinson.[6] The equations estimate predicted FEV1 based on the subject's age, sex, and height. We used percent predicted FEV1, which is the ratio between the observed and predicted FEV1, as our primary outcome variable.

Dan spent a few minutes to train each participant on how to provide peak flow readings so he took quite a few deep breaths that day. They were instructed to give their best effort three consecutive times for each session. The meter electronically stored the best of the consecutive efforts. It was admirable that although he was getting out of breath and getting hoarse, Dan greeted the last participant of the day with the same enthusiasm and trained him with dedication and patience.

At the last station (station E), each participant was asked to complete a daily diary every night before bed, recording self-reported health symptoms, use of rescue medications for breathing (e.g., inhaler), unplanned visits for medical care caused by respiratory problems, and hospital admission caused by respiratory problems that occurred in the prior 24-hour period. Daily diaries also recorded *indirect indicators of exposure*, including time spent within one mile of the landfill (total and outdoors), and perception of odors. The list of odors included: rotten eggs, garbage, sewage, burning or smoke, cigarette or cigar smoke, and cat urine. The first four odors were known to be associated with the landfill; the latter three were not.

A random subset of participants was asked to wear personal H_2S monitoring badges for a 24-hour period each day. This was the only technology that we had available at the time to measure individual exposures to H_2S. Each badge was prelabeled with the participant's ID number. Participants were asked to change badges in the evening when they filled out their daily diary and record the date and time that each badge was changed. Prior to and after use, badges were sealed in plastic bags and kept refrigerated.

The badge color changes were compared to an H_2S color comparator. The color corresponded to parts per million (ppm)·hours. H_2S concentration was determined by ppm·hours divided by the amount of time the badge was worn. Badges worn for 24 hours had a lower detection limit of approximately 20 parts per billion (ppb). One ppm = 1000 ppb.

We placed five continuous real-time ambient air H_2S tapemeters at residential properties around the perimeter of the landfill. Sample inlets were breathing zone height (1 to 5 meters above ground level). The tapemeters provided readings at 5-minute intervals and had a low level range of detection of 2–90 ppb. Tapemeters were checked daily; data were downloaded weekly.

We wanted at least 100 participants. We had 60 participants enrolled by the end of the first day of recruitment, about 30 enrolled the second day, and 22 more enrolled over that weekend. We had one employee from the WRI landfill enrolled as well, although we never saw him after he walked away with our precious resources. We enrolled an employee at the post office next to the Warren Township building a week into the study, bringing the final sample size to 113. In a bid to jeopardize the investigation, the landfill stopped operating on June 13, 2004. The Warren Landfill operators ceased normal operations on day 4 of the study and remained closed until the end of the investigation. Therefore, it is quite possible that the hydrogen sulfide exposures we recorded were lower than they would have been during regular operations.

Planning the study and recruiting participants seemed much less of a challenge than finding ways to keep the participants motivated (Figure 31-4). This study demanded a lot from the subjects—use the badges, fill out the daily diaries, and take peak flow readings over 4 weeks. It was a lot to ask of people, however much they hated the smell of rotten eggs while throwing a barbeque in their backyards. Over the next week, we visited participants' homes to provide additional coaching on the use of the peak flow meter, checked on the badges, and checked the area tapemeters. The people of Warren welcomed us into their homes and, as much as we tried, the visits always took way more than the intended 10 minutes. Somehow, we were considered experts on every

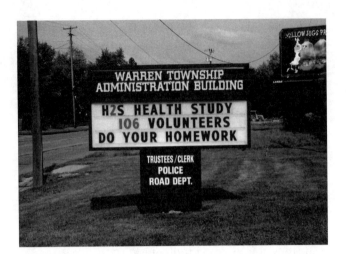

FIGURE 31-4 Township board message to encourage enrolled study participants.

disease in the world. Melting snowcaps, drug companies that made asthma medications, and, of course, the favorite "Fed-bashing." Nothing was off limits. "Hey, you are Indian right? I would love to see an elephant." I found it very amusing that folks in the Western Hemisphere still have this "Indiana Jones" image of India with elephants walking the street. Although I enjoyed these little distractions, I had to politely refocus attention to our study.

As promised, the rest of the team flew back to Atlanta after completing the recruitment. For the next 4 weeks, I was the one-person ATSDR team, making my rounds of participant homes on a weekly basis, downloading the peak flow and FEV1 data onto a computerized database, and collecting the badges. I began enjoying the weekly visits; it is always nice to know the people you are working for. I liked listening to their stories. It was like being in a "small-town America 101" class. Everybody had a story—just like my story.

A typical day for me was an early swim at the YMCA pool, after which I went to my make-shift "office" at the Warren Township building. I spent the rest of the day taking calls and conducting follow-up visits to participant homes. Kay and Debbie (the Township's trustees) stopped by occasionally to check on me, and every now and then I listened to stories about Vietnam and Harleys from a Township war-veteran over lunch on a picnic bench. The only exciting event on the drive back every evening was spotting the sign "Center of the World" right before I took the exit to my hotel. And yes, I googled that to see if it were true, and it wasn't true because I did not find any information to that effect. Finding vegetarian food was a problem and dinner was usually takeaway Chinese food or microwave popcorn that I ate in my room, alone. The highlight of my evening was updating my husband who lived in Chicago—we spoke for hours. We'd been married less than 6 months and were already living in two different cities (I was based in Atlanta). Being away in Warren only made it more difficult, and no training had prepared me for this. I made sure I always had breakfast in the hotel lobby where I could talk to the staff. After 2 weeks, I did not hear much about the landfill, not even from Debbie and Kay, but we could always smell it. However, the media stopped by religiously every week to get an update on the study.

Two major events happened as we entered the midway point of the investigation; only one of these got all the media frenzy though. I celebrated my 30th birthday and, on June 24, 2004, the residents complained about very strong odors and the Ohio EPA hotline was inundated with calls again. Lynn had just flown into Warren the previous evening and we headed out with a handheld real-time monitor to Lovers Lane, the source of the most complaints. One reading over one of the manholes reached levels of 95 ppm. This was 5 ppm less than the NIOSH IDLH (National Institute for Occupational Safety and Health Immediately Dangerous to Life or Health) level of 100 ppm. The odor was so bad that I had to go back to my hotel room that day. The headache and nausea I experienced lasted over the next 24 hours. Inorganic chemistry was certainly not as fascinating as the study of organic molecules, but we all knew the answer when we smelled "rotten eggs" while conducting laboratory experiments—unpleasant as it was. A few years earlier, I had visited a wastewater treatment facility in Cincinnati and it took me days to stop smelling like a "rotten egg" afterwards, but this experience was closest to what the Warren residents had to deal with every day.

The thing about drywall in an anaerobic landfill (like this one at Warren) is that it takes months to years for the bacteria to break it down to the point that hydrogen sulfide is released. You may stop adding construction debris, but the bacteria will continue working on the sulphates, and any rain will continue to create hydrogen sulfide producing leachate pools. Leachate is the liquid that drains or "leaches" from a landfill (Figure 31-5); it varies widely in composition regarding the type of waste that it contains. At a site with large volumes of building waste, especially those containing gypsum plaster, the reaction of leachate with the gypsum can generate large volumes of hydrogen sulfide, which may be released in the leachate and may also form a large component of the landfill gas. Now, although the landfill had scaled back its operations, something had to be done with this leachate. It was suspected that leachate treated with

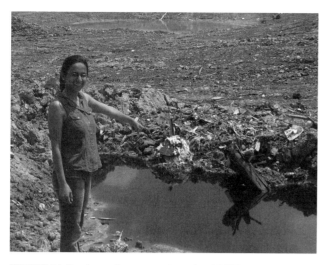

FIGURE 31-5 Leachate pool at the WRI landfill site.

hydrogen peroxide (a typical practice used to degrade hydrogen sulfide gas in landfill leachate) was being illegally dumped through the city's sewer system to the waste water treatment facility. City health officials once again said they would look into this matter, but this event had already triggered the U.S. EPA's interest in this site.

RESULTS

Generally, the ambient hydrogen sulfide levels in the United States range from 0.11–0.33 ppb; Warren had 3–9 times the level for other American cities. Our investigation's hypothesis was that any decreases in pulmonary function and the self-reported health symptoms were associated with elevated levels of hydrogen sulfide in the air around the landfill. Our results weakly supported our hypothesis.

One hundred and seven of the 113 participants completed the study. More than 90% were adults. Forty-six participants performed peak flow measurements, wore personal badges, and filled out daily diaries. An additional 20 volunteers wore personal badges and filled out daily diaries only, while the remaining 41 volunteers only filled out daily diaries. Would we have liked a larger sample size? Yes, but this is the real world and you have to make the most of the cooperation and the data you can collect. So, we were pleased that our participants were motivated enough to complete this 4-week study.

The self-reported health symptoms and odors reported during the study were consistent with those known to result from hydrogen sulfide exposure. The most common symptoms reported daily by high percentages of participants (on average) were eye irritation (39%) and fatigue (38%). Rotten egg odors (28%) and sewage (19%) were the most commonly reported odors daily. Table 31-1 lists Pearson Correlation Coefficients for several outcome variables. The table shows that the correlation between reporting odors and symptoms is high, at 0.80 (p-value <0.001). Days of the week having a higher percentage of badge hits correlated with days with high 24-hour average H_2S levels on the area monitors. Daily 15-minute maximum H_2S levels correlated with the daily percentage of badge hits (r=0.30, p-value 0.04). The other correlation coefficients were not statistically significant.

We also found positive associations between the daily percentages of symptoms reported and (1) the amount of time spent near the landfill, (2) the rate of badge hits, and (3) the rate of odors reported. However, no significant associations were found between percent predicted FEV1 and exposure to H_2S or any of the other air pollutants considered (ozone, particulate matter, sulfur dioxide, and nitrogen oxides). We were looking for very small changes in breathing measurements and the protocol may have been more demanding than we expected.

TABLE 31-1 Pearson correlation coefficients are shown for key outcome variables. The table shows that the correlation between reporting odors and symptoms is high. H_2S levels correlated with the daily percentage of badge hits while reporting symptoms and odors were only mildly associated with H_2S levels.

	Daily H_2S level 15-min max	Daily % badge hits	Daily % symptoms reported	Daily % odors reported
Daily H_2S level 15-min max	1.0	0.30	0.35	0.39
Daily % badge hits		1.0	0.21	0.20
Daily % symptoms reported			1.0	0.80
Daily % odors reported				1.0

LIMITATIONS

The trouble with environmental contaminants like hydrogen sulfide is that the symptoms they cause are very nonspecific. Second, unlike an organism that can be detected in blood or stool, or with a skin swab, the number of biologic monitoring methods available to determine environmental exposures are limited. Third, occupational exposures to contaminants are better documented and controlled with effective manufacturing processes and use of personal protective equipment, but when it comes to community exposures, we are more often than not dealing with low-level chronic exposures! Finally, it is challenging to develop environmental exposure limits for a community exposure because we are dealing with a heterogeneous collection of individuals, including vulnerable populations such as children, the elderly, and immunocompromised patients. This is quite different than trying to develop limits for healthy workers.

Like any other environmental health investigation, our study had its fair share of limitations. For one, hydrogen sulfide in air is usually transient and difficult to monitor. The personal monitoring hydrogen sulfide badges could not measure or detect a 24-hour hydrogen sulfide average below 20 ppb, and we don't know how much above 90 ppb the outdoor air concentrations were—the tape meters could only measure up to 90 ppb of hydrogen sulfide.

While 26% of participants reported being current smokers; 32% said someone else in their home smoked. Eighteen participants reported being currently diagnosed with asthma, and 28 participants reported preexisting chronic respiratory disease. We were looking for very small changes in breathing measurements that would have been even smaller in someone with a preexisting respiratory disease. Some people had problems using the breathing meters—not blowing into the instruments three times in a row, not blowing as hard and fast as they could. These were very difficult meters to use—usually such tests are monitored by a technician.

The maximum 1-hour H_2S average during the 2003 exposure investigation was 4700 ppb, and the maximum 1-hour H_2S during our investigation was 427 ppb. The Warren landfill operators ceased normal operations on day 4 of the study (the timing of this closing was more than a bit suspicious), and remained closed until the end of the investigation. Therefore, it is quite possible that hydrogen sulfide exposures were lower than we would have seen during regular operations. In addition, the exposure investigation was conducted in winter, while we conducted our investigation in summer. Hydrogen sulfide levels are affected by temperature inversions, which occur more frequently in the winter months in Ohio. Hydrogen sulfide is heavier than air and can accumulate in low-lying areas and become trapped under fog closer to the ground during winter.

WAS THIS A SUCCESSFUL INVESTIGATION?

It was no surprise that the landfill resumed operations again on July 23, 2004—a week after we wrapped up our investigation in Warren. But the previous exposure investigation, our health investigation, and the 95 ppm hydrogen sulfide reading on a hot June day had put Warren on the U.S. EPA's radar. Shortly after the U.S. EPA Region V and the Ohio EPA pressured the landfill to clean up the site, the facility closed in 2005 because of the inability to correct numerous regulatory violations and the threat posed to public health. In 2006, the U.S. EPA completed a multimillion dollar cleanup.[7] Upon completion, the maximum value of H_2S detected on the landfill was 43 ppb (compared to 165 ppm in 2005). This investigation led to the passing of a bill changing state regulation of construction and demolition debris landfills in Ohio. It also became a model for a similar investigation by another EIS officer in Florida.

There are about 1,900 active construction and demolition (C&D) debris landfills in the United States, and they continue to increase in number, therefore creating a need for established community-based emission guidelines.[7] In many states, there are no daily cover requirements, air emission controls, or liner requirements. The lack of these engineering controls leads to air emissions of hydrogen sulfide, methane, and other compounds. The ATSDR has been involved in several community health investigations involving H_2S exposures from C&D landfills and has found that many local and state health and environmental agencies are not aware of the health issues surrounding these landfills until community health concerns arise. The ATSDR has established a C&D landfill initiative to focus on community and worker health issues arising from C&D landfills and guidance on how to either avoid problems or take steps to reduce them. A workgroup consisting of members from the ATSDR, the U.S. EPA, and state and local health and environmental agencies share information and data in hope of reducing the need for future health investigations. Prevention is much less costly! Another outcome of the initiative is a guidance document for use by environmental public health officials. Lynn Wilder is the co-lead of this workgroup.

Ideally, we would have liked to see the data support our hypothesis but this was not one of those result-oriented, data-driven investigations. However, in the end, it did what it had to—made a public health impact. At the end of the day, that was all that mattered.

LEARNING QUESTIONS

1. The author identifies several challenges with investigating environmental contaminants. What are these challenges?
2. The author and her colleagues performed a health investigation that she referred to as very demanding on the community participants. What were they asked to do and how did the investigators try to keep the participants motivated to comply with the demands?

ACKNOWLEDGMENTS

Many thanks to Lynn Wider for her recent updates on the ATSDR C&D landfill initiative. This chapter has information from a publication in progress: Wilder LC, et al. Community health outcomes and airborne exposures to hydrogen sulfide from a construction and demolition debris landfill.

REFERENCES

1. Agency for Toxic Substances and Disease Registry. *Health Consultation (Exposure Investigation): Community Exposures to Hydrogen Sulfide, Warren, Ohio.* Atlanta, GA: Agency for Toxic Substances and Disease Registry; 2003.
2. Greenberg M, Hamilton R. The epidemiology of deaths related to toxic exposures in the US workplace, 1992–1996. *Clin Toxicol.* 1998;5:430–432.
3. Agency for Toxic Substances and Disease Registry. *Toxicological Profile for Hydrogen Sulfide.* Atlanta, GA: Agency for Toxic Substances and Disease Registry; 2006.
4. Saadat M, Zendeh-Boodi Z, Goodarzi MA. Environmental exposure to natural sour gas containing sulfur compounds results in elevated depression and hopelessness scores. *Ecotoxicol Environ Saf.* 2006;65(2):288–291. Epub 2005 Oct 5.
5. Venables KM, Farrer N, Sharp L, Graneek BJ, Taylor AJ. Respiratory symptoms questionnaire for asthma epidemiology: validity and reproducibility. *Thorax.* 1993;48(3): 214–219.
6. Hankinson JL, Crapo RO, Jensen RL. Spirometric reference values for the 6-s FVC maneuver. *Chest.* 2003;124(5): 1805–1811.
7. EPA On Scene Coordinator. Warren Recycling, Warren, Ohio—EPA Region V. U.S. Environmental Protection Agency On Scene Coordinator Web site. www.epaosc.org/WarrenRecycling. Accessed September 1, 2009.
8. US Environmental Protection Agency. *Characterization of Building-Related Construction and Demolition Debris in the United States.* Washington, DC: US Environmental Protection Agency; 1988. Report No. EPA530-R-98-010.

PART V

Investigating Hard-to-Reach and Special Populations

CHAPTER 32

Back to School: Using Basic Epidemiologic Data on Asthma in Urban School Children to Improve Respiratory Health

Victoria Persky, MD

Illinois, 1990s to 2010

SCREENING FOR ASTHMA PREVALENCE IN SCHOOLS

In 1994, I was an epidemiologist at the University of Illinois at Chicago School of Public Health and a part-time internist at a community health center on Chicago's west side. My training had been in internal medicine and I had been practicing part-time as a primary care doctor in a West Side underserved neighborhood since 1975. Throughout this time, I had also been studying trends in chronic diseases. My interest in asthma began when physicians from Cook County Hospital suggested we examine asthma deaths in Chicago. Asthma is a complex disease with biologic, environmental, and psychosocial components. Currently, it is estimated that approximately 20 million people in the United States have asthma, 500,000 are hospitalized and 4,000 die from the disease each year.[1] Many of the factors that exacerbate the disease—such as exposure to tobacco smoke, mold, dust mites, pets, pollens, cockroaches, rodents, and dampness—are potentially modifiable.[2] Our research group at the School of Public Health, working with our medical colleagues at County Hospital and using death certificate data, noted substantial increases in asthma deaths in the city beginning in 1976–1978, with substantially higher death rates in persons living in low-income minority neighborhoods.[3,4]

A key issue at that time was whether the higher deaths rates among African Americans were due to differences in prevalence of the disease or in other factors related to severity and/or access to appropriate health care. Surveys of schoolchildren seemed a reasonable way to determine overall prevalence in that age group. We were fortunate to collaborate with other investigators around the world in the International Study of Asthma and Allergies in Childhood, which was surveying children in 155 centers in 56 countries for symptoms of asthma and allergic diseases. Our group performed anonymous surveys for two of the three surveys in the United States—one in Chicago and one in East Moline, Illinois. In East Moline the survey was given to all students in the middle schools and high

> *We were fortunate to collaborate with other investigators around the world in the International Study of Asthma and Allergies in Childhood, which was surveying children in 155 centers in 56 countries for symptoms of asthma and allergic diseases. Our group performed anonymous surveys for two of the three surveys in the United States—one in Chicago and one in East Moline, Illinois.*

schools. In Chicago, the survey was given to a random sample of 7th and 8th grade public and parochial schools in the city with a final 94% participation rate. At that time, we were allowed to use passive consent, which may have contributed to the high participation achieved. Because Chicago had high numbers of both parochial and public schools, we first obtained permission from the archdiocese and from the central Chicago Public Schools (CPS) Administration. Although both surveys were given without personal identifiers, administrators at CPS were concerned about asking any questions other than ones about asthma and respiratory symptoms. Therefore, to obtain data on race/ethnicity and asthma risk factors, we oversampled students in the Catholic schools.

We found high prevalence of symptoms in both East Moline and Chicago, with 16–18% having a diagnosis of asthma. The rates were far higher than appreciated by staff of CPS, who had documented maybe 3–4% of the students having the diagnosis. While 16% of the students overall in Chicago had the disease, these rates varied somewhat by ethnicity and socioeconomic status. Thus, 13% of students in Catholic schools, 17% of students in public schools, 20% of those in schools with more than 98% African Americans, and 22% of those in schools where more than 40% were below poverty level had been diagnosed with asthma. These differences were far less than the differences seen in asthma morbidity and mortality, suggesting that other factors were contributing to the health disparities.[5] The demonstration of such a high burden of disease in this population set the stage for further studies and helped to gain the school administrators' confidence that working with us in subsequent programs could assist in improving the health of their students.

INITIATION OF AN ASTHMA EDUCATOR PROGRAM

Around that time, we also surveyed 9% of the families in the Chicago Head Start program, a national program that promotes school readiness by enhancing early development through education and access to medical and social service resources. Because asthma is often not diagnosed until early childhood, we were interested in whether the 3–5-year-old low-income children served by the Head Start program had already been diagnosed with the disease, and data was not available to guide us with this age group. Funds to support the project were limited. Head Start staff members, however, were enthusiastic about working with us. Specific sites chosen, to some extent, reflected the degree of interest in the staff. The final sample, while not random, was generally representative of the demographic breakdown of Head Start families in the city.[6] We found that 14% of the children, even as early as age 3–5 years, had already been diagnosed with the disease. This percent seemed high to us at the time, but high rates in this age group were subsequently confirmed in studies of children in other cities.[7]

As a result of our findings we held a series of focus groups with Head Start staff, healthcare providers, social service providers, and parents. Most people felt that they could use more education about asthma. With small amounts of outside funding, we held education sessions about common issues relating to asthma for a few hundred Head Start staff. In addition, it appeared that parents of children with the disease often had a better understanding than health professionals of the barriers facing them, as well as creative ways to overcome these barriers. With initial funding, we recruited, hired, trained, and supervised three Head Start parents to work in a pilot study with 60 other families to examine whether a series of home visits, which focused on identification and remediation of factors that exacerbate the disease, could reduce asthma morbidity in their children.

COMMUNITY EDUCATOR PROGRAM IN CHICAGO PUBLIC SCHOOLS

Over time, with additional outside funding from the Chicago Public Schools (CPS) and, subsequently, from the Otho S. A. Sprague Institute and the Illinois Department of Human Services, we expanded our program to involve parents working directly with families and children in Chicago Public Schools. We initially hired, trained, and supervised parents in three schools in the city to work with families with asthma in those three schools. Hiring parents without college degrees within the university system, however, proved cumbersome. In addition, for long-term sustainability as we continued to expand, it seemed reasonable to work with programs that were already established within the school structure. Thus, we decided to work with parents supported by other funds within CPS and train and supervise them, when appropriate, to work with staff and families in the schools on asthma-related issues. Initially, we worked with Parents as Teachers First and subsequently Cradle to Classroom, lodged within the Office of Early Childhood Education at CPS. Parents as Teachers First hired parents to work with other families on preparing preschool children for kindergarten. Cradle to Classroom encouraged pregnant teenagers to stay in school through education in parenting skills and accessing resources.

We trained parents already hired as part of those programs, supervised them on asthma issues, and assisted them in asthma programs. Linking with existing programs was not only cost saving but also allowed us to build upon existing resources at the school, expand ties of these parent–educators with individual school systems and integrate asthma education into ongoing local activities. A major limitation, however, was the decentralization of the supervision—at one point, our nurse was supervising 12 educators at 12 different sites. Regular meetings of the group were helpful and provided opportunities for support and discussion. These meetings, however, did not allow the same level of continuity that occurred when the supervision was on-site. Hiring educators without college degrees within the university system also has limitations. The salary scale is low and, in general, for these tasks, we are not allowed to hire full-time employees who do not have a degree. Nevertheless, benefits of housing educators within the school structure are strong and, although we have decreased the numbers currently being supervised, we have a limited number of educators at schools who assist in education programs, interface with school systems, and link with mobile vans that provide asthma care at the schools.

ESTABLISHING THE CHICAGO ASTHMA CONSORTIUM AND ADOPTION OF INHALER POLICY

In part, as a result of data from our Chicago Asthma Prevalence Study, the Otho S. A. Sprague Institute decided, in 1996, to commit a large portion of its outside funds for 5 years to asthma work in Chicago. Some of those funds went to establish the Chicago Asthma Consortium (CAC), which is a group of individuals and institutions in Chicago committed to decreasing asthma morbidity in the city. My role in the early years of the CAC was to develop a school committee to define and address issues around asthma in Chicago schoolchildren. It was a time of new administration for the Chicago Public Schools (CPS)—an administration that was open to addressing chronic disease issues. Our first task was to form a group of leaders from the schools and the professional asthma community to define issues of importance to schoolchildren. The first issue we dealt with was the ability of children to carry their inhalers.

At that time, children were not allowed to carry their inhalers—they were usually kept in locked drawers in a school office and there was often significant time delay between the onset of symptoms and access to relievers. We worked closely with CPS administration, and within a year (March 1997) achieved a change in policy, allowing students to carry inhalers with appropriate documentation. A similar state rule was signed by the governor in July 2001 and then expanded to all recreational programs. By the spring of 2006, students could have an epinephrine autoinjector (an injectable medication used for acute severe allergic attacks).

CHALLENGES IN IMPLEMENTING THE INHALER POLICY AND IDENTIFICATION OF CHILDREN WITH ASTHMA

These earlier successes were encouraging. We were one of the first large cities to have a self-medication rule and it was instituted fairly quickly. The implementation, however, has been slow. Despite significant support from the central administration, years later there were schools that did not know about the rule and continued education has been necessary. Surveys by the CAC and the American Lung Association of Metropolitan Chicago (currently the Respiratory Health Association of Metropolitan Chicago) in 2003 and 2006 suggested that schools were still enforcing the policy inconsistently, with inhalers locked in many instances in nurses' offices. These findings demonstrate the importance of continuing to perform field surveys even after instituting what should be an effective intervention, because implementation of that intervention may not always be optimal.

Other issues have also been challenging. School nurses still identify less than a third of those with the disease as having diagnosed asthma. At first we thought that adding a question to state physical forms routinely returned to nurses would solve the problem, but the necessity of having physician documentation has continued to be barrier. Dr. Raoul Wolf from La Rabida Children's Hospital (a Chicago hospital that provides care to children with lifelong medical conditions) developed and validated a screening tool (Brief Pediatric

Asthma Screen; BPAS) that several groups, including ours, have been using for more than a decade.[8] These questions address whether the child had

1. previously been diagnosed as having asthma;
2. had an episode of wheezing in the last 12 months;
3. had symptoms after exercise in the last 12 months;
4. had experienced symptoms at night in the last 12 months; and
5. had been to a doctor, an emergency department, or a hospital for wheezing in the last 12 months.

We had hoped that this screening tool might be instituted by the nurses in their routine evaluation of the students, but the chronic understaffing, with one nurse for every 1,000 to 2,000 students, has limited their ability to implement this method. As an alternative, with outside support, our group has sent the screening form home over the years to more than 60,000 families. With approximately 60% return, we identified 13–15% with diagnosed disease and a similar percent with symptoms that could represent the disease, suggesting that prevalence of the disease has not changed substantially in the last decade. With permission from the families (generally about 60–80% of those surveys), we gave the information to the nurses, but because of understaffing, this information has often not been translated to formal identification of the child's asthma in the CPS system.

LINKING CHILDREN WITH ASTHMA AND SYMPTOMS OF ASTHMA WITH APPROPRIATE CARE

A key issue, as we continued screening for asthma, has been follow-up with the families and linking them with appropriate services. We had initially hoped that nurses in the schools could be the case managers for children with the disease, but again, because of understaffing, this has not been feasible. CPS, at one point, attempted to identify a local healthcare provider for each school, but this proved challenging and there are many areas in the city where appropriate health care for asthma is lacking. Two physicians in the late 1990s had a unique solution to the problem—mobile asthma vans working with the schools on identification and treatment of children with asthma in underserved areas of the city (Figure 32-1).

In 1998, the Mobile C.A.R.E. Foundation was incorporated. The Asthma Vans supported by Mobile C.A.R.E. were modeled after those developed in Los Angeles. Unlike those in Los Angeles, Mobile C.A.R.E. is not lodged

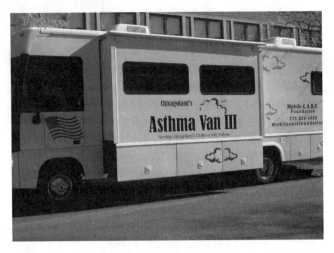

FIGURE 32-1 A Mobile C.A.R.E. Asthma van serving as an outreach tool to assist school children and families with asthma management. Mobile C.A.R.E.

in a public institution, but supported by grants and donations as a stand-alone separate non-profit. The vans are staffed by pediatricians with specific interest in asthma, and supported by nurses and van drivers. They assess students with physical examinations, allergy skin testing, and pulmonary function testing, and follow-up with primary care physicians and patients, if so desired, on a regular basis. They visit each school an average of once a month, and are available by telephone 24 hours a day to assist families in asthma management. Initially, it was thought that the mobile vans might disrupt normal stationary care, but, in fact, they have allowed more in-depth management and coordination in areas of the city not routinely receiving appropriate help. This has proved to be an enormously successful program. Families identified through school screenings, if they desire (approximately 60–80% of those screened), are referred to the vans for further assessment. Currently, there are three vans with the capacity to visit 60 schools, although only two vans are currently in use because of decreased funding.

DEVELOPMENT OF SUSTAINABLE INFRASTRUCTURES

More challenging issues have been centralizing case management and coordinating with individual health providers and social services in the community. Two large programs have been built upon our initial work with the community health educator model. This model is based on the premise that community residents, who often, but not always, are parents of children with asthma, have the best understanding of barriers and ways of overcoming barriers to improving asthma morbidity in their communities. The first project was funded by the Centers for Disease Control and Prevention (CDC); the second was funded by the Merck Childhood Asthma Network. These programs in underserved areas on the south side of Chicago have included screening children in the schools with the BPAS form; linking of those who so desire with school nurses and providers; providing education in schools and the community; and a home visit program in which community educators work with families on the identification and modification of factors affecting asthma. The asthma educators (community residents we trained to work with families with asthma), where needed, have also served as case managers, linking families with appropriate care and services. There is a need for long-term support for stabilization of the systems developed in these and similar programs throughout the country. Ideally, case management should be lodged in stable institutions with long-term support and commitment to asthma in the community. Community clinics are logical, but in the current fee-for-service system, rewards for education are limited, and for home visit programs with community educators, they are almost non-existent. Nursing shortages in many cities are similar to those in Chicago and do not allow for case management within the schools. Case management by educators in community organizations is effective, but relies on outside grant support. There is currently no system for reimbursing community educators without college degrees who operate outside traditional healthcare settings.

CONCLUSIONS

School-based asthma programs have several unique advantages in addressing asthma in underserved populations:

1. They encompass the entire population of children in the targeted area and, thus, provide an opportunity for surveillance of disease, identification of children with symptoms and diagnosed asthma, and serve as the first step in linking those children with appropriate services.
2. Because of their stable infrastructure and presence throughout the city, they also provide an opportunity for education of children, parents, and staff so that the disease can be managed appropriately.
3. Children spend a large part of their day in school. The physical environment in the school also has importance for the disease and the education of students and staff about how to recognize and address issues within the individual schools that can have a direct impact on the student's health.
4. Infrastructures developed for schools with others serving children with asthma can be generalized to other chronic conditions and environmental issues within the community.

Challenges that affect the ability of schools to implement and sustain effective programs still exist:

1. Understaffing of nurses is perhaps the major challenge. Case management must, in many cases, reside in outside agencies with fractionation of services.
2. The lack of integrated tracking systems within schools limits the ability to identify children with asthma, as well as estimates of morbidity from the disease. Chicago, like many other cities, tracks school absences, but not causes of absences. Funding for the schools is tied to attendance and, without data on cause of absence, surveillance and response to factors that affect short-term and long-term attendance is limited.
3. Schools have many priorities that can compete with asthma education programs. Programs must therefore be flexible and adapt to the local situation.
4. Environmental issues in schools are varied and can be severe. Funding for repairs is very limited. Systems must be in place to identify acute and chronic problems, to prioritize them, and to seek additional funding if necessary.

With all these challenges, schools are important factors in children's lives and provide stable institutions in which to address the issues facing families in the inner city.

LEARNING QUESTIONS

1. What epidemiologic data are useful in assessing the burden of asthma in school children and how would you go about collecting such data?
2. What characteristics in schools facilitate the implementation of asthma intervention programs?
3. How can parents be incorporated into school-based interventions?
4. What issues need to be overcome in order to have a successful and sustainable asthma screening and control program in schools?

REFERENCES

1. Moorman JE, Rudd RA, Johnson CA, et al. National surveillance for asthma—United States, 1980–2004. *MMWR Surveill Summ*. 2007;56(8):1–54.
2. U.S. Department of Health and Human Services. *National Asthma Education and Prevention Program Expert Panel Report 3: Guidelines for the Diagnosis and Management of Asthma*. Bethesda, MD: National Institutes of Health; 2007. NIH Publication Number 08-5846.
3. Marder D, Targonski P, Orris P, Persky V, Addington W. Effect of racial and socioeconomic factors on asthma mortality in Chicago. *Chest*. 1992;101;426S-429S.
4. Targonski PV, Persky VW, Orris P, Addington W. Trends in asthma mortality among African Americans and Whites in Chicago, 1968 through 1991. *Am J Pub Health*. 1994;84(11):1830–1833.
5. Persky VW, Slezak J, Contreras MA, et al. Relationships of race and socioeconomic status with prevalence, severity, and symptoms of asthma in Chicago school children. *Ann Allergy Asthma Immunol*. 1998;81(3):266–271.
6. Slezak JA, Persky VW, Kviz FJ, Ramakrishnan V, Byers C. Asthma prevalence and risk factors in selected Head Start sites in Chicago. *J Asthma*. 1998;35(2):203–212.
7. McGill KA, Sorkness CA, Ferguson-Page C, et al. Asthma in non-inner city Head Start children. *Pediatrics*. 1998;102(1 Pt 1):77–83.
8. Wolf RL, Berry CA, O'Connor T, Coover L. Validation of the Brief Pediatric Asthma Screen. *Chest*. 1999;116(4 Suppl 1): 224S–228S.

CHAPTER 33

Sex, Drugs, and Community-Based Ethnography: Field Investigations Involving Difficult-to-Reach Populations Around the World

W. Wayne Wiebel, PhD

Illinois (and around the world), 1980s to 2010

MY ACCIDENTAL CAREER

Far and away the single event that most influenced my career was the appearance of the human immunodeficiency virus (HIV) on the world's stage. Prior to that, I was a relatively obscure substance abuse epidemiologist working for the state of Illinois. The most exciting aspect of my professional life at the time was representing the city of Chicago in attending the twice-a-year Community Epidemiology Work Group Meetings sponsored by Nick Kozel at the National Institute on Drug Abuse. As a matter of happenstance, I had developed a modicum of expertise in relation to subpopulations within American society that sociologists and anthropologists referred to as deviant or stigmatized, psychologists and psychiatrists called abnormal, politically correct public health authorities referenced as being "hidden," and most everyone would agree to as being marginal to mainstream society. This list, which I was proud of in a somewhat maverick fashion, included pornographers, drug addicts and dealers, prostitutes (both male and female), transvestites, sex fetishists, and a large array in types of criminals—most often as a consequence of having to support a drug habit.

How this all came to be is quite a long story, but it certainly had something to do with my fascination for all things exotic, especially people and places sufficiently different from my own experience as to challenge my understandings of the world and those who populated it. In undergraduate school at Northeastern University in Boston, I sampled a variety of majors before settling into the Sociology/Anthropology Department and submerging myself in social psychology, phenomenology, and ultimately symbolic interactionist theory. The Chicago School of Sociology, including the work of George Herbert Mead[1] and his legion of students and followers, became a dominant framework in organizing my own thoughts and considerations about how to make sense of human behavior. Based on symbolic interactionist theory, objects and actions have no independent meaning. Instead, meanings are socially constructed and subject to change over time based upon our experiences and interactions with others. From this perspective, "reality" can be considered a variable, very much dependent upon those doing the defining. As the Thomas theorem stipulates, "If men define situations as real, they are real in their consequences."[2] For me, this was an epiphany in that it shifted the focus of my intellectual curiosity from what might or might not be real to what people believed to be real; precisely because if they believed something to be real, they would act like it was real, and then it would be real in its consequences.

The practical lesson to be gained from symbolic interactionist theory was that a better understanding of people and what they did would require following the proverbial advice of needing to walk a mile in someone else's shoes in order to see the world as he did. I headed off to Northwestern University for graduate school to study under Howard S. Becker, a renowned Chicago School sociologist and qualitative methodologist. Howie Becker was the author of the foremost textbook in the field of social deviance at the time, *Outsiders*,[3] and included in his prolific research portfolio studies based on observations from his own life, including marijuana use among jazz musicians and a life-history interview with a female heroin addict he met in Chicago's jazz scene.

For a fledgling scholar with interests outside mainstream academia, I was convinced at the time that it just could not get much cooler than this. For my master's thesis, I did a study of individuals working in the pornographic movie industry that was in large part made possible by a high school friend's younger sister, who also happened to be a classmate of one of my sisters. As a model in NYC, Marilyn Bridges had her picture taken holding a baby for display on the box of Ivory Snow detergent. Not much later, as Marilyn Chambers, she became the female star of one of the nation's first commercially distributed "Adult" or "XXX" movies, *Behind the Green Door*. Unexpectedly, my research found individuals in the emerging pornographic movie industry to identify more closely with being anti-establishment and other counter-cultural themes than with anything having to do with sex or sexuality. Making sex movies was just a means to an end, which was to challenge the status quo and push the envelope of what was socially accepted. Realizing from a career standpoint that a specialization in pornographic films was not going to take me very far, I shifted interest to illicit drug use and drug users. Topics that were of increasing public health relevance changed with the changing times; we transitioned from rebellious youth and hippies who embraced drug use as a means of expanding consciousness to persons with recognition of a growing toll in causalities from excessive drug consumption and drug dependence.

For my doctoral dissertation, completed in 1983, I wrote up details from an investigation I had conducted under a contract with the National Institute on Drug Abuse (NIDA) on recreational drug users associated with the use of a powerful anesthetic, phencyclidine or PCP.[4] Fortunately for me, I was the only trained ethnographer with experience in drug abuse research at the time George Beschner from NIDA was looking for someone from Chicago to contribute to a planned book. The investigation was to compare ethnographic research on PCP users from six cities across the country. PCP is perhaps best known on the streets as Angel Dust, but that is somewhat geographically based. For example, in Philadelphia, it is most often sold in cigarettes as "Sherms" or "Shermans." Most folk have no idea it is phencyclidine in the cigarettes that makes them high; more often than not, they are told it is embalming fluid. Effects are dissociative and dose-related. Small amounts act as a stimulant; increasing amounts act as a depressant and then a hallucinogen, before knocking you out as intended when used as an animal tranquilizer. Users report feeling like they are walking on clouds or marshmallows and being removed from reality, as if they are watching reality rather than being a part of it. Users also can appear profoundly "stoned," which was the "in" thing among drug users for a while. However, becoming a burnout was inevitable with regular use and the social costs of not being able to act like or experience reality as if you are a participant, ultimately led to the downfall in the drug's popularity. Being lipid soluble like the delta-9-tetrahydrocannabinol (THC) found in marijuana, it was stored in the fat cells and had a very long half-life when used regularly.

The profound pharmacologic action of the drug contributed to some similarities across sites, yet distinct variations were also evident by city. In Chicago, it was particularly noteworthy that the epidemic of PCP use among youth had already peaked and was rapidly declining in prevalence by the time authorities had noticed there was a new drug abuse pattern creating problems for users. The natural history of the outbreak in Chicago concluded as users realized the undesirable side effects associated with regular use. The popularity of the drug then diminished, along with the reputations of those who continued to use. External intervention turned out not to be a significant factor. This was a remarkable finding, given the massive resources beginning to be allocated in the nation's "war on drugs." The notion that problems are most effectively addressed by waging a "war" against them continues to be called to question even to this date, especially in relation to drug problems that, for the most part, seem resilient despite frontal assaults financed by multibillion dollar budgets.

Since then, my work has taken me across the United States and to countries far from Chicago. And, for the most part, it has continued to focus on drug users, sex work, and related public health problems, particularly addiction and infectious disease.

Foremost in career development that made this all possible, was my first job out of graduate school in the mid-1970s. Luckily for me, after completing course work requirements for my doctorate, a position opened at the Drug Abuse Epidemiology Program in the Department of Psychiatry at the University of Chicago (U of C). J. Fred E. Shick, a psychiatrist who had recently completed his residency at U of C, was directing an NIH-funded study of adolescent polydrug abusers in Chicago. In part, the research was to determine if the work of another U of C psychiatrist, Patrick Hughes, involving neighborhood-level interventions targeting outbreaks of heroin addiction could be replicated when redesigned to address adolescent multiple-drug users. Very briefly, Hughes had found heroin-copping areas, the places addicts go every day to purchase heroin, ideal sites to conduct research and offer intervention services. His combined model of research and intervention utilizing ethnographic and epidemiologic methods proved to be most successful. For my part, being hired to work as an ethnographer on this new adaptation of Hughes' groundbreaking work would prepare me for future contributions to public health in ways I could never have imagined. In particular, it would impress upon me the great value to be realized in conducting fieldwork investigations to fully grasp the nature of what most often were referred to as public health or social problems and, further, to plan and assess the effectiveness of interventions to address these problems.

I still look back on those days as some of the best of times in my career. It was 1975 when Fred and I set up a field station on the second floor of a building overlooking the intersection of Clark Street and Diversey Boulevard on Chicago's north side. Although only just finishing his residency in Psychiatry, Fred was already a recognized drug researcher who had helped found the Haight–Ashbury Free Medical Clinic during San Francisco's 1968 "Summer of Love." I, on the other hand, was very much the unseasoned novice in relation to both large-scale, federally funded investigations and the target populations we would end up working with. While I am sure I appeared quite confident to anyone who knew me back then, knowing what I do now, it is scary to realize how little I really did know about conducting investigations on so-called hidden populations. Fortunately, in my trial by fire, I totally immersed myself in the multiple street subcultures of Clark and Diversey and emerged a much wiser young man 3 years later. I have little doubt that almost all of the story that follows about my career in working with marginal groups, including the previously mentioned six cities ethnographic investigation of PCP use, would not have been possible were it not for the experience gained at Clark and Diversey.

Most importantly, over the course of this study, I gained a wealth of practical experience about conducting investigations with marginalized populations that quite simply no amount of reading or instruction from others can replace.

I also learned to be open-minded and nonjudgmental in getting to know folks of almost every imaginable persuasion, be it an addict, drag queen, or pedophile. Prior to this experience, I avoided such folk and for the most part held them in disregard. Yet, many of these people, who at first I considered as only research subjects, grew over time to become true friends. Even now, decades after this study, I am still in contact with a surprising number of the people that I met there who are still alive.

And so it was that on numerous occasions when making introductions in the company of new acquaintances and replying to questions about my work and interests, I recall jokingly assuring folks that although I was a great hit at cocktail parties, the downside of my professional areas of expertise were that there was very little demand for them in the job market. At least, that was the case until AIDS came along and began to decimate these very same subpopulations I had grown to know and developed close understandings with over time.

GOOD TIMES AND BAD TIMES

Like generals and wars, epidemiologists and epidemics are intrinsically related in an ironic fashion such that what can be catastrophic for society-at-large is likely to be a boon to the career of some professionals. In the early 1980s, as recognition of what would eventually become know as HIV and AIDS grew, I was the state drug abuse epidemiologist at the Illinois Dangerous Drugs Commission. Among gay friends, recognition of the threat was rapid and I could not help but be impressed with how quickly and effectively they appeared to mobilize in response. For the other major risk group in America at the time, injection drug users or IDUs, there was no comparable acknowledgment of a threat or any noticeable action being taken on their part to address the epidemic.

The state agency I worked for since 1978 was responsible for a statewide treatment system to help citizens recover from problems related to chemical dependence. Virtually all methadone maintenance patients and a substantial subset of patients in therapeutic communities and outpatient drug-free services had a history of injection drug use. Clearly, we were going to be on the front lines of the epidemic in Illinois, whether state bureaucrats and drug treatment providers wanted to be or not. Working with a friend and colleague at the time, Randy Webber, we set out to revise nursing protocols related to handling patients (so as to integrate universal precautions) and to develop intervention training curricula for treatment providers and clients. Randy and I then scheduled training events at all programs across the state treating IDU clients. During this process it became painfully apparent that we would only be able to reach a small fraction of the at-risk population that needed to hear our prevention education messages. As it was, we were only reaching a small tip of the iceberg in relation to those in need and, at that, we were reaching those least at-risk as a consequence of their being in treatment and attempting to quit using drugs. Unfortunately, our pleas to reach out to active drug users on the streets were to no avail. As far as the agency was concerned, its authority and, hence responsibility, ended within the four walls of the treatment programs it sponsored. For the time being, if external support was to be mobilized, it would have to come from elsewhere.

During this period of time however, there was considerable movement within state and city health departments to respond to the epidemic in progress. I became active in attending meetings and reconnected with Norman Altman, who had managed the polydrug abuse database on the U of C study. Norman was now in the Division of Epidemiology at the University of Illinois at Chicago (UIC) School of Public Health and he invited me to join an informal group of activists who were meeting at each other's homes to discuss AIDS and share thoughts about what could be done. Prevention services targeting sexual transmission in the gay community were increasing by leaps and bounds, but for the most part, folks were at a loss as to what could be done to address the epidemic among IDUs.

The crux of the issue appeared to be what could be done to prevent IDUs from sharing the needles and syringes they used to inject drugs. For the most part, their injecting practices were not well understood. Some thought that the sharing was a matter of necessity. Others believed that injectors shared because they chose to and that it might represent some sort of social bonding ritual. Still others held that it was done unthinkingly, as a matter of habit. Ideally, an intervention strategy should address the reasons injectors shared, and as long as there was uncertainty about this, it would be difficult to assess the relative merits of alternative approaches under consideration. Should there prove to be multiple reasons behind sharing practices, the complexity of strategies proposed to influence the behavior would likely have to increase as well.

Also at issue was the question of whether it was even possible to influence the behavior of drug addicts. After all, they seemingly accepted the risk of dying from an overdose every time they injected. If the addiction to drugs was so powerful as to preclude self-control and the ability to make rational decisions as to how to act, then what hope could there be for prevention education? Even if you could convince them to change their behavior, how could they be reached and effectively educated? IDUs were not only a hidden population, they were a population in hiding. Already distrustful of authorities, what could possibly convince active injectors to risk arrest by revealing themselves, even to those who supposedly wanted to help them? While most public health professionals early in the epidemic were not willing to totally dismiss the potential for controlling the further spread of infection among IDUs, few seemed to hold much hope given the efficiency of bloodborne transmission and the numerous obstacles apparent to even those experienced in working with addicts. It was a worst-case scenario for public health prevention with the potential for the natural history of a bloodborne disease to play out unabated. Drug users were a group primarily defined by their illegal activity, for whom there was little public support and no political support. Furthermore, they had virtually no voice to speak out on their behalf in public forums that might call attention to their plight. The prospects for IDUs to garner their share of limited resources that would be needed to offer protection from this infectious disease epidemic looked bleak at best.

Yet, having already pondered the question of what could be done to effectively intervene in the further spread of HIV among injectors for quite some time, I was ripe with ideas and pleased as could be to find a receptive audience in the group of public health authorities and activists who were meeting informally. I had in mind a strategy for a major initiative and with this newly found support network, the means to accomplish it were readily becoming apparent. However, I would have to leave my job with the state in order to pull it off.

CREATING A COMMUNITY-BASED INTERVENTION

A good 10 years after beginning to work on HIV prevention with IDUs and after not seeing Patrick Hughes for more than 20 years, I bumped into him at a National Institute on Drug Abuse meeting in Washington D.C. in the late 1990s. Introducing myself, lest he did not recognize me, I thanked him for the good fortune of my career and his role in providing the opportunity for me to make a contribution to bettering public health. I am uncertain as to the extent he was aware of his great influence on me because he left the University of Chicago to go to Geneva to work for the World Health Organization about the time Fred Shick was hiring me to replicate his model in working with adolescent polydrug users. As it was, quite a few years had passed since I worked for the University of Chicago and I lost contact with Pat following a number of unsuccessful attempts to reach him. However, when the AIDS epidemic surfaced and began to take its toll among IDUs, I realized that Hughes' now dormant community-based intervention model targeting heroin addicts was exactly what was needed to mount an effective HIV/AIDS intervention for drug injectors.

At the urging of friends in the Chicago Department of Public Health, I developed my plan on paper and submitted the proposal for funding from the Centers for Disease Control and Prevention (CDC). This was not the first time that I had ever written a grant proposal and I received some assistance with the budget and budget justification. What I proposed was about as simple as could be. I adapted Hughes' model combining epidemiology and ethnographic research with community-based intervention to address neighborhood outbreaks of heroin addiction[5] and changed the objective to instead address the spread of HIV among IDUs. The rest, as they say, is history. The small award allowed me to leave my job at the state of Illinois and Norman Altman convinced me to bring the contract to the University of Illinois at Chicago, School of Public Health where he was working. Norman assumed the role of administrator and helped champion the project at the University to make sure we got the necessary support to launch a community-based initiative. That left enough money for three part-time outreach workers to actually implement the planned intervention.

To begin work on the south side of Chicago, I recruited Claude Rhodes. Claude had been a major heroin dealer on Chicago's south side. After stints in jail and drug treatment for his own addiction, he was able to successfully kick his heroin habit. I knew him from my U of C days and watched him progress in his drug treatment career until he eventually became director of one of the state's largest methadone treatment programs. His knowledge of the drug scene on the south side was unrivaled and he had one of the most highly regarded reputations on the street of anyone I have ever met in the addict world. For the north side intervention, I convinced Lenny Haines to join our small team. Len was a dope fiend and heroin dealer that I knew from Clark and Diversey who had entered methadone maintenance therapy after managing a life of addiction for almost 40 years. (Dope fiend was a term heroin addicts preferred to be called as opposed to junkie. This was learned when the Illinois Drug Abuse Program polled addicts about what they called themselves as the state's methadone treatment system was being set up.) Len had stellar street credibility and became a passionate prevention advocate. Finally, to address the bridge population of gay drug injectors, I enlisted a consummate male hustler (street slang for a gay prostitute) who I had met playing pool at a bar frequented by hustlers and their sex work clients or "tricks." Rick greatly impressed me with his concern about AIDS and his eagerness to help out in doing outreach to other gay IDUs. Unfortunately, Rick did not work out as hoped and he was never seen by us again after stealing 8 ounces of cocaine and the Mustang of a guy he'd been living with for a while. How far he made it across country before the coke ran out and/or he was caught by the cops, I never heard. However, an important lesson was learned about the hazards of recruiting staff that may still have one foot planted in lives of addiction and crime.

Thanks to the hard work and dedicated advocacy of the two remaining outreach workers, Claude and Lenny, the project began to be noticed and started to develop a good reputation for its ability to gain access to and educate active drug injectors about HIV/AIDS. In effect, what they were doing was laying the groundwork for what would later become the staged educational sequence of objectives set out in the *Indigenous Leader Outreach Model: Intervention Manual*:[6]

1. Gain access to target group members.
2. Increase HIV/AIDS awareness.
3. Promote individualized risk assessment.
4. Reinforce behavior change.
5. Encourage prevention advocacy.

These objectives laid out the steps to be taken in conducting outreach intervention. Through following them, the success of outreach in preventing HIV transmission was dependent upon the ability of outreach staff to work with clients in identifying viable alternatives to high-risk practices and encouraging the adoption of these practices as risk reduction measures. It worked beyond the expectations of almost everyone involved. Since these early days, the field of HIV prevention targeting IDUs and what is often called "harm reduction" has grown to embrace numerous additional issues, often related to political, legal, and ideological concerns. From my perspective, this is all well and good, although I do hope that it does not ultimately prove to be a distraction from remaining vigilant about HIV prevention. To the extent that those at greatest risk of contracting or transmitting HIV no longer maintain high levels of awareness and concern about AIDS, they surely risk further outbreaks of HIV infection.

INDIGENOUS LEADER OUTREACH AND ETHNOGRAPHIC INQUIRY

At the time we launched our project in 1986, there were only two other significant intervention programs targeting IDUs for HIV prevention in the United States. These were project Health Education Resource Organization (HERO) in Baltimore and the Mid-City Consortium to Combat AIDS in San Francisco. New York City had Don Des Jarlais commencing his impassioned campaign to promote needle and syringe exchange (NEP) as pioneered in Europe, but at the time, little else. Both the Baltimore and San Francisco programs, like Chicago, utilized community-based outreach to access active drug injectors. San Francisco was the first to promote bleach disinfection of used injection equipment in light of our federal government's dogged refusal to fund NEP for decades despite overwhelming scientific evidence and the near universal backing of public health authorities.

At the federal level, it was interestingly the National Institute on Drug Abuse (NIDA) and not the CDC that was first to assume responsibility for mounting a national prevention response to the epidemic of HIV spreading among communities of IDUs. George Beschner was the head of NIDA's Community Research Branch at the time. In his early career, George had worked with gangs on the streets of Manhattan's lower east side and became a devoted proponent of ethnographic fieldwork as a means of understanding the life situations and social dynamics of marginalized populations such as drug users. I had met George when I was hired to do the Chicago portion of his NIDA-sponsored, six-city comparative ethnographic research investigation into PCP abuse (which later became the basis for my doctoral dissertation). If there was to be any hope of mounting a national campaign to prevent the further spread of HIV among IDU, it was the good fortune of the country to have George at the helm. And precisely because of his previous experience in working on emergent problems involving drug use, he fully appreciated the extent to which we still needed to answer fundamental questions about the transmission of HIV through injection before it would be possible to truly roll out a national campaign.

As an aside, recognizing that the sharing of injecting paraphernalia is the key to transmission of HIV and focusing on this to address prevention was something pretty much limited to public health forums. In the mind's eye of the public and media, this reality was by far overshadowed by the fact that drug use was illegal and there was little sympathy for doing anything that was not steadfastly in opposition to such criminal behavior. Consequently, from the perspective of the general public, the simple answer to HIV prevention for IDUs appeared to be the same as drug use prevention for school children, "just say no to drugs." Unfortunately, the practical conundrum of preventing something from happening that is already happening did not occur to most. For those already addicted, just saying no to drugs is about as likely to stop users from using as telling people not to have sex and expecting those already sexually active to stop. Further, such thinking (despite being extremely prevalent) displays no understanding or appreciation for realities surrounding addiction that, by definition, is a chronic, compulsive disorder. At any given time, most addicts have little interest in stopping their use of drugs. The 10% or so who want to stop using drugs experience great frustration and battles in willpower trying to achieve abstinence. In instances when they are successful, numerous attempts and long periods of time are often involved. Psychologically, it is not much different than quitting a tobacco addiction, just illegal and even less socially acceptable. Physiologically, the toll is immeasurably more excruciating. Just saying no to an addiction may appear to be a simple solution, but is, in fact, monumentally difficult to accomplish.

By the late 1980s, contrary to what many even thought possible, a huge budget had been allocated to NIDA's National AIDS Demonstration Research Project

(NADR) and the requisite teams of seasoned researchers had been commissioned to learn what was needed to sow the seeds of HIV intervention in select cities across the country. The huge contribution of NADR's field investigations in furthering understanding about injection drug use and IDUs is chronicled in the 1993 book, *Handbook on Risk of AIDS—Injection Drug Users and Sexual Partners*.[7] Fortunately, Chicago was selected as one of the first-round NADR programs allowing us to at last secure the resources needed to commence a major research and intervention initiative based upon the fledgling success of our pilot project.

> *In keeping with Hughes' original model, our program was designed to inform the development and implementation of an intervention based upon findings from fieldwork investigations incorporating both ethnographic and epidemiologic methods.*

In keeping with Hughes' original model, our program was designed to inform the development and implementation of an intervention based upon findings from fieldwork investigations incorporating both ethnographic and epidemiologic methods. To reflect Chicago's urban ethnic landscape and known concentrations of drug injectors in the city, we decided to rent community-based field stations on Chicago's Black south side, Latino west side, and the racially diverse north side. To head up research and intervention targeting IDUs in each community, advertisements in professional journals sought out seasoned ethnographers. Larry Ouellet, a PhD from Northwestern University (like me) who had been on the faculty of Emory University, was hired to oversee operations on the north side. He eventually assumed responsibility for all of our research activities and then, years later, for the whole program. Wendell Johnson was recruited as the ethnographer responsible for the south side field station in the heart of Chicago's historic IDU subculture, and Antonio Jimenez rounded up the team of three ethnographers to set up programming on the west side.

Not all epidemiologists are familiar with ethnographers, but collaboration with such persons can be very beneficial. An ethnographer studies subcultures in our own society as an anthropologist studies other cultures abroad. An ethnographer is trained in the use of qualitative research methods, as opposed to the quantitative methods associated with other branches of science, and they pursue knowledge inductively rather than deductively (in reference to the logic of scientific analysis). Ethnography is primarily descriptive and exploratory in nature. Qualitative methods generate theory, whereas quantitative methods are typically utilized to test theory.

To complete staffing of the three field station-based teams, each ethnographer was tasked with hiring outreach workers to reflect the composition of IDUs in their community. George Beschner had asked me what I was going to call these workers and I replied, "Indigenous leaders." While not nearly as catchy as San Francisco's Community Health Outreach Workers (CHOWS), at least the name conveyed an accurate description of the people we wanted to fill these positions. Once staffed and trained, the teams set out to increase AIDS awareness and encourage the adoption of viable risk reduction strategies, such as no longer sharing syringes with their friends and trying to avoid situations where they would need to share injection paraphernalia. For their part, the ethnographers conducted their own investigations in the field to better understand injection practice and inform the evolution of effective intervention strategies.

Reflecting back on these early days, at times it felt as if we were some sort of well-lubricated machine, working in total harmony and performing miracles on the street in striving to achieve this monumental goal of halting further transmission of HIV. At other times, it felt as if we were all being cast into a huge, tumbling washing machine with important onlookers screaming their opinions and all manner of advice at us. Yet, however demanding the challenges were that we faced, in stepping back to gain perspective, it was clear we were making great strides in moving forward. Especially in relation to progress with fieldwork investigations, we were way ahead of most other NADR projects in recruiting active injectors as research subjects. Furthermore, we were the only original NADR program to decide to enlist clients in a prospective cohort study that would allow us to assess HIV incidence among our target populations. Much to the credit of ethnographers and outreach staff alike, follow-up rates for active drug injectors over a 4-year period did not differ substantially from many household surveys. And ours was the first cohort study of active IDUs to be successfully attempted in the United States.

It was our good fortune to receive substantial recognition and credit for our early successes. With this, of course, came the opportunity to make further contributions through additional work. The Chicago program was selected as the only one to receive a NIDA contract to replicate our intervention model in three additional cities; Baltimore, Denver, and El Paso. Consistent with our approach, three ethnographers were hired to conduct field work investigations for these new intervention projects: Terry Mason, PhD in Baltimore, Steve Koester, PhD in Denver, and Reyes Ramos, PhD in El Paso.

In Chicago, our first formal ethnographic investigation sought to better understand the role of "shooting galleries," the places addicts go to inject drugs, in contributing to the further spread of HIV. The publication that Larry Ouellet took the lead on, "Shooting Galleries and HIV Disease: Variations in Places for Injecting Illicit Drugs"[8] discovered that instead of being a one-dimensional factor in increasing HIV transmission, shooting galleries could, instead, be seen to have a variable influence on HIV transmission, depending on the type of operation represented. At opposite extremes of the spectrum, there were places like abandoned buildings where IDUs could find a semblance of privacy to inject, and then full-scale, commercial operations where addicts would pay an entrance fee to enter and inject (Exhibit 33-1). In the first variety of gallery, no one was in charge and IDUs could come and go as they pleased. To avoid being caught by police with their "works" (needle and syringe), individuals might seek a hiding place to stash them until they were needed for the next injection. This created an opportunity for a user without works and in need of a "fix" to search, find someone else's equipment to use, and then, perhaps, replace without the original owner ever being aware of what took place. Likewise, such sites often did not have running water, so users would bring in a cup of water to make their injection solutions and then rinse out their works, leaving what was left for whoever might come later and be in need. By our reckoning, this type of shooting gallery represented a high risk for contributing to the additional spread of HIV. Only a year before this, Steve Koester from our Denver project was doing his own ethnographic investigations and published a paper on the hazards of HIV being transmitted through cotton (used to filter injection solutions), cookers (used to heat and dissolve heroin into a solution), and water (used to make injection solutions and to rinse out syringes following injection).[9] This was the first article focusing on something in addition to needles and syringes contributing to injection risk. At the other extreme of the spectrum were the cash galleries that had the potential to be among the safest of places an addict could frequent to inject. At such sites known in the communities served by our intervention, outreach staff would regularly visit to win over the operators who ran the places as HIV prevention advocates. All such operations had rules that addicts were expected to follow and our goal was to make

EXHIBIT 33-1 An understanding of Chicago injection drug users' shooting galleries emerged in the 1980s from this study led by Larry Ouellet, PhD.[8] In Cash galleries, the injection drug user pays for admission and possibly for paraphernalia and services. A Taste gallery involves access through friends and providing a "taste" (small amount) of drugs like a noncash admission fee. A Free gallery has no admission fee.

Free Gallery

- Some privacy is offered.
- No admission is charged.
- No one is in charge.
- It is often found in abandoned buildings or empty apartments.
- Paraphernalia or services are not provided, but might be found there.
- It is not likely a primary location for prostitution.
- It is not likely a primary location for the sale of drugs.
- It is least likely to have a "house doctor" (a person who helps someone to inject).

Taste Gallery

- Some privacy is offered.
- Admission charged is a "taste" of drugs.
- Someone is in charge.
- Volume is usually low, restricted to a close group of friends, but volume could be large and not selective.
- Syringes might be provided, but the syringes are not necessarily new.
- Sex for sale is uncommon.
- It is not likely a primary location for the sale of drugs.
- Person in charge may serve as a "house doctor."

Cash Gallery

- Some privacy is offered.
- It functions like a business.
- A monetary admission fee is charged.
- It is likely to offer a full range of injection equipment and services, including water, a "cooker" (often a bottle cap or spoon) for dissolving drugs in, matches, cotton, and a "tie" (like a tourniquet).
- It rents or sells new and/or used syringes.
- It often has a "house doctor."

sure safe injection practices were integrated into galleries' rules of conduct. Additionally, outreach staff would supply prevention materials, including syringe disposal containers, sterile works, and bleach for disinfection if sterile equipment is temporarily unavailable.

TAKIN' IT TO THE STREETS

As data from the various NADR programs began to pour in, it became clear that it was indeed possible to take positive preventive action in relation to drug injectors and HIV. The CDC took note, with two articles appearing in MMWR,[10,11] and I was invited to testify before Congress. Barry Brown took over the reins of NIDA's demonstration program and turned his sights toward technology transfer and intervention service roll out to cover all areas of the country not already receiving services by the mid-1990s. Our own 4-year prospective cohort study had shown a decrease of more than 80% in high-risk injection practices and a reduction of more than 75% in seroincidence over the course of the study (Figure 33-1).[12]

Thinking back to the time we were just beginning and facing skeptics who doubted anything meaningful could be accomplished for drug addicts, those results tasted pretty sweet and justified all the hard work and dedication of the intervention teams working for the Community Outreach Intervention Projects (COIP) at the UIC School of Public Health.

In recognition of our accomplishments, we were selected by NIDA as one of three scientifically sound prevention strategies proven to be effective in controlling the transmission of HIV among IDUs. We set out to help in developing an intervention manual and training curriculum to facilitate technology transfer. Shortly thereafter, the Secretary of Health and Human Services enacted block grant legislation to encourage all states to adopt one of the three approaches to come out of NIDA's NADR program in order to address the threat of HIV among IDUs in their states. Soon to follow was a Substance Abuse and Mental Health Services Administration (SAMHSA) program to support such efforts. We were quite pleased to learn that out of the first-round states to apply for support from SAMHSA, four out of five chose to replicate the Indigenous Leader Outreach Model (ILOM), the strategy with roots in the Chicago School of Sociology, symbolic interaction theory and the pioneering work of Patrick Hughes in combining epidemiologic and ethnographic methods in an integrated research and community-based public health intervention design.

Would using high-status members of targeted populations (indigenous leaders) to deliver intervention programming prove successful if replicated on a massive scale across the country? Would following a common sense sequence of intervention objectives, including gaining access to target populations, increasing HIV/AIDS awareness, promoting individualized risk assessments, reinforcing behavior change, and promoting prevention advocacy work irrespective of locale or target group characteristics? Would combining ethnographic and epidemiologic methods provide additional insights in both understanding the underlying dynamics of localized epidemics and informing the evolution of appropriate intervention services throughout the course of these epidemics? What we had was substantial evidence to substantiate that the ILOM had the potential to work well in controlling the further spread of HIV. As time would tell, that by no means ensured its effectiveness as applied in many different contexts, both in the United States and abroad.

INTERNATIONAL PERSPECTIVES

By the late 1980s, contacts and exchanges with public health authorities from abroad began to escalate. At first, there was much curiosity about programs in Europe, especially Holland and England, which seemed to be very progressive in addressing the epidemic and were not hindered by prohibitions against the distribution of sterile needles/syringes or concerns that preventing HIV transmission might somehow be misinterpreted as condoning illicit drug use, prostitution, or homosexuality. For a time, we were regularly hosting a series of visitors from Europe and were leveraging whatever opportunities we had to visit over there. Then, the call of Asia beckoned and excited in me a yearning for adventure outside the realm of previous experience. I signed up with Fred Shick to attend the Asian AIDS Conference in Bangkok in 1988 and was pleased to find a world very much unlike

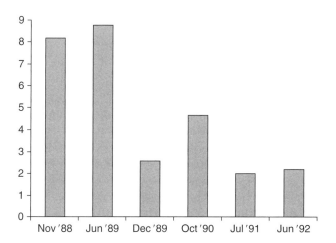

FIGURE 33-1 Seroincidence per 100 person years among a cohort of injection drug users in Chicago [adapted from Wiebel et al, reference 12].

anything I had encountered before. Of further good fortune, the conference abstract submitted on our intervention projects in Chicago, Baltimore, Denver, and El Paso was accepted as a poster presentation.

In my travels to this point, I had relished experiences in Europe, where I developed a deep sense of history from buildings, streets, and architecture that predated by centuries anything that could be found in America. And all of this sense of history could be experienced at a personal level. This was, after all, the homeland of my ancestors. By way of contrast, arriving in Asia, the excitement was increased manyfold by an other worldly impression of everything surrounding me. Not only was this very different and entirely new, it was not related to my background or heritage in any obvious way that I could retrieve from memory or prior experience. Walking around the streets of Bangkok that first day, I was assaulted by the intense tropical heat in combination with sounds, smells, and sights that were both foreign and enticingly captivating.

Putting up the poster the first day of the conference, I noticed one man in particular studying it closely. The poster included a description of the ILOM intervention. He asked a number of pointed questions and said something like, "Wow! I had no idea anything like this was being done back in the States. Is this approach really working?" I answered his questions and then he said, "This is exactly what Thailand needs right now!" He said that he would like to approach the conference organizing committee to make time for me and then asked me if I could make a plenary speech the next day. We exchanged business cards and I found out as a consequence that he was Win McKeithen, United States Agency for International Development (USAID) Director in Thailand. I made the speech, attended a number of meetings that Win arranged, and was introduced to Don Douglas, Program for Appropriate Technology in Health (PATH) Country Director in Thailand. PATH is an international nongovernment organization that does public health related work in a variety of locations around the world (http://www.path.org/index.php). Win asked if I would be willing to launch a pilot project to assess ILOM's intervention potential in Bangkok. When I responded without hesitation in the affirmative, he asked Don if PATH could attend to all of the local arrangements. When Don indicated that he could, I recall questioning for the first time my graduate student belief that it just could not get any cooler than it was for me back then.

We sat down to lay out plans for the pilot project and Win stipulated that we should compare the ILOM to one or more strategies that were more consistent with historical precedent in Thailand. Given the high status accorded older women in Thai slum communities and the fact that they had been successfully utilized in a number of health promotion campaigns, it was decided that they should be enlisted as prevention advocates targeting IDUs and the families of IDUs in one of the comparison projects. For the other comparative project, it was decided that high-status youth from slum communities that addicts lived in could be mobilized as prevention educators to encourage the adoption of safe injection practices.

For our experimental condition, consistent with other ILOM projects, an ethnographer was hired to shed light on Thai injection practices and to inform implementation of the intervention. In this instance, we were fortunate to find a Thai anthropologist who had received his doctorate from the University of California at Berkeley.

Two very important and totally unexpected findings emerged from this pilot initiative. The first hit me like a strike of lightening when I teamed up with the Thai ethnographer and went to one of the slum communities to interview heroin addicts. I was fully dependent upon the ethnographer to translate both the questions I asked and the responses from the IDUs. I told him that I wanted to get a sense of the social hierarchy among IDUs in Thailand, but could not go into detail in the group interview to explain that we had found that higher status individuals tended to work out better as outreach workers in the States in comparison to their lower status counterparts. I began to ask a series of questions to get some sense of the social hierarchy among addicts, but did not seem to be getting any information that would have been helpful to me. I continued on with the questioning and grew frustrated that I was making absolutely no progress in understanding what I was trying to get at. I asked a question about who addicts looked up to in hope of identifying high-status attributes, but again got nowhere. I felt like I was grasping for straws and remember wondering how this guy could have possibly gotten a doctorate in Anthropology from Berkeley and not have a clue about what I was trying to elicit with my questions about social status. Seemingly in tune with my frustration, he shared his interpretation that this group apparently considered the community of addicts to be relatively egalitarian. I was at a loss as to what to ask next, but then got what I thought to be a flash of inspiration. I asked them what characteristics they looked down upon among fellow injectors. The response of, "anyone who stole from others" left me speechless for I do not remember how long. It was like being slapped across the face and feeling humbled in a way that happens only rarely in a lifetime. The response was so outside the realm of what I considered to be possible that I was shocked to the realization that I knew next to nothing about heroin addicts in Thailand. Professor Big Shot, know-it-all about HIV and drug injectors from the United States was all of a sudden wondering what the hell he was doing in Thailand and what, if anything, he could offer to be of assistance to these people.

Dope fiends who looked down upon anybody who stole? I am sure I went to the hotel that night scouring my memory for even a single mention of anyone ever looking down on a fellow addict for being driven to theft in order to secure his next fix of heroin. It boggled the mind. Yet, over the next few days I was able to make sense out of this seemingly incomprehensible statement. As it turned out, heroin in Thailand at the time was both very pure and very inexpensive. It was so pure that overdose deaths were a rarity because it was impossible to stumble across an unexpectedly potent dose that would inadvertently kill an experienced user. And, it was so inexpensive that a dose could be bought for the price of a meal or a pack of cigarettes. That is, it was so inexpensive that even a lazy person would be able to support a habit by street peddling or engaging in some sort of legitimate means of generating income. It was so inexpensive that if they had to resort to thievery, they might be looked down upon by their fellow addicts.

> *While further inquiry offered an answer to the puzzling response I got, a much more important lesson was learned that I would like to share. That is, while confidence and self-assuredness can be positive attributes at times, they can also lead to catastrophic errors in judgment and assumption, especially when dealing with an unfamiliar culture and a population with which you have no previous experience.*

While further inquiry offered an answer to the puzzling response I got, a much more important lesson was learned that I would like to share. That is, while confidence and self-assuredness can be positive attributes at times, they can also lead to catastrophic errors in judgment and assumption, especially when dealing with an unfamiliar culture and a population with which you have no previous experience. I never took the opportunity to revisit this experience with the Thai ethnographer, but I would not be surprised if he wrote me off as just another clueless western expert who had ventured so far astray that he did not even realize that he was lost. The situation is made even more unnerving by the fact that I thought I would be teaching him about addiction because he said he had no previous experience with heroin addicts. Little did I know that the student was a lot more on the ball than the professor when it came to this assignment!

Despite this humbling experience and the consequent realization that I desperately needed help from others more experienced and knowledgeable about Thailand and its drug users, the pilot was launched in relatively short order. With it came the second important and unexpected experience to emerge from this pilot, this time having to do with the eventual outcome of even successful public health intervention demonstrations. In the case of our demonstration pilot, USAID and the Bangkok Metropolitan Administration called an early halt after 6 of the planned 12 months it was scheduled to operate. The ILOM intervention was deemed to be a success because of evidence that addicts were changing their behavior so as to reduce the risk of contracting or spreading HIV. The use of bleach as a disinfectant was rejected as being too time consuming, given the fact that it was only available in powder form there. However, the IDUs participating in the ILOM arm of the demonstration showed a clear willingness to discontinue the sharing of injection paraphernalia. The two control interventions, by way of comparison, seemed to prompt little concern or behavior change among addicts. Apparently the highly respected senior slum women were afraid to directly confront IDUs in their community and they did not feel much more comfortable in approaching the families of the addicts. The other control project that utilized high-status slum youth as health educators likewise was a disappointment. After we learned that these youth looked down upon the IDUs in their community, it was little wonder that they were not successful in rallying recognition of the epidemic threat among addicts or in prompting a change in injection practices.

That left the Bangkok Metropolitan Administration agreeing to adopt the ILOM intervention through the existing methadone programs it operated in slum communities across Bangkok. This led to the first valuable lesson in relation to the potential for rolling out successful intervention strategies within the existing public health system. The lesson learned was that even when successfully pilot tested, a public health demonstration program could fail miserably when implemented in the real world. That is, when the real world quite simply would not allow various necessary conditions to be replicated as intended. On a return visit to Thailand some time following completion of the pilot program, I was taken to meet with the Director of the Bangkok Metropolitan Administration (in which the local health department resided). The Director clearly was most supportive and sincere in his wanting to adopt the ILOM to prevent HIV transmission among Thai IDUs. He explained how the translated training materials were being used to train methadone program nurses to implement the intervention in the communities in which they worked. I explained that up to this point, the indigenous outreach intervention staff utilized by ILOM projects had been ex-addicts or methadone clients who were of high status and possessed the street smarts to engage addicts through outreach in slum communities. It was explained that this would not be possible in Bangkok as there were no pre-existing civil service job categories that could cover this classification of work and type of worker. Dr. Kachit sympathized that the methadone nurses were already over-worked and might be hesitant to undertake outreach assignments in the slum communities, but for now that was the best that could be done. Then I asked about ethnographic oversight to conduct field investigations of addict behavior, assess the success of intervention strategies and supervise implementation of the intervention. Once again he explained that unfortunately there were no existing civil service job classifications for an ethnographer. I had hoped that I might be able to work with USAID, BMA, and PATH more in exploring options for replicating the ILOM in a fashion more true to its intended design, but Thailand had graduated to a Developed Nation status in the eyes of the U.S. government and plans were already underway to close the USAID office in Thailand.

During my visits to Thailand, almost every corner turned led to marvelous new experiences: the fiery food that required you to develop a tolerance to chilies in order for you to experience more than a sense of texture accompanied by the intense incineration of taste buds; a huge district and night market area called Patpong where neon lights and high-decibel blaring music presented a backdrop to relentless, in-your-face hawkers who beckoned passerbys into go-go lounges with scantily clad young ladies and second floor sex shows advertised by the amazing feats reportedly performed for audiences; the embarrassment of being served tea at an official government meeting where the servant shuffled up to me on her knees; the mistake of asking locals to order food and the panic accompanying being served chicken feet and fried insects.

The fun loving but naughty nature of Thais was demonstrated by a government official at a dinner reception when I asked how to order Thai ice coffee and he instructed me to say, "Caffe yen, si nom" (coffee cold with milk). After a feeble attempt on my part, he repeated loudly to all "CAFFE YEN, SI NOM," causing all to burst out in raucous laughter. The joke, of course, had been at my and the waitress's expense, even if in good nature, as he explained that Thai is a tonal language and that with a slight difference in emphasis, imperceptible to me, I had asked the waitress to shake her breasts after ordering iced coffee. My wanderlust was pumping at full speed ahead and, needless to say, I was hooked on Thailand and more than eager to find any additional opportunities for work in Asia.

Fortunately for me, additional opportunities for work in Asia soon followed. Dr. Gary Slutkin was the head of intervention for WHO's Global Programme on AIDS under the leadership of Dr. Jonathan Mann, and then later, Dr. Mike Merson. The Global Programme on AIDS was responsible for coordinating the global response to the HIV/AIDS pandemic. I had met Gary in Geneva while doing some consulting work for the Global Programme on AIDS. Although we had not known each other previously, we shared a bit in common because he was from Chicago and had gone to medical school at the University of Chicago around the same time I was working in the Department of Psychiatry. When he found out I was interested in working in Asia, he asked if I would help out with the Global Programme's fledgling activities there and commissioned me to draft a manual adapting the ILOM to be used in the context of developing countries. This led to opening all sorts of doors and eventually enabled my involvement with UN and WHO projects in Thailand, China, Myanmar, Bangladesh, Laos, India, and the Philippines. I was hired to conduct a post hoc evaluation of the UN's first-round HIV intervention efforts in six Asian countries and later enlisted to train local health authorities in the ILOM for a planned China/Myanmar border initiative. In the process, I was getting a most fascinating introduction to regional public health systems and the HIV/AIDS interface with local populations of sex workers, sex work clients, IDUs, and men who have sex with men (MSM).

From the wealth of epidemiologic data accumulating within the region, there were readily apparent differing epidemic stages and patterns of transmission. Data from a study that I was involved in about the sexual networks of IDUs in Bangladesh and Indonesia years later (in 2004) serves as an example. Characteristics that these countries had in common included substantial poverty, dense and predominantly Muslim populations, and large numbers of injectors among drug using subpopulations.

In Bangladesh, drug injectors' preferred pharmaceutical cocktails contained buprenorphine as a principle ingredient. They were at a relatively early stage of epidemic progression with less than 10% of IDUs being infected with HIV based upon limited available surveillance. On the other hand, in Indonesia, IDUs injected heroin almost exclusively and had experienced an explosive outbreak of HIV infection with more than 50% infected and some of our programs reporting a prevalence in excess of 80%.

What I did not fully appreciate was how much politics, religion, culture, and history influenced not only the situation in each country, but also how each country was responding to this new public health threat. Countries with active civil societies and plentiful non-government organizations (NGOs) had important resources that could be mobilized for purposes of HIV/AIDS intervention. Other countries, like China and Myanmar, had few preexisting NGOs to turn to in orchestrating a response. In some countries, religious issues were seemingly of negligible influence in shaping intervention policy, while in others, like the Philippines, the Catholic Church played a huge role in opposing condom promotion as a preventive measure.

Changing circumstances can also add to complexities. Thailand is often held out as a national example of coordinated and effective response. Yet, Myat Htoo Razak and I were just beginning to launch two HIV-related initiatives targeting drug users in Thailand for Family Health International (FHI) when the prime minister commenced a campaign against drug use that led to the execution of untold numbers of addicts on the streets. We were compelled to halt these projects immediately after it became apparent that our target population might be placing themselves at risk of death as a consequence of participating in our programs. Changing situations created the need for us to change in our approach to work as well. One challenge of working in public health at a regional level is getting to know all about constituent governments and their individual peculiarities. This familiarity represents a very real prerequisite to being able to offer meaningful assistance.

MORE OF THE BEST OF TIMES

By the mid-1990s, I had completed a number of consulting assignments in Indonesia. The easternmost province of Indonesia, then known as Irian Jaya, was the epicenter of the HIV epidemic. Sexual transmission of HIV through sex work was a major factor in underlying dynamics. To better understand the nature of the problem, I joined forces with Iko Safika, PATH provincial representative in Irian. We undertook an investigation of the migratory patterns of sex workers in Irian Jaya, the western half of the second-largest island in the world and home to some of the most primitive and remote areas known to mankind. Preliminary investigation suggested that almost all sex workers in seaside population centers were migrants brought in to service men who themselves were migrant laborers working in natural resource extraction industries. The fact that this region had the highest prevalence of diagnosed AIDS cases and that both the sex workers and their clients were mobile, presented a bleak prospect for containing further spread of infection.

Because no roads link the few population centers on the island, we flew to each destination and interviewed all varieties of sex workers we could identify. Eighty-five women participated in this study. Occupying the bottom half of the social status hierarchy were brothel-based women (56% of the women interviewed). Such individuals affiliated with a group of other women and worked out of a stand-alone building or a complex that might include a large number of buildings and 100 or more sex workers. Most often, these women came from eastern Java and had experienced tragedy in their lives leading up to their introduction to sex workers and, ultimately, a life of sex work. Their backgrounds typically included marriage at a very early age, abuse by spouse and/or family, death or flight of husband, abject poverty, and no potential sources of support. One 45-year-old respondent from a large brothel complex recounted the deaths of her two husbands, the first of lung disease and the second of an accident that she insisted was her full responsibility. The fact that she could not be reasonably held responsible for the deaths was something that she was not willing to consider. Assuming responsibility served to help justify the otherwise unjustifiable. Engaging in commercial sex transactions seemed to be considered a sufficiently shameful and degrading source of financial support that it required a pitifully catastrophic chain of events to approach becoming an acceptable course of action.

In the upper half of the social spectrum were women working out of clubs, discotheques, massage parlors and karaoke venues (32% of the women interviewed). An unanticipated finding among this group was younger women from northern Sulawesi who entered sex work as what they referred to as "an adventure," to accumulate some cash prior to returning home to marry. Moral overtones were largely absent in the personal histories related by these sex workers. The choice to engage in commercial sex was considered to be a practical matter with clear and time bound limitations. Much more so than their brothel-based counterparts, these young adults had specific plans of leaving sex work and returning to more typical lifestyles. This is not to suggest that prostitution was not considered to be stigmatizing by these young women. The fact that they did not like to be referred to as sex workers clearly indicates that they did not consider their choice of occupation to be value free.

Street-based sex workers were the remaining classification we encountered (12% of the women interviewed) and they were one of three types: high class, low class, and transsexuals or "waria." The high-class type often had previously worked in entertainment establishments and often served a higher class of men, such as a businessman or foreigners. In contrast, the low-class sex worker and the "waria" made less money and were often picked up by local men on the streets.

What Iko and I found everywhere we looked were mobile sex workers and mobile sex work clients, almost always in transit and rarely staying any one place for more than 3 months to a year. Most businesses that hired sex workers preferred to bring in new girls rather than renewing contracts with those who had been there a while. For others, a rumor of better money to be made elsewhere was always an invitation to move on to greener pastures. With HIV already introduced within these populations, as reflected in 8% of sex workers from Merauke testing positive during the time we conducted this investigation, it seemed a worst case scenario in the works and prompted us to sound an alarm through the results in our report that we distributed widely, including to relevant public health authorities.

It is especially challenging to prevent HIV transmission in mobile populations because their support networks tend to be transitory and they are often motivated to continue nomadic lifestyles by the need for money. To try to make an impact on this population, you need to work with the fact that everyone is always on the move. Papua is a remote area. Transport there for those without resources to pay for a plane ticket (sex workers and Indonesian labor) is by boat. I suggested that an HIV prevention campaign be mounted to attract the attention of those at risk during the long trip. It is a captive audience and, with a little creativity, a lot of prevention education could be accomplished. For those transiting to work in Papua by flight, it might be best to target the companies that hire them and launch prevention campaigns through their employers.

A unique challenge to prevention planning is that sometimes practices are rooted in locally accepted culture. One fact that most folks back home do not even realize is that there are commercial sex workers across the country that originate from villages that historically raised consorts for sultans that ruled kingdoms across the island of Java. Now, there is only one sultan left that I know about in Java and it has been a long time since anyone has been recruiting consorts for harems, but some of these villages have not changed that much in what they are known best for. That is, they now raise the sex workers that populate all manner of venues across the island. What it is still hard for even me to accept is that the little girls from these villages are expected to grow up to be sex workers and the whole family will rely on the income these young women send home. The thought of having their offspring prematurely marry off before they provided the family with maximum returns would be unthinkable to such villagers.

The year following our study of sex worker migration in Papua, Family Health International (FHI) was awarded the USAID contract for HIV/AIDS support in Asia and I was asked if I was interested in heading up their initiatives targeting drug users. I joined forces with them in 2000, following completion of arrangements back home at UIC to set up a personal services contract. For this assignment in Asia, I was expected to spend about 60% effort in Indonesia, the site where I would be based. By this time, injection drug use had grown to surpass sexual transmission in contributing to new infections (Figure 33-2). I relished the opportunity to see if I could replicate the ILOM and assess its capacity to address a rapidly spreading epidemic in an entirely new context. Dr. Steve Wignall, FHI country director in Indonesia, gave the go-ahead for setting up an Indonesian IDU intervention team. For staff, we were able to recruit some of the country's brightest young activists with a wealth of prior experience in working with NGOs. They were Made Setiawan, Very Kamil, and last, but not least, Ignatius (Gambit) Praptoraharjo. In so many respects, this was the best group I ever had the good fortune to work with overseas. We were in the right place, at the right time, with plentiful resources to help accomplish almost anything we could wish for, as long as it could be justified as addressing Indonesia's intervention needs. This sort of situation just does not happen often enough in a public health career.

I met both Very and Gambit on one of my first consulting assignments to Indonesia. Don Douglas from PATH knew of this nascent community-based NGO in Yogyakarta, central Java called Lentera that he was con-

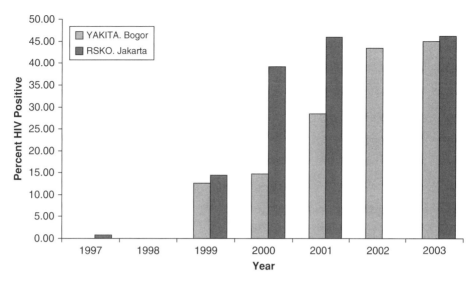

FIGURE 33-2 Trends in the prevalence of HIV infection among injection drug users at two facilities in Indonesia: Yakita (a private therapeutic community drug treatment program) and RSKO (a publicly funded hospital-based national drug abuse treatment program).

sidering giving support for HIV/AIDS prevention programming. The program was staffed by young activists, among them Very Kamil and Ignatius Praptoraharjo "Gambit." As I conducted ILOM training for them, I recall being impressed by how they and Lentera's director, an American ex-pat named Laurel MacLaren, listened intently and asked pointed questions reflecting the fact that they were thinking about what the information might mean to them and eager to learn all they could. Little did I know that not much more than 5 years down the road, we would be working together and that only then would I begin to fully appreciate their personalities and great sense of humor that favorably balanced out the more serious sides I first met. In Jakarta, after work hours our team would regularly get together at my house to hold planning meetings that would identify who would do what in the coming weeks (Figure 33-3). Then, after eating dinner, we would retire to the living room to play pool. Inevitably, I would tire before them and they would play on together until heaven knows what hour of the night. After crashing wherever they could find that was comfortable, they would be off before I woke and I would see them again in a few hours at work, none the worse for wear.

Most importantly, there was something wonderfully synergistic that occurred when my Indonesian colleagues and I worked together. Their devotion and dedication to tasks at hand never seemed to waiver. We were on a mission and whether working together or apart, we never seemed to miss a beat. From the standpoint of an outsider trying to help another country address a major public health challenge, this is about as empowering as it can get for an external consultant. Faced with a different language, different culture, and different expectations and assumptions, achieving intended outcomes is rarely as easy as one would wish. Performance is judged on more than demonstrated expertise in your field(s) of specialization. You have to be a good listener and do a lot of homework to get a firm grasp of both the problem at hand and its local context.

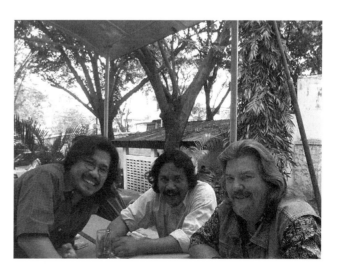

FIGURE 33-3 The author with Very Kamil (far left) and Ignatius (Gambit) Praptoraharjo (center).

Only then can you be prepared for the additional confounding issues, intervening influences, and seemingly irrelevant concerns that threaten to sabotage the best of plans. But for those resilient enough to weather this all and persistent enough to keep on track, the reward of success in being of assistance is possible. Having a team of sharp locals at your side to assist in interpreting situations and help in negotiating the obstacle courses you will face can make matters immeasurably easier and greatly increase the chances of intended outcomes being realized (Figure 33-4).

In wrapping up this description of field investigations associated with my serendipitous career, it seems fitting for me to end my story in Indonesia, where I have written this chapter and I am now sitting in the AIDS Research Center office at Universitas Atma Jaya in Jakarta (Figure 33-5). While still working with FHI, a friend and long-term colleague from the University of Illinois at Chicago (UIC), Judith Levy secured a Fogarty AIDS International Training and Research Program grant in partnership with another long-term friend and colleague, Professor Irwanto from Universitas Atma Jaya. This has enabled some of the promising young scholars with whom I have become acquainted during my work here to be enlisted as Fogarty Fellows and complete their doctoral studies at UIC. Following my return to UIC at contract's end with FHI, Judith Levy secured another NIH grant to assist Indonesia in developing its research capacity to address the HIV/AIDS epidemic. That enabled me to return back here as a Co-Principal Investigator (Co-PI) and prompted the creation of the AIDS Research Center that Prof. Irwanto is

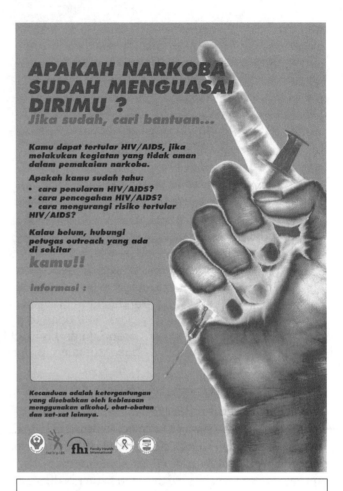

Translation of the poster:

Do you think that drugs have controlled your life?

If so, look for help. . .

If you practice risky drug use, you can be infected by HIV.

Do you know:
- the mode of HIV transmission?
- how HIV transmission can be prevented?
- ways to reduce risk of contracting HIV?

If you need help and information, please contact outreach workers in your neighborhood.

Information:

Addiction is a dependence caused by the habit of consuming alcohol, drugs, and other substances.

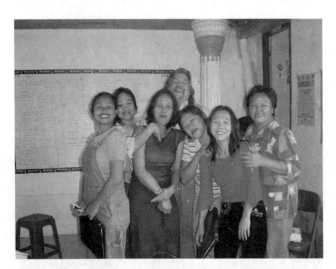

FIGURE 33-4 The author with an indigenous outreach team that targets female sex workers and their clients in Manado, Northern Sulawesi, Indonesia.

FIGURE 33-5 A poster used as one of the information, education, and communication (IEC) materials for an injection drug user intervention in Indonesia. The poster was produced and distributed by Family Health International/Indonesia during 2004 through 2006.

now heading. The research capacity building grant includes three pilot research projects and I am now working on the second one to explore the sexual networks of high-risk populations here as a foundation for developing couples counseling protocols in conjunction with Voluntary Counseling and Testing for HIV. So, at least for the time being, the saga continues. For those of you interested in global health and a desire to participate in field investigations yourselves, a great opportunity for practical learning can be had from affiliating with initiatives like ours that are doing collaborative work with international institutions of higher learning and local public health authorities. May your good fortunes be as abundant as mine have been! (Figures 33-5, 33-6. 33-7)

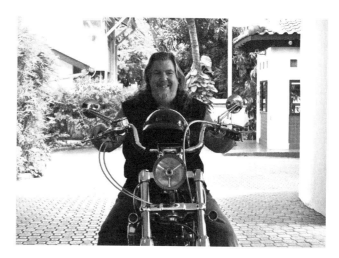

FIGURE 33-7 The author in Indonesia.

LEARNING QUESTIONS

1. What are the distinguishing features of the Indigenous Leader Outreach Model and how could it be applied to other public health problems not covered in this chapter?
2. What are the strengths and limitations of recruiting injection drug users as outreach staff for a program that is targeting injection drug users?
3. Which types of shooting galleries and injection behaviors described in this chapter were relevant to HIV prevention?
4. In Indonesia, the author found "everywhere we looked were mobile sex workers and mobile sex work clients." What was meant by this statement? What are the implications to HIV prevention efforts? How would you overcome this issue of highly mobile persons?
5. Think of a public health problem that you might face at some point in your career. Describe the nature of the problem and develop a series of questions that would help you address the problem in a preliminary field investigation.
6. Discuss the types of strategies that might be adopted to address the public health problem from question 5 and relate how findings from your field investigation might influence your options.
7. What safeguards can you think of to help ensure that your impressions from field investigations and consulting advice are appropriate if you are working in a foreign country?

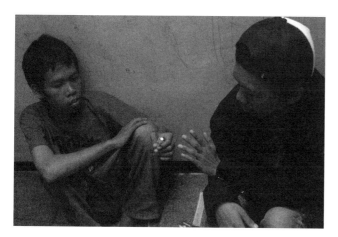

FIGURE 33-6 Educational photo of injection drug users for use in promoting prevention of HIV/AIDS in Indonesia. The target group models photographed have since died of complications of AIDS—a sobering reminder of the public health importance of this prevention work. Photo courtesy of Pusat Penelitian Kesehatan Universitas Indonesia (PPK UI).

REFERENCES

1. Mead GH. *Mind, Self, and Society*. Chicago, IL: University of Chicago Press; 1934.
2. Thomas WI, Thomas DS. *The Child in America: Behavior Problems and Programs*. New York: Knopf; 1928:572.
3. Becker HS. *Outsiders: Studies in the Sociology of Deviance*. New York: The Free Press of Glencoe; 1963.
4. Wiebel WW. Burning out on the Northwest Side: PCP use in Chicago. In Feldman H, Agar M, Beschner G eds. *Angel Dust: An Ethnographic Study of PCP Users*. Lexington, MA: Lexington Books; 1979.
5. Hughes P. *Behind the Wall of Respect: Community Experiments in Heroin Addiction Control*. Chicago, IL: University of Chicago Press; 1977.
6. Wiebel WW. *The Indigenous Leader Outreach Model: Intervention Manual*. Rockville, MD: National Institute on Drug Abuse; 1993. NIH Publication No. 93-3581.
7. Brown BS, Beschner GM, eds. *Handbook on Risk of AIDS: Injection Drug Users and Sexual Partners*. Westport, CT: Greenwood Press, 1993.
8. Ouellet L, Jimenez A, Johnson W, Wiebel W. Shooting Galleries and HIV Disease: Variations in Places for Injecting Illicit Drugs. In Nelken D, Mars G, eds. *Drugs, Crime, and Criminal Justice Volume I*. Sudbury, MA: Dartmouth

Publishing Co.; 1995. Reprint of article in *Crime and Delinquency*. January 1991:37(1):64–85.

9. Koester S, Booth R, Wiebel W. Risk of HIV transmission from sharing water, drug mixing containers and cotton filters among intravenous drug users. *Int J Drug Policy*. 1990; 1(6)28–30.

10. Centers for Disease Control and Prevention. Update: reducing HIV transmission in intravenous-drug users not in drug treatment—United States. *MMWR Morb Mortality Wkly Rep*. 1990;39(31):529, 536–538.

11. Centers for Disease Control and Prevention. Assessment of street outreach for HIV prevention—selected sites, 1991–1993. *MMWR Morb Mortality Wkly Rep*. 1993; 42(45): 879–880.

12. Wiebel WW, Jimenez A, Johnson W, et al. Risk behavior and HIV seroincidence among out-of-treatment injection drug users: a four-year prospective study. *J Acquir Immun Defic Syndr Hum Retrovirol*. 1996;12(3):282–289.

CHAPTER 34

Investigation of Attitudes Toward Immunization in an Old-Order Amish Community

Jonathan S. Yoder, MSW, MPH

Illinois, 2005

INTRODUCTION

On a frigid morning at Chicago's Union Station, a group of travelers attracted attention from the busy commuters hurrying from train to train. They were plainly dressed in solid colored clothing; the women in the group had their heads fully covered with bonnets. The men had full beards without mustaches and wore dark, wide-brimmed hats (Figure 34-1). They were Amish, a Christian sect that avoids many of the modern conveniences of life. Because they did not own automobiles, trains allowed them to travel from their communities to the outside world. Though my appearance was not similar to theirs, I felt a kinship with them and, to some extent, understood their outlook on the world outside their community. Ours was a shared heritage that went back to the early 1900s when my great-grandparents left the Amish church. I grew up in a conservative Mennonite church and community in rural northern Florida that had many of the same customs as the Amish. The adults in our church dressed like the Amish and we lived a simpler life, without distractions, like television, in our home. Farming was an integral part of our culture; I worked on the dairy farms of my grandfather and uncle. Given those experiences, in some ways I understood their view of the world.

As I watched the Amish navigate the busy terminal, I pondered how, except for a small decision by my ancestors, I would share their culture. This was a relatively closed community with little, though definitely some, interaction with the outside world. At work that morning, I internally pondered the question, "What do we know about the health status of the Amish in Illinois?" Answering that question would involve expanding my understanding of public health research, challenging my assumptions of the attitudes and practices of underserved religious communities, and teaching me lessons that impacted my work on the other side of the world.

My life was very different now. I was a Public Health Prevention Service (PHPS) fellow with the Centers for Disease Control and Prevention (CDC) and had recently moved to Chicago with my wife and three young

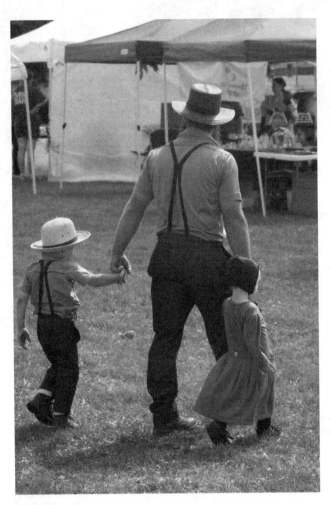

FIGURE 34-1 An Amish father holds hands with his children, a boy and a girl, while walking through an outdoor market. © Ralph R. Echtinaw/ShutterStock, Inc.

children for an assignment with the state of Illinois. I did not plan for a career in public health. After an undergraduate degree in Psychology from Clearwater Christian College, I started graduate school in social work at the University of South Florida, planning to do individual and family counseling. Along the way, a professor convinced me to pursue a master's degree in public health. Following a few years of social work, I was ready to try out a new career and was accepted into the PHPS program, a 3-year CDC fellowship with both federal and state/local public health experience. During my first year of the PHPS program, I worked in Atlanta on waterborne disease surveillance. For the next 2 years, I was assigned to the Illinois Department of Public Health (IDPH) to assist and train local health departments with infectious disease outbreaks and disease surveillance and prevention projects. I had been able to assist with the investigation of outbreaks caused by enterotoxigenic *E. coli*, *Cryptosporidium*, and pertussis, as well as assisting with the development of Hepatitis C prevention plans and communicable disease legislation.

The Amish are descendants of the Swiss Anabaptists, who attempt to live simply and emphasize the importance of community. The Old-Order Amish (hereafter referred to as Amish) are the most distinctive of the various Amish sects, relying on traditional beliefs and practices and rejecting as worldly the majority of modern conveniences. For instance, Amish do not have electricity or phone lines in their homes. They do not own automobiles or use motorized farm equipment. Their transportation is horse-and-buggy and they dress plainly (Figure 34-2). They maintain their own schools, which generally only educate children through the eighth grade. Because of a birth rate of approximately seven children per family and a 90% retention rate for its youth, the Amish population in the United States has increased from 8,200 in the early 1900s to approximately 180,000 now.[1] In Illinois, the largest Amish community surrounds the town of Arthur in the east-central region of the state. Eight additional smaller communities are located throughout central and southern Illinois.[2] Other larger Amish communities are found in Lancaster, Pennsylvania and Holmes County, Ohio, with numerous communities scattered throughout rural areas of the United States. The Amish economy is traditionally centered around the family farm; however, as their population has grown, it has become more difficult to find adequate farming land. Many Amish have developed cottage industries within their community (e.g., woodworking, crafts) or have gone to work for non-Amish employers, likely increasing Amish interaction with the outside world. The Arthur community has a combina-

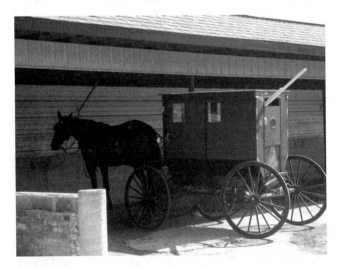

FIGURE 34-2 Amish horse and buggy. Photograph courtesy of Mark S. Dworkin.

tion of family farms, Amish retail shops, Amish-owned industries, and non-Amish business that employed the Amish.

During a meeting with my supervisor (Dr. Mark Dworkin) to discuss projects, he asked if I was interested in doing a project involving the Amish. I mentioned that I had hoped to have that opportunity and we discussed possible areas of study. He mentioned a 1996 pertussis ("whooping cough") outbreak in an Amish community in Whiteside County that ended with many unanswered questions. In that outbreak, local medical providers had diagnosed several cases of pertussis in February 1996 among Amish children and alerted the IDPH. A meeting was arranged with the bishop (the community spiritual leader) and approval was given to start the investigation. Families were interviewed when they came to the local health department and information was collected on ill persons within their family. The vaccine status for family members was ascertained by family report and by checking health department vaccination records. Despite the efforts of the state and local health department, the outbreak continued for 2 months and more than 41 persons became ill. During the outbreak, a wedding in the community brought visitors from Amish communities in Colorado, Arkansas, Missouri, Wisconsin, and other Amish communities in Illinois; spread to those communities was possible, but could not be verified.

> *The size and extent of the outbreak was unknown because community cooperation ended after several weeks. When the elders withdrew support of the investigation, families ceased visiting the local health department, and community members would not talk about the outbreak or any subsequent cases.*

The size and extent of the outbreak was unknown because community cooperation ended after several weeks. When the elders withdrew support of the investigation, families ceased visiting the local health department, and community members would not talk about the outbreak or any subsequent cases. Before the investigation ended, it was clear that the outbreak could largely be attributed to the low vaccination rate found among community members. Among the 41 known cases, only 11 (27%) had any evidence of vaccination. There was also a disparity of vaccination history between males (40%) and females (19%). Because of the abrupt ending of the investigation, these data could not be further explored. Because there were unanswered questions from this outbreak and the risk of vaccine-preventable disease among Amish was unknown, we developed the idea to determine if our health department staff's assumptions about the Amish being anti-vaccine were correct. The answer to that question would greatly influence any public health planning regarding increasing immunization rates in our state (including in populations such as the Amish).

Accessing this population would be a challenge. Because the last contact that the state health department had with them ended abruptly, we recognized that we had to pursue this field epidemiology project with a great deal of forethought. Although I shared a distant heritage with the Amish, I had few ideas about how to understand what the Amish believed about vaccination. Because Amish do not have phones or Internet access, some conventional methods of public health surveys were not available. Additionally, they are often wary of government intervention in their community. This distrust of government is deeply ingrained within Amish cultural memory. When the Amish movement started in 17th century Europe, a key principle was to refrain from government involvement. This belief was further reinforced by their persecution and subsequent expulsion from Europe and their more recent American experiences, such as imprisonment for refusing military service and forced schooling for their children in certain communities. To make a clear distinction between their community and the outside world, most Amish explicitly decline civic activities like voting or jury duty. Amish views on outside government intervention further decreased the likelihood that direct, individual public health surveys (e.g., door-to-door or mailed) would be well-received. These methods might also jeopardize any relationship the local health departments had established with these communities. Complicating government public health relations with this community further, their separate identities both geographically and physically, evident in the separation of their communities and their clear differences in clothing, may cause those in government to hesitate to even approach them when not absolutely necessary because they do not expect the government information or recommendation to be well received.

As I started to research the health issues of the Amish, it was clear that they had been disproportionally impacted by outbreaks of vaccine-preventable diseases. Previous outbreaks of rubella,[3] measles,[4] pertussis,[5] *Haemophilus influenzae*,[6] and polio,[7] as well as increased cases of childhood tetanus,[8] had all been reported among Amish communities. Studies conducted in the context of these vaccine-preventable disease outbreaks made a direct link between the low rate of reported vaccine coverage in Amish communities and their susceptibility to disease outbreaks. The vaccination rates among the Amish impacted by these outbreaks were too low to confer herd immunity within the community, which provided the opportunity for vaccine-preventable disease transmission among community members and placed vulnerable members of the non-Amish community at risk for contracting these diseases. But why were vaccination rates so low in these Amish communities? Did their views of vaccination or church teaching discourage community members from being vaccinated?

When I reviewed available information on the Amish and their view of vaccination, I found some apparently contradictory information. It seemed possible that Amish views on health and health care might contribute to their lack of adoption of vaccination as a means of disease prevention. They consider health as a gift from God and not solely the result of preventive behaviors or medical intervention.[1] Vaccination is not explicitly prohibited by the church; however, it is often not encouraged either. Additionally, the Amish consciously avoid dependence on government assistance and might consider the acceptance of free or subsidized vaccinations to be a form of government welfare. Because Amish children do not typically attend public schools, there are not some of the normal "checkpoints" to ensure that recommended childhood vaccines have been given. Alternatively, the Amish are interested in health behaviors for themselves and their children. As an agrarian culture, they are also familiar with the role of vaccines in preventing diseases among their farm animals. It was possible that other community, family, or individual factors might affect the adoption of vaccination as a preventive health measure.

Dr. Dworkin and I telephoned the local health departments that had public health jurisdiction in Illinois Amish communities. They were also interested in exploring the Amish attitudes and beliefs towards vaccinations. How many of the Amish children were being vaccinated? Were there religious, moral, or logistic barriers to receiving these vaccinations? What could the health department or healthcare providers do to increase the level of vaccination? Because unvaccinated Amish communities can serve as environments where vaccine-preventable diseases persist, putting unvaccinated persons at risk for illness, understanding the Amish view of vaccinations was important to the health of other Illinois citizens as well.

REACHING OUT TO THE AMISH

Because I needed an entry into the Amish community, my first contact was to my aunt and uncle who lived in Arthur, the center of the largest Illinois Amish community. Paul and Carol had lived in the community for decades and had established good relationships with many of their Amish neighbors. Carol provided the name of a local nurse, Dorothy, who provided prenatal counseling and delivered babies for the Amish community. While Dorothy was not Old-Order Amish, she belonged to another Amish denomination in the community. Dorothy had spent time as a nurse in South America where she had seen the devastating effects of vaccine-preventable diseases. This experience made her a strong advocate for vaccinations during prenatal counseling. Her advice to me was that we should discuss our ideas with the Amish medical committee. (I had no idea the Amish had a medical committee.) This committee was developed to assist the Amish, who are primarily uninsured, with accessing the healthcare system. They had negotiated private payment rates with local physicians and hospitals and advised the church on medical matters. I followed this advice and looked for a way to make contact with the deacons on this committee. Fortunately, one of the deacons had a phone at his workplace that we used to contact him; otherwise the communication would have been by mail. He discussed our idea with the other deacons and they agreed to meet me and the state epidemiologist, Dr. Dworkin, at one of their homes so that we could discuss the proposal.

Dr. Dworkin and I drove the three and one-half hours to Arthur to meet with the medical committee to discuss our proposal. We had arrived early, so we walked into a local hardware store in town to spend a little time. Among the batteries, plumbing parts, and paint cans, to our great surprise, we found a genealogic directory that listed all the Amish families in Illinois with the number of children and their ages. This book listed 4,538 persons living in these nine communities; 3,431 (76%) of these persons resided in the Arthur community, which consists of 775 households, including 374 households with children younger than 15 years of age.[2] This information seemed to confirm our assumption that initially focusing on the Arthur Amish community would be the most efficient use of public health resources. It was incredible good fortune to have found this while just browsing in a hardware store to use up some time.

With more time to kill before our meeting, we ate dinner at the local restaurant (interestingly named Yoder's). It was a delicious buffet of simple home-style cooking, such as fried chicken, steamed vegetables, and raspberry crumble. One of the highlights was the homemade peanut butter that was placed on all the tables and tasted great on the local bread. After dinner, as the sun was starting to set, we made the short drive to the deacon's home. We parked by the hitching post and were warmly welcomed into their spacious basement, which also functioned as a Sunday meeting place. We stood around for a short time. While waiting for one more deacons to arrive, two of the deacons were interested in discussing infectious disease threats to their livestock. Last year, several of their workhorses died from West Nile virus and they were keenly concerned with whether the risk had changed in the current year. They had vaccinated their horses for West Nile virus, which I took as a positive sign of their view of the value of vaccinations.

The third deacon and the wives arrived and our meeting began. We were seated around a table with Dr. Dworkin and me at one end. I presented the basic outline of our study and concluded by asking, "Do you have any thoughts or questions?" The silence hung long in the air. As I sat and waited for a response, I realized how silent it really was: no radio or television in the background, no hum of electric motors, no vehicles passing outside. Only the scraping of a chair on the floor upstairs and the clip-clopping of a passing buggy could be heard. Dr. Dworkin and I suppressed the urge to break the silence with more explanation. We had discussed before traveling to Arthur that the Amish may have long silences while considering an issue. We had read of this slow, thoughtful style of communication and had planned ahead not to fill any uncomfortably long silence by blurting out something. It was important to respect their ways and to not seem impatient to them. My sense was that they were seriously mulling over what I had presented; further discussion would be a rude interruption. Finally, the silence was broken. They were curious about our intent and how we would use the information we gathered. "What do you really want to do with the answers to these questions?" they asked. (I had provided a draft questionnaire so they could see the type of information we wanted to gather.) "Would you need to talk to anyone in person or follow up with the answers people gave?" The questions that were asked made it clear that, while they did not oppose conducting a survey in the community, they were wary that this survey was only the first part of a planned government intervention into the community to change their immunization practices. From our understanding of their cultural history, Dr. Dworkin and I recognized their concern and assured them that our only objective was to understand what they thought about vaccines. "Do you plan to publish what you learn here?" they asked. We said it was a possibility; they requested that we discuss any results with the community first and we agreed.

The light inside the basement had become dim. They lit the bare gas flame, which hissed softly and cast a flickering light on our faces. Because it seemed that we had passed a hurdle about the deacons' acceptance of the survey, we asked their advice on the best way to administer the questionnaire. While we were prepared to mail this survey to all 775 Amish households in the Arthur area,[2] they mentioned that the better and less expensive way to proceed would be to include this survey in the weekly newspaper that was delivered to every Amish home. A return envelope with no identifiable information would be included with each survey. Because these results would be completely anonymous, we would not have the ability to follow up on any missing or incomplete surveys. This would be an important but necessary limitation of our study. The medical committee endorsed this approach and offered to introduce the survey and publicly sanction it during the Sunday meetings before the survey arrived. We recognized that this public endorsement was critical to the success of our efforts. As the sun set outside and the business at hand was conducted, we snacked on huge cheese-flavored snacks while we discussed the differences between our city lives and the life of the Amish community.

THE SURVEY

Over the next few weeks, we wrote and rewrote our survey instrument. Although, ideally, we would have pilot tested this questionnaire among a group of Amish people, because of our delicate relationship with them and because we felt fortunate to have been granted permission to circulate this survey at all, we decided to just accept this as a limitation. However, the Amish leaders did review our survey before it was distributed. When we started developing our questions, we kept in mind principles of how to create a good survey or questionnaire.

Questionnaires are the basic information-gathering tools of public health research or outbreak investigations because they provide a standardized form for data collection, comprise the building blocks of the survey database, and allow your work to be used to expand public health knowledge. Questionnaire-development principles have been published in several good review articles on the subject.[9,10] Our survey instrument needed to include questions that were appropriate, ethical, omnicompetent, unambiguous, appropriately coded, unbiased, and piloted; it helped to memorize the acronym AEIOU CUP to remember these guiding principles (Exhibit 34-1).

When we phrased the questions, we kept these principles in mind based on lessons learned from other investigations and reading about questionnaire design:

1. All the words (separately and in context) should be understandable to the respondents (e.g., the question "Did you have dyspnea?" would not be understandable to many).
2. The questions should not be "loaded" (e.g., the question "You don't use drugs, do you?" could bias an interviewee toward a particular answer).
3. The alternatives involved in the questions should accommodate responses that go beyond the choices we give them if we have incomplete knowledge of what they could respond (e.g., use "other, specify____" to capture information if you could have missed something).
4. Avoiding assumptions about the interviewee is important (e.g., asking about additional activities "Did you taste someone else's food? Specify____" rather than just assuming that he or she ate only food from his or her own plate).
5. Consider the frame of reference the respondent is being asked to assume (e.g., are you asking what they did or what they normally do?).

Because there would be no follow-up contact with families to clarify answers, it was especially important that each question was understandable.

After the questionnaire was finalized, a date was set for the survey to be sent to all community households. The primary survey focus was on the 374 households in the community that had children younger than 15 years old; children younger than 15 years would probably still be attending Amish school and be under their parent's care, but soon they would start making decisions for themselves. However, we were also interested in whether adults in the community had been vaccinated and whether the rates of vaccination and attitudes toward vaccination had changed over time. The questionnaire was intentionally short (18 questions that were estimated to take less than 10 minutes to complete). We hoped that this short length would increase both the response and the completion rate, especially given the constraint that no reminder would be sent to participants.

The surveys went out with the community newspaper following the public endorsement by the deacons. We received responses from 345 Amish households including 225 (60%) of the 374 households with children younger than 15 years old and an additional 120 households without children younger than 15 years old. Surprisingly, the results suggested that immunization was relatively well accepted by this community. We found that 84% (189/225) of the households with children reported that all of their children had received vaccinations and an additional 12% (28/225) reported that some of their children had received vaccinations. Only 4% (8/225) reported that none of their children received vaccinations. For the 36 families in which not all of their children had received vaccinations, the most frequently cited reason for not vaccinating (44%; 16/36) was concern about the safety of vaccines. Less frequently cited were personal objections (19%; 7/36) or the belief that vaccination is not an effective disease prevention strategy (14%; 5/36). Only 8% (3/36) cited religious objections as the reason for not vaccinating (Table 34-1). Because we had received responses from 60% (225/374)

EXHIBIT 34-1 Principles for developing an effective questionnaire by using the acronym AEIOU CUP[9]

A: Appropriate—The question asked is the one that leads to the information you need, precisely.

E: Ethical—Do you really need to ask each question? Has informed consent been obtained?

I: Intelligible—Clarity of language is key. You can be too concise or too wordy.

O: Omnicompetent—Questionnaire should be capable of coping with all answers. Try to accommodate all responses by including the category "other" or leaving a space for comments.

U: Unambiguous—The question asked means the same to both the respondent and the interviewer.

C: Appropriately coded—Categories should be exhaustive, but mutually exclusive. For example, the number categories "*1-10, 10-20*" are wrong, "*1-10, 11-20*" are right.

U: Unbiased—Questions should ensure that the interviewer is unlikely to trigger one kind of response.

P: Piloted—Test the questions to iron out design faults or mistakes.

TABLE 34-1 Reasons given for having unvaccinated children among 36 Amish households, Arthur, Illinois*

Reason given	Number of respondents (%)
Vaccines are not safe for my children.	16 (44)
Vaccines are against my personal beliefs.	7 (19)
Vaccination is not an effective way to prevent diseases in my children.	5 (14)
Vaccination is not as important as other daily activities.	4 (11)
Our children are not at risk for becoming ill from any of the diseases prevented by vaccines.	4 (11)
I have religious reasons for not getting a vaccine.	3 (8)
The clinic hours are inconvenient.	2 (6)
I do not want to receive any government handouts.	1 (3)
Vaccines are too expensive.	1 (3)
Getting a vaccine requires inconvenient travel.	1 (3)

*Unknown or undecided responses were excluded from analysis and respondents might have listed more than one reason.

of the households with children, this limited our ability to generalize these findings to the rest of the community. It was unclear whether nonresponders differed from responders in their attitude toward vaccination.

We found several factors that were associated with homes not having all their children vaccinated. These included the interviewee not being vaccinated as a child (OR 4.2; 95% CI 1.1–16.3) or seeking nonemergency care 2 or fewer times in the preceding year (OR 2.6; 95% CI 1.1–6.0). The majority of children's vaccines (74%) were administered in the doctor's office. Contrary to what was found in Whiteside County in 1996, there was no difference in vaccination between boys and girls. Our research about Amish society taught us that it is often a patriarchal society. However, our data challenged that pattern because we found that decisions about the medical care of children were made either jointly (84%) or by mothers alone (13%); fathers made medical decisions in 3% of households. It could be that decisions that were made jointly involved the mother's opinion, but the father's decision. Our data did not determine if that was the case.

The majority of adults (90%, 281/313) who knew their vaccination history reported that they had received vaccinations as children. Younger adult respondents (<45 years old) were more likely to be vaccinated than older respondents (≥45 years old); 96% (194/202) of younger respondents had been vaccinated compared to 78% (87/11) of older respondents. Surprisingly, this high level of vaccination was achieved despite the fact that the vast majority (93%) of respondents were uninsured.

We visited some of the other eight smaller Illinois Amish communities in this region of the state because our goal was to replicate the survey. We learned of a local non-Amish chiropractor with ties to one of these Amish communities. He invited us to meet him at his home to discuss his interaction with the Amish community. At the time, a Chinese scientist from the Jiangsu Province health department was visiting the state health department and Dr. Dworkin, our visitor, and I met the chiropractor at his sprawling estate in the middle of his vineyard. We discussed our study and his interaction with the local Amish community in his kitchen, which looked like it was modeled on a wine tasting destination in northern California. He was very interested in our work and spoke of work he had done in other parts of the world, like Africa. He agreed to take us with him to visit a local Amish family. But first, he had something to show us. He took us upstairs to the "crow's nest." He explained that this is where he shot deer out of his vineyard with his assortment of high-powered rifles. His collection of weapons was impressive and, for the moment, gave us a feeling we were in a Hollywood movie with an uncertain ending. "Would you like to shoot this gun?" he asked our Chinese colleague as he offered it to him. The look of sheer terror on the doctor's face was his reply. Our Chinese doctor was probably concerned that it might not look so good to be found holding a gun; the officials who issued his visa probably did not have that in mind. We politely declined to further examine the rest of our host's hidden gun and knife collection and inquired if we could make the trip to visit his Amish acquaintance. Soon, we departed.

We sat with an elderly Amish widower as he completed our questionnaire. Few Amish families remained in his community; most had moved away in search of better farming land. We realized that the Amish community in that area was too small to provide meaningful results for our survey. In other communities with Amish populations, we were not able to identify key individuals or gatekeepers who could provide access to administer the survey among the local Amish population.

We wondered if the Arthur Amish community was somewhat unique in its approach to medical issues and view of vaccinations. We found much higher percentages of vaccinated children and adults than we expected. Additionally, the primary objections to vaccinations were similar to those expressed by non-Amish parents.[11] We think that these unexpected findings were related to community-specific factors. In the survey, families mentioned that they trusted their local physician and would generally follow his or her advice on vaccinations. The support for vaccinations was further bolstered by a strong advocate, Dorothy, who had a unique position of influence. As a midwife, she gave advice to new mothers on the care of their infants and was a proponent of childhood vaccination because of her international experience seeing the impact of vaccine-preventable diseases in an area where vaccination rates were lower and disease prevalence was higher. The higher rate of vaccination among young adults in our study seemed to indicate that the acceptance of vaccination has increased over time, challenging our assumption of fixed attitudes and practices related to vaccinations. It also demonstrated that individual communities might differ in their view of vaccinations.

During the time we were receiving survey responses, an unvaccinated Amish child in Minnesota was reported with poliovirus with evidence that it was being transmitted to others.[7] While polio had been eliminated from the United States (the last case was diagnosed in 1979 in an Amish person), it was possible that it could be reintroduced. The poliovirus found in Minnesota had, so far, not caused any symptomatic polio cases. There was concern by the CDC and the bordering states that the poliovirus would continue to circulate among persons without immunity to it and could lead to cases of polio among Amish and non-Amish communities in the Midwest and Canada. Surveys performed in Minnesota, Wisconsin, Michigan, Missouri, and Ontario Amish communities as a result of this outbreak[12] revealed that the vaccination rate for poliovirus ranged from 11% to 34%. This level of vaccination was well below the threshold necessary to interrupt transmission of the virus. By contrast, the data from our study demonstrated that the largest Illinois Amish community was likely adequately protected because of their level of vaccination.

CONCLUSIONS

Because we took time to attempt to understand the Amish viewpoint and develop trust with key community gatekeepers, we were able to successfully gather health information from the Amish without damaging the relationship with the local healthcare and public health providers. While the approach to research with other underserved groups is dependent on the circumstances, any efforts should consider that the overall goal is ultimately to improve their health and not merely to gain interesting knowledge about their beliefs and practices. It takes time to learn the cultural and/or religious history of groups; their story holds important clues as to why these groups are underserved. The research done in these settings can either build bridges between public health providers and these groups or it can reinforce long-held misconceptions and prejudices. Because these groups deal with external threats to their identity and existence, public health intervention is often initially perceived as another threat to their way of life. To address this challenge, the person chosen to undertake research and the key informants within the group are important. The researchers should appeal to the group's hopes instead of their fears.

The December evening outside was below freezing as we met later that year in a cozy Amish community center with interested members of the community to discuss the results of our survey. Several of the deacons were there, along with a few dozen Amish and three members of the local health department. The results were greeted with interest and a few questions were asked about what we planned to do with the information we received. There was polite discussion between the health department employees and community members about how to better deliver services to the community. The survey had revealed that most families went to their local doctors for vaccination; it was clear from the discussion that they had developed trust with their physician and relied on his/her recommendation for preventive health practices. As the meeting was ending, the deacons and the local health department discussed how to continue the dialogue about health issues affecting the Amish. One young mother hung around after the meeting. Her newborn baby was swaddled against her body as she gathered her coat for the journey home. "I really want to do what I can for my children's health," she said. "But, I don't always know what information to believe about vaccines. I appreciated coming tonight to learn the concerns that other families have." We stepped outside into a frozen, clear night. Her horse was the only one tethered to the hitching post with the shiny black buggy blending into the inky night. "I never got baby shots when I was a child, but I am reading everything I can about it to see if it is the right thing for my children. Sometimes it is so hard to know the right thing to do." I wished the best to her and her family as she unhitched her horse and prepared the buggy for the 12-mile trip home. Her horse stamped the frozen gravel, exhaled steam from his nostrils, and began the clip-clopping journey home. I was struck again by the main lesson I learned from the experience, a truth that all parents, in some form or another, are on the same quest for understanding that this young mother expressed. We see our future in our children and are willing to examine our beliefs and practices to protect their health.

Within a few weeks of disseminating our findings back to the community, I was in India assisting the World Health Organization with global polio eradication efforts. The lessons I learned from the Amish in Illinois continued to resonate there. Underserved communities had resisted the polio vaccination efforts, primarily because of a mistrust of the public health authorities who were providing the vaccinations. This vaccine refusal had led to increased numbers of polio cases in these communities. Reasons for this mistrust were long-standing and could only be overcome with sustained effort to engage these communities in the decisions about providing vaccines to at-risk children. They did not trust that the goals of vaccination were in their best interest. Gaining the confidence of a skeptical community required a similar strategy of understanding the community's history, communicating a genuine concern for the health of the community's next generation, and demonstrating that the public health community was willing to partner with them to protect the health of their children. My fellowship ended the following summer and I moved to Atlanta to work for the Centers for Disease Control and Prevention on waterborne disease and outbreak prevention. Now, I try to apply the lessons I learned from this investigation in valuing the role of state and local health departments, listening to the viewpoints of diverse communities, developing appropriate questionnaires, and looking for new opportunities for disease prevention.

LEARNING QUESTIONS

1. What are the principles of creating good survey questions?
2. Why do you think the author was successful in performing a survey study in this relatively closed community? If you were trying to perform a similar study in a similar community, how would you gain access?
3. Explain how communication and understanding of culture were important features of this survey study.
4. What are other populations where suspicion of government public health programs or workers could be (or is known to be) a barrier to the success of public health programs? Explain how you might approach these communities and what issues you would consider in order to overcome these barriers.
5. What are some of the methodological limitations of this survey that the authors might report in a presentation or publication of the findings? To what extent do study limitations undermine the usefulness of the results (consider the limitations of this study and possibly a different published study).

The findings and conclusions in this article are those of the author and do not necessarily represent the views of the Centers for Disease Control and Prevention.

REFERENCES

1. Hostetler JA. *Amish Society*. 4th ed. Baltimore: Johns Hopkins University Press; 1993. http://www.amazon.com/Amish-Society-John-Hostetler/dp/0801844428#noop
2. Schlabach L, Schlabach D. *Illinois Directory: Directory of the Illinois Amish*. 3rd ed. Tuscola, IL; 2003.
3. Briss PA, Fehrs LJ, Hutcheson RH, Schaffner W. Rubella among the Amish: resurgent disease in a highly susceptible community. *Pediatr Infect Dis J*. 1992;11(11):955–959. http://www.ncbi.nlm.nih.gov/pubmed/1454439
4. Sutter RW, Markowitz LE, Bennetch JM, Morris W, Zell ER, Preblud SR. Measles among the Amish: a comparative study of measles severity in primary and secondary cases in households. *J Infect Dis*. 1991;163(1):12–16. http://www.ncbi.nlm.nih.gov/pubmed/1984459
5. Etkind P, Lett SM, Macdonald PD, Silva E, Peppe J. Pertussis outbreaks in groups claiming religious exemptions to vaccinations. *Am J Dis Child*. 1992;146(2):173–176. http://www.ncbi.nlm.nih.gov/pubmed/1733146
6. Fry AM, Lurie P, Gidley M, et al. Haemophilus influenzae type B disease among Amish children in Pennsylvania: reasons for persistent disease. *Pediatrics*. 2001;108(4):E60. http://www.ncbi.nlm.nih.gov/pubmed/11581468

7. Centers for Disease Control and Prevention. Poliovirus infections in four unvaccinated children: Minnesota, August–October 2005. *JAMA*. 2005;294:2689–2691. http://jama.ama-assn.org/content/vol294/issue21/index.dtl
8. Fair E, Murphy TV, Golaz A, Wharton M. Philosophic objection to vaccination as a risk for tetanus among children younger than 15 years. *Pediatrics*. 2002;109(1):e2. http://pediatrics.aappublications.org/cgi/content/full/109/1/e2. Accessed October 23, 2009.
9. Stone, DH. Design a questionnaire. *BMJ*. 1993;307(6914):1264–1266. http://www.ncbi.nlm.nih.gov/pmc/articles/PMC1679392/
10. Eaden J, Mayberry MK, Mayberry JF. Questionnaires: the use and abuse of social survey methods in medical research. *Postgrad Med J*. 1999;75(885):397–400. http://www.ncbi.nlm.nih.gov/pmc/articles/PMC1741277/
11. Smith PJ, Chu SY, Barker LE. Children who have received no vaccines: who are they and where do they live? *Pediatrics*. 2004;114(1):187–195. http://www.ncbi.nlm.nih.gov/pubmed/15231927
12. Alexander JP, Ehresmann K, Seward J, et.al. Transmission of imported vaccine-derived poliovirus in an undervaccinated community in Minnesota. *J Infect Dis*. 2009;199(3):391–397. http://www.ncbi.nlm.nih.gov/pubmed/19090774

CHAPTER 35

Performing a Seroprevalence and Ocular Study in Rural Guatemala—Toxoplasmosis, a Chronic Infectious Disease

Jeffrey L. Jones, MD, MPH, and Beatriz López, QB*

Guatemala, 1999 to 2007

Jeffrey L. Jones: In medical school and during my internship, I learned about and managed many severe infectious and metabolic chronic diseases that were largely preventable. During medical school, I was also intrigued by the lectures about outbreak investigations. It seemed that investigation and research could lead to the knowledge needed to prevent suffering from many diseases, and that this is where society should put a strong emphasis to reduce the burden of disease.

My career in public health began with the California Department of Health Preventive Medicine Residency program, which included a master's of public health at the University of California, Berkeley. The residency program involved patient work in public health clinics, and practical instruction in communicable disease control, laboratory science, chronic disease control, state and local health department administration, environmental health, vector control, and toxicology at the California State Department of Health and the Alameda County Health Department (Oakland, California). After public health training, I spent a year working as the health officer of Placer County California, and then applied to the 2-year Centers for Disease Control and Prevention (CDC) Epidemic Intelligence Service (EIS) program to obtain further training in epidemiology and disease investigation. At that time, I planned to complete the EIS program at a state health department and then return to California to work in public health.

Fortunately, I was accepted into the CDC EIS program. During the EIS position recruitment week at the annual spring EIS conference, I reviewed all the state positions and discussed them with former EIS officers. Four former EIS officers that I spoke with (Jeffrey Davis, Jeffrey Sachs, Jeffrey Lybarger, and John Rullan) had done their EIS training in South Carolina and highly recommended it. The supervisors there were Dr. Parker (veterinarian and former EIS officer) and Dr. Heath (public health physician and former EIS officer), who

---

* Química Bióloga (Biological Chemist)

had both completed distinguished careers at the CDC, and Dr. Gamble, a pediatric infectious disease physician from the Medical University of South Carolina in Charleston, who was on the American Academy of Pediatrics Infectious Diseases committee. The EIS program introduced me to the practical aspects of foodborne and other infectious disease investigations, chronic disease risk factor analysis and prevention, HIV/AIDS prevention, environmental sanitation, and environmental toxicology. After EIS, the South Carolina Department of Health and Environmental Control hired me to be state epidemiologist; I worked in this role for 3 years. During this time, I became quite interested in HIV/AIDS surveillance and prevention. At an evening crawfish cookout in a city park in the Garden district of New Orleans during a state epidemiologist's conference, a CDC representative recruited me to work in the Division of HIV/AIDS Prevention in Atlanta.

I became interested in toxoplasmosis while working on opportunistic infections in the Division of HIV/AIDS Prevention at the CDC in Atlanta in the early 1990s. At that time, I coordinated the research for a cohort of more than 50,000 HIV-infected persons located in 10 U.S. cities. Because clinical information was abstracted from patient medical records after hospital and clinic visits, our group was able to follow the progression of HIV/AIDS and determine the importance of infections in causing severe illness. Toxoplasmic encephalitis affected about 7% of HIV-infected persons in the course of AIDS and, without treatment, often caused fatal encephalitis.[1]

Toxoplasma gondii, a protozoan parasite, is the organism responsible for toxoplasmosis. As I learned more about *T. gondii*, I was intrigued by the fact that it is a zoonotic organism that can cross species and infect most warm-blooded animals. Cats are the definitive hosts for *T. gondii* and are the only animals that shed the environmentally resistant form of the organism (called oocysts) in their stool, which can survive months to years in the soil. Humans usually become infected in one of three ways: (1) by ingesting oocysts in soil contaminated with cat feces (for example when changing the cat litter box, or through gardening or handling/eating unwashed fruits and vegetables), (2) by eating raw or undercooked meat from animals that have been infected with *T. gondii*, or (3) by acquiring congenital infection through the placenta when a woman becomes newly infected during pregnancy (Figure 35-1). Once infected, people are generally infected for life; in persons with normal immunity, the organism resides in intracellular cysts in a relatively latent form. Several years ago, I was fortunate in being able to participate in a national serologic survey in the United States, which indicated that nearly one in four persons was infected with *T. gondii*.[2]

T. gondii can cause a number of illnesses in humans. When a pregnant woman acquires a *T. gondii* infection and it is transmitted across the placenta, it can cause mental retardation, blindness, epilepsy, and even death in the fetus (Exhibit 35-1). As mentioned previously, immunosuppressed persons, including those with AIDS, can develop severe encephalitis or other systemic diseases, usually as a result of reactivation of a "latent" infection. People with normal immune function are usually asymptomatic or have symptoms such as lymphadenopathy, fever, and malaise that resolve spontaneously. However, in the United States up to 2% of persons infected after birth can develop eye lesions that can result in loss of vision.[3] There is also ongoing research on whether chronic *T. gondii* infection has an effect on reaction time (psychomotor neurologic transmission time),[4,5] behavior,[6-10] and mental illness.[11,12]

My work in toxoplasmosis and other parasitic opportunistic infections led to my transfer from the Division of HIV/AIDS Prevention to the Division of Parasitic Diseases at the CDC in 1999. Because there are so many different parasites that infect humans, a person interested in biology, zoonotic diseases, and human health could have a hundred lifetime careers and still only touch the surface of what there is to know about parasites. I am constantly humbled by what a one-celled parasite like *T. gondii* can do biologically; for example, evade the immune system well enough to survive for years in most warm-blooded animals. Perhaps it is because much of life evolved from the same primordial soup that parasite survival tricks work on many different species.

In my early years of working with parasitic diseases, the Division maintained a field research station at the University del Valle in Guatemala City, Guatemala. Because I had worked on determining the prevalence of *T. gondii* infection in the United States, I often wondered about the prevalence of infection and disease in other countries. Because of the location of our field station (Guatemala) it was natural to think of that country for a seroprevalence study. We knew very little about the prevalence and characteristics of *T. gondii* infections in Guatemala. There were some data available, but a study of children in various age groups had never been conducted. However, prevalence surveys with blood sampling and testing are expensive and, at the time, we had little funding for international work. Just when I

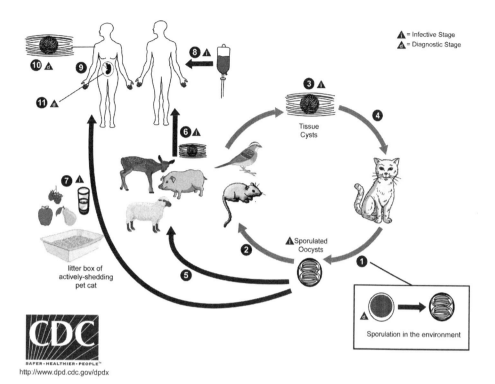

FIGURE 35-1 T. gondii life cycle.

The only known definitive hosts for *Toxoplasma gondii* are members of family Felidae (domestic cats and their relatives). Unsporulated oocysts are shed in the cat's feces (1). Although oocysts are usually only shed for 1-2 weeks, large numbers may be shed. Oocysts take 1-5 days to sporulate in the environment and become infective. Intermediate hosts in nature (including birds and rodents) become infected after ingesting soil, water or plant material contaminated with oocysts (2). Oocysts transform into tachyzoites shortly after ingestion. These tachyzoites localize in neural and muscle tissue and develop into tissue cyst bradyzoites (3). Cats become infected after consuming intermediate hosts harboring tissue cysts (4). Cats may also become infected directly by ingestion of sporulated oocysts. Animals bred for human consumption and wild game may also become infected with tissue cysts after ingestion of sporulated oocysts in the environment (5). Humans can become infected by any of several routes:

- eating undercooked meat of animals harboring tissue cysts (6).
- consuming food or water contaminated with cat feces or by contaminated environmental samples (such as fecal-contaminated soil or changing the litter box of a pet cat) (7).
- blood transfusion or organ transplantation (8).
- transplacentally from mother to fetus (9).

In the human host, the parasites form tissue cysts, most commonly in skeletal muscle, myocardium, brain, and eyes; these cysts may remain throughout the life of the host. Diagnosis is usually achieved by serology, although tissue cysts may be observed in stained biopsy specimens (10). Diagnosis of congenital infections can be achieved by detecting *T. gondii* DNA in amniotic fluid using molecular methods such as PCR (11).

had all but given up on the chance to learn more about toxoplasmosis in Guatemala, I heard that a fellow CDC medical epidemiologist, Dr. Steven Luby (and colleagues), had done a population-based study of drinking water treatment and its relationship to diarrheal disease in 1999 among the indigenous people in rural Guatemala.[13] They found that the incidence of diarrhea was significantly lower with a variety of simple water disinfectant treatments. I knew that Steve did good work because I was his EIS officer supervisor 10 years previously when I was the state epidemiologist in South Carolina. Steve and his colleagues had collected demographic and

EXHIBIT 35-1 Toxoplasmosis, signs and symptoms that can occur

Congenitally Infected Infants

- 70–90% asymptomatic at birth, but many will develop impairment later (including visual impairment, learning disabilities, and mental retardation)
- retinochoroiditis
- hydrocephalus
- intracranial calcifications
- microcephaly
- seizures
- maculopapular rash
- generalized lymphadenopathy
- hepatomegally
- splenomegally
- jaundice
- thrombocytopenia
- deafness

Persons with Normal Immunity Infected After Birth

- 80–90% of persons asymptomatic
- lymphadenopathy
- lymphocytosis
- fever
- sore throat
- malaise
- retinochoroiditis
- rash
- hepatosplenomegaly

HIV-infected and Other Immunosuppressed Persons (Advanced Immunosuppression)

- encephalitis
- pneumonitis
- myocarditis
- systemic toxoplasmosis
- retinochoroiditis
- rash

---

samples from small children's veins is difficult and time-consuming. However, we also wanted to test older children to determine how the rate of infection increased with age and to get an estimate of what proportion of young women are susceptible to *T. gondii* infection as they enter their second decade of life and childbearing years.

Our seroprevalence study would determine the prevalence of *T. gondii* immunoglobulin G (IgG) antibodies in the population evaluated. People infected with *T. gondii* develop IgG antibodies within several weeks of infection. *T. gondii* IgG antibodies generally last for the rest of the person's life, as does the latent infection with *T. gondii* in some of the person's cells (especially muscle and brain cells). It is not possible to accurately determine when a person was infected with *T. gondii* by IgG antibody determination; however, in young children, the infection would not be too far in the past because the children are not very old.

> People infected with *T. gondii* develop IgG antibodies within several weeks of infection. *T. gondii* IgG antibodies generally last for the rest of the person's life, as does the latent infection with *T. gondii* in some of the person's cells (especially muscle and brain cells).

The next challenges in developing a *T. gondii* seroprevalence study were to develop collaboration with the Guatemala field station staff at the University del Valle and to acquire funding to cover testing of specimens, and to cover blood sampling and testing of specimens from older children (3–10 years of age). At this time, spring 2002, I had the opportunity to meet two researchers from the Guatemala field station, Beatriz Lopez and Maricruz Alvarez, when they were visiting the Division of Parasitic Diseases at the CDC. They had worked on the drinking water study with Steve Luby, and he spoke highly of them. Both of these women were charming and competent, and had been trained in microbiology and biochemistry at the University of San Carlos and the University del Valle in Guatemala, respectively. Thus, a collaboration with the Guatemala field station was formed.

Now, I needed to find funding. Fortunately, the Division of Parasitic Diseases has always had supportive directors and branch chiefs. During this time period, Dr. James Maguire was my branch chief. He is a distinguished infectious disease physician who had worked with newborn screening for toxoplasmosis in Massachusetts in the 1980s and 1990s, and was a strong supporter

disease-related risk factor information and blood samples in young children (6 months to 2 years old) during his study, which was done in San Juan Sacatepéquez, one of the municipalities of the Department of Guatemala, located 32 kilometers west of Guatemala City. This information could be very useful for a *T. gondii* infection prevalence study. It is rare to have the opportunity to evaluate a population of children this young for *T. gondii* infection because obtaining blood of investigations that can help define the populations at risk for *T. gondii* infection and risk factors for that infection. Because there were some funds remaining in our branch at the end of the fiscal year, after receiving a proposal that I prepared, Dr. Maguire and the branch leadership agreed to award $17,000 for the study and send me and Marianna Wilson, a laboratorian with expertise in *T. gondii* antibody testing, to Guatemala. Marianna would train the laboratory staff in Guatemala to test the study serum samples for *T. gondii* IgG antibodies. For this study, Mariana had chosen the Platelia Toxo IgG (TMB) enzyme immunoassay (Bio-Rad Laboratories, Hercules, CA), a highly sensitive and specific assay (comparable to the CDC's immunofluorescence IgG assay and the *T. gondii* IgG dye test, which are both known for their accuracy, but more time-consuming and complicated tests to conduct).

Now we had a complete study plan. We would test the approximately 500 serum samples from children aged 6 months to 2 years collected in 1999 by Steve Luby's group. With the remaining funding, Beatriz, Maricruz, and their staff would collect and test serum samples and collect epidemiologic information from an additional 500 children 3 to 10 years old in villages in the same area. A sample of 500 would allow us to determine the *T. gondii* antibody prevalence within +2% (95% confidence, 80% power). Marianna Wilson and I planned to travel to Guatemala for several days to train the staff in *T. gondii* serologic testing (a new test for them) and to visit the areas involved in the study.

Beatriz López: I, and the members of our research team, had always been interested in parasitic diseases, so when we started to talk with Drs. Jones and Maguire about the possibility of working with *Toxoplasma gondii* we were very enthusiastic. We had been involved in the water quality project since the beginning and the idea of taking advantage of the knowledge acquired about the San Juan Sacatepequez population was appealing. We knew that we had a very good team, including the field workers, our laboratory technicians, and the physician in charge of the field work, Dr. Carlos Mendoza. Maricruz and I were in charge of the laboratory component of the water project in Guatemala and presented the idea to the team. We had a great response and everybody was interested in knowing more about this disease that was new for some. They were especially surprised to learn that cats are involved in the life cycle of toxoplasmosis.

Jeffrey L. Jones: Marianna Wilson and I made the trip to Guatemala for 5 days in March 2003. We were hoping to be present when the actual field work (questionnaires and blood sampling) was being done, but these steps had been completed by the time we arrived. Our tasks were to visit the areas involved in the study to better understand the survey methods and population, to make recommendations about data management, and to train the laboratory staff in *T. gondii* testing.

After a three and one-half hour flight from Atlanta, we arrived at a small bustling airport with people moving in all directions at once. Beatriz and Maricruz had set up the Guatemalan "VIP" treatment for our arrival. We were met by a large car with a driver and a guard armed with a machine gun and whisked off to a beautiful hotel in the hills of Guatemala City, with a large inactive volcano in the background (all at the government rate!). Guatemala has endured civil wars over the past decades, but a machine gun escort still felt like overprotection.

It was the dry season and the weather was cool and breezy in Guatemala City (elevation about 1500 meters [4921 feet]), not unlike that of San Francisco and somewhat of a surprise to those of us expecting the tropics. The hotel staff was exceptionally helpful and we had no problem communicating with our limited Spanish. The following day, we met Beatriz and Maricruz at the University del Valle, a nice modern university, but set apart from the city with gates and restricted access. That day, we discussed laboratory testing, data handling, and analysis; then, Marianna and I returned to our hotel for a relaxing dinner looking out a huge picture window at a large perfectly cone-shaped volcano.

The following day, Beatriz and one of the field staff members, Jorge Sincal, took Marianna and me by car out of Guatemala City to the Village of San Juan Sacatepequez and surrounding areas. In our travel through Guatemala City, I saw some very overcrowded impoverished areas with ramshackle houses and what appeared to be very limited sanitation. Seeing these overcrowded urban ghettos led me to reflect on world overpopulation and equitable distribution of resources. Although work in medicine and public health is very helpful to mankind, population and resource management are perhaps even more critical.

Once out of the city, the countryside appeared green and lush in some areas, but somewhat arid along the mountain ridges. The village of San Juan Sacatepequez was picture-book pretty, with a marketplace set up in the town square and indigenous Guatemalan women dressed in brightly colored native dresses. Some did not speak Spanish, but instead Kaqchikel, a language of Mayan ancestry. The food in the open-air market looked very appetizing, but I held myself back in case *Escherichia coli*, *Entamoeba histolytica*, or other organisms that I was not accustomed to were present. I didn't want to acquire a Guatemalan version of Montezuma's revenge.

After visiting San Juan Sacatepequez, we proceeded on to the small rural villages where the survey was conducted. We did see numerous house cats in the area, so there was a source of *T. gondii* (Figure 35-2). I found the villages and inhabitants to be culturally fascinating. Most of the houses were made of thin, rough poles that air could pass between, and had dirt floors and tin or thatched roofs (Figure 35-3). The land where the villages were located on had poor rocky soil, and I wondered why they were not located on more agriculturally suitable land. There was no running water or evidence of latrines. Cooking was done on rock hearths with fires inside the houses (Figure 35-4). Although the material possessions appeared to be minimal, the women were neatly kept and dressed in brightly colored clothing, and the children appeared to be quite happy (we saw very few men). In fact, everyone seemed to be happy and pleasant as they conversed with one of the field staff in Kaqchikel. Later, from the survey results, I discovered that most of the inhabitants had no formal education whatsoever. I was impressed that cultural and family support seemed to keep these people far more satisfied than many relatively wealthy and educated people that I had known in the United States. In the United States, modern society gives most of us plenty to eat, nice houses, and education, but the huge corporate systems can also split up families and blend cultures to the extent that people often lose their social and cultural identities. On one level, "progress" solves many problems of humanity, but on another level, it can cause people to forget where they

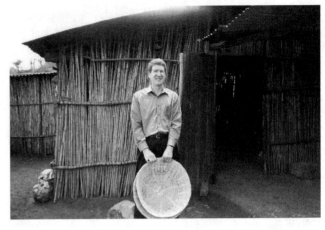

FIGURE 35-3 One of the authors (JJ) in front of a house in a rural village in the San Juan Sacatepéquez area, Guatemala, 2003. Photograph courtesy of the author Jeffrey L. Jones

fit in and what their purpose is. There is probably far more drug use, depression, and crime in many "modern" societies than in these native Guatemalan villages, at least as long as the native cultural values remain.

I saw one small house, not more than 4 by 4 meters, where a family cared for their disabled adolescent daughter. I am not sure of the disability, but because of my background congenital toxoplasmosis came to mind; it was more likely cerebral palsy of some etiology. In spite of the impoverished living conditions, the family seemed to be quite dedicated to their disabled child in providing companionship and care. The child seemed happy and appeared to have a better life than some I had seen in facilities in the United States. Here again, culture and family values appeared to trump progress. Even though many illnesses and disabilities do not have cures, challenges to the comforts of those living with them sometimes do, especially when families provide assistance. This is an observation I had also made over a decade earlier when working with HIV/AIDS programs in the United States.

> *I was impressed that cultural and family support seemed to keep these people far more satisfied than many relatively wealthy and educated people that I had known in the United States. In the United States, modern society gives most of us plenty to eat, nice houses, and education, but the huge corporate systems can also split up families and blend cultures to the extent that people often lose their social and cultural identities.*

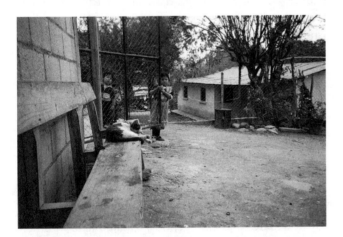

FIGURE 35-2 Cat sleeping on a bench in a rural village in the San Juan Sacatepéquez area, Guatemala, 2003. Photograph courtesy of the author Jeffrey L. Jones

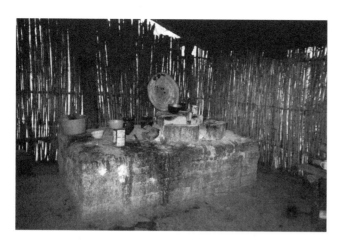

FIGURE 35-4 Cooking area in a house in a rural village in the San Juan Sacatepéquez area, Guatemala, 2003. Photograph courtesy of the author Jeffrey L. Jones

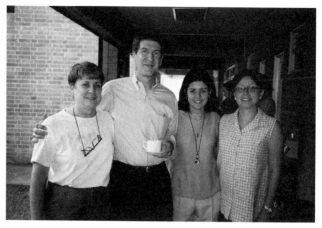

FIGURE 35-5 Toxoplasmosis study research team (left to right: Marianna Wilson, Jeffrey Jones, Beatriz Lopez, Maricruz Alvarez), Guatemala City, Guatemala, 2003. Photograph courtesy of the author Jeffrey L. Jones

The following day, Saturday, we took a short flight from Guatemala City to the ruins of the ancient Mayan city of Tikal in the low-lying tropical Peten District of Guatemala. Tikal still has numerous temples and pyramids set in a vast area of jungle with exotic birds and monkeys. Although it was the dry season for this area, we took our malaria prophylaxis as recommended. I had also previously sprayed my clothes, shoes, and socks with permethrin and was spared the many itchy chigger bites on the feet that Marianna acquired.

I noticed that our Guatemalan tour guide had a large scar on his left forearm and asked him about its origin. He said that he got a sore on his skin from sand fly bites he received in the late evening while sitting outside with his friends at Tikal. Cutaneous leishmaniasis is the technical term. He said that he successfully treated it with the local native treatment of burning the skin lesion with a cigarette. "It leaves a scar," he said, "but I am cured and the lesion has not returned in many years. Everyone here treats it this way."

We returned to Guatemala City where I gave a seminar at the University del Valle (Figure 35-5, after the seminar) and flew back to the CDC in Atlanta the following day. I felt that I had been given a chance to learn about a new culture, but I was not sure how the cultural factors related to *T. gondii* infections and the resulting disease. We saw cats during the trip and the conditions were favorable for exposure to oocysts in the soil and water (tropical environment, rural area, no routine method of water treatment). Village people told us that meat was in somewhat limited supply for them because of cost and that they always cooked it thoroughly, so infection with *T. gondii* from undercooked meat seemed unlikely.

Beatriz López: We had several big tasks on our hands: complete the laboratory analysis of the sera collected in 1999 and organize the second collection of sera and demographic information from 500 older children in similar villages of the San Juan Sacatepequez area. We completed these tasks in a relatively short time, a couple of weeks, with the help and hard work of all the group. Participants were children, 3–10 years old, from families that volunteered to participate in three villages near those involved in the 1999 study. The culture and living conditions were very similar in these villages to those in the 1999 study. A questionnaire specifically designed to inquire about toxoplasmosis-related risk factors was used for this survey in February 2003 and included information about cats and cat feces exposure, pets, diet including meat preparation, soil exposure, and water exposure. The questionnaire was reviewed by epidemiologists, physicians, laboratorians, and veterinarians at the CDC and in Guatemala, then pilot-tested in Guatemala. Trained field workers interviewed the mother or caretaker of each child and completed the questionnaire. We knew that meat was well-cooked in these indigenous villages, so we postulated that cat feces, soil, and water exposure would be the principal risk factors for infection. Some of these villagers had to go to a well or spring to get their water. Sometimes they had to walk long distances.

Our field workers were thoroughly trained. The questionnaire was first piloted with a small group of people. It was very important for the workers to understand the purpose of each question. We gave them probing questions so that they were able to obtain the answers without leading the participants. The workers were aware that sometimes people from these villages are shy, especially woman, so the introduction of the study is one of the most important parts (i.e., the villagers have to understand that the information could help them, and that their participation can influence future health decisions).

The importance of the community worker and researcher partnership cannot be overemphasized. In my work, community workers have been midwives, health promoters, and other community leaders. They were the ones who approached the community to explain the study that we were working on with University del Valle, in collaboration with the Ministry of Health. They conveyed the importance of participating. To do this, they explained how the study could create new knowledge and information about a health condition that could affect them. Their language, style, and trust were all commodities that they brought to the partnership and that we, as researchers, were unlikely to be able to equal. In order to increase participation, a modest incentive was also offered. Usually, it was some plastic ware (such as plastic forks, spoons, and knives) for the mother and a small snack for their children.

Blood samples were drawn using methods similar to those for the water survey in 1999. It sounds easy, but we were really worried about being able to collect blood from the children. This is where trust and knowledge of the community are critical. The help of community leaders (health promoters, midwives, and school teachers) was vital for the study. These leaders were contacted prior to the activity and they accompanied us during the study activities. They understood the purpose of the study and helped explain it to the participants. The team of field workers led by two physicians, Carlos Mendoza and Edwin Ortega, organized the blood sampling and finished in two weeks. Maricruz and I joined them during the sampling. Each day, we returned to the laboratory in Guatemala City and separated the sera in order to do the laboratory testing.

I will not forget the mothers calming their children during the blood sampling in the villages because when the children saw "the doctors," they started to cry and it was like a chain reaction. Nevertheless, they were very cooperative with us. Everybody had something to do. It was like a well-organized factory; one person was at the entrance checking the identification of the participants, another conducting the interview, and a third person giving the children anesthetic for the needle prick. We were assisting the doctors while others were entertaining the brothers and sisters of our subjects. The entertainers (i.e., talented baby sitters) were crucial because the mothers came with the children who were going to participate, and all the brothers and sisters as well. Some cats were wandering around, not aware that they had a big role in this play.

Jeffrey L. Jones: Several months after our visit, the Guatemalan staff had completed the *T. gondii* laboratory testing and we had completed the data analysis at the CDC. The results were interesting from several standpoints. Among the 532 children age 6 months to 2 years, 12.4% were infected with *T. gondii*, a fairly high rate at this young of an age. Among the 500 children 3–10 years old, the prevalence of *T. gondii* infection increased from 24% at age 3 to 43% at age 5, then remained at this level up to age 10. These findings indicate that the children were exposed to sources of *T. gondii* at an early age, but still many of the girls would be vulnerable to new infection (and therefore to transmitting congenital toxoplasmosis) when they reached childbearing age. After analysis, the two principal independent risk factors for infection were drinking well water and not cleaning up cat feces. It is easy to imagine that the unsealed shallow wells in the area could become contaminated if soil containing cat feces washed into them. Because *T. gondii* oocysts are highly resistant to disinfectants such as chlorine, filtering the water is the best method to prevent waterborne exposure. The oocysts are about 10 microns in size, so water filters would need to be appropriate for this particle size (for example, absolute 1 micron filters). After it is shed in cat feces, oocysts take more than 1 day to sporulate and become infectious, so if cat feces are cleaned up daily the risk of infection is reduced. Cats usually shed oocysts for only a few weeks after they become newly infected, but in general, cats do not develop symptoms so it is difficult to determine when they become infected. Therefore, all cat feces should be considered potentially contaminated with *T. gondii*.

Beatriz López: In 2006, I received an email from Jeff. It had been a while since I had heard from him; he was very enthusiastic about pursuing a new study of ocular toxoplasmosis in Guatemala. He mentioned his interest in doing the study with the children originally evaluated in 1999. I also became enthusiastic and luckily we were just in time to apply for a grant from the Guatemalan Commission of Science and Technology. Jeff told me that he had additional CDC funding to supplement a study of ocular toxoplasmosis in Guatemalan children, so I wrote the proposal with Dr. Byron Arana's help. We planned on working with children living in seven villages (Estancia del Rosario, Los Quelex, Los Pirires, Los Ajvix, Las Palmas, San Francisco Las Lomas and Los Caneles) located in the San Juan Sacatepéquez area.

Ocular toxoplasmosis has a fairly characteristic appearance and can be diagnosed (or at least strongly suspected) by ocular examination looking for white-yellow chorioretinal lesions in acute disease or more defined retinal scars from older lesions. It can be treated with drugs such as pyrimethamine and sulfadiazine if active lesions are large or threaten the central structures of the eye, although the efficacy of treatment has not been fully determined. Dr. Silvia Rizzo, an ophthalmologist from Guatemala, and Dr. Gary Holland, a retinal specialist at the University of California, Los Angeles, agreed to help with the study. The census conducted in the seven villages of San Juan Sacatepéquez to locate the children who participated in the 1999 study was revised. The age and name of each child was verified using his/her birth certificate and the databases were updated. Specially trained field personnel conducted the search for the children who had presented seropositive *T. gondii* results in 1999 and their parents or guardians were asked for permission to examine their children and to sign an informed consent form. All households were geo-referenced to facilitate the localization of the children and GPS readings were added to the database.

In 2007, 8 years after the initial 1999 seroprevalence study, a team lead by Nazario López, one of our most loyal field workers who was involved in the project since the beginning, attempted to locate the 66 *T. gondii* IgG positive children from 1999 and evaluate them with eye examinations for ocular toxoplasmosis. Additionally, 104 children who were originally seronegative were included as controls. The controls were chosen to be similar to cases according to the following criteria: they were from the same village (with the same economic and demographic conditions), and the same age. Sera were obtained from all children to establish their serologic status. The selected children received an ocular examination from an ophthalmologist, Dr. Rizzo (Figures 35-6, 35-7); the eye examinations were conducted with indirect ophthalmoscopy. An indirect ophthalmoscope consists of a light attached to a headband, in addition to a small handheld lens, to provide a wide view inside of

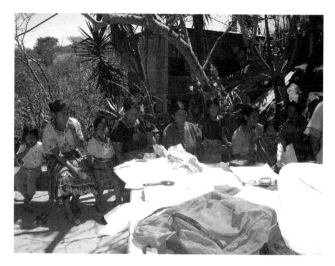

FIGURE 35-6 Mothers and children waiting for children's eye examinations for ocular toxoplasmosis, San Juan Sacatepéquez area, Guatemala, 2007. Photograph courtesy of author Beatriz Lopez

the eye. The retinal lesions were recorded if they were consistent with toxoplasmic retinochoroiditis, i.e., if there were: (1) discrete retinochoroidal scars with variable amounts of pigment at the borders; or (2) discrete foci of white retinal inflammation, either at the border of a retinochoroidal scar or as an isolated lesion. When lesions were observed, we brought the children to Guatemala City where ocular photographs were taken for documentation (Figure 35-8). It was difficult to convince the mothers to authorize the photographs if the

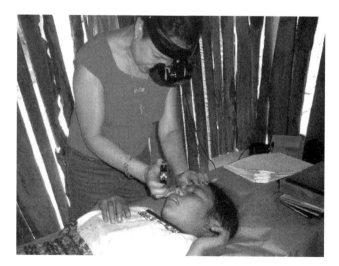

FIGURE 35-7 Ophthalmologic examination using indirect ophthalmoscopy, San Juan Sacatepéquez area, Guatemala, 2007. Photograph courtesy of author Beatriz Lopez

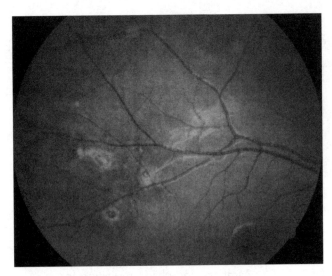

FIGURE 35-8 A 10 year old girl with *Toxoplasma gondii* antibodies since 1999. Ocular photographs of retinal lesions of the left eye, Guatemala City, Guatemala, 2007.

> *It was difficult to convince the mothers to authorize the photographs if the child was asked to go alone, so we brought the whole family to Guatemala City. As you can imagine, it was quite an adventure for these rural indigenous people.*

child was asked to go alone, so we brought the whole family to Guatemala City. As you can imagine, it was quite an adventure for these rural indigenous people. The identified lesions were photographed in an ophthalmologic clinic especially equipped with a Retcam camera. Dr. Holland also reviewed the photographs of the identified lesions.

The children were now 8–11 years old. Ocular examinations revealed that of the 44 children who were located, 4 (9%, 95% confidence limits 4%, 21%) had eye lesions consistent with ocular toxoplasmosis. Compared to the United States, this is a high rate of ocular disease (as previously mentioned, studies in the United States have shown up to 2% with *T. gondii* lesions in infected persons[3]) and provides additional evidence of the importance of *T. gondii* prevention in Guatemala.

Jeffrey L. Jones: Ocular disease is certainly worth preventing, even in the United States. With a lower *T. gondii* prevalence than Guatemala, there are an estimated 1.26 million persons with ocular disease in the United States.[3] Though it would be challenging, it would be enlightening to follow-up the Guatemalan children in our study after another 8–10 years to determine if any additional ocular disease occurs. It is important to note that the results of our ocular toxoplasmosis study may or may not be representative of the Guatemalan population in general. There were problems in locating some of the children and difficulties in obtaining agreement for the retinal photographs; however, it is the first study conducted in Guatemala on this condition and it demonstrates that ocular lesions may be present in numerous children infected with *T. gondii*.

Some questions remain unanswered with respect to the implications of *T. gondii* infections. We think it is necessary to continue with studies of the prevalence of toxoplasmosis in the Guatemalan population for different age groups to define the pattern in which the infection is acquired from the environment. Also, it is important to determine the genotypes of *T. gondii* circulating in the country because they may be a determinant of disease severity. There is still a lot of work to be done on toxoplasmosis in Guatemala in order to have a better understanding of the disease and how to prevent it.

LEARNING QUESTIONS

1. In the 2003 *T. gondii* antibody prevalence study of children 3–10 years of age, what would be the best way to select the study population from the rural villages?
2. In the 2003 *T. gondii* antibody prevalence study of children 3–10 years of age, what are the possible reasons why the *T. gondii* seroprevalence leveled off after 5 years of age?
3. In the 1999 *T. gondii* antibody prevalence study of children 6 months to 2 years old, what could account for seropositivity in children 6–11 months old?
4. Because *T. gondii* is a prevalent infection that can lead to ocular and congenital disease, is there a practical way to prevent it in rural Guatemala? In the United States? During pregnancy?

DISCLAIMER

The findings and conclusions in this report are those of the author(s) and do not necessarily represent the views of the Department of Health and Human Services or the Centers for Disease Control and Prevention.

REFERENCES

1. Jones JL, Hanson DL, Dworkin MS, et al. Surveillance for AIDS-defining opportunistic illnesses, 1992–1997. *MMWR CDC Surveill Summ*. 1999;48(No. SS-2):1–22.

2. Jones JL, Kruszon-Moran D, Wilson M, McQuillan G, Navin T, McAuley JB. *Toxoplasma gondii* infection in the United States: seroprevalence and risk factors. *Am J Epidemiol.* 2001;154(4):357–365.
3. Holland GN. Ocular toxoplasmosis: a global reassessment. Part 1: epidemiology and course of disease. *Am J Ophthalmol.* 2003;136(6):973–988.
4. Havlíček J, Gašová Z, Smith AP, Zvára K, Flegr J. Decrease of psychomotor performance in subjects with latent "asymptomatic" toxoplasmosis. *Parasitology.* 2001;122(Pt 5):515–520.
5. Flegr J, Havlíček J, Kodym P, Malý M, Smahel Z. Increased risk of traffic accidents in subjects with latent toxoplasmosis: a retrospective case-control study. *BMC Infect Dis.* 2002;2: 11.
6. Flegr J, Zitková S, Kodym P, Frynta D. Induction of changes in human behaviour by the parasitic protozoan T*oxoplasma gondii*. *Parasitology.* 1996;113(Pt 1):49–54.
7. Flegr J, Kodym P, Tolarová V. Correlation of duration of latent *Toxoplasma gondii* infection with personality changes in women. *Biol Psychol.* 2000;53(1):57–68.
8. Flegr J, Preiss M, Klose J, Havlíček J, Vitáková M, Kodym P. Decreased level of psychobiological factor novelty seeking and lower intelligence in men latently infected with the protozoan parasite *Toxoplasma gondii* Dopamine, a missing link between schizophrenia and toxoplasmosis? *Biol Psychol.* 2003:63(3):253–268.
9. Lafferty KD. Look what the cat dragged in: do parasites contribute to human cultural diversity? *Behav Processes.* 2005;68(3):279–282.
10. Lafferty KD. Can the common brain parasite, *Toxoplasma gondii*, influence human culture? *Proc Biol Sci.* 2006;273 (1602):2749–2755.
11. Brachmann S, Schroder J, Bottmer C, Torrey EF, Yolken RH. Psychopathology in first-episode schizophrenia and antibodies to *Toxoplasma gondii*. *Psychopathology.* 2005;38 (2):87–90.
12. Brown AS, Schaefer CA, Quesenberry CP Jr, Liu L, Babulas VP, Susser ES. Maternal exposure to toxoplasmosis and risk of schizophrenia in adult offspring. *Am J Psychiatry.* 2005;162(4):767–773.
13. Reller ME, Mendoza CE, Lopez MB, et al. A randomized controlled trial of household-based flocculent-disinfectant drinking water treatment for diarrhea prevention in rural Guatemala. *Am J Trop Med Hyg.* 2003;69(4):411–419.

Index

Numbers
3-(phenylamino)alanine (PAA), 329
9/11, 174–177, 186–187, 273–274, 402
17D vaccine, 221–224, 229–231
74th CDC EPI-AID call, 287
1933 World Fair, 74
1964 outbreak of leptospirosis. *see* leptospirosis
1974 outbreak of cholera. *see* cholera
1976 outbreak of Legionnaires' Disease. *see* Legionnaires' disease
1979–80 outbreak of toxic shock syndrome. *see* toxic shock syndrome (TSS)
1990 outbreak of pork tapeworm. *see* pork tapeworm
1991 outbreak of botulism. *see* botulism
1993 outbreak of cryptopsporidium. *see* *Cryptosporidium* infections
1997 outbreak of hepatitis A. *see* hepatitis A
1999 outbreak of syphilis. *see* syphilis
2001 anthrax investigation. *see* anthrax
2001 outbreak of Ebola. *see* Ebola hemorrhagic fever
2003 outbreak of whooping cough. *see* whooping cough
2006 outbreak of mumps. *see* mumps
2006 World Factbook, 103

A
ABC, 181–184
Aber, Robert, Dr., 45
ACDE (Acute and Communicable Disease Epidemiology), 51
Ackelsberg, Joel, 173–175, 186
acquired immune deficiency syndrome (AIDS). *see* AIDS (acquired immune deficiency syndrome)
activated carbon, 327
Acute and Communicable Disease Epidemiology (ACDE), 51
Acute Communicable Disease Control unit, 73
addiction. *see* drug addiction
Addiss, David, MD, 128–129
Alter, Miriam, 93–95
Admassu, Mekonnen, Dr., 227
adverse events following immunization (AEFI), 222, 230
Advisory Committee on Immunization Practices, 146, 157, 249
Aedes aegypti mosquitoes, 221–222
AEFI (adverse events following immunization), 222, 230
AEIOU CUP questionnaire guidelines, 444
Aeromonas hydrophila, 74–75
aflatoxicosis
  acknowledging experts on, 299
  case-control study of, 291–299
  hypothesis of, 290–291
  preliminary findings on, 288–290
  questions about, 299
  references on, 299
  reports of outbreak of, 287–288
Africa
  aflatoxicosis in. *see* aflatoxicosis
  cholera in, 36–37
  DEG poisoning in, 345
  Ebola hemorrhagic fever in. *see* Ebola hemorrhagic fever
  yellow fever in, 218–221, 241
Africare, 225
Agency for Toxic Substances and Disease Registry (ATSDR), 281, 402–411
AIDS (acquired immune deficiency syndrome). *see also* HIV (human immunodeficiency virus)

blood supply safety and, 69–70
conclusions about, 71
conference on, 112
cryptosporidosis and, 137
early investigations of, 66–68
expanding problem of, 68–69
history in United States, 66
international injection drug users and, 429–437
introduction to, 64
questions about, 71
references on, 71
U.S. injection drug users and, 423–429
AIDS Research Center, 434–435
airborne transmission
of *Aspergillus sydowii* keratitis, 78–79
of Legionnaires' disease, 48
of measles, 85
of mumps virus, 245
of thallium, 396
Akamba people, 292
Al-Ahram Weekly, 106
Alaska, 105
Alaska Division of Public Health, 102
aldicarb, 284
Aldrich, Tim E., PhD, MPH, 349
Alice Hamilton Award, 386
almonds, 14
alopecia. *see* thallium poisoning
Alroy, Gideon, Dr., 95
Altman, Lawrence, MD, 44
aluminum, 395–396
Alvarez, Maricruz, 452–456
amebiasis, pseudo-outbreak of
airborne contamination, 79
automated identification system errors, 79
conclusions about, 77–80
contaminated equipment, media and reagents, 79
control strains, cross-contamination from, 79
detection enhancements, 79
improper testing material and, 79
introduction to, 73–75
investigating, 75–77
laboratory errors and, 77–79
low positive predictive values in, 80
probiotic supplements and, 79
questions about, 81
references on, 80–81
specimen collection techniques in, 77
sporadic cases vs. outbreaks of, 79
transient colonization in, 79
America Online (AOL), 164–168
American Journal of Epidemiology, 386
American Journal of Public Health, 330
American Legion convention, 43–44
American Lung Association, 417
American Media Inc. building, 175, 185
American Poultry Association, 355
Amish communities, immunization in
conclusions about, 446–447
diplomacy in, 442–443
introduction to, 439–442
questions about, 447
references on, 447–448
surveys of, 443–446
ammonia poisoning, 278–284
anaerobic conditions promoting botulism, 102. *see also* botulism

ancient recipes. *see* botulism
And the Band Played On, 69
Anderson, Henry, Dr., 375
Angel Dust (PCP), 422
animal exposure
causing Ebola hemorrhagic fever, 197–200
causing leptospirosis, 22–24, 27
causing toxoplasmosis, 453–456
anthrax
acknowledgements, 188–189
conclusions about, 188
fear of, 273–275
introduction to, 173–174
investigating outbreak of, 49, 174–188
questions about, 189
anti-HBsAg (antibody to hepatitis B surface antigen), 92
antibiotics, 58–59
antibody to hepatitis B surface antigen (anti-HBsAg), 92, 96
antitoxins, 102–103, 106–107
AOL (America Online), 164–168
AOL.com: How Steve Case Beat Bill Gates, Nailed the Netheads, and Made Million in the War for the Web, 168
apes, 197–199
April, 1993, 121–127
Aqua do Vimeiro, 33–34, 38–39
Armstrong, Donald, Dr., 69–70
asbestos, 363–366
Ash, Larry, 73, 75
Asian AIDS conference, 429–430
AskDr.K.org, 169–170
Aspergillus fungus, 287–288, 294
Aspergillus sydowii, 78–79
association vs. causation, 330–332
asthma
Chicago Asthma Consortium on, 417
conclusions about, 419
education programs for, 416–417
inhaler policy for, 417–418
questions on, 419
references on, 420
screening for, 415–416
sustainable infrastructures for treating, 418–419
treating children with, 418
asthma-like respiratory symptoms, 406–407
Asthma Vans, 418
Atlas of Human Parasitology, 73
ATSDR (Agency for Toxic Substances and Disease Registry), 281
Auerbach, David, Dr., 68–69
automated identification system errors, 79
Autumnal fever, 27
Azziz-Baumgartner, Eduardo, MD, MPH, 287, 338

B

Bacillus amyloliquefaciens, 327, 329
Bacillus anthricus. *see* anthrax
Bacillus cereus, 78–79, 276–279, 284
Baine, Bill, 30
Baker, Everett, Dr., 23
baldness. *see* thallium poisoning
Balter, Sharon, 173, 175–176, 182, 186
Bangkok Metropolitan Administration, 431–432
Bangladesh
Demographic and Health Survey, 302
food shortages in. *see* food shortages
injection drug users in, 432–433
toxic exposure in. *see ghagra shak*

banner advertisements, 169
Baroda Medical College, 273
Bartlett, Mary E., 115
bats, 200
Bausch, Daniel G., MD, MPH&TM, 191
BDHS (Bangladesh Demographic and Health Survey), 302
Becker, Howard S., 422
becta-lactamase-resistant antibiotics, 58–59
beer, 135–136, 248
Behind the Green Door, 422
Bellevue-Stratford Hotel, 43–44, 46, 48
Belongia, Edward A., MD, 313
Ben-Porath, Edna, 99
Bergdoll, Merlin, 53
Beschner, George, 422, 426–427
biases
    in case and control selections, 13–14
    in EtO exposure studies, 379–380
    neighbor controls vs., 32
    recall, 279, 284
    selection, 322, 333
    in toxic shock syndrome, 61
    in yellow fever vaccination studies, 235–236
Bin Laden, Osama, 183
biologically plausible hypotheses. *see* tapeworm
bioterrorism
    anthrax as, 173–175, 178–181, 185–188
    fear of, 273–276
    microbiologists and, 204
    preparedness for, 206, 284–285, 402
Bishop, Bonnie, 313–314, 334
Blair, Kathy, 121–122
Blake, Paul, MD, MPH, 12–13, 29, 113
blood supply safety, 69–70
blood transfusions, 68–69
blue food. *see* aflatoxicosis
blue skin. *see* methemoglobinemia
boil-water advisory
    impact of, 131
    invoking, 126–127
    lifting, 138–139
Bong County, yellow fever vaccinations in. *see* yellow fever mass vaccination
Boo, Tom, MD, 261–263, 264–271
Bordetella pertussis. *see* whooping cough
boron, 395–396
bottled water investigation, 33–39
botulism
    antitoxins sources and use for, 106–107
    conclusions about, 106
    faseikh preparation and, 104–106
    forms of, 102
    introduction to, 101
    investigating outbreak of, 103–104
    laboratory findings on, 106
    outbreak of, 102–103
    preliminary control measures for, 11
    questions about, 107
    references on, 107
    religious observances and, 101–102
    symptoms of, 102
BPAS (Brief Pediatric Asthma Screen), 417–419
brain cancer, 351–356
breast cancer, 381, 384–386
Breiman, Rob, 301
Brennan, Muireann, Dr., 221–222, 225, 233

Brief Pediatric Asthma Screen (BPAS), 417–419
Brokaw, Tom, 175–176, 180, 183
bronchopneumonia, 84, 86
Brown, Jennifer, Dr., 226–228, 234, 239–240
Bryant, Juliet, Dr., 228
Bubbles, leptospirosis outbreak at. *see* leptospirosis
bupivicaine, 95
Burgdorfer, Willy, 52
bursa of Fabricius, 352–353

C

C. botulinum, 104–106. *see also* botulism
C. parvum infections, 140–141
C&D (construction and demolition debris) landfills, 403, 406, 410
CAC (Chicago Asthma Consortium), 417
Cairo, outbreak of botulism in. *see* botulism
Caja del Seguro (CSS) hospital system, 338, 341–343
Caldwell, Glenn, Dr., 350
California Department of Health Services, 102
Californiamen.net, 170
cancer clusters
    EtO exposure and. *see* ethylene oxide (EtO) exposure
    follow-up case-control studies of, 362–363
    history of, 349–351
    investigating reports of fair clusters, 351–356
    investigating reports of good clusters, 356–362
    investigating reports of outstanding clusters, 363–366
    questions about, 366
    references on, 366–369
Cancer Registries Amendment Act, 363
carbonated drinking water, 40–41
carboxyatractyloside, 310
Carmichael, Greg, 137
Carney, Tom, 145, 147
Carollton outbreak, 123, 127
Carson, Rachel, 350
Carter, Ken, 145, 147
case-control studies
    of aflatoxicosis, 291–299
    of cancer clusters, 355–356, 362–363, 382
    cohort studies vs., 306–308
    of DEG poisoning, 343–347
    of hepatitis A, 147, 154–155
    of L-tryptophan exposure, 316–319, 321–322, 325–332
    of shigellosis, 113–114
    of syphilis, 166
    of toxic shock syndrome, 57–62
case counts, 10
case definitions
    of aflatoxicosis, 291
    of ammonia poisoning, 279–280
    of *Cryptosporidium* infections, 129–131
    defined, 266
    of Ebola hemorrhagic fever, 197–198
    of eosinophilia-myalgia syndrome, 316–322
    of *ghagra shak* poisoning, 304–308
    of KS-01, 66
    of measles, 84
    of methemoglobinemia, 266
    of mumps, 247
    nonspecific, 333
    of pertussis, 208
    serology vs. surveillance in, 227
    of thallium poisoning, 393
    of toxic shock syndrome, 56
    of yellow fever, 227

Case, Steve, 168
cash galleries, 428
cats and cat feces exposure, 453–456
cattle, 22–24
causes
   associations vs., 330–332
   of *ghagra shak* poisoning outbreak, 306–308
   of leptospirosis outbreak, 27
   of methemoglobinemia outbreak, 269–270
   of thallium poisoning outbreak, 394–397
Cave, Laura, 363–364
CBS, 182, 184
CDC (Centers for Disease Control and Prevention). *see* Centers for Disease Control and Prevention (CDC)
Center for Food Safety and Applied Nutrition, 290
Centers for Disease Control and Prevention (CDC)
   aflatoxicosis, fighting. *see* aflatoxicosis
   AIDS, fighting. *see* AIDS (acquired immune deficiency syndrome)
   asthma, fighting, 419
   cholera, fighting. *see* cholera
   confirmation of diagnoses by, 8
   Division of Bacterial and Mycotic Diseases of, 102
   Division of HIV/AIDS Prevention of, 203, 450–451
   Division of Parasitic Diseases of, 451, 452
   Division of Vector-Borne Infectious Diseases of, 217
   drinking water recommendations of, 40–41
   Enteric Diseases Branch of, 29, 41, 102, 109
   eosinophilia myalgia syndrome, fighting, 316
   Epi Info from. *see* Epi Info database
   Epidemic Intelligence Service of, 5
   Foodborne and Diarrheal Diseases Branch of, 12
   Health Studies Branch of, 337
   Hepatitis Branch of, 150
   injection drug user programs of, 425, 429
   Kenya office of, 291
   Leptospirosis Reference Laboratory of, 26–27
   mumps and, 248
   National Center for Infectious Diseases of, 123
   pneumonia-like illnesses, fighting. *see* Legionnaires' disease
   Public Health Prevention Service of, 439
   Rickettsial Disease Laboratory of, 48
   Special Pathogens Branch of, 191
   toxic shock syndrome, fighting, 56–61
   yellow fever vaccination programs of, 225–233
Centre International de Recherches Medicals de Franceville (CIRMF), 193, 196, 198
CERCLA (Comprehensive Environmental Response, Compensation and Liability Act), 356
Chapin, John, 127
chat rooms, 164–169
chemical foodborne intoxication, 278–284
chemical poisoning of school children. *see* toxic school lunches
Chernivtsi. *see* thallium poisoning
Chernobyl, 390
Cherry, Bryan, 180
Chesney, Joan, 52
Chesney, Russ, 52
Chicago Asthma Consortium (CAC), 417
Chicago Public Schools (CPS), 416–418
Chicago School of Public Health, 415
Chicago School of Sociology, 421
chicken farms, 351–356, 362–363
chicken tenders, 277–284
child care facilities. *see also* school children
   cryptosporidosis at, 136

   hepatitis A in, 146, 149, 157
   shigellosis at, 110–113
children's hair loss. *see* thallium poisoning
China
   DEG poisoning in, 345–346
   injection drug use programs in, 432–433
   leptospirosis in, 27
chlorine, 126
cholera
   bottled water investigation of, 37–39
   Faro District investigation of, 35–37
   interviews in role of hypothesis generation for, 13
   introduction to, 29–30
   Lisbon investigation of, 30–35
   questions about, 42
   references on, 42
   Tavira investigation of, 35–37
   wrapping up, 39–41
Chorba, Terry, 91
CHOWS (Community Health Outreach Workers), 427
Christian Scientists, 83–88
Church of Christ, Scientists, 85. *see also* Christian Scientists
CIRMF (Centre International de Recherches Medicals de Franceville), 193, 196, 198
citric acid, 268–269
CIVPOL, 227
Clark and Diversey intersection, 423
class I-reportable diseases, 83
Cline, Barney, 192
clinical features
   of *Cryptosporidium* infections, 129–131
   of eosinophilia myalgia syndrome, 322
   of leptospirosis, 27
   of thallium poisoning, 389
   of toxic shock syndrome, 59
close contacts, defining, 210–211
closing businesses, 12
cluster busters, 350
clusters of cancer cases. *see* cancer clusters
CNN, 347
coagulants, 141
cocklebur seedlings, 310–311. *see also* ghagra shak
Cohen, Neal, 178, 187–188
coherence, 330–331
cohort studies
   of EtO exposure. *see* ethylene oxide (EtO) exposure
   of *ghagra shak* poisoning, 308
   of injection drug users, 427–429
   justification for, 12–13
   of water park attendants, 13
COIP (Community Outreach Intervention Projects), 429
cold chain system, 222–223, 230
coliforms, 125
Collapse, 298
college campuses, 84–87, 247–248, 256–257
colonic irrigation, 74–75
Columbia River, 22–23
Columbia University, 330
Communicable Disease section, IDPH, 275–277
communications
   among surveillance stakeholders, 274
   in bioterrorism preparedness, 285
   breaking down barriers to, 67
   with community, 199
   in hepatitis A outbreaks, 147
   inter-agency, 206–208

Internet, 228
with laboratories, 213–215
with media, 212
in mumps outbreaks, 249
objectives of, 5, 151
on prevention, 15
of risks, 181, 188
community-based interventions, 109–114, 425–426
Community Health Outreach Workers (CHOWS), 427
Community Outreach Intervention Projects (COIP), 429
Comprehensive Environmental Response, Compensation and Liability Act (CERCLA), 356
computerized tomography (CT) scans, 115–116
confidentiality
in cancer cluster research, 351
in hepatitis A outbreaks, 153
of HIV/AIDS patients, 136
of names, 15
in syphilis outbreaks, 167
confirmed vs. laboratory confirmed cases, 9–10
Congo, Ebola hemorrhagic fever in. *see* Ebola hemorrhagic fever
Connor, Julius, Dr., 152, 160
consistency, 330–331
construction and demolition debris (C&D) landfills, 403, 406, 410
contaminated equipment, 79
control measures
existing, 14–15
for methemoglobinemia, 262–264
new, 14–15
preliminary, 11–12
Conway, Judy, 206–208
Cook, Robin, 401
cooked crabs, 13
cooling towers, 51–52
Cope, Lewis, 313
Copeland, Jefffrey, 177
Coptic Christians, 103–106
counting cases, 10
Cox proportional hazards model, 382
CPS (Chicago Public Schools), 416–418
Craigslist, 169
Cronauer, Adrian, 177
cross-contamination, 79, 99, 188
cross-species transmission, 27. *see also* animal exposure
Cruz, Miguel, 340–342
Cryptosporidium infections
on April 5, 1993, 121–122
on April 6, 1993, 122–123
on April 7, 1993, 123–127
boil-water advisory for, 138–139
businesses preventing, 135–136
case definitions for, 129–131
in children and childcare settings, 136
clinical characteristics of, 129–131
coagulants in water plants and, 141
conclusions about, 142–143
early logistics fighting, 127–128
emergency department surveillance of, 131
genotyping and, 140
HIV infection and, 136
human amplification of, 141–142
infrastructure improvements fighting, 142
introduction to, 13
laboratory-based active surveillance and testing for, 129
magnitude of outbreak of, 131–135
Milwaukee Water Works South Plant in, 137–138
mortality and, 136–137
nursing home surveillance, 131
outbreak and investigation, generally, 127
point-of-use filters and, 139–140
policy impacts, 142
post-outbreak transmission of, 139
questions about, 144
raw water sources and, 128–129
references on, 143–144
review of MWW data in, 128–136
sanitary vs. storm sewers and, 141
South Plant intake grid and, 140–141
in special populations, 136–137
standards and, 142
studies and investigations, additional, 139–140
surveillance data and, 15–16
surveillance methods for, 138
swimming pool-related, 139
testing and, 142
theories on massive outbreaks of, 140–142
unusual clusters of, 138
in visitors to Milwaukee, 135
in water supply, 137
weather conditions and, 140–141
CSS (Caja del Seguro) hospital system, 338, 341–343
CT (computerized tomography) scans, 115–116
cutaneous anthrax, 174, 177–179, 185. *see also* anthrax
Cuvette Ouest region, 199
cyanosis. *see* methemoglobinemia
cyberspace, tracking outbreaks through. *see* syphilis
cysticercosis, 115–119

D

Darrow, Bill, Dr., 67–68
Davis, Jeffrey P., MD, 51, 54–55
day care facilities. *see* child care facilities
DDRR (Disarmament, Demobilization, Reintegration, Rehabilitation), 233
de Bock, Steven, 230
De Cock, Kevin, Dr., 289
Dean, Andy, 53
death certificates, 378
DEG (diethylene glycol) poisoning. *see* diethylene glycol (DEG) poisoning
Delbeke, Isabelle, 198
Delphi surveys, 139
delta-9-tetrahydrocannabinol (THC), 422
Denko K.K., 323, 326–330, 332–334
Department of Homeland Security, 274
Department of Inspections and Appeals, 268
Departments of Health (DOH)
California, 102, 449
Florida, 49
Minnesota, 314–316, 320, 323–325
New York City. *see* anthrax
Ohio, 404
Polk County, 155
South Carolina, 450
U.S., 299, 402, 458
Virginia, 167
Wisconsin. *see* Wisconsin Division of Health (DOH)
Des Moines, Iowa, 145
Des Moines Register, 147, 149, 250
descriptive epidemiology, 197–198
detection enhancements, 79
Dhaka, 301–304

diagnoses
    confirming, 8
    laboratory, 126, 193, 210
    rapid, 110–112, 285
    serologic, 116
    verifying, 73–80
dialysis-related outbreaks, 94–95
Diamond, Jared, 298
diarrheal outbreaks
    cholera and, 29, 35
    Cryptosporidium causing. *see Cryptosporidium* infections
    determining cause of, 3
    drinking water and, 451
    E. coli and, 11–12
    hepatitis A and, 151
    legal means for preventing, 5
    in pseudo-outbreak of amebiasis, 77
    shigellosis and, 110–113
Dietary Supplement Health and Education Act (DSHEA), 334
diethylene glycol (DEG) poisoning
    arrival at site of outbreak of, 340–341
    case-control study of, findings, 344–346
    case-control study of, generally, 343–344
    case-control study of, impacts, 346–347
    initial reports of, 337–338
    investigating outbreak of, 341–343
    preparing to investigate, 338–340
    questions about, 347
    references on, 347
difficult-to-reach populations and HIV. *see* HIV (human immunodeficiency virus)
dinitrobenzene, 270
dioxin poisoning, 398
Disarmament, Demobilization, Reintegration, Rehabilitation (DDRR), 233
Disease Outbreak News, 222, 225
Division of Food, Drugs, and Dairies, 276–277, 281
Division of Health, Wisconsin. *see* Wisconsin Division of Health (DOH)
Division of HIV/AIDS Prevention, 450
Division of Narcotics Enforcement (DNE), 148
Division of Parasitic Diseases, CDC, 66, 451, 452
Division of Public Health, Alaska, 102
(DOH) Departments of Health. *see* Departments of Health (DOH)
dope fiends, 425, 431
Douglas, Don, 430, 433
Drug Abuse Epidemiology Program, 423–424
drug addiction
    HIV and. *see* human immunodeficiency virus (HIV)
    of injection drug users in U.S., 421–429
    of injection drug users internationally, 429–437
    to methamphetamine, 145–148, 153–161
DSHEA (Dietary Supplement Health and Education Act), 334
DT104, 274
Duffy, Joseph, Dr., 315
Dworkin, Mark S., MD, MPH & TM, FACP
    Amish community and, 441–445
    on outbreak investigations methodology, 7–16
    on overview of outbreak investigations, 3–6
    on toxic school lunches, 273–281, 283–285
    on whooping cough. *see* whooping cough

E
E. coli, 11, 78–79, 203
East Moline, Illinois, 415–416

Ebola hemorrhagic fever
    case definition of, 197–198
    conclusions about, 200–201
    descriptive epidemiology for, 197–198
    end of outbreak of, 199–200
    friction in community over, 199
    initial assessment of outbreak of, 194–196
    introduction to, 191–192
    isolation wards controlling, 196
    laboratory confirmation of, 193–194
    nosocomial transmission of, 198–199
    questions about, 202
    recognition of outbreak of, 193–194
    references on, 201–202
    reservoir of virus, hunting for, 199–200
    responses to outbreak of, 192–193
EBT (1′-ethylidenebis(tryptophan)), 329
Eddy, Mary Baker, 85
Education and Research Center (ERC), NIOSH, 401
education programs
    about *ghagra shak* poisoning, 311
    during anthrax scare, 181
    for asthma care, 416–419
    on cancer clusters, 353
    as control measures, 12
    for *Cryptosporidium* infections, 128
    for hepatitis A prevention, 158–159
    for mumps prevention, 247–248
Egoz, Nahum, Dr., 95–96
Egypt, botulism outbreak in. *see* botulism
Ehlert, Bob, 313
EIS (Epidemic Intelligence Service). *see* Epidemic Intelligence Service (EIS)
elementary school children. *see* school children
Eleven Blue Men, 270
ELISA (enzyme-linked immunosorbent assay), 194
Elliott, Larry, 379
Elsah, Illinois, 84
emergency department surveillance, 131
emergency rooms, 156
emergency yellow fever mass vaccination. *see* yellow fever mass vaccination
EMS (eosinophilia myalgia syndrome). *see* eosinophilia myalgia syndrome (EMS)
Engstrom, Jinx, 317, 334
Entamoeba hystolytica, 73–77
Enteric Diseases Branch, CDC, 29, 41, 102, 109
Enterococcus durans, 78–79
environmental investigations
    of ammonia poisoning, 278
    of anthrax outbreak, 177–181
    of epizootics, 200
    human exposure to toxins in, 339
    introduction to, 11
    of methemoglobinemia outbreak, 267–268
    of toxic school lunches, 281–283
Environmental Protection Agency (EPA)
    in anthrax investigation, 188
    in *Cryptosporidium* infection investigation, 125
    on EtO exposure, 386–387
    on hydrogen sulfide exposure, 409–410
    of Ohio, 403, 410
    as regulatory agency, 402
    on superfund sites, 356
enzyme-linked immunosorbent assay (ELISA), 194
eosinophilia myalgia syndrome (EMS)

association vs. causation in, 330–332
case-control study of, 325–326
clinical and pathological features of, 322
conclusions about, 334
ethics and, 332–334
L-tryptophan, Peak E chemical constituent in, 328–329
L-tryptophan, Showa Denko K.K. manufacturing, 326–328
L-tryptophan, testing for contaminants in, 324–325
L-tryptophan use, community survey of, 322–323
L-tryptophan use, other studies of, 329–330
L-tryptophan use, tracebacks, 323–324
litigation and, 332–334
looking for cases of, 320–322
in Minnesota, 314–316
in New Mexico, 313–314
questions about, 335
references on, 335–336
scientific debate on, 332–334
weekend study of, 316–320
eosinophilic fasciitis, 322
EPA (Environmental Protection Agency). see Environmental Protection Agency (EPA)
Epi-Aids
for aflatoxicosis, 287–288
for hepatitis A, 154
for hydrogen sulfide exposure, 402–404
for Legionnaires' disease, 52
Epi Info database
2002, 266
introduction to, 11
version 6.04, 280
in whooping cough investigation, 209
in yellow fever mass vaccinations, 235
epidemic curves, 266
Epidemic Intelligence Service (EIS)
on aflatoxicosis, 298
in aflatoxicosis investigations. *see* aflatoxicosis
in anthrax investigations, 173
Bacterial Meningitis and Special Pathogens Branch of, 109
Belongia in, 314
Blake in, 29
in cancer cluster investigations, 352
Davis in, 51
Division of Parasitic Diseases of, 117
Dworkin in, 203
in echinococcosis investigations, 116
focus of, 297
guidelines of, 41
Hepatitis Branch of, 91, 93
introduction to, 5
Jones in, 449–450
Klausner in, 163
in Legionnaires' disease investigations. *see* Legionnaires' disease
Lohff in, 262
Pratap in, 402
training program of, 19–20
Venereal Disease Control Division of, 65
Weber in, 102
in yellow fever vaccinations, 217
Epidemic Scorecard, 219–220
epidemics, defined, 3–4
epidemiologic analyses, defined, 10–11
epidemiology
as basis of public health, 49
descriptive, 197–198, 278–279
EIS training in field, 19–20

of leptospirosis outbreak, 27
in outbreak investigation generally, 7–16
"quick and dirty" investigations, 150
"shoe-leather," 29, 315
tool kit for, 4–6
uncertainty in, 80
epinephrine autoinjector, 417
epizootics, 200
ERC (Education and Research Center), NIOSH, 401
erythromycin, 213
eschar. *see* anthrax
Escherichia coli, 11, 78–79, 203
ethics, 332–334
ethnographic inquiries, 426–428
ethylene oxide (EtO) exposure
acknowledging experts on, 387
assessing, 378–380
cohorts of, 377–378, 384–386
epilogue to studies of, 386–387
history of, 373–374
medical device manufacturing industry, enlisting, 374–375
medical device manufacturing industry, studies by, 382–384
preliminary feasibility studies of, 374
references on, 387–388
results of studies of, 380–382
vital status of, 378
walkthrough surveys on, 376–377
ethylidenebis(tryptophan) (EBT), 329
EtO (ethylene oxide) exposure. *see* ethylene oxide (EtO) exposure
European Longitudinal Study of Pregnancy and Childhood, 398
exclusion criteria, 13
exposure. *see also* intoxications
dates of, 10
to EtO. *see* ethylene oxide (EtO) exposure
evaluations, 403
to hydrogen sulfide, 403–404, 407–410
indirect indicators of, 407
sites of, 11
to thallium. *see* thallium poisoning
via animals. *see* animal exposure

F
Factor, Stephanie, 183
Family Health International (FHI), 433–436
Faro District, 35–37
faseikh, 104–107
FBI (Federal Bureau of Investigation), 175–180, 183
FDA (Food and Drug Administration). *see* Food and Drug Administration (FDA)
fecal leukocytes, 76–77
fecal-oral disease transmission, 75
fecal-percutaneous transmission, 160
Federal Bureau of Investigation (FBI), 175–180, 183
Federal Food, Drug, and Cosmetic Act, 339
FELTP (Field Epidemiology and Laboratory Training Program), 291–294
FEV1 (forced expiratory volume in the first second of expiration), 407–409
FHI (Family Health International), 433–436
field epidemiologic investigations
of aflatoxicosis, 289–297
of hepatitis A, 154–161
of measles in Amish communities, 441–447
of toxic school lunches, 275–280
training in, 19

Field Epidemiology and Laboratory Training Program (FELTP), 291–294
Field Epidemiology Training Program (FETP), 340
filtering water at point of use, 139–140
fish preparation, 104–107
Fitin, Professor, 397
Florida
  anthrax cases in, 174–176, 181, 185
  Department of Health, 49, 174
  KS-01 in, 68
Fogarty grants, 393, 436
follow-up case-control studies, 362–363
Fonte do Bispo, 36–37, 40
Fonte Santa Isabel, 34
Food and Drug Administration (FDA)
  in aflatoxicosis investigation, 289–290
  in botulism investigation, 105
  communicating with, 15
  DEG testing by, 342
  on dietary supplements, 334
  on L-tryptophan, 314, 316–318, 323–324
  in methemoglobinemia investigation, 268
  on toxic shock syndrome, 61
Food Safety and Inspection (FSIS) laboratory, 279
food shortages
  cocklebur seedlings, 310–311
  ghagra shak, defined, 308–310
  ghagra shak, foregoing, 311
  ghagra shak, hypothesis, 306–308
  ghagra shak, toxic levels of, 310
  hypotheses, developing, 304–306
  outbreaks associated with, 302–303
  questions about, 312
  references on, 312
  rice crops and, 302
  toxic exposure hypothesis in, 303
Foodborne and Diarrheal Diseases Branch, CDC, 12
foodborne illness
  aflatoxicosis. *see* aflatoxicosis
  botulism, 102
  hepatitis A, 148–152
  investigating generally, 11
  methemoglobinemia. *see* methemoglobinemia
  in school lunches. *see* toxic school lunches
forced expiratory volume in the first second of expiration (FEV1), 407–408
Fort Bragg fever, 27
Fox, Kim, 138
Francis, Byron, MD, 87
Fraser, David, MD, 44
free galleries, 428
Frisby, Holly, 136
frozen strawberries, 149–150
FSIS (Food Safety and Inspection) laboratory, 279, 283
fulminant hepatitis B. *see* hepatitis B

G
Gabon. *see* Ebola hemorrhagic fever
galleries for shooting drugs, 428
Gallo, Robert, 70
gastric acid, 29–30
gastroenteritis, 11–12
gay population
  AIDS in, 65–71
  drug injectors among, 423–425
  Entamoeba hystolytica among, 74

hepatitis A in, 158–159
syphilis outbreaks among, 164–169
Gbehleygeh district, 228–231
Gblah village, 232
gender ratios, 198
genotyping, 140
geographic information systems (GIS), 351
ghagra shak
  causing outbreak, 306–308
  as cocklebur seedlings, 310–311
  defined, 308–310
  hypotheses, developing, 304–306
  questions about, 312
  recommendation to not eat, 311
  references on, 312
  toxic levels of, 310
GIS (geographic information systems), 351, 362–363
Giuliani, Rudy, 178
Gleich, Gerald, Dr., 314, 321, 324–325, 328
Global AIDS Program (GAP), 289
Global Programme on AIDS, 432
glowing blue. *see* aflatoxicosis
gonorrhea, 65
Good Morning Vietnam, 177
Google Scholar, 386
Gottlieb, Michael, Dr., 66
Gottstein, Bruno, 116
Gradus, Steve, Dr., 121–122, 125–126, 129
Greenfield, Bruce, Dr., 314
grey mullet, 104–106
Griffin, Patricia, Dr., 109–113
Grimson, Roger, 353
Guatemala, toxoplasmosis in. *see* toxoplasmosis
Gulf War, 101
Gurley, Emily S., MPH, 301, 311
Gweley village, 231

H
H5N1 (bird flu), 303
Hadler, Steve, 91, 97
Haifa, Israel, 93–96
Haines, Lenny, 425
hair loss. *see* thallium poisoning
Haitian Americans, 68–70
Halperin, William, Dr., 375
Handbook on Risk of AIDS—Injection Drug Users and Sexual Partners, 427
handwashing campaigns, 110–113, 155–157
Haney, Ann, 128
HANs (health alert networks), 250
Harkin, Tom, Senator, 158
Harvard Medical School, 99
Harvard School of Public Health, 375
Hayes, Richard, Dr., 375
hazardous waste, 356–357
HBc (hepatitis B core antigen), 92
HBsAg (hepatitis B surface antigen), 91–92
HBV (hepatitis B virus). *see* hepatitis B virus (HBV)
Head Start program, 416–417
health alert networks (HANs), 250
health care workers, deaths of, 195
Health Education Resource Organization (HERO), 426
health effects investigations, 403
Health Industry Manufacturers Association (HIMA), 375
Health Insurance Portability and Accountability Act (HIPAA), 351–352

health maintenance organizations (HMOs), 73–76
Health Studies Branch (HSB), CDC, 337–339
Health Studies Program, 314
Heath, Clark, Dr., 350
Hedberg, Craig, 323–324
hematopoietic neoplasms, 382–384, 387
hemoglobin, 264
hemophilia, 68–70
Henderson, Alden, 402, 404
heparin locks, 96–98
hepatitis A
   conclusions about, 162
   field epidemiologic investigation of, 154–161
   introduction to, 145–154
   questions about, 162
   references on, 162
hepatitis B core antigen (HBc), 92
hepatitis B surface antigen (HBsAg), 91–92
hepatitis B virus (HBV)
   overview of, 91–99
   questions about, 100
   references on, 99–100
hepatitis D virus, 94
hepatomyoencephalopathy, 306
HERO (Health Education Resource Organization), 426
heroin addicts, 425, 430–431
Hershow, Ronald C., MD, 88
Hertzman, Phil, Dr., 314
HIDTA (High Intensity Drug Trafficking Area of the Midwest), 161
high-performance liquid chromatography (HPLC) fingerprints, 324–325, 328
Hill, Austin Bradford, Sir, 330
Hill, Bradford, 310
HIMA (Health Industry Manufacturers Association), 375, 384
HIPAA (Health Insurance Portability and Accountability Act), 351–352
Hippocrates, 245
HIV (human immunodeficiency virus)
   aflatoxicosis and, 294
   appearance of, 421
   career in study of, 421–423
   community-based interventions for, 425–426
   Cryptosporidium infections and, 136
   drug injector interventions for, 429, 435–437
   emergence of, 423–425
   ethnographic inquiries into, 426–428
   indigenous leader outreach and, 426–428
   injection drug users, in U.S., 423–429
   injection drug users, internationally, 429–437
   international perspectives on, 429–433
   questions about, 437
   references on, 437–438
   sex workers and, 433–437
   syphilis and, 166–170
   toxoplasmosis and, 451
   Women and Infants Transmission study of, 99
HMOs (health maintenance organizations), 73–76
homosexuality. *see* gay population
The Hot Zone, 192
hotlines, 152
Howard Avenue Purification Plant, 123–126
Hoxie, Neil, 131
HPLC (high-performance liquid chromatography) fingerprints, 324–325, 328
Hryhorczuk, Daniel, MD, MPH, 389

HSB (Health Studies Branch), CDC, 337–339
HTLV-III, 70
Hughes, Patrick, 423, 425, 427
Huhn, Gregory, MD, MPH&TM, 217, 277
human immunodeficiency virus (HIV). *see* HIV (human immunodeficiency virus)
human-to-human transmissions, 220–221
hunger. *see* food shortages
Hunter's Lodge, 290, 292
hunting, 197–198
Hussein, Saddam, 101
Hutin, Yvan, MD, 145, 147, 155, 160
hydrogen sulfide exposure, 403–404, 407–410
Hydromet, 397
hypocalcemia, 59
hypotheses
   aflatoxicosis, 290–291
   ghagra shak, 304–306
   in outbreak investigations, 11
   thallium poisoning, 390–391

I
IARC (International Agency for Research on Cancer), 373–375, 386
ICDDR,B (International Centre for Diarrhoeal Disease Research, Bangladesh), 301–302
ice, 127, 137
iceberg effect, 398
ICP (inductively-coupled plasma) atomic emission mass spectroscopy, 268
IDLH (National Institute for Occupational Safety and Health Immediately Dangerous to Life or Health), 408
IDP (internally displaced persons) camps. *see* internally displaced persons (IDP) camps
IDPH (Illinois Department of Public Health). *see* whooping cough
IDPH (Iowa Department of Public Health). *see* methemoglobinemia; mumps
IDUs (injection drug users). *see* injection drug users (IDUs)
IEDCR (Institute of Epidemiology, Disease Control and Research), 301–308
IG (immunoglobulin), 146
IHC (immunohistochemical) staining, 176–177
Illinois
   Dangerous Drugs Commission, 423–424
   Department of Children and Family Services, 86–87
   Department of Public Health. *see* whooping cough
   measles in, 83–87
   State Board of Education, 281–282
   whooping cough in. *see* whooping cough
ILOM (Indigenous Leader Outreach Model), 429–432, 434–435
Imm, Ivan, 127
immunization in Old-Order Amish communities. *see* Amish communities, immunization in
immunoblot assays, 116
immunodeficiency. *see* AIDS (acquired immune deficiency syndrome)
immunoglobulin G (IgG) antibodies, 452
immunoglobulin (IG) shots, 146–150
immunohistochemical (IHC) staining, 176–177
incident command system, 252–256
Indigenous Leader Outreach Model (ILOM), 426–432
Indigenous Leader Outreach Model: Intervention Manual, 425
Indonesia, 99, 432–436
inductively-coupled plasma (ICP) atomic emission mass spectroscopy, 268
Industry Wide Studies Branch (IWSB), 374

infant botulism, 102. *see also* botulism
infants congenitally infected with toxoplasmosis, 451
Infectious Diseases of Man, 20
influenza, 9, 85
Information Collection Rule, 142
inhalation anthrax, 174–177, 183, 185. *see also* anthrax
inhaler policy, 417–418
injection drug users (IDUs)
    internationally, 429–437
    in U.S., 424–429
insomnia, 313–314, 320
inSPOT.org, 169
Institute of Epidemiology, Disease Control and Research (IEDCR), 301–308
Institute of Medico-Ecologic Problems, 391–392
Institute Pasteur, 70
Internal Revenue Service (IRS), 384
internal review boards (IRBs), 351
internally displaced persons (IDP) camps
    yellow fever in, 218, 228
    yellow fever vaccinations in, 222, 233–240
International Agency for Research on Cancer (IARC), 373–374
International Centre for Diarrhoeal Disease Research, Bangladesh (ICDDR,B), 301–302
International Day of Reflection on the Genocide in Rwanda, 239
International Study of Asthma and Allergies in Childhood, 415–416
Internet Sexuality Information Services, Inc. (ISIS-Inc.), 169
Internet tracking. *see* syphilis
intoxications. *see also* noninfectious causes
    with aflatoxin, 287–288
    with ammonia, 278–284
    with carboxyatractyloside, 310
    with diethylene glycol, 338–339
    with ethylene oxide. *see* ethylene oxide (EtO) exposure
    with L-tryptophan, 327–329
    with methemoglobin, 251–270
    with thallium compounds, 397
intravenous (IV) drugs, 68. *see also* injection drug users (IDUs)
investigating outbreaks. *see* outbreak investigations overview
investigating pseudo-outbreaks. *see* amebiasis, pseudo-outbreak of
Iowa
    hepatitis A in. *see* hepatitis A
    mumps in. *see* mumps
    toxic shock syndrome in, 60
Iraq, 101
IRBs (internal review boards), 351
irrigation water, 21–24
IRS (Internal Revenue Service), 384
ISIS-Inc. (Internet Sexuality Information Services, Inc.), 169
isolation
    Ebola and, 196
    fear of, 196–199
    mumps and, 248
Israel, hepatitis B in. *see* hepatitis B virus (HBV)
Istre, Greg, 74
IV (intravenous) drugs, 68
Ivasiuk, Volodymyr, 391
IWSB (Industry Wide Studies Branch), 374, 375

J

Jack in the Box hamburgers, 203
Jaffe, Harold W., MD, 65
Jakubowski, Walt, 137–138
James A. Farley Post Office, 183–185
Japan, 323

jaundice, 291, 294–296
Jennings, Charles E., 80, 205–206, 209
Jersey County Health Department, 84–87
Jewish communities, tapeworm in. *see* tapeworm
Jimenez, Antonio, 427
Johns Hopkins University, 349
Joliet, Illinois. *see* toxic school lunches
Jones, Jeffrey L., MD, MPH, 449–458
Jones, John Paul, Dr., 374
Journal of Rheumatology, 334
Journal of the American Medical Association, 75
Juranek, Dennis, Dr., 123, 137

K

Kamil, Very, 434–435
Kansas, 245
kapchunka, 105–106
Kaposi's sarcoma (KS), 66–68
Kaslow, Dick, 52
Katzer, Christian, 198
Kazmierczak, Jim, 121–123, 126
Kearney, Angela, 225–226, 240
Keene, William, PhD, 11
Kentucky, shigellosis in. *see* shigellosis
Kenya, aflatoxicosis in. *see* aflatoxicosis
kheshuri lentils, 308
Khmer refugee camps, 91
Kilbourne, Ed, Dr., 314–315
Kim, Andrea, 166
Kinnikinnick River, 128–129
Klausner, Jeffrey D., MD, MPH, 161
Kozel, Nick, 421
Kramer, Nola, 84
KS (Kaposi's sarcoma), 66–68
KS/OI Task Force, 66–68
Ksiazek, Tom, 191
Kulwicki, Allen, 138

L

L-5 hydroxytryptophan, 320
L-tryptophan. *see* eosinophilia myalgia syndrome (EMS)
La Rabida Children's Hospital, 417
laboratory analysis
    of botulism, 106
    confirming cases, 9–10
    of *Cryptosporidium* infections, 129
    of Ebola hemorrhagic fever, 193–194
    errors in, 77–79
    guidelines for, 5–6
    of leptospirosis, 22, 26–27
    in outbreak investigation generally, 11
    of toxic school lunches, 279–280, 283–285
    of toxic shock syndrome, 55
    of toxoplasmosis, 456
Lake Michigan, 123, 140–141
Lancet, 52
landfills
    acknowledging experts on, 411
    assessing investigation of, 410–411
    community health and, 401–403
    investigating, 404–409
    limitations in studies of, 410
    problems in, 403–404
    questions about, 411
    references on, 411
    results of studies of, 409

Langmuir, Alexander, Dr., 349–350, 352
Laraway Elementary School, 274–281, 283
Lassa fever, 201
LaVenture, Martin, 51
Layton, Marci, MD, 173–177
leachate pools, 408
lead poisoning, 395
LeChevallier, Mark, 139
legal issues, 167, 332–334
legally mandated control measures, 5
Legionella species, 4
Legionnaires' disease
    introduction to, 43
    investigating outbreak of, 43–48
    personal reflections on, 49
    questions about, 50
    references on, 49–50
    in Wisconsin, 51–52
Lehman, Herman, Dr., 350
lentils, 308
leptospirosis
    causative organisms in, 27
    epidemiology of, 27
    history of disease in, 27
    introduction to, 19–20
    laboratory studies of, 26–27
    lessons from, 28
    notes about, 28
    outbreak of, 20–26
    questions about, 28
    references on, 28
Leptospirosis Reference Laboratory, 26–27
lesbian population, 168. *see also* gay population
leukemia. *see* ethylene oxide (EtO) exposure
Level 4: Virus Hunters of the CDC, 402
Levine, Deb, 169
Lewis, Lauren Seymour, MD, MPH, 298–299, 337
Lexington, Kentucky. *see* shigellosis
Liberia, yellow fever in. *see* yellow fever mass vaccination
Libreville, 194, 199
life table analysis system (LTAS), 382–383
Likimani, Sopiato, Dr., 295
Lindblade, Kim, Dr., 292
Linnwood Avenue Purification Plant, 123–125
Lisbon, cholera in, 30–35
lisinopril, 341–347
Littlefield, Abraham, Dr., 349
Lohff, Cortland, MD, MPH, 261–264, 267–271
López, Beatriz, QB, 449–458
Los Angeles, 65–68
lot quality assurance sampling (LQAS) surveys, 238–240
low positive predictive values, 80
LQAS (lot quality assurance sampling) surveys, 238–240
LTAS (life table analysis system), 382–383
Luby, Steven, Dr., 301–303, 306, 451–452
Lucht, Roland, 209
Lyme disease, 52, 80
lymphatic-hematopoietic neoplasms, 377, 381–384, 387
lymphoid tumors, 382–384

M

M. fortuitum, 78–79
M. tuberculosis, 78–79
MacKenzie, Bill, MD, 123–126, 131
MacMahon, Brian, Dr., 375
magnetic resonance images (MRIs), 116–117
magnitude of outbreaks, 131–135
Maguire, James, Dr., 452–453
Maharaja Sayajirao University, 273
mail distribution, 183–188
maize. *see* aflatoxicosis
Makokou, 194–200
Maks, Nuhu, Dr., 228
malaria, 195, 198, 218–219
Manhattan Eye, Ear, and Throat Hospital (MEETH), 185–186
Marburg virus, 200–201
March, C. Ralph, 87
Marfin, Tony, Dr., 217, 225–227, 233
Mason, Terry, 428
MAT (Microscopic Agglutination Test), 22–23, 26–27
Matte, Tom, 183
Mayeno, Arthur, 324–325, 328–329
Mayer, James, Dr., 313
Maynard, James, 91
Mayo Clinic, 314–315, 321
Mayo Clinic Proceedings, 315
Mayoun, Julien, 195
McDade, Joseph, PhD, 48
McGeehin, Michael, Dr., 339–340
McKeithen, Win, 430
MDH (Minnesota Department of Health), 314–316, 320, 323–325
Mead, George Herbert, 421
measles, 83–89
measles, mumps, and rubella (MMR) vaccine, 245–246, 248–251, 256–257
Médecins Sans Frontièrs (MSF)
    in Ebola investigations, 192
    in Liberia, 218, 222
    in yellow fever vaccinations, 230, 233–235, 238–240
media, anthrax attacks on. *see* anthrax
media coverage
    on averting epidemics, 159–160
    confidentiality and, 153
    of donating blood, 158
    of frozen strawberry contamination, 150–151
    of hepatitis A outbreak, 147–149
    of human elements, 154
    of mumps epidemic, 249–250
    of public health issues, 151–152, 155, 161
    of syphilis outbreak, 167–168
    of vaccination campaigns, 158
    of whooping cough outbreak, 212
medical device manufacturing industry, 374–375, 382–384
medical record abstraction, 9
medical wards, hepatitis B in. *see* hepatitis B virus (HBV)
"Medico-Ecologic Problems of Women and Children" conference, 392
MEETH (Manhattan Eye, Ear, and Throat Hospital), 185–186
Mekembo, 194–199
memos of understanding (MOUs), 375
men having sex with men (MSM)
    AIDS in, 65–71
    Entamoeba hystolytica among, 74
    hepatitis A in, 157–159
    syphilis among. *see* syphilis
Mengue, Abessolo, Dr., 200
meningococcal meningitis, 11–12
Menomonee River, 128–129
menstrual toxic shock syndrome, 57–63
Merck Childhood Asthma Network, 419
mercury poisoning, 398
mesothelioma, 363–366

methadone clinics, 425
methamphetamine users, 145–148, 153–161
methemoglobinemia
  causes of, 269–270
  conclusions about, 269–271
  control measures for, 262–264
  environmental investigation of, 267–269
  epidemiologic investigation of, 265–267
  laboratory investigation of, 268–269
  overview of, 264
  questions about, 271
  references on, 271
  reports of outbreak of, 261–262
  starting investigation of, 262–264
  tracebacks and, 267–268
methomyl-contaminated salt, 284
methylene blue, 262, 270
Metropolitan Transit Authority, 187–188
Mexico, pork tapeworm in, 117–119
Microscopic Agglutination Test (MAT), 22–23, 26–27
Mid-City Consortium to Combat AIDS, 426
Midwest High Intensity Drug Trafficking Area (HIDTA), 161
Miller, Barry, Dr., 221–222
Milwaukee Journal, 56
Milwaukee River, 128–129, 140–141
Milwaukee Water Works (MWW)
  North Plant, 123–125, 139
  review of data on, 128–136
  South Plant. *see* South Plant
Milwaukee, Wisconsin. *see Cryptosporidium* infections
Ministry of Health and Family Welfare, Bangladesh, 301–302
Minnesota
  Department of Health of, 314–316, 320, 323–325
  in eosinophilia myalgia syndrome investigation, 314–316
  toxic shock syndrome in, 53–60
Mitsui Toatsu Chemicals, Inc., 326, 329
MMR (measles, mumps, and rubella) vaccine, 245–246, 248–251, 256–257
MMWR (Morbidity and Mortality Weekly Report)
  on AIDS, 66, 68–70
  on EMS epidemic, 332–333
  on hepatitis, 92
  on injection drug users, 429
  on L-tryptophan, 318
  on mumps epidemic, 249–254
  on pertussis outbreak, 204
  on toxic shock syndrome, 57–60
Mobile C.A.R.E. Foundation, 418
Mohle-Boetani, Janet, MD, MPH, 109
Moline, Illinois, 215
mononuclear leukemia, 374
Monrovia, 218, 226
Montagnier, Luc, 70
Montgomery, Susan, Dr., 226–227, 233
Moore, Anne, PhD, MD, 117
Morawetz, John, 379
Morbidity and Mortality Weekly Report (MMWR). *see MMWR (Morbidity and Mortality Weekly Report)*
Morgan Processing and Distribution Center (P&DC), 184
Mori, Kay, 76
mosquito-borne diseases, 220–221
Motta, Jorge, Dr., 340
MOUs (memos of understanding), 375, 382
MRIs (magnetic resonance images), 116–117
MSF (Médecins Sans Frontièrs). *see* Médecins Sans Frontièrs (MSF)
MSM (men having sex with men). *see* men having sex with men (MSM)
Mujica, Oscar, 340–342
Mullin, Sandy, 181
mumps
  on college campuses, 248
  communication issues, 248–250
  history of, 245–246
  introduction to, 245
  Iowa outbreak of, generally, 246–248
  questions about, 258
  references on, 257–258
  vaccine efficacy, 251–257
Muslims, 101–104
MWW (Milwaukee Water Works). *see* Milwaukee Water Works (MWW)

N

Nabeta, Alfred, 234
NADR (National AIDS Demonstration Research Project), 426–429
Nairobi, 288–289
Nannis, Paul, 126
narcotics, 153
NASCAR events, 138
Nash, Denis, 180
nasopharyngeal swabs, 209–210
National AIDS Demonstration Research Project (NADR), 426–429
National Cancer Institute (NCI), 349, 375
National Center for Environmental Health (NCEH), 314, 337–339, 344
National Death Index (NDI), 378
National Environmental Public Health Tracking (NEPHT), 365–366
National Health Interview Survey (NHIS), 407
National Immunization Days, 240
National Institute for Occupational Safety and Health Immediately Dangerous to Life or Health (IDLH), 408
National Institute of Occupational Safety and Health (NIOSH)
  in anthrax investigation, 184
  Education and Research Center of, 401
  on EtO exposure, 373–380, 382–387
National Institute on Drug Abuse (NIDA), 421–429
National Institutes of Health (NIH), 70, 320
National Public Health Laboratory of Kenya, 289
National School Lunch Program (NSLP), 275–276
natural disasters, 49
NBC, 175–183
NCAA hockey tournaments, 138
NCEH (National Center for Environmental Health), 314, 337–339, 344
NCI (National Cancer Institute), 349, 375
NDI (National Death Index), 378, 384
necrotizing fasciitis, 203
needle and syringe exchange (NEP), 426
NEJM (New England Journal of Medicine). *see New England Journal of Medicine (NEJM)*
Nelson, Kenrad E., MD, 19
NEP (needle and syringe exchange), 426
nephelometric turbidity units (NTUs), 122, 125–126, 137–138
NEPHT (National Environmental Public Health Tracking), 365–366
neurocysticercosis, 115–118
New England Journal of Medicine (NEJM)
  on amebiasis, 74
  on EtO exposure, 380, 386
  on toxic shock syndrome, 57, 61

New Mexico, 313–314
New York City
    9/11 in, 49
    AIDS in, 66–68
    anthrax outbreak in. *see* anthrax
    mumps outbreak in, 246
New York Post, 182–184
New York Times
    on anthrax outbreak, 178
    on Epidemic Scorecard, 219–220
    on L-tryptophan, 318–320
    on Legionnaires' disease, 44
    on mumps epidemics, 250
    on syphilis outbreak, 168
NGOs (non-government organizations). *see* non-government organizations (NGOs)
Nguku, Patrick, Dr., 292
Nguyen, Kathy, 185–188
NHIS (National Health Interview Survey), 407
NIDA (National Institute on Drug Abuse), 421–429
NIH (National Institutes of Health), 70, 320
Nimba County, 222, 227–232
NIOSH (National Institute of Occupational Safety and Health). *see* National Institute of Occupational Safety and Health (NIOSH)
Njapau, Henry, Dr., 297
non-government organizations (NGOs)
    in Ebola investigation, 192
    injection drug use programs by, 433
    in yellow fever vaccinations, 222, 228
non-Hodgkin's lymphoma, 382–384
noncausal associations, 330
nonhuman primates, 197–200
noninfectious causes. *see also* intoxications
    cancer clusters and. *see* cancer clusters
    ethylene oxide exposure. *see* ethylene oxide (EtO) exposure
    landfill toxins, 403–409
    thallium poisoning, 394–397
Norquist, John, 126–127
North Plant, 123–125, 139
nosocomial transmission, 195–199
NSLP (National School Lunch Program), 275–276
NTUs (nephelometric turbidity units), 122, 125–126, 137–138
nursing home surveillance, 131

O
O-group 139. *see* cholera
Oak Valley Elementary School, 274–275, 280, 283
Occupational Safety and Health Act, 374
Occupational Safety and Health Administration (OSHA), 374, 386
ocular studies in Guatemala. *see* toxoplasmosis
ocular toxoplasmosis, 456–457. *see also* toxoplasmosis
OFDA (Office of Foreign Disaster Assistance), 233
Office of Early Childhood Education, 417
Office of Foreign Disaster Assistance (OFDA), 233
Office of Management and Budget (OMB), 385
Ogooué Ivindo Province, 193, 198
Ohio
    Department of Health, 404
    Environmental Protection Agency of, 403–404, 410
    Warren City Health Department in, 401
OIs (opportunistic infections), 66
OLC (Our Lives Count), 403
Old-Order Amish communities. *see* Amish communities, immunization in
OMB (Office of Management and Budget), 385

onset of illness dates, 10
Onsongo, Mary, 290
oocysts, *Cryptosporidium*, 136–142
opportunistic infections (OIs), 66
oral vs. written communications, 15
Orihel, Tom, 73
Orthodox Jewish communities, 116
OSHA (Occupational Safety and Health Administration), 374, 386
Osler, William, Dr., 219
Osterholm, Mike, Dr., 315–316, 320–325, 334
Otero, Hansel, Dr., 218–220, 234
Ouellet, Larry, 427–428
Our Lives Count (OLC), 403
Outbreak, 401
outbreak investigations overview
    additional studies, 12–14
    analyses, performing additional, 13–14
    conclusions about, 16
    control measures, 11–12, 14–15
    counting cases in, 10
    diagnoses, confirming, 8
    environmental investigations, 11
    epidemiologic analyses, 10–11
    hypotheses, 11
    introduction to, 3–6
    laboratory investigations, 11
    observations, 12–13
    outbreaks, defined, 3–4
    prevention information and findings, 15
    questions about, 6, 16
    references on, 16
    surveillance data, 15–16
    teams for, 8–9
    tentative case definitions, 9–10
    verifying outbreaks, 7–8
Outokumpu Corporation, 396
Outsiders, 422
oxygen, 264

P
P. aeruginosa, 77, 79
P. Leiner Nutritional Products, 323
P values, 36–37
P&DC (Morgan Processing and Distribution Center), 184
PAA (3-(phenylamino)alanine), 329
PAC (polyaluminum chloride), 123–125
PAHO (Pan American Health Organization), 340, 398
Pan Am Flight 103, 101
Pan American Health Organization (PAHO), 340, 398
Pan American Zoonoses Center (PAHO/WHO), 116
Panama, EMS in. *see* eosinophilia myalgia syndrome (EMS)
Panama Ministry of Health (MOH), 338–342, 346–347
Papua, 434
Parasites in Human Tissues, 73
Patel, Alpesh, MBBS, MPH, CERC, CPHA, 273–281, 283–285
PATH (Program for Appropriate Technology in Health), 430–433
Patient O, 68
Payne, Thomas, 44
PCP (Angel Dust), 422, 426
PCP (*Pneumocystis carinii* pneumonia), 66
PCR (polymerase chain reaction) testing
    for anthrax, 177–180
    for Ebola hemorrhagic fever, 194, 200
    for mumps, 247
    for whooping cough, 209–210
    for yellow fever, 220

Peak E (eosinophil), 328–329
pediatric cancer, 360
Pediatric Clinic, Chernivtsi, 392–393
penicillin, 166–167
Persky, Victoria, MD, 415
pertussis, 9–10. *see also* whooping cough
Peters, C.J., 192
Petersdorf, Robert, Dr., 65
pharmaceutical companies, 151
pharmacies, 209
phencyclidine (PCP), 422
PHPS (Public Health Prevention Service), 439–440
PIDVS (Program on Infectious Disease and Vaccine Sciences), 301
Pirie, Phyllis, Dr., 322
Plan B, 170
PlanetOut, 168
Plasmodium falciparum malarial epidemic, 401
Platelia Toxo IgG (TMB) enzyme immunoassay, 452
pleural cancer clusters, 363–366
Pneumocystis carinii pneumonia (PCP), 66
pneumonia, 48, 84
point-of-use filters, 139–140
polio, 446–447
Polk County, 145, 149, 152–161
polyaluminum chloride (PAC), 123–125
polymerase chain reaction (PCR) testing. *see* PCR (polymerase chain reaction) testing
Pond, Bob, 139
Pope Paul VI, 43
poppers, 67
pork tapeworm. *see* tapeworm
pornographic industry, 422
Portugal, cholera in. *see* cholera
post-outbreak transmissions, 139
postal service, 183–188
Pott, Percival, 349
Poundstone, John, Dr., 109, 111–112
poverty. *see* food shortages
power lines, 362–363
Praptoraharjo, Ignatius (Gambit), 434–435
Pratap, Preethi, PhD, 401
predictive performance, 330–331
preliminary feasibility studies, 374
Preston, Richard, 192
prevention information and findings, 15
primary cases, 10
primates, 197–200
Principia College, 83–88
probable cases, 9–10
probiotic supplements, 79
Proctor and Gamble, 60
Proctor, Mary, PhD, MPH, 123, 131
Prodanchuk, Mukola, Dr., 391–395
Program for Appropriate Technology in Health (PATH), 430–433
Program on Infectious Disease and Vaccine Sciences (PIDVS), 301
ProMED, 222, 225, 241
prophylaxis for whooping cough, 210–211, 213
proton-induced X-ray emission spectroscopy, 396
pseudo-outbreak of amebiasis. *see* amebiasis, pseudo-outbreak of
Pseudomonas cepacia, 206
psittacosis, 45, 48
Public Health Prevention Service (PHPS), 439–440
public relations, 166–167
pulses. *see* aflatoxicosis
punch, contaminated. *see* methemoglobinemia

Q

Quad City Times, 214
quarantine. *see* isolation
"quick and dirty" investigations, 150
Quinlisk, Patricia, MD, MPH, 145–147, 245, 261, 269–271

R

radiation poisoning, 394
Rahman, Mahmudur, 302–303
Ramadan, 101
Rambam Medical Center, 93–99
random digit dialed phoned surveys
    RDD 1, 129–131
    RDD 2, 131–134
    RDD 3, 134
rapid response teams (RRTs), 203–205
Rather, Dan, 182
raw water sources, 128–129
Reagan, President Ronald, 69
religious fasting, 101
religiously exempt persons. *see* measles
Rely tampons, 60
Rentz, Danielle, PhD, 339–344, 346
Republic of Congo, Ebola in. *see* Ebola hemorrhagic fever
Resource Conservation and Recovery Act, 357
respiratory health. *see* asthma
restaurants, 151–159
retinochorioidal scars, 456–457
Reynolds, Mary, 196
Rhodes, Claude, 425
rice crops, 302
Rickettsial Disease Laboratory, 48
risk factors, 9
Rizzo, Silvia, Dr., 456–457
Rock Island County, whooping cough in. *see* whooping cough
Rockette, Howard, Dr., 375
Rosenberg, Mark, 33, 56
Roueché, Berton, 270
Rous avian sarcoma virus, 352–355
RRTs (rapid response teams)
    Patel and Dworkin on, 273–274
    in toxic school lunch investigation, 275, 277–280
    in whooping cough investigation, 203–205
Rubin, Carol, Dr., 287, 297, 337–339, 344–346

S

Salmonella
    food handlers and, 5
    outbreaks of, 3
    primary vs. secondary cases of, 10
    serotype enteritidis, 14
    types of, 8
Salmonella typhimurium, 274
salt curing, 104–105
salt vs. saltpeter, 270
SAMHSA (Substance Abuse and Mental Health Services Administration), 429
sample sizes, 238
San Francisco, syphilis in. *see* syphilis
San Juan Sacatepequez, 453–455
Sandburg, Carl, 245
sanitary vs. storm sewers, 141
SARS, 219–220
Save the Children, 222
SCE (sister chromatid exchange) rates, 374

Schantz, Peter M., VMD, PhD, 115
Scheff, Peter, Dr., 396
Schell, Wendy, 51, 135
Schier, Joshua, Dr., 339–344
school-based asthma programs, 419
school children. *see also* child care facilities
    asthma among. *see* asthma
    cryptosporidosis among, 136
    hepatitis A exposure among, 149–150
    leptospirosis among. *see* leptospirosis
    shigellosis among, 110–113
    toxic lunch foods of. *see* toxic school lunches
scleroderma, 320, 322
screening for asthma, 415–416
secondary cases, 10
Sedmak, Gerald, Dr., 121
SEERStat Software, 363, 385
Sejvar, James, Dr., 342
Sencer, David, Dr., 67
Seratia marcesans, 79
serologic testing, 210
seroprevalence of *T. gondii*. *see* toxoplasmosis
serotype G mumps virus, 246
sewage treatment, 129
sex and HIV. *see* HIV (human immunodeficiency virus)
sex workers, 433–437
Sexually Transmitted Disease (STD) Prevention Section, 163
sexually transmitted diseases (STDs), 65–68
SFM4M chat room, 164–168
Sham-el-Nessim holiday, 101–106
Shandera, Wayne, Dr., 66
Shands, Kathy, 56–57
sharing information, 6
shellfish, 31, 35
Shick, J. Fred, 423
shigellosis
    conclusions about, 114
    initial investigation and recommendations, 110–111
    initial response, 111–112
    introduction to, 109–110
    questions about, 114
    references on, 114
    second phase of investigation, 112–114
Shilts, Randy, 69
shooting galleries, 428
Showa Denko K.K., 323, 332–334
sick room facilities, 85
Silent Spring, 350
Singh, Ajaib, Dr., 121–122
single overriding communication objectives (SOCOs), 5, 151, 405
Sioux City Journal, 147
Siouxland, 147, 154
SIRs (standardized incidence ratios), 363, 385
sister chromatid exchange (SCE) rates, 374
Smith, Tom, Dr., 375
SMRs (standardized mortality ratios), 363, 380–383
social deviance, 422
social mobilization for mass vaccinations, 222–223
Social Security Administration, 376–378, 384
SOCOs (single overriding communication objectives), 5, 151, 405
sodium nitrate, 270
sodium nitrite, 268–270
software for statistical analysis, 10–11
Sorvillo, Frank, PhD, 73
Sosa, Nestor, Dr., 342–344, 347

South Carolina, 357, 363–366
South Plant
    filtration at, 137–138
    intake grid, 140–141
    refurbishing, 139
    treatment capacities of, 123–126
Soviet Ministry of Health, 389, 394
Spain, 320
Speakes, Larry, 69
special populations, 136–137
specificity in cause and effect, 330–331
specimen collection techniques, 77
sporadic cases vs. outbreak, 79
St. Luke's Hospital laboratory, 121–122, 126
Stallones, Reuel, 61
standardized incidence ratios (SIRs), 363
standardized mortality ratios (SMRs), 363
staphylococcal enterotoxins, 53–59, 62
Staphylococcus aureus, 276, 284
Stapleton, Margaret, MSPH, 113
Star Tribune, 313
statistical receptor modeling method, 396
Stayner, Leslie, PhD, 373, 387
STD (Sexually Transmitted Disease) Prevention Section, 163, 167
STDs (sexually transmitted diseases), 65–68
Steele, James H., Dr., 116
Steenland, Kyle, PhD, 373, 387
steps of outbreak investigations, 7–8
Strassburg, Marc, 75
strawberries, 149–150
strength of associations, 330–331
subpopulations, 421
Substance Abuse and Mental Health Services Administration (SAMHSA), 429
subways, 187–188
Superfund, 356, 402
surveillance data, 7, 15–16, 138
surveys of Amish communities, 443–446
Susser, Mervyn, 330–331
sustainable infrastructures, 418–419
swimming pool-related outbreaks, 139
swine influenza, 43, 83
Swisher, Kara, 168
Sylhet Medical College Hospital, 303–305
syphilis
    conclusions about, 170
    implications of cyberspace and, 169–170
    introduction to tracking through cyberspace, 164
    outbreak of, 164–169
    questions about, 171
    references on, 170–171
    as sexually transmitted disease, 65

T
T. gondii. *see* toxoplasmosis
Taenia solium, 115–119
tampons, 57–62
tapemeters, 403
tapeworm
    introduction to, 115–116
    investigating outbreak of, 116–118
    questions about, 119
    references on, 119
    uniqueness of outbreak of, 119
Tapper, Michael, Dr., 186

taste galleries, 428
Tavira investigation, 35–37
Taylor, Bill, 53
Taylor, Charles, 217–218
Teale, Kevin, 145, 147
TECRA immunoassay, 279
telephone reports, 7
Telfer, Jana, 343
tentative case definitions, 9–10
terrorism, 101–102, 107. *see also* bioterrorism
Thacker Stephen B., MD, MSc, 43
Thailand
    Family Health International in, 433
    hepatitis B in, 91
    injection drug users in, 430–432
thallium poisoning
    causes of, 394–397
    conclusions about, 398
    hypotheses, developing, 390–391
    introduction to, 389–390
    investigating outbreak of, 391–394
    questions about, 398–399
    references on, 399
    testing hair, nail, blood and urine samples for, 397–398
THC (delta-9-tetrahydrocannabinol), 422
Thompson, Tommy, 174–175
ticks, 52
Tikal, 454–456
time-weighted averages (TWAs), 374
TMB (Platelia Toxo IgG) enzyme immunoassay, 452
Todd, Jim, 52–56
Toms River cluster study, 365
TOPOFF II (top officials, second exercise), 274
Tormey, Mike, 75
toxic exposure hypothesis, 310
toxic exposures. *see* intoxications
toxic oil syndrome, 320
toxic school lunches
    conclusions about, 285
    environmental investigation of, 281–283
    epidemiologic investigation of, 278–279, 280–281
    field investigation, November 25, 2002, 275–277
    field investigation, November 26, 2002, 277–280
    field investigation, November 27–28, 2002, 280
    introduction to, 273–274
    laboratory investigation of, 279–280, 283–285
    notification of, 275
    questions about, 285
    references on, 285–286
toxic shock syndrome (TSS)
    case control studies, impact of, 61–62
    case control study of, CDC, 59–60
    case control study of, initial Wisconsin, 57–59
    case control study of, tri-state, 60
    case definition of, 56
    introduction to, 51–52
    laboratory studies of, 55
    management of, 55
    outbreak of, 52–53, 57
    personal reflections on, 62–63
    questions about, 64
    references on, 63–64
    reporting, 55–56
    U.S. Department of Health and Social Services on, 54–56
    Wisconsin team study of, 57–59, 62–63
toxidromes, defined, 390

Toxoplasma gondii. *see* toxoplasmosis
toxoplasmosis
    cultural factors and, 453–456
    defined, 450–451
    introduction to, 449–450
    laboratory analysis results, 456
    prevalence studies of, 451–453
    questions about, 458
    references on, 458
    treating children with, 456–458
tracebacks, 14, 267–268
transient colonization, 79
Trent, Lisa, 383–384
Trute, Wendy, 205, 214
tryptophan poisoning. *see* eosinophilia myalgia syndrome (EMS)
TSS (toxic shock syndrome). *see* toxic shock syndrome (TSS)
TSST-1 toxin, 62–63
tuberculosis, 19
Tulane School of Public Health and Tropical Medicine, 201
Turkey, 310
TWAs (time-weighted averages), 374
Twin Cities, 322–325

U
UAB (University of Alabama, Birmingham), 350
Uganda, 200
UHL (University Hygienic Laboratory), 246–247, 268–269
Ukrainian Academy of Medical Sciences, 398
Ukrainian Environmental Health Project, 398
Ukrainian Ministry of Health, 389, 394
The Ukrainian Weekly, 389–390, 398
UNICEF (United Nations Children's Fund)
    in thallium poisoning investigation, 391
    in yellow fever vaccinations, 217–222, 225–233, 235–241
United Nations, 432
United Nations Mission in Liberia (UNMIL), 227–228
United States Agency for International Development (USAID), 233, 430–432
United States, AIDS in. *see* AIDS (acquired immune deficiency syndrome)
United States Pharmacopeia (USP), 324
University del Valle, 451–453, 455
University Hygienic Laboratory (UHL), 246–247
University of Alabama, Birmingham (UAB), 350
University of California, 166
University of Chicago, Drug Abuse Epidemiology Program, 423–424
University of Illinois
    Chicago School of Public Health at, 415, 425
    in thallium poisoning investigation, 396, 398
University of Minnesota, 322–323
University of Washington, 170
University of Wisconsin Survey Research Institute, 131
UNMIL (United Nations Mission in Liberia), 227–228
unsolved investigations, 48
urban school children with asthma. *see* asthma
U.S. Agency for International Development, 102–103
U.S. Department of Agriculture, 15, 279
U.S. Department of Health and Human Services, 299, 402, 458
U.S. Embassy in Cairo, 102
U.S. Food and Drug Administration (FDA). *see* Food and Drug Administration (FDA)
U.S. National Institutes of Health, 70
U.S. Naval Medical Research Unit 3, 103
U.S. Public Health Service, 70
USA Today, 150, 250

USAID (United States Agency for International Development), 233, 430–433
USP (United States Pharmacopeia), 324
Utah, 59–60

V

vaccinations
   in Amish communities, 441–447
   for hepatitis A, 146, 149, 157–161
   for measles, 87
   for polio, 446–447
   religious groups opposed to, 88
   for whooping cough, 211, 216
   for yellow fever. *see* yellow fever mass vaccination
verifying outbreaks, 7–8
veterinary medicine, 115–116
Vibrio cholerae O-group. *see* cholera
Vimeiro Thermal Springs, 33, 38–40
viral encephalitis, 304
viral hemorrhagic fevers, 219
Virginia Department of Health, 167
vital status, ascertaining, 378
vomiting with unconsciousness, 308–309

W

Wadden, Rick, Dr., 396
walkthrough surveys, 376–377
Wall Street Journal, 168
Wamsley, Jay, 344
Wand, Phil, 56
Warren City Health Department, 404
Warren, Ohio, 401
Warren Recycling Incorporated (WRI), 403
Washington State Health Department, 20
Wassilak, Steven G. F., MD, 86–87
water parks, 13
water supply, detecting, 137
waterborne outbreaks, 121. *see also Cryptosporidium* infections
watery diarrhea, 129–134
Watts Retreat cancer cluster, 356–363
weather conditions, 140–141
Webber, Randy, 424
Weber, J. Todd, 101
websites, 169, 252
wedding party. *see* methemoglobinemia
weighted multiple regression models, 379–380
Weil, Adolph, 27
Weil's Disease, 27
Weisfuse, Isaac, 181
Weiss, Don, MD, MPH, 173
Welch, Pat, 206–209
well water, 13
West Nile virus, 217, 274
Westinghouse, 238
WFO (World Food Programme), 234
white powder, 175, 177–178
WHO (World Health Organization). *see* World Health Organization (WHO)
whooping cough
   age factors in, 211–212
   in Amish communities, 441
   close contacts, defining, 210–211
   communication issues and, 212–215
   conclusions about, 215–216
   introduction to, 203–207
   questions about, 216
   references on, 216
   surveillance of, 207–210
Wiebel, W. Wayne, PhD, 421
Wignall, Steve, 434
Wilder, Lynn, 411
Will County Health Department, 274–277
Wilson, Marianna, 452–455
Wisconsin, cryptosporidosis in. *see Cryptosporidium* infections
Wisconsin Department of Health and Social Services. *see* Wisconsin Division of Health (DOH)
Wisconsin Division of Health (DOH)
   Cryptosporidium infections and, 121–128, 131–136
   Sexually Transmitted Disease program staff of, 129
   toxic shock syndrome and, 51–53, 54–56
Wisconsin Epidemiology Bulletin, 51
Wisconsin Laboratory of Hygiene (WSLH), 53–57
Wisconsin team study of TSS, 57–59, 62–63
Wong, Marie, 179
Wong, Otto, Dr., 375, 382–384
World Bank Environmental Mission, 396, 398
World Food Programme (WFO), 234
World Health Organization (WHO)
   in aflatoxicosis investigation, 298
   in cholera investigation, 32, 39–40
   in DEG poisoning investigation, 340
   in Ebola investigation, 192, 197
   in EtO exposure investigation, 373
   Global Programme on AIDS of, 432
   on polio, 447
   on thallium poisoning, 390–392, 395
   on yellow fever vaccinations, 220–222, 225–229, 233–240
World Trade Center attacks, 49, 173
Worthington, Julie, PhD, MPH, 349
wound botulism, 102. *see also* botulism
WRI (Warren Recycling Incorporated), 403
written communications, 15
WSLH (Wisconsin Laboratory of Hygiene), 53–57

X

X. strumarium seed poisoning, 310

Y

Yakita, 434
yellow fever mass vaccination
   aftermath, 223–225
   in Bong County, 233–238
   CDC response to, 225–233
   cold chain system for, 222–223
   conclusions about, 241
   controlling outbreak with, generally, 222
   introduction to, 217–218
   lot quality assurance sampling for, 238–240
   operations for, 222
   outbreak and, 218–222
   questions about, 243
   reassessing treatment of, 233–238
   recommendations for treating, 240–241
   references on, 242–243
   social mobilization for, 223
Yoder, Jonathan S., MSW, MPH, 439

Z

Zaki, Sherif, 177
Zayglay village, 232
Zoegeh district, 228–231